Nursing Knowledge & Practice

Foundations for Decision Making

SECOND EDITION

Edited by

Maggie Mallik MPhil BSc(Hons) DipN(Lond) CertEd RGN

Associate Director of Nursing – Clinical Education, Salisbury Healthcare NHS Trust, Salisbury and Assistant Head of Practice Education, IHCS, Bournemouth University, Bournemouth, UK

Carol Hall PhD BSc(Hons) DipN(Lond) DipAdEd Dip(Res)M RGN RSCN

Senior Health Lecturer, School of Nursing, The University of Nottingham, Queen's Medical Centre, Nottingham, UK

David Howard PhD MEd RMN RGN CertEd DipN(Lond)

Senior Health Lecturer (Mental Health) and Director, MSc Organisational Leadership in Health and Social Care, The University of Nottingham, County Hospital, Lincoln, UK

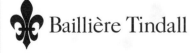

Baillière Tindall

EDINBURGH LONDON NEW YORK OXFORD PHILADELPHIA ST LOUIS SYDNEY TORONTO 2004

First edition 1998
Second edition 2004

ISBN 0 7020 2697 2

British Library Cataloguing in Publication Data
A catalogue record for this book is available from the British Library

Library of Congress Cataloging in Publication Data
A catalog record for this book is available from the Library of Congress

Note
Medical knowledge is constantly changing. Standard safety precautions must be followed,
but as new research and clinical experience broaden our knowledge, changes in treatment
and drug therapy may become necessary or appropriate. Readers are advised to check
the most current product information provided by the manufacturer of each drug to be
administered to verify the recommended dose, the method and duration of administration,
and contraindications. It is the responsibility of the practitioner, relying on experience and
knowledge of the patient, to determine dosages and the best treatment for each individual
patient. Neither the Publisher nor the editors or contributors assumes any liability for any
injury and/or damage to persons or property arising from this publication.

The Publisher

your source for books,
journals and multimedia
in the health sciences
www.elsevierhealth.com

The
Publisher's
policy is to use
**paper manufactured
from sustainable forests**

Printed in China

Contents

Contributors vii
Editors' introduction ix
Acknowledgements xi
How to use this book xiii
Abbreviations xv

1. Communication 1
   Paul Crawford and Brian Brown

2. Safety and risk 25
   Kate Beaumont

3. Resuscitation and emergency care 45
   Roderick Cable and Helen Swain

4. Infection control 75
   Rachel Peto

5. Handling and moving 105
   Eileen Aylott

6. Homeostasis 127
   Helen Dobbins, Gary Adams and Diane Hewson

7. Nutrition 153
   Lindsey Bellringer

8. Stress, relaxation and rest 175
   David Howard

9. Medicines 199
   Carol Hall

10. Pain 221
    Karen Jackson

11. Aggression 245
    Paul Linsley

12. Death and dying 263
    Linda Wilson

13. Hygiene 281
    Maggie Mallik

14. Skin integrity 305
    Kerry Lewis and Lorraine Roberts

15. Sexuality 329
    Steve Eastburn

16. Confusion 353
    Moonee Gungaphul

17. Mobility 367
    David Nichol and Sam Annasamy

18. Continence 391
    Alison Kelley

19. Rehabilitation 423
    Janet Barker

Glossary 443

Index 449

Contributors

Gary Adams BSc(Hons) RGN PGDipAdEd PhD MRSC
Lecturer, Insulin Diabetes Experimental Research School of Nursing, Faculty of Medicine and Health Sciences, The University of Nottingham, Nottingham, UK

Sam Annasamy MA BEd RGN ACP ONC CertEd RNT DN(Lond)
Lecturer, School of Nursing, The University of Nottingham, Queen's Medical Centre, Nottingham, UK

Eileen Aylott BSc(Hons) Dip/HE RN
Practice Educator, Salisbury District Hospital, Salisbury, UK

Janet Barker PhD BSc(Hons) SRN RMN PGDipAdEd
Senior Health Lecturer (Mental Health), The University of Nottingham, County Hospital, Lincoln, UK

Kate Beaumont RGN DPSN MA DipClinicalRisk
Patient Safety Manager, National Patient Safety Agency, London, UK

Lindsey Bellringer BSc(Hons) RGN
Practice Educator, Salisbury District Hospital, Salisbury, UK

Brian Brown PhD BSc
Senior Lecturer, Faculty of Health and Community Studies, De Montfort University, Leicester, UK

Roderick Cable RGN BSc (Nursing) DipAdEd RNT
Lecturer, School of Nursing, The University of Nottingham, Queen's Medical Centre, Nottingham, UK

Paul Crawford PhD BA(Hons) DPSN PGCHE RMN
Senior Lecturer in Mental Health, School of Nursing, The University of Nottingham, Derby, UK

Helen Dobbins MA
Lecturer, School of Nursing, The University of Nottingham, Queen's Medical Centre, Nottingham, UK

Steve Eastburn MSc BSc(Hons) RGN NDNCert DipAdEd
Health Lecturer (Adult Nursing), The University of Nottingham, County Hospital, Lincoln, UK

Moonee Gungaphul MSc BSc(Hons) CertEd RGN RMN DND
Health Lecturer (Mental Health), The University of Nottingham, County Hospital, Lincoln, UK

Carol Hall PhD BSc(Hons) DipN(Lond) DipAdEd Dip(Res)M RGN RSCN
Senior Health Lecturer, School of Nursing, The University of Nottingham, Queen's Medical Centre, Nottingham, UK

Diane Hewson BN(Hons) RN(Child) ENB998 (Teaching and Learning in Clinical Practice) ENB147 (Renal Nursing)
Practitioner Health Lecturer, School of Nursing, The University of Nottingham, Queen's Medical Centre, Nottingham, UK

David Howard PhD MEd RMN RGN CertEd DipN(Lond)
Senior Health Lecturer (Mental Health) and Director, MSc Organisational Leadership in Health and Social Care, The University of Nottingham, County Hospital, Lincoln, UK

Karen Jackson MSc PG DipAdEd RGN RSCN NDN(Cert)
Senior Lecturer, School of Nursing, De Montfort University, Leicester, UK

Alison Kelley BSc(Hons) RGN DipN(Lond) DipNEd(Lond)
Health Lecturer, School of Nursing, The University of Nottingham, Queen's Medical Centre, Nottingham, UK

Kerry Lewis MSc BA PGCE RGN
Health Lecturer, School of Nursing, The University of Nottingham, Pilgrim Hospital, Boston, UK

Paul Linsley MMedSci BMedSci RMN RGN ADIP(Acute Psych) PGDipEd CertMHS
Health Lecturer (Mental Health), The University of Nottingham, County Hospital, Lincoln, UK

Maggie Mallik MPhil BSc(Hons) DipN(Lond) CertEd RGN
Associate Director of Nursing – Clinical Education, Salisbury Healthcare NHS Trust, Salisbury and Assistant Head of Practice Education, IHCS, Bournemouth University, Bournemouth, UK

David Nichol BA DipEd RGN RNT FETC ONC
*Health Lecturer, School of Nursing, The University of
Nottingham, Queen's Medical School, Nottingham, UK*

Rachel Peto BSc(Hons) RGN ENB176 (Operating Department
Nursing) DPSN
*Health Lecturer, School of Nursing, The University of
Nottingham, Queen's Medical Centre, Nottingham, UK*

Lorraine Roberts BSc(Hons) RGN CertEd
*Health Lecturer, School of Nursing, The University of
Nottingham, Pilgrim Hospital, Boston, UK*

Helen Swain RGN RSCN BSc(Hons) MSc DipEd
*Health Lecturer, School of Nursing, The University of
Nottingham, Queen's Medical Centre, Nottingham, UK*

Linda Wilson MA RGN OND CTCert CertEd
*Health Lecturer (Adult Nursing), The University of
Nottingham, Grantham and Kesteven Hospital,
Grantham, UK*

Editors' introduction

The original idea behind the first edition of *Nursing Knowledge & Practice* arose from our experiences of teaching student nurses within the Diploma in Higher Education curriculum. We identified that students found it difficult to integrate the theoretical aspects of the course into daily nursing practice, issues subsequently identified by two major reports into nurse education: the Peach Report (Department of Health 1999) and Making a Difference (UK Central Council 1999). This book took a radical approach by integrating the knowledge base from subject areas within the nursing curriculum through a focus on the needs of service users. It was emphasized that such needs were paramount within the primary domain of knowledge and decision making across all fields of nursing practice.

Knowledge derived from the practice experience is an important element of being a nurse. In fact, the preoccupation of the new student when in the practice setting is firmly focused on learning how to do nursing and also on being able to cope with the interpersonal experiences involved. Evaluating what has been learned about nursing is now encouraged through recording and reflecting over a wide range of practice experiences.

For students to reflect critically on situations, they should be able to connect observed behaviours and subjective impressions to a substantiated and well delineated knowledge base. The first edition of this book became a resource for students to debate existing theory and observations from a variety of practice situations. From this, they could propose new solutions to the nursing care problems they met. Such development of critical thinking skills further assisted students to interpret and integrate data from several perspectives to arrive at their own 'truths' about their experiences in practice.

We expect the use of the second edition to build on this original success as a key text within health and social care. To facilitate this, contributors have relocated issues raised within their chapters in the context of contemporary practice and stakeholder interests. They have drawn extensively on current best evidence, including research, policy and substantial internet-based resources, reflecting UK and international perspectives. The content has thus been updated to meet the demands of nursing in the 21st century, while retaining the emphasis on the influence of evidence in practice. The inclusion of key websites is a new feature that will support readers in pursuing contemporary evidence that underpins competency based practice.

With the above issues in mind, our continuing commitment is to provide a book that:

- enables readers to integrate knowledge from theoretical and practical learning to make competent decisions in nursing practice
- provides foundation knowledge relating to the needs of practitioners and service users, and is applicable across all fields of nursing
- motivates readers to seek out and appraise current evidence critically and constructively.

Furthermore, it is the intention of this new edition to:

- encourage the development of personal knowledge through the development of portfolio evidence
- evaluate personal development and competency in practice through the use of reflection, and in preparation for clinical supervision
- develop skills for practice by utilizing both the content and the references to supportive resources within this book.

BOOK STRUCTURE

In this second edition, changes have been made that reflect comments from our reviewers and readers and learners. We acknowledge their valuable input in shaping the changes made to this text.

We have not placed the chapters within labelled sections, as in the first edition, thus encouraging the individual reader to use the book in a flexible way to suit their own teaching or learning needs.

This second edition includes a new chapter on communication: while in the first edition we embedded appropriate communication skills within each chapter, we consider this aspect of nursing to be so fundamental to good practice that we have identified key skills and theories within this chapter. This is further emphasized by placing the chapter at the beginning of the book.

Two chapters presented in the first edition – 'Stress and anxiety' and 'Sleep and rest' – have been integrated into one chapter, 'Stress, relaxation and rest'. It begins by examining factors underpinning the concepts of stress and relaxation. From this knowledge base, strategies for managing stress, both in your own life and in others', and methods of promoting relaxation and rest are identified and discussed.

The chapter previously called 'Environmental safety' has been renamed 'Safety and risk', and has been extensively updated to include the many current quality assurance frameworks which now guide all practitioners in reducing risk to their clients and themselves.

All other chapters have retained their original titles and have been updated and revised to meet the needs of the contemporary learner.

Maggie Mallik
Carol Hall
David Howard

Salisbury and Nottingham 2004

References

Department of Health 1999 Making a difference: strengthening the nursing, midwifery and health visiting contribution to health and healthcare. Department of Health, London

UK Central Council for Nursing, Midwifery and Health Visiting 1999 Fitness for practice. UK Central Council for Nursing, Midwifery and Health Visiting, London

Acknowledgements

We wish to acknowledge our anonymous reviewers and the pre-registration nursing students who took part in the publisher-organized focus groups. We value their critical commentary on the first edition of this book as well as their suggestions for improvements.

We thank all the contributors to our first edition who were willing to update and refocus their original chapters and to add new material where appropriate. We welcome and acknowledge our new contributors, who have had to shape their knowledge and expertise to suit the structured framework of this book or have had to reshape and update the material of a previous contributor.

Acknowledgement goes to Ninette Premdas, Katrina Mather, Claire Wilson, Gail Wright, Anna Hodson, and the rest of the team at Elsevier for their advice and support during the whole process of completing this second edition.

This second edition could not have been completed without the love and continual support of our families: our partners Penny Howard, Rich Hall and Alan Mallik, and our children, Simon and Peter Howard, James and Rachel Hall, and Catherine Mallik.

How to use this book

Each chapter is structured into the following four sections

- **Subject knowledge**, which incorporates two subdivisions:
  - Biological knowledge
  - Psychosocial knowledge
- **Care delivery knowledge**
- **Professional and ethical knowledge**
- **Personal and reflective knowledge.**

In addition, each chapter is designed to contain a number of features that will guide you around the topic as well as encourage you to reflect on your learning and your experiences in practice.

At the start of each chapter

- A **Key issues** list provides a succinct menu of topics covered within the chapter for quick and easy reference.
- The **Introduction** and **Overview** provide a guide to the chapter, indicating how and why this topic is an important component of nursing practice.

Within the chapter

Each chapter contains a number of different types of information and activities that are highlighted within the text. They are designed to help you reflect on your own knowledge, consider the basis of nursing decisions and demonstrate the evidence base for practice.

Reflection and portfolio evidence

Reflection is a very important process to develop in order to aid your learning. You can learn from your practice experience and also from your reactions to the knowledge presented in texts and the classroom. The main focus of the reflective exercises in this text is on yourself and your reactions and how these interact with the particular situation observed or reflected upon. There are many models that can be used to guide and structure your reflections. You will be advised and supported in the use of any one of these models by your teacher or education facilitator. Many of the exercises will focus on dilemmas where there is no right or wrong answer but one that is negotiated to suit the specific situation. You may find these exercises particularly useful as a basis for discussion and debate in a group. Writing up your reflections in a 'reflective diary' or 'learning journal' helps to fix the knowledge gained and allows you to review your learning experiences over time.

These exercises also offer helpful suggestions and hints as to what can be included in your Portfolio of Evidence of Learning.

Decision making exercises

Decision making exercises are generally related to material presented in the chapter; however, they may ask you to complete further work that will take you outside the scope of the text. Founded on the philosophy of problem based learning where you are given a short scenario, critical incident or case study from practice (broadly defined), you are requested to review information already obtained from whatever source, collect further information and then make decisions as to what actions you would take, supporting this with the rationale for your actions.

Guidance may be given, and helpful references, but some exercises will be open-ended as textbooks and articles go out of date quickly. It is important to do a literature search for up-to-date and local material that may be relevant to the topic being explored.

There is an assumption that you are able to use the appropriate internet and library facilities to find the relevant material. These are skills you should develop and maintain throughout your professional career.

Finally, discussion with your peers, teachers and practitioners will help you to focus your learning within the exercises.

Evidence based practice

Brief summaries of a research study or several studies are presented in order to provide support for evidence based practice. Although this is not explicitly stated in the book, you are encouraged to obtain a copy of the full report, read and critically appraise the study. You should also link these studies with your practice experiences, where you can. Research evidence, where at all possible, is from studies completed from the late 1990s onwards; however, you must remember that these research briefings can quickly become out of date, so they should act as the starting point for further investigation.

Case studies

In the **Personal and reflective knowledge** section of each chapter you will find four case studies. These are designed to show how core nursing knowledge is relevant across all the four branches of nursing. Each case study provides an opportunity for you to consider nursing decisions and to appreciate how knowledge from different sources is integrated in nursing practice. They may also act as a stimulus for you to explore in more depth issues related to your chosen branch of nursing. You may also wish to read them before reading the chapter.

At the end of each chapter

A **Summary** section at the end of each chapter provides a reminder of the key content of the chapter and can be used to evaluate the learning gained through reading the chapter.

An **Annotated further reading and websites** section provides guidance on sources of relevant information if you wish to pursue particular interests further. Each suggested item has a brief commentary explaining why it has been recommended. These resources are in addition to the extensive list of **References**.

Abbreviations

ABPM	ambulatory blood pressure measurement
ACLS	advanced cardiac life support
ADH	antidiuretic hormone
ADL	activities of daily living
ADP	adenosine diphosphate
AED	advisory external defibrillator
AIDS	acquired immune deficiency syndrome
ALS	advanced life support
APN	advanced practice nurse
ATNC	Advanced Trauma Nursing Course
ATP	adenosine triphosphate
BAC	British Association of Counselling
BCA	back care adviser
bd	twice a day, usually morning and evening
BLS	basic life support
BMI	body mass index
BMR	basal metabolic rate
BNF	British National Formulary
CA	care assistant
CAPE	Clifton assessment procedures for the elderly
CASU	Controls Assurance Support Unit
CBT	cognitive behavioural therapy
CCTV	closed circuit television
CDSC	Communicable Diseases Surveillance Centre
CHD	coronary heart disease
CHI	Commission for Health Improvement
CINAHL®	Cumulative Index to Nursing and Allied Health
CNST	Clinical Negligence Scheme for Trusts
CoA	coenzyme A
COHSE	Confederation of Health Service Employees
COPD	chronic obstructive pulmonary disease
COT	College of Occupational Therapists
CPN	community psychiatric nurse
CPR	cardiopulmonary resuscitation
CPS	Crown Prosecution Service
CSP	Chartered Society of Physiotherapists
DLF	Disabled Living Foundation
DoH	Department of Health
DRE	digital rectal examination
ECG	electrocardiograph
EEG	electroencephalograph
EHR	Electronic Health Records
EPR	Electronic Patient Records
ERC	European Resuscitation Council
FBAO	foreign body airway obstruction
GP	general practitioner
HAI	hospital acquired infection
HDL	high density lipoprotein
HIV	human immunodeficiency virus
HSAC	Health Services Advisory Committee
HSE	Health and Safety Executive
ICNP	International Classification for Nursing Practice
ICU	Intensive Care Unit
IDDM	insulin dependent diabetes mellitus
IHD	ischaemic heart disease
ILCOR	International Liaison Committee on Resuscitation
IV	intravenous
LDL	low density lipoprotein
LREC	Local Ethics Research Committee
MDMA	3,4-methylene-dioxymethamphetamine (ecstasy)
MDRTB	multidrug resistant tuberculosis
MMR	measles mumps rubella
MRSA	methicillin resistant *Staphylococcus aureus*
MS	multiple sclerosis
NBE	National Back Exchange
NDE	near death experience
NHS	National Health Service
NHSLA	National Health Service Litigation Authority
NICE	National Institute for Clinical Excellence
NMC	Nursing and Midwifery Council
NMSC	non-melanotic skin cancer
nocte	at night
NPSA	National Patient Safety Agency
NRL	natural rubber latex
NSF	National Service Framework
PALS	paediatric advanced life support

PALS	Patient Advice and Liaison Services	RN	registered nurse
PCA	patient controlled analgesia	RPST	Risk Pooling Scheme for Trusts
PCT	Primary Care Trust	SIDS	sudden infant death syndrome
PEA	pulseless electrical activity	SOLER	sit squarely – open posture – lean forwards – eye contact – relax
PHLS	Public Health Laboratory Service		
PN	parenteral nutrition	tds	three times a day
PRN	*pro re nata* – when necessary	TENS	transcutaneous electric nerve stimulation
PTSD	post-traumatic stress disorder	TILER	task – individual – load – environment – resources
PVS	persistent vegetative state		
qds	four times a day	UKCC	United Kingdom Central Council for Nurses, Midwives and Health Visitors
RDA	recommended daily allowance		
REM	rapid eye movement	UTI	urinary tract infection
RIDDOR	Reporting of Injuries and Dangerous Occurrences Regulations	VAC	vacuum assisted closure
		VF	ventricular fibrillation

Chapter 1

Communication

Paul Crawford and Brian Brown

KEY ISSUES

SUBJECT KNOWLEDGE
- Models of communication
- The biological basis of communication
- Language acquisition
- Non-verbal communication
- Psychosocial factors influencing communication
- The role of culture in narratives of health and illness

CARE DELIVERY KNOWLEDGE
- Counselling and developing a therapeutic relationship
- Interviewing and assessment
- Giving information, teaching and promoting health
- Keeping records of care
- Communication difficulties

PROFESSIONAL AND ETHICAL KNOWLEDGE
- Professional and legal aspects of record keeping
- Confidentiality and access to records
- Complaints and communication
- Patient advocacy

PERSONAL AND REFLECTIVE KNOWLEDGE
- Reviewing the use of language in nursing
- Four case scenarios related to the four branches of nursing

INTRODUCTION

The ways in which people communicate have profound effects on those around them. It is over 50 years since Peplau (1952) took the first steps in redefining nursing as an interpersonal, interpretive process (Tilley 1999). Peplau provided one of the first manifestos for the study of nursing as a communicative process:

> nurses – like other human beings – act on the basis of the meaning of events to them, that is, on the basis of their immediate interpretation of the climate and performances that transpire in a particular relationship. At the same time, the patient will act on the basis of the meaning of his illness to him. The interaction between nurse and patient is fruitful when a method of communication that identifies and uses common meanings is at work in the situation. (Peplau 1952: 283–284)

The impact of this view of the nursing encounter has been profound over the last 50 years and there has been an explosion of research and theory on communication processes in health care. Indeed, a search of the CINAHL® (Cumulative Index to Nursing and Allied Health) database yielded nearly a thousand citations in response to the terms 'nursing' and 'communication'. Consequently, it is important for practitioners to understand the major trends and topics in the study of communication, in order to incorporate this knowledge within professional practice.

Communication is a powerful life-changing activity and very different results can emerge from the process of caring for others depending on how communication is performed. Inadequate inter- and intraprofessional communication has been consistently cited as a cause for concern by Ombudsman Reports on the National Health Service in the UK (Ombudsman 2003) and various studies have found poor communication in health care to be the largest source of patient dissatisfaction (Caris-Verhallen et al 1999). As Fredricksen (1999) notes, how nurses speak, write, gesture, use signs and images and respond to the spoken, written and non-verbal communication of other people will have a great impact on the quality of care. In fact, care and communication are often one and the same thing.

This chapter addresses a variety of facets of the communication process in health care. Whereas the study of language is a lifetime's work, the examples and the ideas presented here serve to demonstrate the importance of language in the life of an effective and compassionate practitioner.

OVERVIEW

Subject knowledge

In subject knowledge, the theory and modes of communication are introduced. The biological basis of communication is outlined through describing the sensory organs and the interpretation of language and non-verbal signals in the brain. Insight into ideas about how and why human beings come to be language users is an important area to understand. Knowledge of the rich and versatile range of gestures, sounds and facial expressions which go to make up face-to-face communications is important for nurses. Finally, modes of communication that are used by health professionals to both care for, and control, clients will be discussed.

Care delivery knowledge

There are various aspects to communication in care delivery, from questioning, interviewing and assessing patients to information giving, teaching and promoting health. At the heart of all communication should be general counselling skills and the means of developing a therapeutic relationship. In addition, care professionals need to keep accurate and appropriate records and be able to deal with a variety of communication difficulties. In performing these activities, however, it is important to consider how language can be used to comfort, socialize and establish roles as well as to restrict and punish individuals.

Professional and ethical knowledge

In this section, legal and ethical issues concerning record keeping are considered. The implications of good and bad record keeping are contrasted and the implications for service users, care workers and professionals are discussed. The quality of care that clients receive can depend on adequate communication so in the final section of this chapter, the nurse's role in client advocacy within this context is examined.

Personal and reflective knowledge

This chapter will enhance awareness of the importance of language in nursing and provide a basic understanding of what it takes to be a critical and sensitive communicator. This section helps you to reflect on the implications of issues raised within this chapter for your day-to-day practice. On pages 21–22 are four case studies, each one relating to one of the branch programmes. You may find it helpful to read one of them before you start the chapter and use it as a focus for your reflections while reading.

SUBJECT KNOWLEDGE

CONCEPTUALIZING COMMUNICATION: MODELS AND THEORIES

Communication is at the heart of all individuals' interpersonal lives – that is how they relate to others – and also their internal worlds of thoughts and feelings. Most people move freely in and out of these two realms of dialogue throughout their waking hours. Indeed, humans are always communicating – to themselves or to others. If they are not speaking, writing or gesticulating, then they are likely to be receiving messages from others. Thus, it is impossible to switch off communication since everything individuals do, even silence, sends out messages.

Reflection and portfolio evidence

Sit quietly for a few minutes and think about all the different kinds of communication going on around you.

- What do you hear, see, think and feel?
  As you do this, you will be experiencing the internal monologue of your own thoughts, and external verbal and non-verbal exchanges of other people. You will remind yourself that communication is the most important or central human activity.
- Extend this exercise by spending 5 or 10 minutes observing the kinds of communication that take place in your practice area. You may wish to repeat this activity at different times of the day or in different clinical situations. If applicable, record your findings in your portfolio.

In considering communication within health and social care, the first task is to consider the various ways in which scholars have attempted to define and model the communication process. How people send and receive messages and the kinds of messages involved is very complex. A number of scholars have tried to build models or metaphors of the communication process.

MODELS OF COMMUNICATION

Early beginnings: the one–way flow

One of the oldest 'folk models' of communication sees it as a kind of conduit, where the thoughts are translated into words and the language transfers the thoughts bodily from one person to another. This began with Shannon & Weaver's (1949) model of communication, where an information source passes the message to a transmitter and the message then passes down a channel (originally, a telephone wire) and reaches the destination or recipient. This kind of thinking is also found in Lasswell's (1948) classic formula 'Who says what to whom in what channel with what effects.' These metaphors of communication tend to see communication as being rather like the transport of goods, services and people (Carey 1989).

Communicating as a transaction: the two-way flow

In contrast to the one-way flow model, some researchers and theorists have proposed two-way or transactional models of communication (Ratzan et al 1996). Two-way communications are the preferred model in nurse–patient exchanges because they involve dialogue between sender and receiver where shared meaning and mutual understanding can be more easily developed. In other words, they involve a feedback loop (Kreps 2001).

Cognitivist models

In these models of language it is easy to see how communication may be subject to psychological factors: in this way they are cognitivist models. Language is believed to be shaped by the individual speaker's intentions, mental representations, the 'hard-wiring' of their language faculties, and decoded in terms of the receiver's interpretative frameworks to make sense of any message (Chomsky 1993, Fodor 1998). Thus, in this model, any communication can be influenced by beliefs, values, assumptions and prejudices. Additionally, perceptual differences and distortions among individuals can affect communication. Any social event or situation will yield a variety of interpretations depending upon who perceives it. In this view the language is a window into the mind and what we say or write reflect a variety of preceding cognitive, emotional and neurological states.

The contexts and intentions of communication

Another way of making sense of communication is to consider the context and purpose for sender and message, following the Russian linguist Roman Jakobson (1960). In this tradition, theorists are also interested in how the context or circumstances in which individuals find themselves determines the meaning of any message. People are believed to engage in a good deal of 'recipient tailoring' to make the speech suit the situation (Brown & Fraser 1979).

Language as action: the theory of speech acts

All communication is a kind of action, that is, it has a purpose – promising, warning, threatening, praising, apologizing and so on (Searle 1979). Communication is fundamentally an activity; it is a way of doing things and getting others to do them. In Habermas's (1995) theory of communicative action, humans establish their persona or identity through communication with others. Sumner (2001) notes that these communicative actions in nursing can, if successful, lead to a sense of fulfilment and validation for client and carer.

Language as a construction yard: co-constructing realities through language

In contrast to the above humanistic models of communication, there are other ways of conceptualizing the process of communication. To some students of communication in health care, language is a way of constructing reality in healthcare encounters. In this sense language is a kind of construction yard where versions of reality can be created (Potter 1996). As Fox (1993) demonstrated, a patient who has just undergone an operation may be in a great deal more pain than before the intervention, yet it is the job of the medical team to put a favourable gloss on this often unhappy situation. They do this by focusing on upbeat topics like the number of days until discharge, or until the stitches can come out.

This construction yard model of communication may sound abstract, but it is a useful way to think about the process of communication in nursing. For example, Bricher (1999: 453) describes how trust can be constructed between nurses and sick children. As one of her respondents said: 'I show them a photo of my dog and they realize … that you've got a backyard and a dog too, … not just this person that sticks suppositories up.' Within children's nursing, this focus can be particularly valuable in that trust allows the treatment to be undertaken with a minimum of distress, and even when a distressing procedure is undertaken, the relationship can be re-established quickly.

Reflection and portfolio evidence

Think of a recent communication that you have made. The task in this exercise is to think about it in relation to the various models we have presented.

1. The transmission model – what was transmitted to the other person or people by you? What did they transmit to you? What were you thinking at the time? What do you suppose they were thinking? To what extent was it a transaction?
2. The contextual model – how did the context influence the communication?
3. Communication as action – what were you trying to achieve in the interaction? What were you trying to get the other people to do? What were they trying to get you to do?
4. Language as a construction yard – did the communicative event construct or formulate reality in a particular way? Why? What alternative formulations of reality might there have been?
5. If appropriate write up an account and analysis of an episode of communication you had with a patient and/or a colleague.

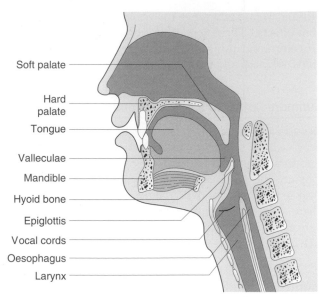

Figure 1.1   Normal anatomy of the head and neck. (After Kristen Wienandt; email: kristen@medartdesign.com with kind permission)

So far this chapter has presented a variety of theories related to communication, and sketched out a number of different research approaches, demonstrating what language may do in health care. But how did human beings become technically competent as communicators in the first place?

THE BIOLOGICAL BASIS OF COMMUNICATION

Communication is founded in human anatomy and physiology. In speech, several parts of anatomy are involved: mouth, nose, pharynx, epiglottis, trachea and lungs (Fig. 1.1). These combine and relate to produce particular kinds of sound that make up the medium for conveying messages to others. But beyond direct speaking mechanisms, other parts of the body support and bring about communication. From the ears and eyes to complexes of muscles and the nervous system, individuals are able to do such things as type on a keyboard, write, or produce and receive a vast range of verbal and non-verbal messages. Moreover, this activity is facilitated by a variety of neurological processes. The next section examines these in a little more detail, beginning with a summary of mechanisms of speech.

Mechanisms of speech

To speak is to articulate sound by pushing air out of the lungs, through the trachea into the larynx where vocal cords take up one of two positions. When the vocal cords are drawn together like a stiff pair of curtains, the air from the lungs has to push them apart, and this causes a vibration, which can be experienced by placing a finger on the top of the larynx and producing sounds like [z]. Sounds made this way are described as 'voiced'. When the vocal cords are left apart though, air passes silently to make 'voiceless' sounds such as [s] or [f].

In its journey onwards, the air passing through the larynx moves into the mouth and/or nose. Consonant sounds, for example [m] in *mother* or [p] in *pretty*, are formed by changing the shape of the oral cavity, notably with the tongue. Try out the following articulations and determine which sounds are 'voiced' or 'voiceless':

Alveolars   Sounds like [t] in *tap* or [n] in *nit* are made with the tip of the tongue on the alveolar ridge at the front of the hard palate.

Alveopalatals   Sounds like [ch] in *child* and [sh] in *shampoo* are made by placing the tongue at the front of the palate.

Bilabials   Sounds like [b] in *bat* or [p] in *put* are made by using both the upper and the lower lip.

Dentals   Sounds like [th] in *think* or *bath* are made by placing the tip of the tongue behind the upper front teeth.

Glottals   Sounds like [h] in *house* or *who* are made when the space between the vocal cords or glottis is open but the sound is not shaped or manipulated by the mouth.

Labiodentals   Sounds like [f] in *fat* and [v] in *vampire* are made with the upper teeth and lower lip.

Velars   Sounds like as [k] in *cold* or *keen* and [g] in *gun* are made by pressing the back of the tongue against the velum (soft palate) at the back of the mouth. The sound [ng] in *tongue* or *bang* is formed by lowering the soft palate to let air through the nasal cavity.

Of course, these are just the positions and shapes taken in the mouth to produce sounds, but this manipulation is done in particular ways. Thus there are:

Affricates   when sounds like [ch] in *chop* are made by the friction of obstructing the release of air that has been briefly stopped.

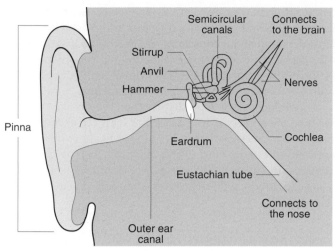

Figure 1.2 The anatomy of the ear.

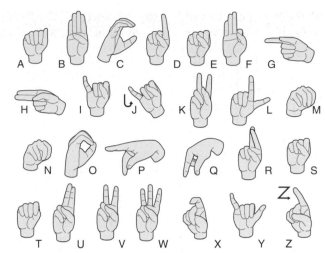

Figure 1.3 The alphabet in sign language.

Approximants   when sounds like [w] in *wet* or [y] in *yes* are made with the tongue moving forward.

Glottal stops   when the glottis is briefly closed and released as when people speaking Cockney say *bitter* or *matter* without pronouncing the 'tt' part in the middle.

Nasals   when sounds like [m], [n] or [ng] as in *boring* are made when air is directed out through the nose.

Stops   when sounds such as [p], [b], [d], [t], [k] or [g] are produced by briefly stopping the passage of air in the mouth cavity and letting it go.

Many of the sounds produced in this way form words, but a significant proportion form what have been termed 'guggles' or paralinguistic cues – the expressions of surprise, support, 'um hmm', 'ah ha' and so forth, which may be used to support and encourage a speaker or to indicate that a person wishes to interrupt. They are an informative part of the 'music' of conversation. Indeed, they may be important in conveying emotion. Whilst these may have some similarities across cultures there is often some difficulty in reading them accurately when the speaker and hearer are from very different linguistic or cultural communities (Scherer et al 2002).

Once the sounds have been made, of course they must be perceived for communication to take place. In the ear sound waves – a kind of 'compression wave' in the air – are converted into nervous impulses and enter the brain via the cochlear nerve. The basic anatomy of the ear is shown in Figure 1.2.

Sound waves enter via the pinna and outer ear canal and vibrate the eardrum or tympanum. This transmits vibration via the bones of the ear – the hammer, anvil and stirrup – to the cochlea which is rich in nerve endings that are able to detect the minute deformations in the tissues caused by the vibrations and turn them into nerve impulses. These impulses then pass along the auditory nerve to the midbrain and then to the auditory cortex of the temporal lobes. Whereas the processing of sound into meaningful units of communication is not well understood, it may be that different brain cells or groups of cells specialize in the recognition of certain kinds of sounds.

Communication difficulties and disabilities

If the sensory processes themselves are impaired, this can lead to difficulties with communication. There are a variety of techniques which can be used to compensate for these impairments. Deaf people can use a number of strategies in communicating: speech, gestures, formal sign language (see Fig. 1.3), finger spelling, writing, reading, lip reading and using hearing aids.

There are a variety of aids to help visually impaired people communicate. These include: glasses, braille, large print, books and magazines on tape, dark lined writing paper, or even a grooved writing board, through to electronic aids such as label readers or voice recognition phone diallers.

One critical aspect of non-verbal communication is the interpretation of facial expressions of emotion, and children with learning difficulties have been found to be less accurate than non-disabled children in making such interpretations. As Bandura (1986) has pointed out, the ability to read the signs of emotions in social interaction has important adaptive value in guiding actions toward others. Presumably, deficits in this area play a significant role in the social difficulties experienced by children with learning disabilities (Dimitrovsky et al 1998).

Message interpretation in the brain

The ability to use language is located in the brain, and debate has ensued about the locality for this specific function. The role of Broca's area in the human brain in the production of speech and Wernicke's area in understanding the significance of content words in speech has been appreciated since the 19th century (Dronkers 2000) (see Fig. 1.4). These two areas are linked by a bundle of nerve fibres called the *articulate fasciculus*. These two main areas have been studied closely, not least in relation to various forms of brain damage and how such lesions affect language production. Damage to Broca's area is related to difficulty in producing speech, while damage to Wernicke's area is related to speech comprehension difficulties. In addition, a part of the motor cortex, close to Broca's area, controls the muscles that articulate the face, tongue and larynx – all key to language production – which when damaged also affect communication.

If a client were to hear a word and repeat it, this suggests a simple transmission of a word being heard and understood in Wernicke's area, which transfers a signal via the articulate fasciculus to Broca's area, where production of the word is set up with a signal being sent to the motor cortex to put it out in a physical form by moving particular muscles, etc. Yet there is evidence that a large number of different areas of the brain are used for the production of spoken utterances (Posner & Raichle 1997) and that different areas of the brain are activated for different aspects of speech. Hence, a rich variety of anatomical and physiological mechanisms and senses lie

---

Decision making exercise

How can people with sensory impairments be assisted to communicate in health care settings? This is particularly crucial as people usually enter health care because something is wrong and there may be strong emotions evoked. Think about different techniques and how you might decide on what to do and what strategy to employ.

In the case of deafness, cochlear implants are an increasingly popular treatment. These involve the implantation of a device with a microphone and electrodes which stimulate the cochlear nerves directly and can provide some measure of hearing. Unfortunately these do not suit everyone, and up to 30% of people so treated give up. Think about the practical help a nurse could give to someone in this situation.

There are communication issues that may require help but people may also be angry at the previous failures of treatment. How might you build rapport or a working therapeutic relationship with a person in this situation?

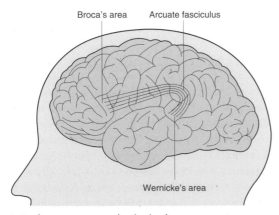

Figure 1.4   Language areas in the brain.

---

behind human communication, and scientists are still examining this complex phenomenon, just as they still have much to understand about consciousness itself. Thus, in contrast to a localized view of language functioning in particular parts of the brain, it appears that this human skill is wrapped up with interdependent aspects of brain function.

Sometimes people's predispositions may make them less likely to interpret cues in a particular way. For example those who are apt to be cynical or hostile are likely to misattribute happiness (Larkin et al 2002). Research has also revealed gender differences in the accuracy of decoding facial expressions of emotion, with males being less accurate than females (Pell 2002).

LANGUAGE ACQUISITION

It is extraordinary how children acquire language. As well as becoming competent users of a complex syntax, on average, English-speaking children acquire a vocabulary of about 60 000 words by the age of 18. The early stages of children's communicative learning are outlined in Table 1.1.

During periods of peak vocabulary development, this must mean learning a new word on average every 2 hours at some points during childhood. This has led some theorists, such as Chomsky (1976) and Pinker (1994) to suggest that there are somehow 'hard-wired' cognitive and neural structures that enable the grammar and lexicon to be learned so readily; in Chomsky's phrase, a 'language acquisition device'. This is debatable, however, and some critics charge Chomsky and Pinker with paying insufficient attention to the sheer diversity of the world's languages, or with not considering how difficult it is to explain language in evolutionary terms (Allott 2001). At the present state of knowledge, communication is far more than biology can explain. Whilst

---

Table 1.1   Language development in children

Child's age	Communication development
0–4 months	Babies start to coo and produce vowel sounds. Will make sounds back when spoken to
6 months	Laughing. Will start to make consonant sounds like d, p and m
6–12 months	Laughing, smiling babbling. Multi-syllable speech such as uh-oh, da-da. Points to objects of interest
12–24 months	Development of vocabulary – about 50 words by 18 months, or 100 by 24 months
2–3 years	Builds sentences such as 'doggy go home'. Acquires concepts such as 'in', 'under' or 'behind'
3–5 years	Development of vocabulary and syntactic ability (the grammatical arrangement of words). Can phrase requests. Sentences get longer. Working vocabulary of about 2300 words by the age of 5 and ability to comprehend 8000 words

biology identifies the mechanics, as it were, it can say little about the ways in which communication is employed.

Broadly speaking, messages are conveyed through our use of a rich and versatile language system. It is difficult to find a shared natural language system anywhere in the world that does not have these features. Even languages that were once believed to be 'primitive' such as sign language (which was supposed to have a more limited range of expressiveness and to be confined to a more limited visual domain) have repaid recent study with fresh insights about their syntactic and expressive complexity (Neidle et al 2002). This also highlights the way that for most hearing cultures gesture, facial expression and style of expression are vitally important too. Therefore it is worth examining the issue of non-verbal communication in more detail, as an awareness of these issues will enable nurses to become flexible and efficient communicators.

NON-VERBAL COMMUNICATION

Much of human communication is delivered through non-verbal channels or 'body language' and is not dependent on sound. Through their gestures, postures and facial expressions, people convey rich messages to others. The vocabularies here are enormous. Early attempts to study these phenomena identified about 20 000 different facial expressions (Birdwhistell 1970), which, when combined with gestures and movements yield about 700 000 different possibilities, which may or may not be meaningful (Pei 1997).

Non-verbal communication involves a variety of issues (Patterson 1983). Some of its functions are relational and concern how an individual feels towards another person. That is, it might express feelings about the other person, such as liking or disliking; it can establish dominance or control; or it can be used to express intimacy, perhaps by touching and mutual eye contact. Non-verbal signals can be used to regulate interactions, by signalling the approaching end of an utterance or the desire to speak, or it may facilitate goal attainment, for example by pointing. Facial expressions add to this visual richness, especially through changes to the eyes and mouth. In interaction in contemporary Western cultures participants typically spend about 60% of the time gazing at one another and these gazes typically last about 3 seconds (Argyle & Ingham 1972). Mutual gazes take up 30% of the time, with the actual gaze lasting about 1 second (Kleineke 1986). The eyes often signal that a person is ready to speak or to end communication. The use of body space – how close people position themselves to others (proximity) – and the shape or posture they adopt affect how messages are sent and received. Whether individuals touch others and how they do this, and what clothes they choose to wear, are used to signal messages such as status and bring yet more dynamics to communication. The issue of how well-attuned a health care professional is to the client's communicative preferences is therefore important. If health care professionals make decisions or communicate in a way that fails to account for clients' cultural beliefs and preferences, then the client's self-care, adherence to advice and overall outcome may well be poorer (Stewart et al 1999).

In an information-rich society, much communication relies on visual images from film and television to photography and art. Most people use a wide spectrum of all these forms of communication in addition to verbal and written language. Sometimes verbal and non-verbal communications amplify one another. At other times, though, such as when people say they are OK but their bodies indicate otherwise, they create more ambiguous communications.

Decision making exercise

Think of different styles of communication associated with different kinds of emotional tone. How would you speak and act if you were being:

- Bullying?
- Nervous?
- Confident?
- Humorous?

Evidence suggests that people who are being abused would often like to talk to a health professional about it, but are unsure of how to broach the subject (McAfee 2001). Imagine that you had a client whose physical symptoms suggested that she came from an abusive family situation.

- How could you make it easier for her to disclose the problem? Bear in mind that people in such a situation might not necessarily disclose this in response to a direct question.
- Think about how you could use style of speech, vocabulary, delivery, facial expressions and gestures, or even the seating arrangements in the room to make it easier for the client.
- What systems should be in place to support you in dealing with this client?

Graphical communication

Drawing and graphical communication can be an important tool in the hands of nurses and their clients. Indeed, it may be especially useful when communicating with people from different language groups or with people who suffer sensory or communicative impairments. For example, there are cases of people who have been severely communication-impaired following a stroke who have become functional communicators once more through drawing (Rao 1995). Some authors have also noted the way that drawings provide a useful window into the emotional lives of children who have suffered a traumatic event such as bereavement (Clements et al 2001, Wellings 2001).

PSYCHOSOCIAL FACTORS INFLUENCING COMMUNICATION

Communication takes place in a whole range of social settings or environments, involving people with a variety of identities and outlooks. Communication is affected by variables such as age, gender, social class, culture and ethnicity that can influence its content and style. Although this makes sense intuitively, it has been rather difficult to reliably identify specific markers or interpersonal differences in speech style (Hogg & Vaughan 2002), perhaps because people are extremely flexible and usually competent in several different speech styles. A person may be able to speak some version of the 'received pronunciation' or formal, official language in which a good deal of institutional business is done, yet at the same time may use a dialect or less formal language such as slang socially. In addition, the kind of language used, rules or laws of social behaviour, the social status and power relations of participants, and the kinds of roles or life scripts that they have adopted may equally affect communication.

Decision making exercise

Observe some interaction between consultant and nurse or nurse and patient. Look at the way they communicate. Observe who is in charge and note how this is manifested.

- How could you use this observation in your practice?
- For example, a patient adopting a 'sick role' may communicate in a very passive, dependent way. How would you counteract this tendency?
- If a consultant dominates a multidisciplinary team meeting, what might you as a nurse do to change the balance of power?

The speech style of a person in a powerless position tends to involve the use of features such as:

- 'intensifiers', e.g. 'very', 'really' and 'so'
- 'hedges', e.g. 'kind of', 'sort of', 'you know'
- rising intonation, which makes a declaration sound like a question
- polite forms of address (Lakoff 1975).

Power can be associated with the ability to interrupt and take control of the 'floor' in conversation (Reid & Ng 1999). Nearly 30 years ago, Zimmerman & West (1975) noted that 98% of interruptions were by men. More recently, although the situation has become more equitable, men are still more likely to interrupt, especially when interaction is studied in field settings and when there are more than three people present (Anderson & Leaper 1998).

Evidence based practice

Interruptions can be considerably more than a nuisance. Individuals who interrupt a good deal may be doing this as part of the Type A behaviour pattern, characterized by loud speech and frequent interruptions, as well as a rapid speech rate, hard-driving hurried behaviour, impatience and hostility. The Type A behaviour pattern has been associated with an increased likelihood of heart disease, originally by Friedman & Rosenman (1959), with the interest in speech styles being pursued by other researchers more recently (de Pino-Perez et al 1999). Indeed, Ekman & Rosenberg (1997) note that as well as rapid and aggressive speech, Type A behaviour is associated with more facial expressions of glare and disgust. Thus, communicative style can be a valuable clue that a person's lifestyle may be making them more vulnerable to illness. Friedman & Rosenman were cardiologists and their initial ideas were stimulated by noting that the edges of the seats in their consulting rooms wore away. Eventually they deduced that this was to do with the 'edge of the seat' stance of their impatient patients.

Gender differences in speech styles are not innate in any obvious sense, but reflect status differences in situations. We may anticipate changes in the pattern of gender differences as greater social, economic and occupational equality is achieved. In the meantime, Fairclough (1989) argues that nurses, among others, should be aware of 'how language contributes to the domination of some people by others' and suggests that being conscious of this 'is the first step towards emancipation' (Fairclough 1989: 1).

Awareness of language and communication thus involves an awareness of the diverse range of biological, personal and social factors that have an impact on the speech styles in use in health care. Moreover, becoming aware of these factors can enable nurses to work to change the situation to the benefit of clients and nurses themselves.

USING LANGUAGE IN HEALTH CARE

An individual's capacity for communication does not remain static, but changes over the lifespan, and adult communicators will be concerned with how to be efficient and effective communicators and avoid the pitfalls of communicating in limited, negative or harmful ways. The notion that language might be harmful is of particular importance in the context of health care, where the overriding premise is to promote human well-being (Crawford et al 1998). Language may not always work in the client's interests, however. It is important, therefore, to be aware that some styles of communication are more contentious and the role they can play in facilitating the oppression of clients, as well as healing them, requires careful examination.

Language, ideology and power

Nursing communication takes place in a context informed by wider political and economic directives, and involves communication with other health care professionals, such as doctors, psychologists, occupational therapists, administrators and managers, as well as clients and their families. As such it is caught in a web of powerful conceptions and ideologies of what society should be like, how it is constructed and what is important. Moreover, according to Fairclough (1989), nursing is shaped by equally powerful ideologies of bureaucratic 'cost-effectiveness' and 'efficiency', and nurses' training tends to promote acquisition of communication or social skills 'whose primary motivation is efficient people-handling' (Fairclough 1989: 235). At times, this may mean that nurses are communicating in a way that is incompatible with their profession's or their own value systems, but which has more to do with economics, politics and the public image of the institution for which they work.

Kinds of talk in health care settings

Language can be a means of socializing a client into a particular kind of role, as a patient, a victim, as someone who is in pain or as someone who is incapable. There has been a good deal of research about the role of language styles and plot structures in enabling the roles of health care professionals and patients to be performed in health care settings.

Evidence based practice

Proctor et al (1996) studied how nurses in a trauma centre in a US hospital talked to injured patients. By video-taping interactions between nurses and patients in pain, the authors identified what they called the Comfort Talk Register. The register involved different kinds of talk with specific pragmatic functions. The researchers identified holding on, assessing, informing and caring functions:

- *Holding on* was conducted through the use of phrases like 'Big girl', 'You're doing great', 'Count to three'. This served to praise, to let the patient know they can get through, to support, to instruct or distract the patient.
- *Assessing* involved 'How are you?' questions or giving the patient information – 'You're in the emergency room'. These involved getting information, explaining the situation or validating and confirming the patient's input.
- *Informing* were statements like 'It's gonna hurt' or 'We'll be inserting a catheter', i.e. warning the patient or explaining procedures.
- *Caring* included statements like 'Relax' or 'OK sweetie' or 'It does hurt, doesn't it?', i.e. reassuring, empathic or caring comments (Proctor et al 1996: 1673).

The authors suggest that because these features of comfort talk are regularly used, the talk has a rhythmical, sing-song quality and is mainly used to get patients to endure the situation a little longer. The researchers highlight the importance of the style and content of communication in the commencement of courses of treatment.

Reflection and portfolio evidence

Observe two or three clinical situations or events and imagine that you are watching a play or television drama.

- What is the plot? Who is/are the main character(s)?
- What differences can you find in the way the different clinical situations proceed?
- Do they have different endings?
- How active was the patient in the way the 'drama' unfolded?
- Do they seem to have a particular formula or any dramatic motifs or features? Do they have: formulaic expressions – 'What seems to be the trouble?'; complications and difficulties; happy endings?
- Where appropriate and maintaining confidentiality, include one of these 'dramas' along with your critical commentary in your portfolio.

The negative use of communication

As nurses deal with clients, a number of features of their language can be a source of complaint. When caregivers are interacting with elderly clients, they have been observed using high-pitched baby talk, controlling institutional talk, short utterances, simple grammatical structures, interrogatives (questions) and imperatives (commands) (Ambady et al 2002). Moreover there is some evidence to suggest that this use of patronizing speech styles does not depend on the status of the patient – the confused are no more likely to be patronized than those who are alert and oriented. Rather, the speech style seemed to depend on the attitudes of the caregiver (Caporael et al 1983). The features of speech and non-verbal behaviour – for example high pitch, pats on the shoulder and expressions like 'That's a good girl' – are not only perceived by the elderly patients themselves as patronizing, but are also seen to be unfavourable by observers (Ryan et al 1994). It is important, therefore, that those working with elderly people are aware of the tendency of caregivers to talk in these ways and that some instruction on these matters is incorporated into the education of caregivers (Ryan et al 1994).

Evidence based practice

Albert Robillard (1996), a sociologist who suffers multiple disabilities, movingly describes the effects of patronizing talk. He illustrates people's responses to his anger at this kind of mistreatment thus:

The response of my interlocutors to my visible anger ranges from 'I did not know you could hear', 'I didn't know you could think!', 'Most of my patients are stroke victims and have trouble understanding me' to 'Oh, I am sorry, I won't do it again.' Most react to my outburst by ignoring me, leading me to see the ignoral as a further documentary reading of my symptomatology by my interlocutor.

It is a toss-up if my harsh reaction will change the course of interaction. Frequently those who say 'I did not know you could ...', or 'I am sorry, I will not do it again' go back to exclusionary practices in a few moments. (Robillard 1996: 19)

Much can be learned from attempting to make sense of people's complaints about health care, however bizarre they might seem at first.

Institutional care encourages dependency, by means of both open (overt) and secret or disguised (covert) strategies on the part of care staff (Ryan & Scullion 2000). Although the situation is changing slowly, being a 'good patient' traditionally involves being passive, compliant and docile. The language of the institution is thought to be more important in producing dependency than the disability itself. Moreover, despite the ethic of care in such institutions, the experience of being cared for is often profoundly dehumanizing:

Older residents must adapt to a new set of routines, expectations and rules, frequently compromising or abandoning their own lifetime preferences, habits and needs. Further, they must make these adaptations from the socially inferior or less powerful role of resident or patient. (Ryan et al 1994: 238)

The examples of 'comfort talk' and 'secondary baby talk' in therapeutic encounters illustrate the way that language is a tool for socialization in health care settings. The role of language may be to offer comfort and to enlist clients in the rituals of health care in a way that might ultimately benefit them. At the same time it is important to be aware of how the role of language might just as easily be to patronize or incapacitate the client and place them in a position where they are disadvantaged and disabled by the communicative style adopted. This should highlight the importance of language as a tool for the clinician and encourage reflection on the ways in which language use might harm or heal clients.

THE ROLE OF CULTURE IN NARRATIVES OF HEALTH AND ILLNESS

Most fundamental ideas about medicine are embedded in culture and language. Within the UK in the 21st century, most people think that they know what a sick person is. Everyday complaints like the common cold and gastrointestinal upsets have a set of symptoms that are expected to co-occur. As sufferers or healers, people tended to look for distinct patterns in illness. However, history suggests that the way illness is defined today depends a great deal on fairly recent changes in patterns of sickness and health. Contemporary illnesses are different from those described in the 18th century – people no longer claim to suffer from 'seizures of the bowels' or 'rising of the lights'. Nevertheless, in all centuries, the coherence of an illness is an important part of the sufferer's experience of it.

The concern with narratives emerges from the everyday observation that when we find out about someone, we usually do so by means of a story that they tell or which someone else tells about them. These stories are important because they do not merely describe experience but constitute or make it.

Nurses narrate both their own stories of care and the stories told to them by clients. This does not mean that the stories nurses tell are pure fictions. What it does mean is that much of what happens between nurses and patients is to do with narration. This idea has been developed in psychology, sociology, anthropology and in the study of medical and nursing activities and the experiences of clients.

Reflection and portfolio evidence

Consider how much of your work depends on the stories you tell about yourself and about those for whom you care. To make this exercise a little more concrete, you might like to think about the following examples: physical problems – broken femur, appendicitis; psychological problems – depression, anxiety; life course changes – birth, hospice care.

● What kinds of events are these problems likely to involve?
● What might one encounter as a nurse?
● How do these 'stories' about clients' problems influence the kind of care we make available?
● Write up your experiences for your portfolio and discuss with your peer group or personal tutor.

Narratives also reflect the interests of the teller. For example, Hyden (1995) describes how in cases of domestic violence, male perpetrators favour words that emphasize purpose (why they acted as they did) whereas female partners emphasize agency (how they were beaten) and the physical and emotional consequences. This kind of storytelling reveals another important feature – the communicators are often at pains to manage their 'stake' and 'interest' in the piece. A critical comment about a patient may be prefaced with the claim 'I usually try to be on the patient's side, but ...'. Everyday speech is littered with similar examples. Homophobic comments are often accompanied by statements like 'Some of my best friends are gay' or potential accusations of ethnic prejudice are headed off with 'I'm not racist but ...'.

In terms of the tales of illness that nurses are likely to encounter, it is important to consider the role that culture has in helping to make sense of these phenomena. In European or North American white majority cultures, the degree of correspondence between the stories told by clients and professionals makes it easy to take the signs, symptoms, syndromes and illnesses for granted. However, it is important to realize that if the cultural frame of reference is moved a little, the problems people express may seem to be at odds with dominant Western medical notions of health and illness.

Evidence based practice

Sachs's (1983) account of Turkish women resident in Sweden highlights how you need to consider cultural differences in the way people define or explain their illness states:

> In the forty days after childbirth known as the lohusa period, a woman is liable to contract albasmasi. This condition, characterized by the woman seeing everything in red, turning hot and getting cramps as well as choking, is one of the most feared reactions connected with childbirth. All women have heard of it and been in touch with it one way or another in Kulu (a region of Turkey). Albasmasi is an illness with specific symptoms. When a case has been established, it is only the personal and folk sectors of health care that can provide treatment. A scientific doctor will not be consulted. The Kulu women know that only their own experts can cure a person from albasmasi and that scientific doctors have not even heard of the illness. (Sachs 1983: 86)

Cross-cultural issues are becoming increasingly important in health care as global migration changes the cultural map of the world (Choi 2002). In the case of unusual or exotic complaints such as albasmasi, debate might revolve around the extent to which albasmasi is similar to postnatal depression, and whether benefits from the traditional treatment might be akin to the placebo effect or Euro-American concepts of psychotherapy.

Carr & Vitaliano (1985: 244) ask whether disorders are particular to specific cultures or 'simply culturally determined variants of universal forms of psychopathology like depression'. However, this sort of debate, about whether one culture's illnesses and treatments can be recast in those of another, misses the point. To a practitioner confronted with a client who describes their problems in unfamiliar terms, it is often of secondary importance whether a 'better' approximation to their problems might be found in a Western textbook. The exhortation from governments, policy makers and educators is that health care assessments should be undertaken in the client's own terms. That means that nurses must sometimes act more like anthropologists exploring cultures, ways of seeing and feeling and formulations of reality with which they are unfamiliar.

Decision making exercise

Consider the comments of a woman of South Asian parentage speaking after her nephew had died in an accident: 'My heart is weak. I am ill with too much thinking ... the blood becomes weaker with worry ... I have the illness of sorrows' (Fenton & Sadiq-Sangster 1996).

- Can this account be repackaged by the interviewer as depression, or does labelling what she is suffering as depression lose some of the culturally important information which could lead to her being helped?
- Do existing forms, records and checklists that you use in your practice allow for the inclusion of such accounts? If not, why not?
- How could health care practice be broadened to include more of the experience of other cultures?

Scientific terms used to describe mental and physical illnesses can have a metaphorical quality (Sontag 1979), that is, they may be applied to objects to which they are not literally applicable. People's descriptions of symptoms are burdened with other meanings even when they are talking about apparently clear-cut areas such as alcoholism or agoraphobia. Migliore (1993) describes the way Sicilian-Canadians use the idea of 'nerves' to 'express feelings of concern and distress over their social situation. They translate social problems into the metaphorical language of psychic and somatic distress' (Migliore 1993: 343). 'Nerves' operates both as a sort of illness, and as a device for metaphorically expressing personal and social problems. Metaphors of illness may be especially powerful. Some theorists such as Lakoff (1987) argue, even more radically, that metaphor influences not only how we perceive reality but that it can also structure how we experience that reality.

The lens of language formulates people and their problems in various ways, depending upon the kinds of frames (Goffman 1974) the actors are working with. For example, studies of doctor–patient interaction suggest that there are complex rules governing the shift from an interpersonal frame of reference to a biomedical one. Coupland et al (1994) noticed that the health professional sometimes asked two 'How are you?' questions. One came at the very start of the encounter and was a kind of sociable device, whereas the other came a little later and signalled that it was time to begin an account of the symptoms. Language crucially informs the way that diagnoses are achieved and 'progress' is accomplished. This has important implications for ethnic sensitivity in nursing practice, as the dominant understandings of progress or desirable outcomes in Euro-American medicine and psychiatry will not necessarily be shared by other cultures. Understanding the language of health care is important in making sense of the critiques of medicine and psychiatry offered from anti-racist or feminist positions, where the frameworks and inferential structures of mainstream medical and psychiatric care are argued to embody white, male, middle class assumptions and values (Parker et al 1995).

Thus, the frame, script or linguistic formulation within which the client and his or her problems are formulated may have important practical consequences for their future. In this respect, it is important that nurses remain vigilant about the potential for oppression in everyday healthcare language and communication, and the frameworks for understanding and problem solving that are embedded in everyday practice.

CARE DELIVERY KNOWLEDGE

Much of nursing is about communicating in day-to-day spoken and written interactions with other members of the healthcare team, patients and relatives. This might take place in such activities as counselling and building a therapeutic relationship, assessment and care planning, information giving, teaching and health promotion, record keeping, and dealing with communication difficulties. Each of these areas in care delivery will be explored further.

COUNSELLING AND DEVELOPING A THERAPEUTIC RELATIONSHIP

This section examines some of the basic types and styles of communication needed for general counselling and building therapeutic relationships.

Listening and gaining rapport

In order to develop a therapeutic relationship with patients, it is vital to remember the finer aspects of courteous communication that are often taken for granted in daily life, but are complained about bitterly when someone does not use them. For example, it is important to properly meet and greet clients in a respectful way. This may mean, for example, addressing them by a formal name such as 'Mrs Brown' and only using informal first name terms if invited to. For most clients brought up in a Western culture, an appropriate non-verbal performance should include facing the client

with an open posture (not arms folded), leaning slightly towards them, with regular but not fixed eye contact, and maintaining a relaxed demeanour. By adopting such a stance and by attending to a person and actively listening in a genuine way to what they have to say (rather than thinking about what you are going to say next), or simply giving time to share your 'presence' with them, you will begin the process of gaining rapport or bonding with the client.

When listening to clients it is important to use an appropriate level of verbal prompts such as 'Yes', 'Go on', 'I see' or 'OK' and non-verbal prompts such as nodding, smiling, etc. These signal that you are interested in what they are saying. Again, avoid fiddling with objects while conversing, or looking away or over the patient's shoulder.

The process of gaining rapport will be further enhanced by demonstrating that you are a 'warm', authentic individual who is not going to judge in a negative fashion what they have to say, and that your attitudes and values are driven by 'unconditional positive regard' – you do not compromise or restrict your esteem or valuation of the patient even when their values, morals or behaviour do not agree with your own. Finally, fundamental to this whole process of gaining a client's trust and creating a therapeutic relationship, is empathy – attempting to enter into and understand what it might be like being a particular patient, in particular circumstances, in conversation with you.

Reflection and summarizing

One of the common ways that reflection on the content of what others say is facilitated by paraphrasing. Rather than 'parrot-phrasing', in which what the other person said is merely repeated, paraphrasing involves restating in brief what was said in order to:

● clarify they were heard accurately
● provide an opportunity to reflect on what was said (the content)
● encourage further development of ideas or issues.

It is often also helpful to reflect back or acknowledge feelings or emotions that were expressed verbally and non-verbally during the conversation. This can deepen the sense of empathy and may help to review areas in the individual's life that need addressing. By summarizing the content of a conversation it is possible to draw together the key aspects of what was communicated. This can help to bring a shape to what may have been an unstructured discussion, and may lead to exploring possible solutions to problems. Once rapport is established, negotiating solutions can occur in a creative process of formulating new approaches or strategies, and where unhelpful thinking or behaviours can be challenged and reframed into a new, more helpful perspective.

Thus, a key aspect of assessing and probing for solutions occurs through questioning.

Questioning

The process of questioning is central to many aspects of communication. Although there are several forms of questions that can be used, these can be categorized into two major groups: open and closed. Closed questions are designed to obtain simple 'Yes' or 'No' responses. In contrast, open questions allow greater exploration of ideas and exchange of information.

For example, if you ask a client, 'Are you in pain?' (closed question) the answer would usually be 'Yes' or 'No'. However, if you asked 'What is the pain like?' (open question) you would normally receive a longer account or response.

In asking questions, it is important to pay particular attention to topic areas that may be particularly sensitive and where questioning may come across as intrusive. Where topics are sensitive, for example in relation to sexual health or other potentially embarrassing areas of care, then issues of privacy and framing any questions in a suitably polite form need to be addressed.

Asking too many questions, particularly in a quick-fire series, should be avoided as this can be uncomfortable and intrusive, particularly where rapport has not been fully established or developed. It may also be stressful, particularly if the individual is confused or anxious, and lacking in emotional warmth. Finally, it may come across as rude and increase frustration. Equally, it is best to avoid questions beginning with 'why' because this tends to suggest that judgement is being passed on what an individual has or has not done.

Closure

Ending a period of communication is as important as beginning one. In other words, attention needs to be paid to clarifying what has been discussed and decided upon in terms of any goals that have been set, and when further meetings will take place. In situations that occur over a longer period, such as counselling, clients may become dependent on the relationship and steps need to be taken to outflank this difficulty by setting out a clear contract of involvement from the start, indicating any time limitations, and highlighting the desirability of preserving the autonomy and independence of the person throughout.

Models for counselling

There are a wide variety of theoretical models available to guide nurse counselling and analyse communication approaches. Such models can be investigated as part of a nurse's commitment to continuing professional development, not least as part of portfolio keeping. An excellent introduction is Heron's (1990) six category intervention, where he identifies two sets of interventions: those that are authoritative or nurse-directed (prescriptive, informative, confronting) and those that are facilitative or enable patients

to develop themselves in some way (cathartic, catalytic, supporting). In brief:

- prescriptive – directing, delegating, advising
- informative – factually informing, explaining
- confronting – challenging patient perspectives, attitudes or behaviour
- cathartic – encouraging expression of emotions
- catalytic – promoting further self-discovery
- supportive – valuing, accepting.

This framework can be used to reflect upon communication exchanges and shape subsequent interactions.

INTERVIEWING AND ASSESSMENT

Communication is very important in relation to assessment and care planning. In the UK, health and social care policy is increasingly focused on supporting people in their own homes rather than in hospital or nursing home environments. Good interprofessional communication is therefore vital to ensure a quality seamless service for the patient between home, health and social care organizations.

Assessment of vulnerable people

Assessment, even with very vulnerable or frail older adults, should include the client as an active collaborator in the assessment process. The UK's Better Service for Vulnerable People agenda (Department of Health 1997a) has called upon local authorities to review their practice of multidisciplinary assessment of people with complex needs. Assessment should also provide care plans that help users achieve their personal goals (Department of Health 1998).

The assessment process

It can still be the case that users and carers have to repeat their stories to several different health and social care professionals and often face various assessments with a lack of co-ordination between agencies. This leads to different assessment records being compiled with separate questionnaires and interview schedules peculiar to different professional groups (Health Committee 1999). However, there are increasingly more examples of interagency patient-held records so as to maximize not only the availability of a range of information to interested professionals, but also give the client a greater sense of ownership over their plan of care (Dunstan 1999). Nolan & Caldock (1996) make some suggestions as to how the assessment process can best be carried out (Fig. 1.5).

As should be clear, all of these criteria (Fig. 1.5) are based on good communication and an acknowledgement of the central role of the client's perspective in the assessment process.

This notion of enabling clients to express their views and including these views in the delivery of care underlies much

1. Empower both the user and carer – inform fully, clarify their understanding of the situation and of the role of the assessor before going ahead.

2. Involve the user and carer, make them feel that they are full partners in the assessment.

3. Shed your 'professional' perspective – have an open mind and be prepared to learn.

4. Start from where the user and carer are – establish their existing level of knowledge and what hopes and expectations they have.

5. Be interested in the user and carer as people.

6. Establish a suitable environment for the assessment, which ensures there is privacy, quiet and sufficient time.

7. Take time – build trust and rapport, and overcome the brief visitor syndrome; this will usually take more than one encounter.

8. Be sensitive, imaginative and creative in responding – users and carers may not know what is possible or available. For carers in particular, guilt and reticence may have to be overcome.

9. Avoid value judgements whenever possible – if such judgements are needed, make them explicit.

10. Consider social, emotional and relationship needs, as well as just practical needs and difficulties. Pay particular attention to the quality of the relationship between user and carer.

11. Listen to and value the user's and carer's expertise or opinions, even if these run counter to your own values as a professional.

12. Present honest, realistic service options, identifying advantages and disadvantages and providing an indication of any delay or limitations in delivery of the service.

13. Do not make assessment a 'battle' in which users and carers feel they have to fight for services.

14. Balance all perspectives.

15. Clarify understanding at the end of the assessment, agree objectives and the nature of the review process.

Figure 1.5 Suggestions for the assessment process. (Reproduced by kind permission of Blackwell from Nolan & Caldock 1996.)

of contemporary healthcare policy in the UK (Department of Health 1997a). The National Service Framework for Mental Health (Department of Health 1999), for example, emphasizes the inclusion of clients' voices, with client groups being surveyed, focus grouped and consulted about all aspects of their care. The contemporary trend then, 50 years after Peplau (1952), is that the interpersonal nature of nursing is now embedded in policy.

Reflection and portfolio evidence

In your practice placement review the documentation and interactions that take place during the assessment of a patient/client.

- Reflect on how helpful the assessment process is in allowing the patient control over the subsequent plan of care.
- Review whether it is the approach of the individual professional that is of primary importance rather than the particular documentation used for assessment.
- Comment on the level of 'interprofessional' assessment achieved through the model in use.
- Record your findings in your portfolio.

GIVING INFORMATION, TEACHING AND PROMOTING HEALTH

The role of the nurse is increasingly one of being a teacher, health promoter and giver of information. Mackintosh (1996) notes that there are a number of aspects to this:

> [it] involves social, economic and political change to ensure that the environment is conducive to health. Health promotion not only encompasses a nurse educating an individual about his health needs, but also demands that the nurse plays her part in attempting to address the wider environmental and social issues that adversely affect people's health. (Mackintosh 1996: 14)

Despite this expanding role, as Whitehead (2003) notes, there is little systematic evaluation of whether this activity has been effective. Nevertheless it is possible to offer some guidance on the basis of what we know already about effective health communication in terms of educating others.

- Determine individual learning styles, adopting a flexible approach to presentation of material to suit the learner. This may result in individual learning, learning in groups and/or through experience, such as doing exercises and activities. The latter increase learner involvement and aid memory for what was taught.
- Establish and maintain effective learning environments. This means paying attention to when and where teaching takes place. For example, trying to teach in a noisy, public area is not ideal. Yet nurses often need to teach 'on the hoof' as it were, weaving this aspect of their work into or alongside busy clinical activities, and therefore need to be flexible.
- Plan and structure learning activities. Where possible, it is best to set out learning objectives and outcomes for any teaching, paying attention to time limits and resources. Most people find it hard to concentrate for long periods, so it is best to break down any teaching into 'bite-size' chunks, with sufficient breaks.
- Use appropriate resources to support learning. There are various resources available to enhance teaching. For example, think about using 'Powerpoint', audiovisual materials, the Internet, and so on.
- Where possible provide handouts for any session, with suggested reading, and follow-up questions.
- It is desirable to undertake evaluations to determine whether the intervention is suitable for the clients' needs and values, and whether the intervention is being understood, appreciated, and whether it is leading to changes in the clients' health status (Whitehead 2003).

KEEPING RECORDS OF CARE

Nursing practice is constructed by a variety of texts, such as procedure manuals, nursing policy documents, videos of nursing procedures, diagrams of techniques and the nursing process itself which forms a kind of backbone to nursing language. Berg (1996) notes that texts such as records in medicine have a circular relationship with medico-nursing work. The structure of the medical encounter often corresponds to the structure of the forms that have to be filled in and the narrative structure of patients' problems. This frequently happens in research where the questions asked determine the sorts of responses elicited. In understanding the pervasiveness of a particular structure of storytelling we have to understand a great deal more about the narrative structure of care as a whole.

In many clinical settings, including those studied by Berg (1996), the records made by doctors are accorded a higher status than those made by nurses. The medical record is considered to define reality in a way that nursing records are not. Berg (1996) shows how doctors include or exclude information that arises from the practitioner–patient relationship in a highly selective and elaborative way. Because the records exist as printed forms with predefined categories, they aid in the process of detailing the patients' problems in ways that are medically relevant. Summarizing reduces the unruly, unauthorized complexity of patients' talk of distress and imposes another, medically approved frame of reference.

In settings where nurses have a more active authorial role, much of what Berg (1996) observes about the medical records' constitutive and organizational roles can be extended to the nursing record. Nursing keeps its own records which constitute reality in its own terms and direct subsequent nursing action to deal with that reality.

Decision making exercise

In an older adult healthcare setting, you are allocated to look after two patients who have recently been admitted. You note from the verbal handover given by the nurse on the previous shift that one patient has acute physical problems combined with lack of support being available from relatives or friends. The second patient, who is physically fit but very confused with loss of short-term memory, has a very worried daughter who wishes to care for her mother at home but is becoming increasingly stressed.

- Reflect and decide on what images you received of your two patients from the verbal handover and how these influenced your first encounter with these patients and the carer.
- Review the models of care inherent in the documentation you might use for assessing and planning care for these two patients.
- Decide whether these models will help you fully assess the different needs of both these patients.
- How will you ensure that the patient and carer are involved in the assessment process?
- What factors will determine how care is prioritized through interprofessional working and patient centred record keeping?

One way of gaining insight into how written communication frameworks mediate the relationship between health professionals and patients is to imagine what would happen if all the records in all hospitals and health centres were to vanish overnight. Berg (1996) demonstrates that the record is not just an auxiliary feature of clinical life but that it is

a material form of semi-public memory: relieving medical personnel's burden of organizing and keeping track of the work to be done and its outcomes. The medical or nursing record is a structured distributing and collecting device, where all tasks concerning a patient's trajectory must begin and end. The simple ticking of a box, or the jotting down of some words set organizational routines in motion. (Berg 1996: 510)

The records enable staff to make sense of their patients.

Evidence based practice

Berg (1996) highlights the way that health care has a kind of 'paper life' in the records that are kept. The records are public repositories which store the actions of professionals for inspection or auditing.

Other kinds of material are included in records, such as photography, especially in wound care (Russell & Gray 2002). There is also a growing body of research on record keeping itself (Gerrish et al 1999, Sharma et al 2002). Research is likely to be more productive if researchers understand the social life of records, rather than merely bemoan the fact that they are incomplete. One way to improve the situation has been highlighted by Crow & Harmeling (2002) where records are redesigned to reflect the assessment procedures that practitioners use, and correspond to the way they deal with their patients. Thus the information is collected in a way which is intuitive and fits easily into the diagnostic and treatment process, rather than seeming like an extra burden.

Computer based records

Managers and service planners have attempted to increase the productivity of record takers by introducing computer-aided documentation systems. Increasingly, information will be created, stored, and disseminated electronically as work progresses towards implementation of the Electronic Patient Records (EPR) and Electronic Health Records (EHR) (Department of Health 2000).

Despite some favourable reports that recording information in this way is faster and more comprehensive, the introduction of computers into care situations has not always been a success. Bedside terminals may be scarcely used (Marr et al 1993) and despite the implementation of guidelines on record keeping there are often major omissions by the staff, such as the date, or whether important diagnostic information has been taken into account (Sharma et al 2002).

The modernization agenda in the NHS increasingly involves patients as partners in care and even recording care should be, where possible, a joint venture.

The drive towards quality documentation may be difficult for some nurses. Howse & Bailey (1992) highlight nurses' lack of confidence in their writing skills and their difficulty in articulating what exactly is done in nursing practice. Yet comprehensive, accurate recording of what is 'out there' – the often complicated context of patient care – will always be difficult to pin down in language. Indeed, studies of 'telling the truth' (Nash 1985) and telling factual accounts (Potter 1996) suggest that there are a great many social rituals and language forms involved in these apparently straightforward practices. Adding more detail suggests that the writer or speaker is trying to be convincing. It does not necessarily correspond to what you would have seen if you had been there in the first place. Therefore the drive towards accuracy and completeness can only take us so far. It is important to be aware of these limitations.

Reflection and portfolio evidence

The process of record making in health care is often repetitive and not always patient centred. It is worth thinking about healthcare records at different levels: organizational policy requirements; design of forms or computer data entry systems; kinds of descriptions of patients that are entered; the way the records are used; how patients can be encouraged to say the right things to the healthcare professionals so as to influence what they write; the current use of patient centred multiprofessional records; audited care pathways.

- Review the type of record keeping you have observed in your various practice placements.
- Using the information above, critically comment on these records and add to your portfolio.

COMMUNICATION DIFFICULTIES

Everyone experiences minor communication difficulties from time to time. Take, for example, how sound production can be hampered when you have a sore throat, a mouth ulcer, or after receiving local anaesthetic at the dentist, or even when your mouth is very dry. Nurses may be called upon to work with clients with more serious communication difficulties. The nature of many illnesses is such that the client's ability to communicate is impaired, for example, and most obviously, in the case of loss of consciousness. Yet even under these circumstances, there are reports of people remembering conversations around them whilst they were apparently comatose or anaesthetized, thus highlighting the importance of ensuring that communication is appropriate. Or disorders of speech may be due to problems with

---

Reflection and portfolio evidence

Nurses working in Intensive Care Units have been the subject of much research into the patterns of communication that occur with their heavily sedated and ventilated patients and they are very aware of the need for appropriate communication. Review and reflect on your experiences of communicating with patients who had difficulties.

- Reflect on how much time you spent with a patient who had communication difficulties in comparison to a patient who was able to respond normally.
- Reflect on what communication patterns/styles are more effective if the patient can hear but is unable to speak to you (e.g. patient following a stroke).
- If a patient has hearing difficulties review what alterations you would make to your way of communicating.
- Review your current knowledge of hearing aids such as those supplied by audiologists.
- Record your learning as appropriate in your portfolio.

---

anatomical mechanisms for speech (*dysarthria*). A variety of speech and language problems arise when people suffer strokes or dementia, or have learning difficulties, sensory impairments and mental health problems, all of which may impair a person's communicative abilities. In strokes, for example, it is common for the sufferer's comprehension or expression of speech to be disturbed (*dysphàsia*).

Amongst clients who are conscious, and attempting to recover their communication abilities, a good deal of the communication therapy may well be undertaken by a speech therapist, but often nurses will be the front line carers for such clients. There are a number of reports in the literature of nurses being able to screen patients for difficulties with chewing, drinking and swallowing (Cantwell 2000, Dumble & Tuson 1998) which may require more specialist interventions and yield improvements in communication.

As well as the technical issues of identifying impairments, nurses may be key to developing new ways of dealing with people whose communication is problematic. Bradshaw (1998) described how clinic staff developed a communication programme for a man with profound hearing loss, learning disabilities and challenging behaviour. As a result of changing their communicative actions so that there was greater use of signing and gesturing that involved a greater range of communicative functions, staff noted that the communication skills of the man significantly improved. Staff attitude appeared to change as they then saw him as being challenged rather than as challenging.

Teaching the client and their relatives, friends and informal caregivers how to enhance the communication environment can be achieved successfully. Tye-Murray & Schurm (1994) describe how communication enhancement with individuals suffering from hearing loss can involve the rest of their family and social circle, so that 'frequent communication partners' are enabled to use more effective strategies such as clearer speaking behaviours, message tailoring and verbal repair strategies. This kind of training can also include professional carers. A variety of techniques, such as diaries and logs, can be used to help identify areas of particular difficulty and suggest strategies for improvement. On the other hand, sometimes the client and their regular communication partners can become so skilled at communicating with each other that the client has great difficulty interacting with anyone else. This may present difficulties if the client needs to go into hospital and cannot be attended by their usual carers (Erber & Scherer 1999).

Evidence based practice

This idea that communication is concerned with the reciprocal and mutually constitutive interactions between clients and their carers is important. According to Sundin et al (2001) identity is established through relationships, and the loss of a person's ability to communicate threatens their sense of self. Once people's communicative ability has been impaired, perhaps through a stroke, social relationships become much more difficult. In Sundin et al's (2001) study of the professional carers of people who had been disabled through stroke, they detected a tendency to see the patients as fragile and vulnerable; at the same time it was felt to be important to support them in a way which sustained their dignity and did not make them feel even more disabled. Equally, important parts of the caring practice with these communication-impaired patients involved developing relationships, developing feelings of closeness and sensitivity often involving non-verbal communication. This was seen to be achievable by spending time with the patient as a companion, not necessarily just attending to the mechanics of care. Communication, in this case, was seen to be essential to the well-being of the patients but was not possible through the normal medium of speech; instead it was accomplished through the medium of presence, trust and security.

PROFESSIONAL AND ETHICAL KNOWLEDGE

Once interactions with clients have been undertaken, the next stage is to make some account of what has occurred. As well as providing information for day-to-day clinical care, records are important in resource management, self-evaluation, audits of performance, care, quality assurance and research (Currel & Wainwright 1996). The 1999 Audit Commission report, *Setting the Record Straight: A Study of Hospital Medical Records*, criticized the poor standard of NHS

record keeping and strongly recommended that corrective action should be taken. Even though the nursing literature is full of exhortations to complete high quality records (Pennels 2002), there is good evidence that both doctors and nurses are not adhering to these criteria. The question thus arises of how policy makers, managers and practitioners are to improve the situation. Under the Clinical Governance agenda, audits are currently used to monitor performance and give advice on practice improvement (see Ch. 2 on safety and risk).

Evidence based practice

Moloney & Maggs (1999) conducted an extensive review of all the reports in the literature and a number of unpublished sources concerning record keeping and care planning, and found that despite the massive investments in such systems there was sadly little evidence that they led to better patient outcomes. In the current state of knowledge, the authors doubt whether we know enough to make worthwhile decisions about the viability of moving to IT based systems of record keeping rather than the traditional paper based variety.

PROFESSIONAL AND LEGAL ASPECTS OF RECORD KEEPING

Although record keeping is a vital facet of nursing there are problems surrounding their use. The patterns of care involved are complex and the record is only ever a partial account of what has transpired between client and nurse. In order to ensure the legal adequacy of records in the UK, the Nursing and Midwifery Council recommends:

- *a full account of your assessment and the care you have planned and provided*
- *relevant information about the condition of the patient or client at any given time and the measures you have taken to respond to their needs*
- *evidence that you have understood and honoured your duty of care, that you have taken all reasonable steps to care for the patient or client and that any actions or omissions on your part have not compromised their safety in any way*
- *a record of any arrangements you have made for the continuing care of a patient or client.*

The frequency of entries is determined both by professional judgement and local standards and agreements. You will need to exercise particular care and make more frequent entries when patients or clients present complex problems, show deviation from the norm, require more intensive care than normal, are confused and disoriented or generally give cause for concern. You must use your professional judgement (if necessary in discussion with other members of the health care team) to determine when these circumstances exist. (Nursing and Midwifery Council 2002: 9)

Written communication is dictated by the nursing process of assessment, planning, implementation and evaluation. Despite having this framework, documentation is often problematic for nurses. Not only are they under pressure to record those nursing interventions that can easily be costed, but they must also adhere to the Standards for Records and Record Keeping published by the Nursing and Midwifery Council's predecessor, the United Kingdom Central Council (1993), so as to demonstrate that their duty of care has been fulfilled.

Reflection and portfolio evidence

How helpful are the following nursing entries in patient records: 'Slept well'; 'Good appetite'; 'Up and about'; 'No complaints'; 'No change', 'Resting comfortably'? Have a look through some nursing records of patients, perhaps even those that include entries made by you.

- Can you find other examples of 'weak' entries that provide little information?
- What factors are influencing the way nurses make entries in records?
- In your view, what kinds of records would be more useful?
- How might entries in nursing notes be improved?
- Discuss and record your findings in your portfolio.

The ideal for a record which is universally intelligible and follows a common nursing language has been developed in the International Council of Nurses's International Classification for Nursing Practice (ICNP). This is a document designed to provide a common means of describing phenomena and activities in nursing (International Council of Nurses 1999) and contains three elements, namely

1. Nursing phenomena or nursing diagnoses.
2. Nursing actions or nursing interventions.
3. Nursing outcomes (Kisilowska 2001).

In terms of how clinicians, especially nurses, feel about record keeping, Allen (1998) noted that the nursing staff she observed and interviewed were positive about record keeping in general because of its link with the nursing process and because it represented professionalism. On the other hand, her participants were sometimes critical as they felt that they were encouraged to provide details in each patient's care plan concerning issues such as bowel movements and health education; details that they felt were not relevant in every case and sometimes problematic when the patient read the records.

CONFIDENTIALITY AND ACCESS TO RECORDS

Williams et al (1993) observed that whilst the patient was becoming the centre of all NHS activity, the documentation of care had not developed in tandem to reflect this. Patient records are usually episode focused, provider based, and emerge in numerous different forms throughout their lifetime, even when describing a single experience of ill health. In the UK a good many records are kept about patients in a number of different places. An individual might have records at the GP's surgery, held by health visitors and district nurses, at the hospitals they attend and other documentation relating to social services.

A further question concerns what kind of information from the record should be disclosed to different professional groups. The Caldicott Report, *Review of Patient Identifiable Information* (Department of Health 1997b), raised concerns about the general lack of awareness of confidentiality and information security requirements throughout the NHS at all levels. The Committee was also concerned at the NHS's ability to limit access to patient information to those who truly need to know.

Evidence based practice

The UK's Audit Commission (1999) discovered that records are often difficult to use because they are

- incomplete
- structured in a variety of different ways with only half of them having any kind of index or guide to the contents.

This makes the information difficult to navigate for the user. Indeed, some clinicians appeared to spend as much as 20% of their time at work locating information in records.

All NHS staff have a common law duty of confidence to patients and a duty to maintain professional ethical standards of confidentiality. Everyone working for or with the NHS who records, handles, stores or otherwise comes across patient information has a personal common law duty of confidence to patients and to his or her employer (Department of Health 2002). The duty of confidence continues even after the death of the patient, or after an employee or contractor has left the NHS. The duty of confidence to an employer regarding company/NHS Trust information is included in the terms and conditions of the job and the contract of employment. Public breaches of confidentiality in relation to individual patients and/or of NHS Trust information can result in disciplinary procedures being taken against the employee (as defined in the Data Protection Act 1998). The patient can take legal action against the individual within the remit of negligence in a 'duty of care' (McHale et al 1998).

However, this duty of confidentiality is not an absolute duty and can be subject to an overriding public interest. This ruling is often applied to the result of research where it is necessary to consider whether any public interest in the research outweighs the duty of confidence, having regard to all the circumstances. A Local Research Ethics Committee

(LREC) must first approve any research using patient records. Currently three areas have special regulations and include: those diagnosed with sexually transmitted diseases (including HIV and AIDS); information related to human fertilization; and information on abortions.

Access to records by clients

The Access to Health Records Act 1990 permitted patients to have access to manual health records made after the Act came into force in 1991. The later Data Protection Act 1998 permits access to all manual health records whenever made, subject to specified exceptions. Although initially professional groups were unhappy with patient access, on the basis of paternalistic arguments such as: lack of understanding by the patient; professionals being less candid in their reporting; and that the knowledge gained was not in the best interest of the patient, there is now recognition of the patient's right of access (McHale et al 1998). This is also contained in the Human Rights Act 2000.

With the modernization agenda in the NHS, the climate has been reversed and the latest initiative, as part of partnership working, is to include the patient in all correspondence between a hospital consultant and the patient's GP, the 'copy letters' project, and to allow patients to browse their own records on a computer terminal (NHS 2003).

COMPLAINTS AND COMMUNICATION

As society becomes better informed, access to Internet information on health care becomes more easily available to all, and consumer satisfaction becomes a 'right' in Western democratic societies there is an inevitable rise in expectations of good quality health care. If not satisfied with the service offered, patient and patient groups will complain, holding all types of professionals to account. The media have become involved and cases of negligence by any professional group now come under increasing public scrutiny (McHale et al 1998).

Complaints against nurses are increasing internationally (Beardwood et al 1999). Rather than necessarily reflecting any deterioration in the standard of nursing, this is attributed to changes in the culture of Britain and North America, where the public are increasingly reminded of their rights and status as citizens yet are faced with cost cutting and restrictions in the available care. Professional councils on both sides of the Atlantic are encouraging patients to register their complaints, and are streamlining the process. In 2001 the UK Central Council (and its successor the Nursing and Midwifery Council) for the first time began publishing reports from its professional conduct committee. This body oversees complaints from the public, employers or the police, and a complaint which is upheld can result in nurses being removed from the UK's register (Nursing Ethics 2001).

Physical and verbal abuse of patients remain the most common reasons for removal from the register, accounting for 28% of cases in 2000–2001, highlighting once again the centrality of communication issues to the level of satisfaction clients and other professional groups have with the service that nurses provide. Further, according to the UK Central Council (2001), many of these complaints originate in the nursing home sector, where staff may be working long hours and are in contact with clients with whom communication is difficult. Indeed, one of the cases in the UK Central Council's 2001 report concerns a nurse who was alleged to have shouted at residents in a nursing home. A good deal of the argument centred on whether, as she maintained, the communications were 'loud' and 'jovial', or whether they were 'angry' as other witnesses at the hearing contended.

While nurses, like everyone else, can never guarantee the meanings of their spoken or written words, they need to reduce the scope for misinterpretation and remain vigilant when considering the meanings of their own and other people's speech and writing. The power of language to construct the world in which we live makes it important for nurses to monitor health care language as it affects the lives of others. Paying attention to what is spoken and written about patients or clients is vital if nursing is to continue its tradition of advocacy. Vital parts of effective nursing practice involve a critical interest in how we talk to and write about those in our care; or how patients give accounts of themselves; or how other professionals describe them. Effectively, caring is about communicating carefully.

In writing, we should be concerned about how healthcare professionals represent those in their care and whether they linguistically 'incarcerate' or 'restrain' them by using judgemental words and phrases and even jumping to conclusions, which may be untrue and may damage the client. For example, a GP's referral letter to a Community Mental Health Nurse described a client as a 'young prostitute' with an 'inadequate personality'. On visiting the client at home, the nurse found no evidence that she was either a 'prostitute' or 'inadequate', but was merely complaining of tiredness (Crawford et al 1995). This incident highlights the often difficult issue of how to challenge communications which we feel are prejudicial, damaging or unethical. Rather, to fail to challenge in such a situation is to permit potential damage or harm to those for whom we stand as advocates. It is thus worth describing in a little more detail what it means to think of nursing as a process of advocacy.

PATIENT ADVOCACY

Advocacy has been linked to the nurse's role in the UK since the late 1980s and is believed to be desirable because it furthers nursing's endeavours on behalf of the patients or clients (Grace 2001). The Oxford English Dictionary (1989: 194) defines an advocate as 'one who pleads, intercedes or speaks for or on behalf of, another: a pleader, intercessor, defender'. This kind of definition emphasizes how the advocate may represent another through language. In the legal profession, the assumption is that a legal professional will be able to act solely and diligently on behalf of their client. Nurses on the other hand have a rather more ambiguous role. As Grace (2001) argues, there is little consensus as to what advocacy entails in nursing, as well as a concern that nurses are using this role as a tool to serve their own self-interests and make themselves appear more professional (Mallik & Rafferty 2000). Moreover, nurses are sometimes in an awkward position when they do try to advocate on behalf of patients because they are often constrained by their employment situation, and 'rocking the boat' too much might result in personal and professional isolation and even job loss (Mallik & McHale 1995). Grace (2001) argues that rather than merely concentrating on the situation of patients or groups in the immediate practice setting, nurses should embrace an advocacy role that includes broader issues of national health policy and funding. Not all policy makers are amenable to this kind of bottom-up persuasion, but it might be possible via more indirect routes, perhaps by mobilizing public opinion.

In addition, there are other frameworks for providing advocacy in health care. These include self-advocacy, agent advocacy and independent advocacy, all of which have a long tradition of providing support for clients in the mental health field, the disabled, people with chronic illnesses, the elderly, and ethnic minority groups accessing health care (Teasdale 1998). These pressure groups and individual agents are included in the current policy framework that has established Patient Advice and Liaison Services (PALS) in all NHS Acute Trusts in the UK (Department of Health 2003).

Decision making exercise

When on your practice placement in an acute hospital, investigate the current provision of the PALS service. Find out how the service is accessed by patients and where possible have a discussion with the person leading that service. Many managers of this service have been recruited from the nursing profession. After your investigation:

- Decide on whether this service helps you in any situation where you have concerns about a patient's care or treatment.
- Will this service deal with all issues? If not, what are its limitations?
- If there is a pattern of mistreatment or inadequacy in the services to patients, is there any other mechanism through which you can raise your concerns?

In practice, when we ask nurses about their experiences of advocacy, the findings tend to show that those nurses with an interest in the matter see advocacy as very strongly bound up with ideas about what it means to be a nurse and what a therapeutic relationship involves; indeed, nurses in Snowball's study held 'a philosophy of nursing which encompasses advocacy as a role responsibility both of professional practice and personal humanity' (Snowball 1996: 73). Moreover, in Snowball's study, there appeared to be an interest amongst the participants in working with colleagues and other interested parties to promote patients' well-being, again highlighting the importance of communication, both inter- and intraprofessionally. However, in much research on advocacy, the overall finding is that nurses tend to advocate at an individual level – concerned with the needs of particular patients – and not necessarily at the level of the whole organization or in terms of the resources which a society makes available for the clients of health services (Chafey et al 1998, Grace 2001, Mallik 1997).

PERSONAL AND REFLECTIVE KNOWLEDGE

AWARENESS OF THE USE OF LANGUAGE IN NURSING

Language enables you to describe and potentially transform aspects of your work. Progress and growth are the positive outcomes of reflective practices, embodied in increased choices and increased professional awareness. The past few years have seen an increasing reflection on what it means to be a nurse and what the effects of nursing activity are. The considerable increase in the number of conferences, seminars and journals for nurses bears witness to the urgency of critical inquiry that is currently taking place within nursing. By first reflecting critically on your own language you may gain the right, and indeed the skills, to challenge the language of others. Reflective practice, as championed by Schon (1983) and as discussed in the introduction to this book, is based on the belief that people can actually effect change through the raising of consciousness about their activities.

The quality of your care will improve as you develop effective communication skills. For example, a nurse describes a particular piece of interaction in the following terms:

I said something like 'How are you doing Paul?' When he predictably answered 'Fine' I could easily have gone out the door and on with my work, but just by the way he answered I could tell he had much more to say. I asked Paul if he would like me to stay awhile and he replied that he would ... For almost an hour I just listened to Paul as he talked about his life, his achievements, the risks he had and hadn't taken and his hopes for his limited future ... When I stood up to go, his eyes met mine and we thanked each other in silence. (Perry 1996: 9)

This extract shows a number of important things about caring work. Firstly, it is not wholly about catering to the patients' physical needs; their desire for company and companionship may be especially important. Secondly, it highlights the importance of probing beyond the initial appearance of the interaction – the patient's assertion that he is 'fine' – to create an experience which is rewarding to both nurse and patient. This example highlights the importance of being aware of the value of communication in order to add to patients' quality of life. Of course, often nurses will not be able to allocate an extended block of time for this kind of communication, but they should strive to give as much time as possible to empathic communication and interaction. This may be done in and around completing a variety of other nursing tasks.

CASE STUDIES INVOLVING THE USE OF LANGUAGE

In the following exercises we have selected some examples that highlight the role of language in health care. The questions are provided in an attempt to get you thinking about the centrality of language to different aspects of health care, from the initial description of health problems through to rehabilitation and therapy.

Case study: Adult

Margaret is 38 years old and is suffering from systemic lupus erythematosus, a disorder of the connective tissues, primarily affecting women in their 30s and 40s. It may involve arthritis, and problems with the kidneys, heart and brain. One day she opens up and begins to talk about her condition: 'If you have lupus, I mean one day it's my liver; one day it's my joints; one day it's my head, and it's like people really think you're a hypochondriac if you keep complaining about different ailments ... It's like you don't want to say anything because people are going to start thinking, you know, 'God, don't go near her, all she is ... is complaining about this.' And I think that's why I never say anything because I feel like everything I have is related one way or another to the lupus but most of the people don't know I have lupus, and even those that do are not going to believe that ten different ailments are the same thing. And I don't want anybody saying, you know, [that] they don't want to come around me because I complain.'
(*Adapted from Charnaz 1991: 114–115*)

- How is Margaret making sense of her illness experience?
- What kinds of difficulties is she having in her working and social life?
- When you hear the term illness, what kinds of things does it make you think of? Does Margaret's account fit with your own ideas of illness?
- How could Margaret tell others about her condition in a way that might make her life easier?
- Try to write a few responses to Margaret and ask a mentor or peer to review these. For example, you may wish to focus on Margaret's account of how the illness has affected her notion of selfhood.

Case study: Mental health

Crystal is in his mid-40s and has been diagnosed as suffering from schizophrenia since his late teens. He lives in a hostel in the community and spends most of his day on the street. He has no friends and although he receives regular visits from a community nurse, he has failed to take his oral medication to control his symptoms. He experiences command hallucinations that tell him to actively waste other people's time. One morning he is overheard crying out 'Help me. The Time Wasters are coming to get me. They're going to tear me apart!' (*Adapted from Crawford 2002*)

- Which of the following would be the best response and why?
  1. 'Don't worry about it. I'm sure they wouldn't do that.'
  2. 'I don't think that will happen. Do you fancy a cup of tea?'
  3. 'You must feel really frightened. Tell me more about these "Time Wasters".'
  4. 'Can you prove that these 'Time Wasters' are coming to get you?'
- If you met Crystal for the first time how would you begin to build up rapport with him?
- What would you say to Crystal if you visited his flat and saw lots of tablets lying around on the floor?

Case study: Child

Donald is 12 years old and has been experiencing severe pain postoperatively. He is on a patient controlled analgesia (PCA) pump, but he still complains of pain to his mother. His mother is upset about this, and is becoming frustrated because she does not understand how the pump works, and does not feel able to seek further information from nursing staff. Each time nursing staff enter the room, she complains that her son's pain is not properly controlled. During handover, she seeks out the nurses and tells them that Donald is in so much pain that he is crying loudly. One of the nurses tells her 'We'll go and see', to which the mother replies, 'Can't you take my word for it?' (*Adapted from Simons et al 2001*)

- How might you communicate empathy for the mother witnessing Donald's pain?
- How might you go about educating and providing information for Donald and his mother?
- To what extent does the emotional state of Donald's mother make this kind of education difficult? How can we get round this problem?
- What weight should you attach to your own opinion about the level of pain Donald is experiencing, compared to that of Donald's mother, or Donald himself? How can you come up with a nursing strategy that satisfies everyone?
- Under what circumstances might you be sceptical of information provided by Donald's mother?

Case study: Learning disabilities

Janet is 16 years old, lives in a community residential unit and has a learning disability that means she is unable to give informed consent. According to staff, Janet needs to be chaperoned because she is young and attractive, very immature and adores being kissed and cuddled. In the past, this has led to difficult situations when Janet has struck up friendships with other people, and staff are concerned that she is not abused. (*Adapted from Deeley 2001: 25; a further useful and evocative account of the sexuality of young women with learning difficulties and sexuality is provided by McCarthy 1999*)

- What sorts of difficulties over sexuality might a young woman in Janet's situation face?
- What ways are there of making the issue of sexuality and people with learning disabilities easier to talk about for staff and clients?
- What communication strategies would you use to foster more independence for Janet despite staff concerns for the need to chaperone her?
- How might you respond verbally and non-verbally to any show of affection by Janet?
- To what extent could a person in Janet's situation be empowered to make her own informed choices about relationships and sexuality?
- How might it be possible for you to help Janet avoid abusive and exploitative situations without being intrusive or over-controlling?

Summary

This chapter has drawn together theoretical concepts relating to communication and applied this knowledge in relation to the practice of caring for individuals. It has included:

1. The biological theoretical basis of communication, models of communication, language acquisition and non-verbal communication.
2. Psychosocial and sociocultural factors influencing communication.
3. Consideration of factors influencing nurses' decision making in using communication in care delivery.
4. Professional and ethical dimensions of communication, the importance of maintaining records, issues of confidentiality and the role of the nurse as an advocate for the patient.
5. The use of communication in addressing and managing complaints and the dissatisfied client.

Knowledge illuminated within this chapter has been combined with evidence from other referenced sources and applied within a range of situations. Suggestions have been made for portfolio development in relation to the development of communication skills.

Annotated further reading and websites

Crawford P, Brown B, Nolan P 1998 Communicating care: the language of nursing. Stanley Thornes, Cheltenham
This book will assist its readers to acquire a critical view of their use of language in professional practice. The authors synthesize theoretical studies and critical analysis of a wide range of examples of good and bad use of language, in order to guide nurses towards models of good practice. Full consideration is given to the changing nature of the health care environment, and to the need to address ethical, legal and professional issues beyond the fundamentals of patient–nurse interactions.

Teasdale K 1998 Advocacy in health care. Blackwell Science, Oxford
An informative book on advocacy which outlines the advocacy frameworks in relation to all patient/client groups, such as self-advocacy, external advocacy and advocacy for special needs groups, as well as giving an overview of the development of patient advocacy as a nursing role.

http://www.mhas.info/
Modernizing the Hearing Aid Services in the NHS is part of a government plan to upgrade the current service offered to patients in the UK. Targets have been set for the next 5 years and this new website provides up-to-date information on progress.

http://www.ombudsman.co.uk
Provides the Ombudsman's annual reports on the main areas of patient complaints, many of them related to failures in communication within healthcare teams.

http://www.nmc-uk.org
The website introduces this body as follows: 'The Nursing and Midwifery Council is an organisation set up by Parliament to ensure nurses, midwives and health visitors provide high standards of care to their patients and clients.' It has taken over from the old UK Central Council and is concerned to promote good practice and to deal with complaints.

http://www.doh.gov.uk
The Department of Heath has a useful website providing a good deal of information on policy and practice. Many documents can be downloaded free of charge, including reports, research, legislation and a great deal more.

http://www.nhs.uk
The NHS website allows access to valuable information on all reports and guidelines related to services within the NHS that are referred to in this chapter. In addition, there is now a National Knowledge Service, accessible from the NHS main site.

References

Allen D 1998 Record keeping and routine nursing practice: the view from the wards. Journal of Advanced Nursing 27:1223–1230

Allott R 2001 The natural origin of language. Able, Hemel Hempstead

Ambady N, Koo J, Rosxenthal R et al 2002 Physical therapists nonverbal communication predicts geriatric patients' health outcomes. Psychology and Aging 17(3):443–452

Anderson K J, Leaper C 1998 Meta-analysis of gender effects in conversational interruption. Sex Roles 39(3–4):225–252

Argyle M, Ingham R 1972 Gaze, mutual gaze and proximity. Semiotica 6:32–49

Audit Commission 1999 Setting the record straight: a review of progress in health records services. Audit Commission, London

Bandura A 1986 Social foundations of thought and action: a social cognitive theory. Prentice-Hall, Englewood Cliffs

Beardwood B, Walters V, Eyles J et al 1999 Complaints against nurses: a reflection of 'the new managerialism' and consumerism in health care. Social Science and Medicine 48(3):363–374

Berg M 1996 Practices of reading and writing: the constitutive role of the patient record in medical work. Sociology of Health and Illness 18(4):499–524

Birdwhistell R 1970 Kinesics and context: essays on body movement communication. University of Pennsylvania Press, Philadelphia

Bradshaw J 1998 Assessing and intervening in the communication environment. British Journal of Learning Disabilities 26(2):62–66

Bricher G 1999 Paediatric nurses, children and the development of trust. Journal of Clinical Nursing 8:451–458

Brown P, Fraser C 1979 Speech as a marker of situation. In: Scherer K R, Giles H (eds) Social markers in speech. Cambridge University Press, Cambridge, pp 33–108

Cantwell J 2000 Pressures, priorities and pre-emptive practice. Speech and Language Therapy (Winter): 16–19

Caporael L, Lukaszewski M, Culbertson G 1983 Secondary baby talk: judgements by institutionalised elderly and their caregivers. Journal of Personality and Social Psychology 44(4):746–754

Caris-Verhallen W M C M, de Gruitjer I M, Kerkstra A et al 1999 Factors related to nurse communication with elderly people. Journal of Advanced Nursing 30(5):1106–1117

Carey J 1989 Communication as culture. Routledge, London

Carr J E, Vitaliano P P 1985 The theoretical implications of converging research on depression and the culture bound syndromes. In: Kleinman A, Good B (eds) Culture and depression. University of California Press, Los Angeles, pp 137–156

Chafey K, Rhea M, Shannon A M et al 1998 Characterisation of advocacy by practicing nurses. Journal of Professional Nursing 14(1):43–52

Charnaz K 1991 Good days, bad days: the self in chronic illness and time. Rutgers University Press, New Brunswick

Choi H 2002 Understanding adolescent depression in ethnocultural context. Advances in Nursing Science 25(2):71–85

Chomsky N 1976 Reflections on language. Fontana, London

Chomsky N 1993 Language and thought. Moyer Bell, London

Clements P T, Benasutti K M, Henry G C 2001 Drawing from experience: using drawings to facilitate communication and understanding with children exposed to sudden traumatic deaths. Journal of Psychosocial Nursing and Mental Health Services 39(12):12–20

Coupland J, Robinson J D, Coupland N 1994 Frame negotiation in doctor–elderly patient interactions. Discourse and Society 5:89–124

Crawford P 2002 Nothing purple, nothing black. Book Guild, Lewes

Crawford P, Nolan P, Brown B 1995 Linguistic entrapment: medico-nursing biographies as fictions. Journal of Advanced Nursing 22:1141–1148

Crawford P, Brown B, Nolan P 1998 Communicating care: the language of nursing. Stanley Thornes, Cheltenham

Crow J L, Harmeling B C 2002 Development of a consensus and evidence based standardised clinical assessment and record form for neurological inpatients. Physiotherapy 88(1):33–46

Currell R, Wainwright P 1996 Nursing record systems, nursing practice and patient care (Protocol). In: Bero L, Grilli R, Grimshaw J et al (eds) Collaboration on effective professional practice module of the Cochrane database of systematic reviews. The Cochrane Collaboration, Oxford, pp 47–61

Deeley S 2001 Professional ideology and learning disability: an analysis of internal conflict. Disability and Society 17(1):19–33

Department of Health (1997a) Better services for vulnerable people, EL(97)62, CI(97)24. Department of Health, London

Department of Health 1997b The Caldicott Committee: report on the review of patient-identifiable information. Department of Health, London

Department of Health 1998 Partnership in action: new opportunities for joint working between health and social services – a discussion document. Department of Health, London

Department of Health 1999 A National Service Framework for Mental Health. Department of Health, London

Department of Health 2000 Good practice guidelines for general practice electronic patient records. Available: http://www.doh.gov.uk/gpepr/ guidelines.pdf 24 May 2003

Department of Health 2002 Statutory instrument 2002 no. 1438: The Health Service (control of patient information) regulations.

Available: http://www.doh.gov.uk/ipu/confiden/instrument.pdf 24 May 2003

Department of Health 2003 Patient advice and liaison services. Available: http://www.doh.gov.uk/patientadviceandliaisonservices/downloads.htm 24 May 2003

de Pino-Perez A, Meizoso M T G, Gonzalez R D 1999 Validity of the structured interview for the assessment of Type A behaviour. European Journal of Psychological Assessment 15(1):39–48

Dimitrovsky L, Spector H, Levy-Shiff R, Vakil F 1998 Interpretation of facial expressions of affect in children with learning disabilities with verbal or nonverbal deficits. Journal of Learning Disabilities 31(3): 286–292, 312

Dronkers N F 2000 The pursuit of brain–language relationships. Brain and Language 71:59–71

Dumble M, Tuson W 1998 Identifying eating and drinking difficulties. Speech and Language Therapy Practice (Winter):4–6

Dunstan C 1999 From assessment into action: changing process and culture. British Geriatrics Society Newsletter (May):19–21

Ekman P, Rosenberg E L 1997 What the face reveals. Oxford University Press, Oxford

Erber N P, Scherer S C 1999 Sensory loss and communicative difficulties in the elderly. Australian Journal on Ageing 18(1):4–9

Fairclough N 1989 Language and power. Longman, Harlow

Fenton S, Sadiq-Sangster A 1996 Culture, relativism, and the expression of mental distress: South Asian women in Britain. Sociology of Health and Illness 18(1):66–85

Fodor J A 1998 In critical condition: polemical essays on cognitive science and the philosophy of mind. MIT Press, Cambridge

Fox N J 1993 Discourse, organisation and the surgical ward round. Sociology of Health and Illness 15(1):16–42

Fredricksen L 1999 Modes of relating in a caring conversation: a research synthesis on presence, touch and listening. Journal of Advanced Nursing 30(5):1167–1176

Friedman M, Rosenman R 1959 Association of specific, overt behaviour pattern with blood and cardiovascular findings. Journal of the American Medical Association 169:1286

Gerrish K, Clayton J, Nolan M et al 1999 Promoting evidence based practice: managing change in assessment of pressure damage risk. Journal of Nursing Management 7(6):355–362

Goffman E 1974 Frame analysis. Harper & Row, New York

Grace P J 2001 Professional advocacy: widening the scope of accountability. Nursing Philosophy 2:151–162

Habermas J 1995 Moral consciousness and communicative action. MIT Press, Cambridge

Health Committee 1999 Session 1998–1999: The relationship between health and social services. First Report, vol. 1. Report and proceedings of the committee. HMSO, London

Heron J 1990 Helping the client: a creative practical guide. Sage, London

Hogg M A, Vaughan G M 2002 Social psychology, 3rd edn. Prentice Hall, London

Howse E, Bailey J 1992 Resistance to documentation: a nursing research issue. International Journal of Nursing Studies 29(4):371–381

Hyden M 1995 Verbal aggression as prehistory of woman battering. Journal of Family Violence 10:55–71

International Council of Nurses 1999 International classification for nursing practice, beta version. International Council of Nurses, Geneva

Jakobson R 1960 Closing statement: linguistics and poetics. In: Sebeok T A (ed) Style in language. MIT Press, Cambridge, pp 350–377

Jha A, Tabet N, Orrell M 2000 To tell or not to tell: comparison of older patients' reaction to their diagnosis of dementia and depression. International Journal of Geriatric Psychiatry 16(9):879–885

Kisilowska M 2001 Reorganized structure and other proposals for the ICNP development. International Nursing Review 4:218–233

Kleinke C L 1986 Gaze and eye contact: a research review. Psychological Bulletin 100:76–100

Kreps G 2001 The evolution and advancement of health communication inquiry. In: Gudykurst B (ed) Communication yearbook, vol. 24. Sage, Thousand Oaks, pp 231–253

Lakoff G 1987 Women, fire and dangerous things: what categories reveal about the mind. University of Chicago Press, Chicago

Lakoff R 1975 Language and woman's place. Harper & Row, New York

Larkin K T, Martin R R, McClain S E 2002 Cynical hostility and the accuracy of decoding facial expressions of emotions. Journal of Behavioural Medicine 25(3):285–293

Lasswell H 1948 The structure and function of communication in society. In: Bryson L (ed) The communication of ideas. Harper & Row, New York, pp 37–53

McAfee R E 2001 Domestic violence as a women's health issue. Women's Health Issues 11(4):371–376

McCarthy M 1999 Sexuality and women with learning disabilities. Jessica Kingsley, London

McHale J, Tingle J, Peysner J 1998 Law and nursing. Butterworth Heinemann, Oxford

Mackintosh N 1996 Promoting health: an issue for nursing. Quay, Dinton

Mallik M 1997 Advocacy in nursing: perceptions of practising nurses. Journal of Clinical Nursing 6(4):303–313

Mallik M, McHale J 1995 Support for advocacy. Nursing Times 91(4):28–30

Mallik M, Rafferty A M 2000 Diffusion of the concept of patient advocacy. Journal of Nursing Scholarship 32(4):399–404

Marr P B, Duthie E, Glassman K S et al 1993 Bedside terminals and quality of nursing documentation. Computers in Nursing 11(4):176–182

Maynard D 1991 The perspective display series and the delivery and receipt of diagnostic news. In: Boden D, Zimmerman D H (eds) Talk and social structure. Polity Press, Cambridge

Migliore S 1993 'Nerves': the role of metaphor in the cultural framing of experience. Journal of Contemporary Ethnography 22(3):331–360

Moloney R, Maggs C 1999 A systematic review of the relationships between written manual nursing care planning, record keeping and patient outcomes. Journal of Advanced Nursing 30(1):51–57

Nash J 1985 Social psychology: society and self. West, St Paul

Neidle C, Kegl J, MacLaughlin D et al 2002 The syntax of American Sign Language: functional categories and hierarchical structure. MIT Press, Cambridge

NHS 2003 IT questions and answers. Available: http://www.nhs.uk/nhsmagazine/primarycare/it_qa.asp 24 May 2003

Nolan M, Caldock K 1996 Assessment: identifying the barriers to good practice. Health and Social Care in the Community 4(2):77–85

Nursing Ethics 2001 News. Nursing Ethics 8(1):81–82

Nursing and Midwifery Council 2002 Guidelines for records and record keeping. Nursing and Midwifery Council, London

Ombudsman 2003 Reports. Available: http://www.ombudsman.co.uk 24 May 2003

Oxford English Dictionary, 2nd edn. 1989 Clarendon Press, Oxford

Parker I, Georgaca E, Harper D et al 1995 Deconstructing psychopathology. Sage, London

Patterson M L 1983 Nonverbal behaviour: a functional perspective. Springer, New York

Pei M 1997 The story of language, 2nd edn. Lippincott, Philadelphia

Pell M D 2002 Evaluation of nonverbal emotion in face and voice: some preliminary findings on a new battery of tests. Brain and Cognition 48(2–3):499–504

Pennels C 2002 The importance of accurate and comprehensive record keeping. Professional Nurse 17(5):294–296

Peplau H 1952 Interpersonal relations in nursing. Putnam, New York

Perry B 1996 Influence of nurse gender on the use of silence, touch and humour. International Journal of Palliative Nursing 2:7–14

Pinker S 1994 The language instinct. Morrow, New York

Posner M I, Raichle M E 1997 Images of mind. Scientific American Library, New York

Potter J 1996 Representing reality. Sage, London

Proctor A, Morse J M, Khonsari E S 1996 Sounds of comfort in the trauma centre: how nurses talk to patients in pain. Social Science and Medicine 42(12):1669–1680

Rao P R 1995 Drawing and gesture as communication options in a person with severe aphasia. Topics in Stroke Rehabilitation 2(1):49–56

Ratzan S C, Payne J G, Bishop C 1996 The status and scope of health communication. Journal of Heath Communication 1:25–41

Reid S A, Ng S H 1999 Language, power and intergroup relations. Journal of Social Issues 55:119–139

Robillard A B 1996 Anger in the social order. Body and Society 2(1):17–30

Russell F, Gray D 2002 Accountable wound care: the role of photography in record keeping. Practice Nurse 13(7):306–312

Ryan A A, Scullion H S 2000 Family and staff perceptions of the role of families in nursing homes. Journal of Advanced Nursing 32(2): 626–634

Ryan E B, Meredith S D, Shantz G B 1994 Evaluative perceptions of patronizing speech addressed to institutionalized elders in contrasting conversational contexts. Canadian Journal on Ageing 13(2):236–248

Sachs L 1983 Evil eye or bacteria: Turkish migrant women and Swedish health care. University of Stockholm, Stockholm

Scherer K R, Banse R, Wallbott H G 2002 Emotion inferences from vocal expression correlate across languages and cultures. Journal of Cross Cultural Psychology 13(1):74–92

Schon T 1983 The reflective practitioner. Basic Books, New York

Searle J 1979 Speech acts: an essay in the philosophy of language. Cambridge University Press, London

Shannon C E, Weaver W 1949 The mathematical theory of communication. University of Illinois Press, Champaign

Sharma S, Downey G, Heywood R 2002 Guidelines: are they adhered to in clinical practice? Journal of Clinical Governance 10(2):71–75

Simons J, Franck L, Roberson E 2001 Parent involvement in children's pain care: views of parents and nurses. Journal of Advanced Nursing 36(4):591–599

Snowball J 1996 Asking nurses about advocating for patients: reactive and proactive accounts. Journal of Advanced Nursing 24:67–75

Sontag S 1979 Illness as metaphor. Allen Lane, London

Stewart A L, Napoles-Springer A, Perez-Stable E 1999 Interpersonal processes of care in diverse populations. Millbank Quarterly 77(3):305–339

Sumner J 2001 Caring in nursing: a different interpretation. Journal of Advanced Nursing 35(6):926–932

Sundin K, Norberg A, Jansson L 2001 The meaning of skilled care providers' relationships with stroke and aphasia patients. Qualitative Health Research 11(3):308–321

Teasdale K 1998 Advocacy in health care. Blackwell Science, Oxford

Tilley S 1999 Altschul's legacy in mediating British and American psychiatric nursing discourses: common sense and the 'absence' of the accountable practitioner. Journal of Psychiatric and Mental Health Nursing 6:283–285

Tye-Murray N, Schurm L 1994 Conversation training for frequent communication partners. Journal of the Academy of Rehabilitative Audiology 27:209–222

UK Central Council 1993 Standards for records and record keeping. UK Central Council, London

UK Central Council 2001 Professional conduct annual report. Nursing and Midwifery Council/Central Council for Nursing Midwifery and Health Visiting, London

Wellings T 2001 Drawings by dying and bereaved children. Paediatric Nursing 13(4):30–31

Whitehead D 2003 Evaluating health promotion: a model for nursing practice. Journal of Advanced Nursing 41(5):490–498

Williams J G, Roberts R, Rigby M J 1993 Integrated patient records: another move towards quality for patients. Quality in Health Care 2(2):73–74

Zimmerman D H, West C 1975 Sex roles, interruptions and silences in conversations. In: Thorne B, Henley N (eds) Language and sex: differences and dominance. Newbury House, Rowley, pp 105–129

Chapter 2

Safety and risk

Kate Beaumont

KEY ISSUES

SUBJECT KNOWLEDGE
- Exploration of the concept of internal and external environments
- Basic human requirements for life
- Hazards to human safety
- Psychological and social concepts of risk
- Risk concepts in health care
- Environmental and occupational safety
- Health promotion in relation to safety

CARE DELIVERY KNOWLEDGE
- Safety of the individual
- Learning from adverse events and 'near misses'
- Safe systems of care
- Risk assessment
- Planning and implementing a strategy for risk management
- Safe equipment and safe substances
- Implementing strategies for a safe environment

PROFESSIONAL AND ETHICAL KNOWLEDGE
- Interprofessional working
- Upholding the law and maintaining standards
- Statutory requirements
- Professional requirements
- The consent process
- Ethical dilemmas in risk management

PERSONAL AND REFLECTIVE KNOWLEDGE
- Case studies applying principles of safety and risk in branches of nursing

INTRODUCTION

A safe environment is something many of us take for granted. Florence Nightingale highlighted the importance of ensuring that patients were safe when she stated in her instructions to nurses, *Notes on Nursing*, that nursing should 'Do the patient no harm.' She also offered advice on the design of hospital wards in an attempt to ensure an optimum environment for hospital patients (Nightingale 1863). Over 140 years later, the Department of Health, in conjunction with the National Patient Safety Agency, has reiterated Florence Nightingale's ideal, whilst recognizing that no harm may be optimistic ('In a service as large and complex as the National Health Service, things will sometimes go wrong'); its draft document *Doing Less Harm* (Department of Health and National Patient Safety Agency 2001) has become one of the building blocks of risk management in the NHS in the UK.

However, to view the promotion of a safe environment as simply something nurses can do for their patients is simplistic. This perspective, alone, fails to recognize the sociological components of maintaining a safe environment, that is, the need for patients (and nurses) to be aware of potential threats to health within their personal environments and to behave in a safe manner. Nursing has a responsibility to understand and promote both the concept of maintaining patient safety in care environments and the notion of safe patient behaviour through health promotion.

Risk management is inextricably linked to and sits under the overarching umbrella of Clinical Governance. The government in 1997 formally introduced the concept of Clinical Governance to the NHS (Department of Health 1997). It has been defined in various ways (British Medical Association 1999, Department of Health 1998, NHS Executive 1999) but in effect is a new term for concepts already in place in health care in disparate amounts; concepts such as clinical audit, clinical guidelines, evidence based practice, continuing professional education, continuous quality improvement, risk management and complaints procedures. In essence it is:

a system through which NHS organizations are accountable for continuously improving the quality of their services and safeguarding high standards of care by creating an environment in which excellence will flourish. (Department of Health 1997: 7)

The key to effecting the implementation of good Clinical Governance lies in eradication of the blame culture that runs through the NHS, both in clinical and managerial circles. Not until the fear of blame has gone will health staff feel safe to report the mistakes and 'near misses' that allow learning and improvement to take place.

Although patients have always featured as a prime concern with regard to health and safety, the safety of the nurse at work has not always received as much attention. The last 100 years has seen many legislative attempts at improving the health of the worker in society. Many people, including health service workers, were not given legal protection whilst at work until the last decade. For many, the establishment of the Health and Safety at Work Act 1974 was the first real opportunity for ensuring safe working premises and practices. The NHS became subject to the new law, but avoided the need for implementation because of Crown Immunity. After a number of well publicized incidents of poor standards, this immunity was finally lifted by the NHS (Amendment) Act 1986.

Today, the provision and maintenance of an optimum environment for both patients and healthcare staff is a major concern. Laws, regulations, local procedures and policies at European, national and local levels offer guidance for safe practice. Under these acts, nurses have a responsibility to ensure that the workplace is a safe place for themselves and their patients. Some nurses, in particular occupational health nurses and those who represent unions with regard to health and safety, have additional responsibility to ensure that the workplace of the workforce is a safe place for all employees.

This chapter explores issues in the provision of a safe environment for patients and carers. Safety in the care environment includes the introduction of risk management, exploring the roles of both the nurse and patient. Health and safety at work is a key feature of the day-to-day management of a workload and the relationship between professional practice and the law is illustrated. The scope of this chapter presents a broad overview as other chapters in this book contain sections that focus on specific areas of safety such as handling and moving (see Ch. 5), infection control (see Ch. 4) and medicines (see Ch. 9). Food safety will be addressed under nutrition (see Ch. 7) and stress arising from multiple external environmental sources will be explored under stress, relaxation and rest (see Ch. 8). The functions and maintenance of the body in dealing with environmental threats are addressed under homeostasis (see Ch. 6).

OVERVIEW

Subject knowledge

The concept of 'environment' and the meanings of internal and external environment are explored. Threats to safety that are either part of the natural world or human-made are outlined.

In the psychosocial knowledge section, our interaction with the world around us is considered and there is discussion about the basic human needs for maintaining safety and well-being. Behavioural issues are addressed, with a particular reference to factors that may compromise safety. These factors include theories of risk behaviour and individual and societal non-compliance in maintaining a healthy environment.

Care delivery knowledge

Ways to facilitate an optimum environment for patients are explored in relation to the planning of safe care for the individual as well as the need to minimize hazards in the care environment. Emphasis is placed on risk assessment and on adverse event and 'near miss' reporting and investigating, as the key components of effective risk management.

Professional and ethical knowledge

This section touches on interprofessional team working but addresses in more depth the requirement for nurses to maintain professional and statutory requirements. There is a review of the many external agencies that set standards for the management of risk in the NHS today. Consideration is given to some ethical dilemmas within risk management, which may provide a stimulus for further discussion and deliberation.

Personal and reflective knowledge

Throughout the chapter you will be encouraged to apply information reflectively through exercises and by considering examples. In this final section case studies from the four branches of nursing help you reflect further and apply the knowledge you have gained.

On page 42 there are four case studies, each one relating to one of the branch programmes. You may find it helpful to read one of them before you start the chapter and use it as a focus for your reflections whilst reading.

SUBJECT KNOWLEDGE

BIOLOGICAL

A SAFE ENVIRONMENT

It is important to clarify what is meant by the 'internal' and 'external' environments, for it is within these domains that threats to well-being and safety take place. Although both have potential dangers for human life and well-being, they are discretely different, both in the likely risks to safety and in the way in which threats may be managed.

For the purposes of this chapter, the internal environment can be described as the functions and workings of the human body. The body's ability to maintain a homeostatic (stable) internal environment is essential to well-being (see Ch. 6). The essential consideration of the internal environment in relation to health and safety is concerned with its interaction with the external environment and the effects which may result. The external environment is the world surrounding the human body. In order to function, the human body has essential requirements, which must be met externally. Conversely the actions of individuals can influence the safety and ambience of the external environment for all who live in it. Both environments are highly dependent upon one another for their own maintenance.

Basic needs of human life

The basic requirements of living are well known. Physiological needs include:

- air
- water
- food
- shelter.

Without these basic needs, higher order psychological needs such as belonging and esteem cannot be easily achieved (Maslow 1970). Over thousands of years of development, however, an increasingly complicated way for meeting basic needs has developed. This has resulted in modifying the external environment to suit our needs.

Table 2.1 The environmental system (adapted from Purdom & Walton 1971 by kind permission)

Life support	Activities	Residues and waste
Air	Home	Solids
Water	Work	Liquids
Food	Recreation	Gases
Shelter	Transportation	

Environmental hazards			
Type	Example	Type	Example
Biological	Animal	Psychological	Stress
	Insect		Boredom
	Microbiological		Anxiety
			Discomfort
			Depression
Chemical	Poisons and toxins		
	Allergens		
	Irritants	Sociological	Overcrowding
			Isolation
			Anomie
Physical	Vibration		
	Radiation		
	Forces and abrasion		
	Humidity		

Table 2.1 illustrates how individuals interact within the external environmental system. It demonstrates how components essential for life support are taken from the external environment and how the two environments interact through activities of living. Waste and residues are contributed to the external environment as a byproduct of human existence.

Throughout life activities, individuals may find threats to safety both to and from the external environment. These are also summarized in the categories outlined in Table 2.1.

POTENTIAL HAZARDS IN MEETING BASIC REQUIREMENTS FOR LIVING

Air

The air that we breathe usually contains 21% oxygen and 78% nitrogen with the other 1% being made up of trace gases such as carbon dioxide, xenon and neon. If the oxygen concentration were to drop below 16%, anoxia would develop resulting in effects on the brain and other body functions. If the oxygen level decreased further to 6%, life could not be sustained and immediate loss of consciousness results from exposure to a zero oxygen atmosphere.

Air can also act as a vehicle for microorganisms, allergens, waste gases and dust, all of which enter the body via the lungs (Harrington & Gill 1992). These pollutants may cause damage or illness if present in sufficient quantity or if an individual develops an allergic response to them. Air quality is particularly compromised in large urban areas when the temperature rises and there is little wind movement. Threats to health have been acknowledged in the increasing rates of respiratory disease, especially in young children (Brunekreef et al 1997, Clancy et al 2002, Karol 2002). There is evidence to suggest that children exposed to lead in exhaust fumes arising from the increased use of the car in our society have exhibited symptoms (such as decreased intelligence) consistent with the expected neurological sequelae identified in those with high levels of lead exposure via other sources such as contaminated drinking water (Maas et al 2002).

Water

Life for individuals without water can be measured in days, but it is not only individuals who suffer if water is in short supply. A civilization cannot develop or prosper without sufficient water to grow crops, develop industries or establish communities for people to live in. Water for human consumption must be clean and free from toxins and microorganisms.

In developing countries and in areas affected by war or disaster the greatest risk to the population may be contamination of the drinking water, resulting in life-threatening infections such as cholera and amoebic dysentery. In developed countries, most residents have access to water purification systems that have been in place for many decades (Ineichen 1993). We have now become preoccupied with water contaminants arising from the original source of the water and from the old (sometimes lead) pipework through which water is delivered to each household. Water companies are being urged by their regulating body to produce cleaner water at a time when water demand is growing with increasing ownership of dishwashers and washing machines. This has led to the introduction of water metering and a proposed 'smart card' for the prepayment of water in the UK. In these initiatives, water is paid for by volume rather than by the traditional method, which used a standard rate. Measures such as these, however, are controversial, since those most in need of clean water for health and well-being could be those least able to afford it under this scheme (Cohen 1996).

Preoccupation with contamination of supplies among the wealthier population has spawned a large water bottling industry. This development in the provision of water for drinking, however, is not without problems, as it is not suitable for everyone. Small babies cannot physically manage the increased mineral content found in many bottled waters due to renal immaturity. Care is required in educating parents about the provision of water for consumption by infants and young children.

In nursing, there are occasions when water must be sterile. This is especially important when water is being used for the preparation of feeds for those who are immunosuppressed as a result of illness. Infants require sterile feeds because they have not developed resistance to infective organisms. Sterile water is also essential where water is used to irrigate wounds or in the preparation of medication via infusion, to protect patients from absorbing harmful contaminants.

Food

For dietary provision to be considered safe, it must be free from contaminants such as harmful bacteria (e.g. *Salmonella*, *Escherichia coli*) or disease (e.g. bovine spongiform encephalopathy) (Irani & Johnson 2003) which may be passed to humans. Additionally, food should be in adequate supply,

and this is not always the case in the developing world or in some instances in developed countries such as the UK. Within nursing, providing adequate nutrition for clients is important to promote healing and recovery. Health promotion is also important to prevent malnutrition and obesity.

Although the main impact of nutrition on health is discussed in greater detail in Chapter 7, it is important to recognize that modern systems for developing food sources need to be monitored closely. Contamination of food at any stage in the external food chain processing will be a potential threat to the well-being of the internal environment.

Shelter

Shelter is essential for survival. It provides protection from both excessive heat and cold, from the weather and from other environmental hazards. However, shelter should be safe for the resident and should not itself be contributory to disease. These two aspects are surprisingly difficult to achieve within the home and institutional setting.

Evidence based practice

Poor housing has been linked to increased levels of limiting long-term illness, respiratory and infectious diseases, accidents, psychological problems and perceived poor general health and even increased mortality (Gielen et al 1995, Hunt & McKenna 1992, Packer et al 1991). Peat et al (1998), Williamson et al (1997) and Verhoeff et al (1995) have demonstrated that dampness in houses leads to increased levels of house dust mites and fungal spores and this increases an individual's risk of respiratory or allergic symptoms. There is an increased risk of cough and wheeze in children living in a home with damp or mould.

Care institutions are often work settings and there is an increasing interest in how the design of individual workplace buildings can have an effect on the health of the individual workers within the building (Raw & Goldman 1996). Sick building syndrome (SBS) has been linked to a group of symptoms developed by people in certain buildings, notably office blocks. Symptoms of SBS include physical and behavioural problems such as irritation of the eyes, nose, throat and skin, headaches, lethargy and lack of concentration. Features of the buildings that appear to cause problems are associated with the air conditioning systems, office layouts, windows and light, furnishings and decorations (Raw & Goldman 1996).

ENVIRONMENTAL HAZARDS

As we have seen above, an individual's basic needs can be threatened by insufficiency or excess or poor management

---

Decision making exercise

What information about 'sterile' feed preparation would you need to offer Julie, a new mother, who wishes to bottle feed her baby?

● How would she ensure that the feeding implements are sterile?

● How would she ensure that the water she is using is safe for her baby?

● Where would you obtain information to give to Julie?

leading to the occurrence of identified hazards to health such as food poisoning or respiratory illness.

Potential hazards in our environment may be naturally occurring or result from human-made conditions, including the production of wastes and residues. Production of waste is unavoidable within communal societies and with modern technology and the production of consumer goods. Safe waste removal and disposal strategies are of vital importance to the survival of a community. Within nursing the type of waste is different from that produced domestically or industrially because of its clinical nature. Sharps and dressings need to be treated separately from paper and glass, because of the risks to health associated with cross-infection. Policies for the safe disposal of clinical waste and environmental policies ensure the safe disposal of clinical and non-clinical waste in care settings.

Reflection and portfolio evidence

In nursing, the disposal of clinical waste is an essential component of providing safe care.

In your next practice placement, identify how waste disposal is managed. Look especially at the management of sharps and of infected waste and linen, but do not forget to consider the day-to-day management of waste produced in the work setting.

- Identify and list any policies or protocols guiding waste disposal.
- Describe how optimum safety is maintained in relation to disposal of sharps.
- Critically comment on the evidence you have collected and add to your portfolio.

Apart from waste products, other hazards can seriously compromise the safety of the internal and external environments. They may be categorized into the following five groups:

- biological
- chemical
- physical
- psychological
- sociological.

Biological hazards

Biological hazards are concerned primarily with the entry of disease-producing infectious agents into the body, thus causing a risk to the stability of the internal environment. Such organisms include bacteria, viruses and fungi as well as parasites, which may additionally carry harmful pathogens.

Chemical hazards

Chemical hazards are not new: the gaining of knowledge into which plants are safe to eat and which liquids are safe to drink must have been fraught and littered with many accidents. Even though our predecessors may not have known the finer physiological details of any particular poison, they would have learnt to avoid it. Chemical agents may be synthetic or derived from natural substances and can affect the internal or the external environment beneficially or detrimentally. The most important consideration related to chemical hazards is regarding knowledge about the substance and the judicious application of this knowledge in using chemical substances safely and effectively. It is important to consider the impact of improper use or exposure to substances by patients. Nurses have a large role to play in caring for the public who may have become poisoned by chemicals.

Landrigan & Garg (2002) describe the potential chronic effects of toxic environmental exposures on children's health. Children have unusual patterns of exposure to environmental chemicals, and they have vulnerabilities that are quite distinct from those of adults. Increasingly, children's exposures to chemicals in the environment are understood to contribute to the causation and exacerbation of certain chronic, disabling diseases in children including asthma, cancer, birth defects, and neurobehavioral dysfunction. The protection of children against environmental toxins is a major challenge to modern society (Landrigan & Garg 2002). There is also a nursing role in the management and education of the public in maintaining a safe home environment for themselves and their families.

Physical hazards

Physical hazards are all around us and may cause disease, disability or fatality, and are manifest in many different ways. Certain dusts can be dangerous to the internal environment if they are inhaled and then absorbed, while other powders can be used therapeutically in the form of inhalers. Temperature in the external environment can also be a physical hazard. Extreme external temperatures can lead to a loss of the internal homeostatic balance (see Ch. 6). Contact with an extreme hot or cold source can cause extensive physical damage (burning) and potentially, death.

Electromagnetic radiation, which includes X-rays, ultraviolet and infrared light, and microwaves, can cause skin burns, an elevation in temperature and fatality with prolonged exposure. Understanding of the dangers related to uncontrolled exposure to these radiations is vital for nurses since controlled ionizing radiation such as X-rays and gamma rays can be used beneficially to produce radiographic pictures and in the treatment of neoplastic disease (cancer).

Human inventions such as equipment and machinery can cause accidents as well as offering the intended benefit. Modern machinery, including all nursing equipment, is being continually made safer as it is evaluated through use. Equipment that is used inappropriately or without regard to the manufacturer's instructions may provide a hazard to safety, even if it is functioning correctly technically. In the community, everyday machinery such as motor vehicles, drills or gardening equipment can be dangerous if not used appropriately.

Accidents

The above hazards are associated with a risk of accident or an undesirable interaction between the internal and external environment. The risk may be higher if an individual is unable to physically meet the demands of the world in which he or she is living, for example an elderly frail individual may be more likely to fall, or a small child may tumble while trying to reach an object from a high shelf. Additionally, accidents may occur if the individuals are unable to appreciate the effect of their behaviour either as a result of their stage of cognitive development or because of their disease process. Such examples would include a baby who becomes burned as a result of pulling a cup of hot tea from a nearby table onto herself because she is too young to understand the hazard associated with such contact with extremes of heat. Another example is an individual with senile dementia who wanders out into a busy road and is knocked down by a car because he is confused about his environment.

Accidents are a major concern for health carers. According to the Royal Society for the Prevention of Accidents, in 1998 there were an estimated 4300 people killed in home and garden accidents in the UK. About 172 600 people suffered serious injuries and were detained in hospital. An estimated 2.84 million attended an accident and emergency unit with respect to a home accident. This total includes over 1 million children (under 15) injured.

Some accidents can be prevented if carers are aware of the hazards and able to offer health and safety education. Patients and their families need to understand clearly the outcomes of risky behaviour and the implications that may arise. This requires imaginative education for the most vulnerable groups to communicate this information in a way that can be easily understood and accepted.

PSYCHOSOCIAL

PSYCHOLOGICAL AND SOCIAL HAZARDS

Psychological and social hazards are closely linked to human interactions with the environment. The next section explores the influence of psychosocial factors in the promotion of a safe and healthy environment.

There are many ways in which individuals strive to understand risks in their daily lives and factors influencing how they may act in the light of such perceptions (Bloor 1995). Fallowfield (1990) suggests that quality of life and therefore ultimately perceived health and well-being is directly related to the quality of the environment in which life exists. The environment must not only satisfy physiological needs, but also psychological and sociological needs. Fallowfield (1990) further identified four areas where the perception of life quality is paramount as follows:

- psychological – related to the perception of mental well-being
- social – related to involvement in social activities
- occupational – related to functional ability to achieve work (paid or voluntary)
- physical – related to pain, comfort, sleep, physical ability.

These areas are useful for exploring factors associated with determining life quality. However, it should be remembered that the way you view something may be very different from the way another person may perceive it. Culture, social class, gender, age, level of education, and emotional state should be acknowledged. Toxic effects from drugs and general level of health are also important.

Decision making exercise

Mrs James, a widow who lives alone, has been admitted with a severe chest infection that has made her acutely short of breath. She is frail and appears undernourished. You read in her medical history that she has suffered numerous falls at home, twice requiring admission to hospital and once resulting in a fractured neck of femur, requiring surgery. On arrival to the ward you are involved with her immediate nursing needs and are very busy assisting the medical team in her care. However, Mrs James remains agitated and anxious. Further discussion leads you to establish that she has left home without feeding her cat. She is also depressed about her admission, commenting that none of her friends will visit her as they do not have transport to make the journey.

1. Which of the areas identified by Fallowfield (1990) in Mrs James's environment are causing concern to (a) the medical team and (b) Mrs James?
2. What effect does this difference in priorities have in relation to Mrs James's health and well-being?
3. As Mrs James's nurse you are responsible for assessing and planning her care needs. Try to formulate a risk assessment within your nursing assessment for Mrs James, remembering to consider her physical as well as psychological needs.
4. Consider the possible differences in priority of needs between you as the nurse and Mrs James as the patient and try to ensure you incorporate both perspectives in your assessment.

Finally, there may be differences in the perception of priorities between patients and their carers. A knowledge of these differences can be critical in facilitating the provision of appropriate care.

PSYCHOLOGICAL STRESS

Stress can alter an individual's perceived environment, which can ultimately become hazardous.

The main issues associated with psychological stress and its effects on the internal environment are addressed elsewhere (see Ch. 8). However, it is important to consider how the effects of stress on an individual can impact on his or her immediate external environment.

RISK PERCEPTION

Risk perception is different from the knowledge of a danger, as it does not necessarily cause people to worry. Risk perception may result from the personal orientations that guide an individual to make commitments consistent with one specific political culture and inconsistent with others. At the same time cultures may select those individuals who support their way of life. Individuals may choose what to fear in supporting their preferred way of life (Royal Society Study Group 1992). For example, a religious sect propounding a particular set of beliefs may attract new members who are sympathetic to the views of that sect. Gabe (1995) identifies that in this sense risk cannot be objectively 'measured', but must be viewed as a social construct. This draws from the original anthropological work by Douglas (1966), which addressed questions about why different cultures select different risks for particular attention using beliefs to rationalize behaviour. Given that such interpretations of risk perception are valid, then points of cultural difference are extremely important in nursing. If a patient has different social expectations and selects different risks from the nurse's social expectation then a true assessment could be difficult and treatment could fail to meet the expectations of both parties. There may even be open conflict between the patient and health professional. For instance, Jehovah's Witnesses can present a challenge because they may refuse to receive blood transfusions. Where patients are severely ill and unable to give informed consent to treatment or where children require urgent blood transfusion, nurses may then face moral dilemmas in respecting the cultural beliefs of such individuals while acting in their best interest to maintain their safety.

Finally, individuals may react differently in different environments. A perception of risk and knowledge of danger are important in the care setting because patients may rely on the nurse to protect them (Simpson 1991). Those who are particularly vulnerable include:

- Children and people with a learning disability, who may not perceive risks to their well-being as they are unable to understand them.
- People with a mental health problem whose perception of danger may be reduced as the result of their illness or because of the treatment they are receiving.
- People who are critically ill and unable to determine dangers.

Within the hospital setting most patients are away from their known environment and are therefore unable to perceive risks in what amounts to an 'alien' environment. It is the responsibility of the nurse to ensure that individuals are aware of hazards wherever possible and are protected by either their own action or action on their behalf by the nurse. The nurse's role is to ensure the safety of the environment by assessing the potential risks and facilitating action for change.

Risk – the possibility of injury or loss – must be in the minds of all who deliver health care, in every clinical episode and in the planning of all health care delivery. The roots of risk management lie in risk assessment and implementation of ensuing preventative action plans and in the reporting, analysis, investigation and prevention-planning of adverse events. Engaging in preventative risk management activity, in addition to the reactive process of adverse event management, will enable the identification of many things that could go wrong, as part of a systematic approach to risk assessment (Department of Health and National Patient Safety Agency 2001).

An understanding of 'systems failures', in which errors are not attributed to individuals but to processes, is essential in recognizing the causes of error. Reduction in risk will only be achieved where risk management goes hand in hand with quality improvement and within an 'open and fair' culture. An open and fair culture is one in which disciplinary action is not normally invoked when a mistake occurs and is reported. It is well recognized that deficiencies in systems of care will not be readily identified unless those involved in the system feel safe to report a mistake or near miss. Whenever a risk is identified, the care delivery system that incorporates the risk must be broken down to reveal the weaknesses and changes or improvements made, to reduce or remove the chance of the weakness leading to harm.

Even before a risk has been identified, assumptions about safety of a system of care should be replaced with an explicit expectation of safety and traditional methods of care delivery reviewed to ensure their evidence base and quality. Reason (1997) describes these 'accidents waiting to happen' as latent risks. It is against the latent risks within our systems of health care, as well as the obvious risks, that nurses, who are at the forefront of care delivery, must contribute to safeguarding their patients and colleagues.

PSYCHOSOCIAL HAZARDS IN THE WORK ENVIRONMENT

Up to this point there has been an emphasis on the individual's responsibility within their personal environment and some discussion in relation to the behaviour of people when interacting within the healthcare environment. It is important to recognize that the organization has some influence in creating a safe and healthy environment. According to Cox & Griffiths (1996: 128) a 'safe' environment might be relatively easy to define, but perceptions of a 'healthy' work environment are usually narrowly focused on physical threats to health. These authors argue that healthy work can be defined as 'work that does not threaten but which helps maintain and enhance physical, psychological and social well-being'.

A 'hazard' has been defined as an event or situation that has the potential to cause harm (Cox & Griffiths 1996). Besides the physical hazards referred to in the previous section, the International Labour Organization (1986) has defined psychosocial hazards arising from interactions between job content, work, organizational, management and environmental conditions, and the employee's competencies and needs. Those interactions that can be defined as hazardous influence the health of employees through their 'perceptions' and 'experiences' of these conditions (Cox et al 1995, International Labour Organization 1986). Exposure to psychosocial hazards in particular is often chronic and cumulative, except when a particular acute, traumatic incident occurs. Table 2.2 outlines the common psychosocial hazards associated with the work environment and the conditions that define the potential level of hazard for the individual employee.

Table 2.2 Psychosocial hazards in the work environment (from Cox & Griffiths 1996)

Category	Conditions
Content of work	
Job content	Lack of variety or short work cycles, fragmented or meaningless work, underuse of skills, high uncertainty
Workload and work pace	Work overload or underload, lack of control over pacing, high levels of time pressure
Work schedule	Shift working, inflexible work schedules, unpredictable hours, long or unsocial hours
Interpersonal relationships at work	Social or physical isolation, poor relationships with superiors, interpersonal conflict, lack of social support
Control	Low participation in decision making, lack of control over work
Context of work	
Organizational culture and function	Poor communication, low levels of support for problem solving and personal development, lack of definition of organizational objectives
Role in organization	Role ambiguity and role conflict, responsibility for people
Career development	Career stagnation and uncertainty, underpromotion or overpromotion, poor pay, job insecurity, low social value of work
Home work interface	Conflicting demands of work and home, low support at home, dual career problems

It is important to remember the synergistic nature of the physical and psychosocial hazard in the work environment. Significant interactions can occur between the different types of hazard and their consequent effects on the health of the individual (Levi 1984). Stress in the workplace, from whatever cause, may inadvertently lead to risk taking behaviour by the individual worker.

MANAGEMENT OF HAZARDS AND DANGERS

When it comes to dealing with safety issues, particularly in the workplace environment, there have been three common approaches to the problem (Landy 1989) as follows:

1. The 'engineering' approach assumes that by modifying the environment or the equipment used, safety can be enhanced and accident rates reduced. Modifying the environment should include both physical and psychosocial factors.
2. The 'person psychology' approach in which the psychologist attempts to identify particular individual characteristics that might lead a person to be more accident-prone or to take risks. Within this particular approach the focus is on training programmes that will highlight individual behaviour and will attempt to influence change in unsafe behaviour.
3. The 'industrial–social' approach makes the assumption that unsafe behaviour is linked to group motivation. Individual motivation is linked with conditions in the environment that might support unsafe behaviour, for example it might be that taking risks is considered the 'macho' thing to do or that safe behaviour takes a lot more energy than careless behaviour. The focus in this approach is to try and change group behaviour so that people prefer safe practices (Landy 1989).

Each of the above three approaches can be applied to reduce risks and promote health in other environments besides the workplace. It is interesting to note that although health promotion approaches (Naidoo & Wills 2000) recognize the multiple factors that influence the health status of an individual, they often focus on changing individual behaviour.

For individuals in society, the desire to manage hazards relies on many factors. It is possible to relate to Bandura's concept of self-efficacy (Bandura 1977) which suggests that to make behavioural changes (and thus promote personal safety), the individual needs to have an awareness or risk perception of the danger or threat, to have the competence and incentive to change in order to avert the hazard and a feeling that change would be beneficial with few adverse consequences. According to Naidoo & Wills (2000), Bandura's model (Bandura 1977) has been incorporated into Becker's health belief model (Becker 1974), which focuses on demonstrating the functions of personal beliefs in decision making regarding health.

When exploring 'how' individuals may change their behaviour to avert hazards to their external or internal environment, nurses must also be aware about 'why' individuals behave the way they do. They must also be aware that individuals may not carry out their stated intentions (Ajzen & Fishbein 1980). The nurse's role in health education and promotion of safety is reliant upon the patient's willingness to listen, understand and comply with the information he or she is being offered. Health professionals must present information in a way that is appropriate to the patient's needs and sensitive to the patient's likely reaction if it is to be successful.

The main factors influencing an individual's response to health advice include:

- readiness
- motivation
- maturity
- level of education (Akinsola 1983).

Readiness

Human beings will only respond positively when they are physically, socially and psychologically ready to respond. For instance, the parent of an acutely ill 2-year-old child may not be ready to learn what caused the child's illness until the physical condition of the child improves; or elderly patients may be reluctant to mobilize independently in hospital because the floor is too slippery or they are unsure of the ward layout.

Motivation

To gain a better patient outcome, patient involvement and active participation are essential. Motivation requires an explanation about the importance of treatment and the use of equipment. Teaching patients with newly diagnosed diabetes mellitus to test their own blood sugar and to give their own insulin will mean that they can regain their self-esteem by being independent. Gaining someone's involvement in his or her treatment requires the individual to have some insight into the illness. This can be difficult if the nature of the illness affects perception, as in some mental illnesses in which the individual has no insight or if there is apathy due to low self-esteem.

Maturity

Because of differences in the maturity of individuals, carers need to be able to choose their words carefully so as not to either patronize clients or relatives or use words or concepts that are inappropriate. Careful consideration also has to be given to people with learning disabilities or adolescents who appear physically more mature than their chronological age. Although they may appear adult, their perceptions and experiences and understandings may be limited. Initiatives, such as 'A campaign with street cred' (Lowery 1996) have successfully targeted teenagers with asthma, aiming information and support directly at the adolescent

age group in order to resolve risk-taking problems associated with poor compliance. If patients are not used to medical terminology, using complex ideas or words can leave them frustrated and isolated. It is wise to avoid the use of medical jargon.

Theories of risk taking are of interest to psychologists and health educators alike because they can help to explain major barriers to the effective provision of healthcare advice. Campaigns to encourage individuals to stop smoking or to reduce the number of people drinking and driving cars are two examples where individuals may be aware of the risk to safety in their own (and others) environment, but still persist in risk taking behaviour.

Decision making exercise

Staff Nurse Baker has just completed five shifts on day duty and is just about to finish her final shift before taking 2 days off work. When leaving the ward she is approached by the ward manager who asks her to fill in for a colleague who is 'off sick' that night. Staff Nurse Baker agrees as she welcomes the idea of earning some extra money for her holidays. Her manager also emphasizes that she can find no one else to complete the shift. During the night shift, one of Nurse Baker's patients slips to the floor when attempting to sit on the commode, which had been by her bedside. She is unhurt and Nurse Baker attempts to move her from the floor back to the commode. The client is 66 kg and feeling weak due to her illness.

- Identify the potential risk factors to Nurse Baker's health through her decision to complete the night shift.
- Decide on what factors may motivate Nurse Baker in how she copes with her client's fall.
- Decide on what staff training or health promotion strategy is needed in this situation for all of the workforce involved in the incident.

CARE DELIVERY KNOWLEDGE

Risk management in nursing falls within two main remits, firstly the safety of the individual patient or client and secondly, in partnership with the multidisciplinary team, ensuring safe systems of care.

PATIENT SAFETY

There is a need to assess individual patients in relation to their own safety and the safety of others. This is an essential part of nursing care and is important in all branches of nursing. The need for cognitive understanding of risk and physical compatibility within the environment has already been illustrated in relation to accidents in the community and these features are equally applicable in the care setting. In caring for children these two considerations are particularly important. For clients with learning disabilities, an assessment of individual ability and understanding is essential in order to ensure a safe environment for care. It cannot be assumed that an individual will behave in a way consistent with someone of a similar chronological age. Nurses in mental health have to assess and plan care for their patients ensuring the safety of the patient and other patients within the care setting, and their own personal safety. Nurses are also becoming involved in ensuring that patients who are released into the community do not pose a hazard to themselves or anyone else (Noak 1997). Finally, in caring for adults, there is a need for all of the above, because adult individuals develop to different stages of maturity both physically and psychologically, and the effects of disease can impair individual ability to maintain a safe environment. Adults have uniquely different motivations for their behaviours, which may not necessarily be predictable or rational.

Ensuring patient safety while receiving care is ultimately an employer's responsibility in all settings, but nurses have a direct role in ensuring the implementation of safe care for their patients. Since patients are all individuals they all bring different situations to the care setting. Fear or anxiety may mean a patient is not willing to comply with planned procedures of care regardless of how content they may have appeared with the negotiated plan. For example, a patient with a stroke may not like the hoist used to transfer him or her from the bed to the chair. There will always be dilemmas about how patients should receive intervention that is appropriate and safe. Discussing interventions with the patient can air anxieties, and in this case finding a different lifting system that the patient would feel happier with could be safer for all concerned.

Other examples include critically ill patients who may have numerous devices for treatment and monitoring equipment around them; in such a case the nurse should endeavour to make the area as safe as possible. If there is a lot of electrical equipment, extension sockets should not be used as the number of electrical items could overload the socket and result in a fire. Oxygen cylinders and wall points must have 'No smoking' signs in view to make everyone aware of the danger.

In general, the nurse identifying a risk must ensure that action is taken. Further investigation may reveal that the problem has already been recognized and a solution is being sought; a policy decision may be required; or the solution may have cost implications and the money has yet to be found. The nurse has a responsibility to establish the current position and if necessary to facilitate change for improvement. Change must be implemented with the co-operation of all staff to ensure maximum benefit. If working with managers and staff to resolve a risk to the patient is ineffective, then advice may be required from outside agencies with a remit for the facilitation of health and safety at work. A safe policy for practice should exist and be readily available for most of the procedures that a nurse will perform with a patient.

Evidence based practice

The 2002 National Confidential Enquiry into Perioperative Deaths (NCEPOD) Report, based on a sample of deaths within 3 days of an intervention, revealed that over 80% of the patients who died were urgent or emergency admissions. In this situation, there has often been no formal assessment of comorbidities, and many otherwise remedial conditions go uncorrected. The report states:

There needs to be more teamworking. This involves not only consultants working together but also trainees, nurses, managers, professions allied to medicine and sometimes patients themselves.

One of the key points of the report, in relation to postoperative care, is the vital need for maintenance of accurate fluid balance charts by nursing staff, stating that medical staff should review these daily.

A LEARNING ENVIRONMENT

It is vital that we learn from events where things have gone wrong. Generally, these events can be called adverse events (for example, a needlestick injury) or, if the event caused or may have caused harm to a patient, a patient safety incident or prevented patient safety incident.

The value of structured investigation into the causes of patient safety incidents (or adverse events), and prevented patient safety incidents (or near misses) locally, and of learning from incidents reported nationally and internationally, is now well recognized. To this end nurses and other health workers, in all healthcare settings, have a duty to report any act or omission arising during health care, that could have or did lead to unintended or unexpected harm, loss or damage. Those events that did lead to harm are referred to as patient safety incidents. Those incidents that did not lead to harm, but could have done so, are termed prevented patient safety incidents. In fact prevented patient safety incidents are invaluable as tools that provide 'free lessons' and should not be wasted. These terms have been developed by the National Patient Safety Agency in place of the terms 'adverse healthcare event' and 'healthcare near miss' first set out in the document *Organization with a Memory* (Department of Health 2000). The person who notices the event should complete a report at the time and not assume someone else will do so. It is important that the reporting system is entirely separate from the disciplinary process, except when an event involved malicious or criminal activity or where it was part of an activity which contravened the individual's professional code of conduct. The reasons for passing on information about errors and potential errors is to allow safer systems of care to be developed. New guidelines, care pathways, policies or additional training are some of the measures that can be introduced in response to adverse events, to reduce the risk of errors in the future. Incident report forms are disclosable in the event of litigation or external inquiry; it is therefore vital to ensure details are accurate and factual and do not apportion blame or give opinions.

Examples of patient safety incidents include the following:

- delay in diagnosis or wrong diagnosis
- administration of the wrong drug or incorrect quantity of the right drug (an incorrect prescription intercepted before administration would be regarded as a near miss)
- healthcare associated infection.

Prevented patient safety incidents should be graded according to the actual impact, the likelihood of recurrence and the most likely consequence of the event if it were to occur again. Scoring of these factors allows a risk category to be established. The National Patient Safety Agency (NPSA) was set up in the UK in 2001 to aid learning from errors in health care and to allow the sharing of lessons learned. The agency will request anonymous reports from NHS sites, on all patient safety incidents, and will collate information to enable learning across the NHS. The NPSA will also work to find solutions to recurring themes, such as inadvertent administration of high dose potassium and wrong site surgery. The following is suggested as a matrix for grading incidents at a local level; however, the NPSA will only require data relating to the initial impact of the incident and not the future likelihood of occurrence.

Patient safety incidents can be graded according to the initial impact as:

- death (including unexpected death)
- major (including procedure involving wrong body part)
- moderate (including healthcare associated infection that may lead to semi-permanent harm)
- minor (including healthcare associated infection that may result in non-permanent harm)
- none (no obvious harm).

The consequence if the event were to recur might be considered to be the same as when the initial event happened or could differ, but the same grades can be used. The likelihood of recurrence can be rated as:

- almost certain
- likely
- possible
- unlikely
- rare.

Using a grading matrix the potential future risk can be evaluated as high, moderate, low, or very low, which should lead to a level of investigation and prevention planning

commensurate with the risk level (Department of Health, National Patient Safety Agency 2001).

It is also mandatory to report some events to various agencies, including to the Medical Device Agency, the Mental Health Act Commission, the Health and Safety Executive and the Medicines Control Agency. Feedback from these agencies is by means of hazard notices, safety notices and alerts and should be used to identify similar latent risks within individual organizations.

Investigation of adverse events

Root cause analysis is one of the most popular methods of investigating adverse events (Roberts 2002). It is a technique pioneered outside health care some 20 years ago, but in recent years has begun to be adapted for use in health care. The essential requirement of root cause analysis is to keep asking the question 'Why?' until you are satisfied that all of the contributing factors have been teased out.

Trends in adverse events are used as important tools in risk management and are accessed from databases holding adverse event reports. The information may assist the exploration of root causes of events, by revealing patterns, times, staffing levels, etc. One example might be analysis of adverse medication events showing a peak in 'missed doses' in the afternoon. Asking 'Why?' might reveal that this coincides with a set visiting time, and 'Why?' again, that the nurse is repeatedly interrupted by relatives asking questions. Reduction in error may be achieved through introduction of a simple 'Do not disturb' sign, requesting visitors to ask a different nurse or to wait until the nurse administering medications has finished.

SAFE SYSTEMS OF CARE

The second remit for nurses in risk assessment is more general and interprofessional and relates to the care environment. The outcome of risk assessment must be the identification and implementation of risk management strategies to ensure that particular risks are eliminated or adequately controlled. However, there is evidence that accidents do happen and that many result from the failure of control systems, such as policy failure, deficient working practices and inadequate communication, as well as poorly defined responsibilities and staff working beyond their competence.

RISK ASSESSMENT

Nurses need to know what the risks are and develop appropriate control systems. Risk assessment is not a 'once and for all' activity; it must be revised as changes occur such as new equipment, revised systems of work and different approaches to patient care.

Defining a risk

Before carrying out the risk assessment, a distinction must be made between 'hazard' and 'risk'. You will have already seen that a hazard can be defined as something with the potential to cause harm (Griffiths 1996). A risk can be defined as the likelihood that the harm from a particular hazard is realized. The relationship between risk and hazard can be illustrated by the use of glutaraldehyde, which is a hazard in nursing. The risk of industrial asthma resulting from inhalation of glutaraldehyde is high if it is used in areas without adequate ventilation and personal protective clothing (i.e. inappropriately). However, with effective ventilation and a defined safe system of work, the risks associated with glutaraldehyde can be reduced, although it still remains a hazard.

Reflection and portfolio evidence

Some risks and hazards associated with common problems affecting nurses are moving and handling clients, back injury in nursing, verbal violence to nurses by patients, pathogens, nosocomial disease and injury from assault. In your practice placement complete the following exercise.

- Decide from the above list which of these are hazards and which are risks.
- Use your examples to decide whether the hazards identified have acceptable or unacceptable risks.

Other risks might affect patients, staff, visitors or everyone within the environment. Find out what method of documentation of risk assessment is used in your current placement. After discussion with other staff members:

- Try to decide what you think are the 'top three' risks to patients, staff or visitors in your working environment.
- Use the recognized documentation to make an initial assessment and scoring of these three risks.
- Establish an action plan aimed at risk reduction or removal for each of the risks assessed.
- Add your findings to your portfolio evidence.

PLANNING AND IMPLEMENTING A STRATEGY FOR RISK MANAGEMENT

Planning care relates to the promotion of a safe environment for clients. There are two levels to planning: firstly, planning care in relation to the safety of the individual client, and secondly, planning daily work in relation to controlling of risks or hazards in the environment.

Issues in planning related to patients

The need for a hospital admission may bring about physical hazards associated with the strangeness of the environment and an unknown ward layout. Patients may demonstrate anxiety and an unnatural response as a result of their situation. The nurse should identify and address these problems when making the assessment of a client's needs and in negotiating a safe and acceptable plan of care. Talking with the patient about how best to address his or her needs is an important starting point, since compliance with a safe plan for care is critical. An example could relate to a hospital 'no smoking' policy. If a client usually enjoys cigarettes at home and will not entertain giving up smoking in hospital, it is not helpful to include in the nursing care plan that smoking is prohibited. For the client, this may lead to anger and frustration and potential non-compliance, either overtly or covertly. In a setting where there are inflammable substances (such as oxygen) this can create a serious risk both for the client and all others in the vicinity. It is safer to negotiate a plan with the client which agrees where cigarettes can be smoked safely, also ensuring that the client is able to gain access to this area. Information can also be given about the hazards of smoking in no-smoking areas, and there may be an opportunity for health education, leading to a reduction in smoking.

Reflection and portfolio evidence

In your next practice setting, look at a patient's plan of care. Take a particular note of any assessment that includes areas where safety may require interprofessional care planning.

- What measures would you plan for this patient?
- How do your ideas compare with those of the care team?
- Have both psychological and physical safety issues been addressed?
- Has the plan been updated to incorporate any changes in the patient's situation?
- Record your findings as a 'managing risk case study' in your portfolio.

Risk and hazard control in the care setting

The key questions in identification of risk (Roberts 2002) are:

- What can go wrong?
- How frequently can it go wrong?
- What would be the effect?
- What can be done to stop it happening?

Risk management is promoted by the NHS Controls Assurance Support Unit (CASU) and provides a framework for the assessment, analysis, prioritization, treatment and review of risks. A register of identified risks should be compiled in every area. This should include the date the risk was identified, the risk itself, the impact (consequence) the risk would have, the chance (likelihood) of the risk happening and the risk score (consequence × likelihood). In addition, the register should also provide information on the person assigned as responsible for the risk, what action needs to be taken to minimize the risk, what residual risk (if any) remains and the continuing monitoring action plan. The Australian/New Zealand Risk Management Standard 4360:1999 is the standard used by CASU.

Decision making exercise

Managers opened an acute mental illness admission ward on the fourth floor of a general hospital to replace the admission facility of the local psychiatric hospital, which was due to close. The ward was previously used as an acute surgical ward and there were numerous cubicles, several exits, and the windows opened without restriction and were not glazed with safety glass. Shortly after the ward opened, the managers were surprised by the occurrence of a number of suicides.

- How might a risk assessment have identified potential hazards in this situation?
- Using methods of hazard control, how could you address the hazards of poor observation from cubicles, exits and windows?
- Find out what the National Patient Safety Agency's position is on suicides achieved through hanging from non-collapsible shower rails.
- What measures should be taken to prevent this? Are these measures applicable to all healthcare settings? If not, how would you ensure the safety of 'at-risk' patients?

Safe equipment

In order to ensure an optimum working environment for nursing, it is important that all equipment in use is well maintained and all practices are safe and without risks to health as outlined by Section 2(2)(a) of the Health and Safety at Work Act 1974. This is a general requirement, defined by the Health and Safety at Work Act as including machinery, equipment and appliances used at work, as well as the establishment of safe systems or practices while working.

In caring for clients, nurses use a wide variety of equipment. The following criteria apply to the way in which all equipment is used:

- Equipment must meet all the current health and safety standards.
- Equipment must be regularly inspected and serviced.
- The system of work must be safe.
- Repair and maintenance operations must have a safe system of work identified.
- Personal protective equipment should be provided if required.

A safe system of work needs to be identified for repair and maintenance operations themselves and this can have implications for nurses. For instance, the safe decontamination of equipment before maintenance must be specified. This may be especially important in areas where equipment has been used with clients carrying infectious organisms. At a simple level, working with children for instance, this may mean that there should be a procedure for cleaning toys safely after a child who has an infection such as diarrhoea and vomiting has used them, before checking their safety for offering to another child. It also implies the appropriate cleaning of equipment or even rooms after use by patients.

Managing safe handling and storage of substances

Within nursing practice, handling of potentially hazardous substances may be a regular occurrence. Issues related to the safe handling of substances are addressed in Section 53 of the Health and Safety at Work Act and are developed further by the Control of Substances Hazardous to Health (COSHH) Regulations 1988.

COSHH Regulations 1988

This was the most significant piece of health and safety legislation after the Health and Safety at Work Act 1974. It applies to all work where people (including nurses) are exposed or liable to be exposed to substances hazardous to health. The regulations give both a general description of the types of substances that are hazardous to health and a specific list of materials currently regarded as hazardous. There are 19 regulations, which include key duties such as assessment and training and a related Approved Code of Practice is given for each regulation.

Any 'substance' should be regarded as hazardous to health in the form in which it occurs in the work activity, whether or not its mode of causing injury to health is known and whether or not the active constituent has been identified. A substance hazardous to health is not just a single chemical compound but also includes mixtures, for example of compounds, microorganisms or allergens. The Approved Code of Practice further defines what is hazardous. Among the key points are that:

- different forms of the same substance may present different hazards, for instance when a solid is ground into dust
- impurities may create hazards
- fibres of a certain size or shape can be hazardous.

There is also a summary of duties of employer under the COSHH Regulations, which states that the employer must:

- assess the risks
- assess the steps needed to meet the regulation
- prevent or at least control exposure

- ensure controls are used to monitor exposure
- provide health surveillance
- examine and test control
- inform, instruct and train employees and non-employees (Brewer 1994).

The storage of substances on a ward or unit should follow the principles of 'good housekeeping' to improve safety. This may mean storing glass bottles on the back of a low shelf to avoid breakages, or keeping the stock of substances to a minimum to avoid stock expiring and the dangers of major spillages. There should be procedures and policies in relation to the handling of substances and these should be readily available.

Decision making exercise

A 5-gallon container of glutaraldehyde is knocked over accidentally and its contents spill over the clinic room floor. A nurse tries to mop it up, but is overcome by a coughing fit and is off sick for 3 months.

- Using the summary of the Control of Substances Hazardous to Health (COSHH) Regulations 1988, what questions could be asked in attempting to establish liability?

PROFESSIONAL AND ETHICAL KNOWLEDGE

INTERPROFESSIONAL WORKING

Initiatives to minimize risk are best formulated and actioned through a team approach. However, all members of the team may not necessarily share the same interests, values, beliefs and reasons for being a part of the team and may therefore not always support the same objectives. A clash of objectives and interests may be a significant hurdle to the implementation of any risk reduction strategy. Effective risk management presupposes the creation of a healthcare team which through patient focused care strives for quality improvement and above all safety. Doctors still exercise considerable control over the workplace and all that goes on within it, since they ultimately have responsibility for patients in their care. Whilst there is often resistance to any proposed change, the nature and reasons for resistance need to be understood and respected, encouraging a shared ownership of any improvement strategy. Nurses must work with their health colleagues, valuing and sharing the expertise that each profession brings to patient care, if they are to achieve successful changes in practice and improve the quality and safety of health care.

Reflection and portfolio evidence

- Find out what method of reporting patient safety incidents is used in the healthcare setting in which you are working.
- Using a standard report, try writing an adverse event report about a patient for whom you have been caring, imagining that the patient has been given intravenous antibiotics intended for a different patient.
- You later identify that the patient who received the antibiotics is actually documented as being allergic to penicillin and the antibiotic he received was in fact penicillin. What steps should you take?
- Record your findings in your portfolio.

UPHOLDING THE LAW AND MAINTAINING STANDARDS

There are many laws that relate to the provision of health care and in addition there are professional and patient standards, regulations, rules, guidelines and expectations, which all govern the way health professionals must work. Some of the laws, for example the National Health Act 1977 and the Health Act 1999, impose upon carers a duty of quality. Case law also sets ever-increasing standards of care amidst a climate of the requirement for increasing patient involvement. The key issues for nurses are statutory requirements and professional requirements. Local policies and guidelines are often formed on the basis of these requirements and therefore serve to assist health professionals in meeting the standards of care required of them.

Evidence based practice

Gershon et al (1995) surveyed 1716 American care workers about their compliance with universal safety precautions. They found that compliance varied according to activity, but was overall strongly correlated to several key factors, including perceived organizational commitment to safety and perceived conflict of interest between the workers' need to protect themselves and the need to provide care for their patients. Risk taking personality, perception of risk, and knowledge and training were also noted to be influential factors.

Statutory requirements

Statutory requirements are laid down in legislation as Acts of Parliament. The key legislation that governs the way all health professionals must work is the Health and Safety at Work Act 1974. The Act aims to secure the health, safety and welfare of persons at work and to protect members of the

Management of Health and Safety at Work Regulations 1992

Manual Handling Regulations (Health and Safety Executive) 1992

Workplace (Health, Safety and Welfare) Regulations 1992

Health and Safety (Display Screen Equipment) Regulations 1992

Provision and Use of Work Equipment Regulations 1992

Personal Protective Equipment (PPE) at Work Regulations 1992

Figure 2.1 The 'six-pack' regulations for health and safety: UK interpretations of the European Community directives.

public from risks that might be created by the work of others. European Union Directives (nicknamed the 'six-pack'; Fig. 2.1) came into force in 1993 and the Management of Health and Safety at Work Regulations 1999 form the legal framework for health and safety in the UK today. It is a criminal offence to fail to discharge any of the duties laid down in the Act and subsequent regulations, whether by intention or neglect. It is therefore vital that all nurses familiarize themselves with both the Act and subsequent regulations.

One set of regulations, Reporting of Injuries, Diseases and Dangerous Occurrences Regulations (RIDDOR), is of particular importance in relation to adverse event reporting. Accidents and Incidents covered by the regulations, must be reported directly to the Health and Safety Executive, using a statutory reporting form. This is usually the responsibility of a designated person (e.g. the Health and Safety Officer or Risk Manager) but the legal requirement for this highlights the necessity for nurses to ensure all adverse events are reported in a timely manner.

Decision making exercise

The following scenario could be used for a debate between two teams, one team representing the plaintiff and one the employer.

You are the defendant in a court case based on the Health and Safety at Work Act 1974, after you received a back injury from slipping on a wet floor. Although the floor dryer was broken and had been sent for repair, the cleaners did possess warning cones to advise employees about wet floors. There were none in evidence on the day that you slipped. The onus of proving that an employer has not fulfilled the statutory obligation by being 'reasonably practicable' is placed on the defendant (i.e. you). The court would then have to decide what is or was reasonable or practicable in your case.

- Decide how you could convince a court that the employer had broken the law.

Professional requirements

The Nursing and Midwifery Council (NMC) requires nurses to maintain a safe environment for their patients. This is

8   As a registered nurse, midwife or health visitor, you must act to identify and minimize the risk to patients and clients.

8.1   You must work with other members of the team to promote healthcare environments that are conducive to safe, therapeutic and ethical practice.

8.2   You must act quickly to protect patients and clients from risk if you have good reason to believe that you or a colleague, from your own or another profession, may not be fit to practise for reasons of conduct, health or competence. You should be aware of the terms of legislation that offer protection for people who raise concerns about health and safety issues.

8.3   Where you cannot remedy circumstances in the environment of care that could jeopardize standards of practice, you must report them to a senior person with sufficient authority to manage them and also, in the case of midwifery, to the supervisor of midwives. This must be supported by a written record.

8.4   When working as a manager, you have a duty toward patients and clients, colleagues, the wider community and the organization in which you and your colleagues work. When facing professional dilemmas, your first consideration in all activities must be the interests and safety of patients and clients.

8.5   In an emergency, in or outside the work setting, you have a professional duty to provide care. The care provided would be judged against what could reasonably be expected from someone with your knowledge, skills and abilities when placed in those particular circumstances.

Figure 2.2 Risk management issues from the Nursing and Midwifery Council's (2002) *Code of Professional Conduct*, with kind permission.

illustrated within the Code of Professional Conduct (Nursing and Midwifery Council 2002) in which risk management features as one of the shared values of all the UK health care regulatory bodies. It states that nurses must: 'act to identify and minimize risk to patients and clients'.

Professional requirements are the standards required of all health professionals and can be used to regulate activities, to discipline individuals and increasingly, in the assessment of professional liability and medical negligence. Negligence can be defined as breaching a duty to use reasonable care and causing an injury to another. Compensation for injury (which may be psychological as well as physical) as the result of the action of a health professional is usually pursued through the civil law but may also come under the jurisdiction of the criminal courts. It is currently mainly doctors that face charges of negligence, but increasingly this is a pressure that nurses, particularly given their rising professional accountability and extended roles, are meeting in providing patient care. It is incumbent upon all health professionals and the health provider to have a duty of care to every patient. The Nursing and Midwifery Council (2002) has somewhat controversially extended the scope of this duty of care in its recently revised Code of Conduct, Part 8.5 (Fig. 2.2).

External agencies and standards

In terms of risk management, numerous external agencies set their own standards and requirements, with which healthcare providers must demonstrate compliance. It is important for nurses to have some knowledge of these agencies and the standards they set, as they form the basis of the way risk is managed in the NHS.

Controls Assurance

Controls Assurance is a process designed to provide evidence of effective systems within NHS organizations. The process is one of self-assessment against set standards, which results in the NHS organization providing an assurance statement of its compliance. Risk management is one of the core standards within Controls Assurance. The Controls Assurance website and the Department of Health Controls Assurance website addresses are listed at the end of this chapter.

Clinical Governance

Clinical Governance is a system designed to ensure both quality and effective health care. It is defined in *A First Class Service: Quality in the New NHS* (the 1998 White Paper; see NHS Executive 1999) as: 'A framework through which NHS organizations are accountable for continuously improving the quality of their services and safeguarding high standards of care by creating an environment in which excellence in clinical care will flourish.' Clinical Governance is in fact a risk management system that integrates quality with safety.

Commission for Health Improvement

The Commission for Health Improvement (CHI) is an independent body, created under the Health Act 1999, whose aim is to improve standards of care through a rolling review programme of Clinical Governance arrangements throughout the NHS. In addition to providing national leadership in the development of the principles of Clinical Governance, the commission conducts 4-yearly inspections, which are increased to 2-yearly for organizations that fail to meet the standards required. The government can also instruct the Commission to carry out an extraordinary inspection of a trust where it has serious concerns about clinical practice or patient safety. The government has emphasized the key role of nurses, midwives and health visitors in ensuring that high quality health care is established and maintained. In 2002, CHI became CHAI, that is the Commission for Health and Audit Improvement.

Clinical Negligence Scheme for Trusts

The Clinical Negligence Scheme for Trusts (CNST) was established by the Department of Health in 1995, in response to the increasing incidence of clinical negligence litigation against NHS trusts. A special health authority, called the NHS Litigation Authority (NHSLA), administers the scheme. Although membership is not compulsory, the scheme has been adopted by most trusts and is similar to having an insurance policy. Regular contributions mean that much of the cost of claims is met through the scheme. CNST provides a financial incentive to trusts to have well-developed risk management programmes, as a staged reduction in contribution costs is given to trusts that achieve CNST standards. External assessment ascertains the level at which a trust is succeeding in managing its risk (level 0, 1, 2, 3). The standards represent best practice, developed in co-operation with the healthcare professions and therefore form the goals of risk management.

Risk Pooling Scheme for Trusts

The NHSLA also operates a 'non-clinical insurance scheme' for trusts. This is called the Risk Pooling Scheme for Trusts (RPST) and operates in a similar manner to CNST, with separate external assessment of achievement of standards. RPST standards now form the risk management standard of Controls Assurance, which avoids prior duplication and overlap.

Other standards

Other standards being set include those set by the National Institute for Clinical Excellence (NICE), which is another special health authority, with direct responsibility to the Secretary of State for Health. NICE reviews specific areas of health care and uses panels of experts to form guidelines for best clinical practice. The Essence of Care benchmarks best practice for nurses and other staff in various aspects of care, such as in nutrition, tissue viability, privacy and dignity.

The Care Standards Act 2000 allows the government greater control over the independent sector, in a similar way that the Health Act 1999 regulates the NHS. A Care Standards Commission has been given the authority to develop and maintain minimum standards throughout the independent sector.

Decision making exercise

You may like to discuss some or all of this exercise with practice colleagues or your tutor.

You are at work when the fire alarm sounds. The fire doors shut automatically.

- What would your action be?
- Staff and visitors continue to go through the doors and do not respond to the alarm. How would you deal with this situation?
- You are advised by the fire officer that the ward should be evacuated. While you are making arrangements for evacuation a patient has a cardiac arrest.
- What would be the priority? The patient who has arrested or the other patients?
- What action would you need to take in both cases?
- What questions may you need to ask (a) at the time? (b) afterwards?

THE CONSENT PROCESS

Gaining patient consent to treatment is a process largely overseen within risk management, and the NHS Litigation Authority in the Clinical Negligence Scheme for Trusts sets out standards of good practice. An overview of the consent process is therefore included within this chapter.

In 2001, the Department of Health introduced a number of guidance documents on consent, as well as a 'model' consent policy and consent forms (Department of Health 2001). These are required to be adopted in all NHS trusts. This has the advantage of ensuring that the transient population of health professionals is familiar with consent procedures and documentation in every NHS hospital in the UK.

Consent is a patient's agreement for a health professional to provide care and must be 'informed', meaning that the patient must give agreement based on a sound understanding of the nature and consequences of the care offered, or indeed the consequences of not agreeing. For consent to be valid, the patient must:

- be competent (mentally able) to take the particular decision
- have received sufficient information to take it
- not be acting under duress.

Whilst a patient must agree to every act of nursing care, this can usually be a verbal agreement, whereas for significant procedures, it is essential for health professionals to document clearly both a patient's agreement to the intervention and the discussions that led up to that agreement. This means that informed consent must be a two-stage process; the information stage and the agreement stage. The process may take place at one time, or over a series of meetings and discussions, depending on the seriousness of what is proposed and the urgency of the patient's condition. In most cases where written consent is being sought, treatment options will generally be discussed well in advance of the actual procedure being carried out. The health professional carrying out the procedure is ultimately responsible for ensuring that the patient is genuinely consenting to what is being done: it is they who will be held responsible in law if this is challenged later. However, teamwork is crucial to the way the NHS operates and participation in the consent process may be delegated to other members of the healthcare team. Where an anaesthetist is involved in a patient's care, it is their responsibility (not that of a surgeon) to seek consent for anaesthesia, having discussed the benefits and risks.

Consent to treatment of children and adults who lack mental capacity is complex and requires specialist knowledge. For guidance on this and for further information, health professionals should consult the *Reference Guide to Consent for Examination or Treatment* (Department of Health 2001), available on the Department of Health website, the address of which is listed at the end of this chapter.

ETHICAL DILEMMAS IN RISK MANAGEMENT

The government seeks to meet its objective of standardizing quality in health care through Clinical Governance. The Department of Health states as the official view that Clinical Governance is necessary to overcome regional variations in the quality of health care. One of the functions of NICE is to develop the standardization of treatments throughout the UK. Evidence based guidelines on the most appropriate treatments for a range of medical conditions are drawn up by NICE, which also bases its recommendations on cost as well as clinical effectiveness. Whilst the government's objective is to end the so-called 'postcode' prescribing lottery, Harpwood (2001) points out that NICE, as a public body is subject to the Human Rights Act 1998, and must therefore not act in a manner that is incompatible with the rights in the European Convention on Human Rights. She comments that it might be possible for an individual who believes that a NICE recommendation denies him the right to life-saving treatment to bring a challenge under the Act. This might prove an interesting ethical and legal challenge.

Following the tragic events at Bristol Royal Infirmary, where there was found to be an unacceptably high mortality rate in paediatric cardiac surgery, the Bristol Inquiry made many recommendations (see annotated website). The inquiry sought to identify any professional, management and organizational failures and to recommend action to safeguard future patients and secure high quality care across the country. 'Whistleblowing' is the term given to raising concerns about the professional competency of colleagues. As a result of the inquiry, NHS trusts are being encouraged to require employees to pass on such information and must establish mechanisms of protection for those that do. Many trusts are therefore establishing 'raising concerns' policies, which allow concerns to be expressed in a confidential manner. There are ethical dilemmas surrounding whistleblowing, for whilst essential that incompetent or unsafe health professionals are prevented from doing harm, policies may be open to abuse by aggrieved or malicious members of staff. In addition, it may prove very difficult to afford career protection to a person who in good faith reports a concern about the practice of a colleague.

Greater openness on the part of the NHS, in terms of publication by the government of league tables, surgical success rates, waiting list times and death rates may present a negative picture to a patient awaiting surgery in one of the worse-faring trusts. This raises concerns and debates about equity and fairness in access to quality health care.

Doctors wishing to safeguard against litigation might in the course of the process of informed consent reasonably advise patients of even the smallest risks to a procedure, which may stop some patients going ahead with a beneficial operation. Empowering patients to weigh up the relative benefits and risks of a procedure also highlights the need for patient advocacy for those more vulnerable patients who are not willing or unable to give informed consent.

PERSONAL AND REFLECTIVE KNOWLEDGE

Within the scope of your role as a learner in health care it is important to maintain your own health and safety and promote that of your patients and clients. Occupational health departments provide support and help for all workers and should be accessed for advice whenever you have concerns about your own health.

Risk and safety go hand in hand and are everybody's business. It can be argued that the most crucial role for the nurse is as set out in Part 8 of the Nursing and Midwifery Council's (2002) Code of Professional Conduct: to act to identify and minimize the risk to patients and clients and above all else, as Florence Nightingale said, 'Do no harm.'

CASE STUDIES APPLYING PRINCIPLES OF SAFETY AND RISK

Case study: Mental health

Jeremiah Jacobs is 62 years old. He has lived in a large rural hospital for the mentally ill for the last 30 years and is diagnosed as having moderate learning disabilities and schizophrenia. Jeremiah remains in a long-term care facility because as yet no appropriate community facility has been found. In the hospital where he lives many patients have been moved into community homes and wards have been closed. The hospital is now a small facility where all clients are well known by the resident staff. Jeremiah enjoys sitting on the main ward corridor trying to trip passers-by up. As everyone knows him, they know to keep out of tripping distance. One day a visitor comes into the hospital and is tripped up by Jeremiah. The visitor sustains a number of bruises and sues the hospital.

- Do you think the visitor will be successful in her claim?
- Who was responsible for ensuring the visitor's safety?
- Which section of the Health and Safety at Work Act 1974 may be referred to in this case?
- Decide how you could have prevented this situation from arising.

Case study: Adult

Mrs Smith is a 95-year-old woman who has arrived at the Accident and Emergency Department after a fall at her home. She had been found by neighbours after crying out for some hours. On arrival in hospital Mrs Smith is cold and in pain and appears confused. She is to have a radiograph of her femur as a fracture is suspected. A nurse takes Mrs Smith to the Radiography Department and then goes on a coffee break. Mrs Smith attempts to get off the trolley while left alone in the radiography department and falls again.

- Using the information gained from this chapter write down the questions that you think should be asked, in the event of an inquiry into the incident. For example, did the nurse inform the radiographer that the patient was there? If not, why not? If yes, why was there no one with her?

- Were the trolley sides up or down? What system of work is there for transferring patients from the Accident and Emergency Department to the Radiography Department? Is there one? Was it followed?

Case study: Child

As a school nurse you are attempting to reduce the number of home accidents among schoolchildren. This means that you plan to attend the children's school and talk to a group of 5–7-year-olds about the types of accidents that may occur in the home.

- What factors may influence the way in which you help to ensure that the children can participate actively in their own risk assessment and hazard management?
- Decide on a plan of action that could help get the safety message across to this group.
- Who is ultimately responsible for ensuring your safety while you are visiting the school to talk to the children? Which section of the Health and Safety at Work Act 1974 would apply in this instance?

Case study: Learning disabilities

Benny Wong is a 25-year-old Chinese man with moderate learning difficulties. He is unable to care independently for himself and tends to be noisy and aggressive at times. Benny's parents are elderly and although they have been caring for him at home they have recently been finding him an increasing challenge. Benny has now been accepted into a community home, which provides full-time care for a few clients with learning disabilities. For Benny the move is a great change since he is used to living with his Chinese-speaking parents in a quiet house in a small village where he is well known to the community. His new home is in a suburban estate close to a main road.

- Using the principles of risk assessment, identify the hazards that may be a problem for Benny in his new home.
- Try to decide what the main safety risks are for Benny.
- Now decide what strategies may be appropriate for tackling the risks that you have identified.
- Finally, identify what barriers may need to be overcome in making Benny safe in his new home.

Summary

This chapter has sought to draw together the concepts of a safe environment and safety for the individual. It has included:

1. Basic human needs and the problems that might arise from a lack of or substandard level of achievement of these needs.
2. An overview of the hazards that might be encountered in the environment and the risks associated with the effect of these hazards.

3. Examination of ways that health professionals might seek to reduce the likelihood of materialization of risk for their patients.
4. Principles of careful risk management, both proactive and reactive that are applicable to all health care settings, demonstrated by case study exercises in the four branches of nursing.
5. An insight into health and safety, thereby including health workers in the wide context of risk.
6. The current and rapidly evolving agenda for patient safety in the UK, which is based on the need to prevent occurrence and recurrence of adverse healthcare events.
7. A brief overview of the consent process.

Annotated further reading and websites

Akass R 1994 Essential health and safety for managers: guide to good practice in the EC. Gower, Cambridge
A book covering, for employees and especially for employers, the ways to comply with the demands needed.

Garrick B J, Gekler W C 1991 The analysis, communication, and perception of risk. Plenum, New York
This book deals extensively with the problems associated with people's understanding of health and safety.

Health and Safety Commission 1992 Monitoring Strategies for Toxic Substances, *Guidance Note EH42*. HMSO, London
This guidance handbook covers essential thoughts behind all safe practice by using assessment as a tool.

Rogers R, Salvage J 1989 Nurses at risk: a guide to health and safety at work. Heinemann Nursing, Guildford
A book specifically for nurses, giving the principles of health and safety.

www.chi.nhs.uk
This is the website of the Commission for Health Improvement. It gives reports from inspected NHS Trusts in the UK.

http://www.casu.org.uk and http://www.doh.gov.uk/riskman.htm
These are the websites for Controls Assurance.

www.doh.gov.uk/bristolinquiryresponse
This provides useful reading on the Bristol Inquiry and lessons learned, which might be said to have generated the emphasis on risk management in the UK today.

www.doh.gov.uk/essenceofcare
The Essence of Care Standards used in the UK for benchmarking quality of nursing and interprofessional care can be found at this Department of Health website.

www.doh.gov.uk/consent
This site gives information about the consent process, the reference document, *Reference Guide to Consent for Examination or Treatment* and the Department of Health model consent policy and forms.

www.nice.org.uk
This is the National Institute of Clinical Effectiveness website and publishes current guidelines on best practice in a variety of clinical fields.

www.phls.co.uk/publications/index.htm and www.doh.gov.uk/haicosts.htm
These websites provide a useful resource for information on hospital acquired infection rates.

http://www.npsa.org.uk
This website highlights the activities of the National Patient Safety Agency, which is dedicated to analysing reports on adverse events and near misses among NHS patients, introducing preventative measures and bringing the patient safety movement to a national level.

http://qhc.bmjjournals.com
This is the website of the *Quality and Safety in Health Care* journal. Based in the UK, it offers online access to the results of research on patient safety improvement. Although most material on the site is free only to subscribers, it offers tables of contents for all issues of the journal, abstracts of all articles and direct access to Medline for further online journal searching.

www.rospa.org.uk
The website of the Royal Society for the Prevention of Accidents. This is a useful site if you wish to research accident statistics for project work.

References

Ajzen I, Fishbein M 1980 Understanding attitudes and predicting social behavior. Prentice Hall, Englewood Cliffs
Akinsola H Y 1983 Behavioural science for nurses. Churchill Livingstone, Singapore
Bandura A 1977 Social learning theory. Prentice Hall, Englewood Cliffs
Becker M H (ed.) 1974 The health belief model and personal health behavior. Slack, Thorofare
Bloor M 1995 The sociology of HIV transmission. Sage, London
Brewer S 1994 Royal College of Nursing safety representatives' manual. Royal College of Nursing of the UK, Southampton
British Medical Association 1999 Clinical Governance: GPC guidance. British Medical Association, London

Brunekreef B, Janssen N A, De Hartog J et al 1997 Air pollution from truck traffic and lung function in children living near motorways. Epidemiology 8(3):298–303
Clancy L, Goodman P, Sinclair H et al 2002 Effects of air pollution control in Dublin, Ireland: an intervention study. Lancet 360(9341):1210–1214
Cohen P 1996 Water companies threaten to return to Victorian times. Health Visitor 69(7):259
Consumer Protection Act 1987 HMSO, London
Control of Substances Hazardous to Health (COSHH) Regulations 1988 HMSO, London
Control of Substances Hazardous to Health (COSHH) Regulations 2002 HMSO, London

Cox T, Griffiths A 1996 Assessment of psychosocial hazards at work. In: Schabracq M J, Winnubst J A M, Cooper C L (eds) Handbook of work and health psychology. John Wiley, Chichester, pp 127–143

Cox T, Griffiths A, Cox S 1995 Work-related stress in nursing: managing the risk. International Labour Organization, Geneva

Department of Health 1997 The new NHS: modern dependable. Department of Health, London

Department of Health 1998 A first class service: quality in the new NHS. Department of Health, London

Department of Health 2000 Organization with a memory. Department of Health, London

Department of Health 2001 Reference guide to examination or treatment. Department of Health, London

Department of Health and National Patient Safety Agency 2001 Doing less harm. Department of Health, London

Douglas M 1966 Purity and danger: an analysis of concepts of pollution and taboo. Routledge, London

Electricity at Work Regulations SI 635 1989. HMSO, London

Fallowfield L 1990 The quality of life: the missing measurement in healthcare. University College London Press, London

Gabe J 1995 Medicine, health and risk: sociological approaches. Blackwell, Oxford

Gershon R R M, Vlahov D, Felknor S A et al 1995 Compliance with universal precautions among healthcare workers at three regional hospitals. American Journal of Infection Control 23(4): 225–236

Gielen A C, Wilson M E, Faden R R et al 1995 In-home injury prevention practices for infants and toddlers: the role of parental beliefs, barriers and housing quality. Health Education Quarterly 22:85–95

Harpwood V 2001 Negligence in healthcare: clinical claims and risk. Informa, London

Harrington J M, Gill F S 1992 Occupational health, 3rd edn. Blackwell, Oxford

Health and Safety at Work Act 1974 HMSO, London

Health and Safety (Display Screen Equipment) Regulations SI 2792 1992 HMSO, London

Health and Safety (First Aid) Regulations SI 917 1981 HMSO, London

Health and Safety Information for Employees Regulations SI 682 1989 HMSO, London

Hunt S, McKenna S 1992 The impact of housing quality on mental and physical health. Housing Review 41:3

Ineichen B 1993 Homes and health: how housing and health interact. Spon, London

International Labour Organization 1986 Psychosocial factors at work: recognition and control. International Labour Organization, Geneva

Irani D N, Johnson R T 2003 Diagnosis and prevention of bovine spongiform encaphalopathy and variant Creutzfeldt–Jakob disease. Annual Review of Medicine 54:305–319

Karol M H 2002 Respiratory allergy: what are the uncertainties? Toxicology 181–182:305–310

Landrigan P J, Garg A 2002 Chronic effects of toxic environmental exposures on children's health. Journal of Clinical Toxicology 40(4):449–456

Landy F 1989 Psychology of work behaviour, 4th edn. Brooks Cole, Pacific Grove

Levi L 1984 Stress in industry: causes, effects and prevention. International Labour Organization, Geneva

Lowery M 1996 A campaign with street cred to target teenagers with asthma. Nursing Times 92(42):34–37

Maas R P, Patch S C, Parker A F 2002 An assessment of lead exposure potential from residential cutoff valves. Journal of Environmental Health 65(1):9–14, 28

Maastricht Treaty 1992 HMSO, London

Management of Health and Safety at Work Regulations SI 2051 1992 HMSO, London

Manual handling operations regulations, SI 2793 and guidance on regulations, L23 1992 HMSO, London

Maslow A H 1970 Motivation and personality, 2nd edn. Harper & Row, New York

Naidoo J, Wills J 2000 Health promotion: foundations for practice, 2nd edn. Baillière Tindall, Edinburgh

National Health Service Executive 1999 Clinical Governance: quality in the new NHS. NHS Executive, London

National Health Service Management Executive 1994 Risk management in the National Health Service. National Health Service Management Executive, London

NHS (Amendment) Act 1986 HMSO, London

Nightingale F 1860 Notes on nursing: what it is and what it is not. Harrison, London

Nightingale F 1863 Notes on hospitals, 3rd edn. Longman Roberts & Green, London

Noak J 1997 Assessment of the risks posed by people with mental illness. Nursing Times 93(1):1–8

Nursing and Midwifery Council 2002 Code of Professional Conduct. Nursing and Midwifery Council, London

Personal Protective Equipment (PPE) at Work Regulations SI 2966 1992 HMSO, London

Packer C N, Stewart-Brown S, Fowle S E 1991 Damp housing and adult health: results from a lifestyle study in Worcester, England. Journal of Epidemiology and Community Health 22:85–95

Peat J K, Dickerson J, Li J 1998 Effects of damp and mould in the home on respiratory health: a review of the literature. Allergy 53:120–128

Provision and Use of Work Equipment Regulations SI 2932 1992 HMSO, London

Purdom P, Walton X Y 1971 Environmental health. Academic Press, London

Raw G, Goldman L 1996 Sick building syndrome: a suitable case for treatment. Occupational Health 48(11):388–392

Reason J 1997 Managing risks of organizational accidents. Ashgate, Aldershot

Reporting of Injuries, Diseases and Dangerous Occurrences Regulations SI 2023 1985 (amended 1995) HMSO, London

Roberts G 2002 Risk management in healthcare, 2nd edn. Witherby, London

Royal Society Study Group 1992 Risk analysis perception and management. Royal Society, London

Safety and Health at Work: the report of the Robens Committee 1972 HMSO, London

Safety Representatives and Safety Committee Regulations SI 500 1972 HMSO, London

Single European Act 1987 HMSO, London

Simpson G C 1991 Risk perception and hazard awareness as factors in safe and efficient working: report for the Commission of the European Community. British Coal Corporation, Eastwood

Social Security Regulations 1979 HMSO, London

Verhoeff A P, Van Strien R T, Van Wijnen J H et al 1995 Damp housing and childhood respiratory symptoms: the role of sensitization to dust mites and molds. American Journal of Epidemiology 141:103–110

Wall P G, Ryan M T, Ward L R et al 1996 Outbreaks of salmonellosis in British hospitals. Journal of Hospital Infection 33(3):181–190

Williams H C, Strachan D P, Hay R J 1994 Childhood eczema: disease of the advantaged? British Medical Journal 308:1132–1135

Williamson I, Martin C, Macgill G et al 1997 Damp housing and asthma: a case control study. Thorax 52:229–234

Workplace (Health, Safety and Welfare) Regulations SI 3004 1992 HMSO, London

Chapter 3

Resuscitation and emergency care

Roderick Cable and Helen Swain

KEY ISSUES

SUBJECT KNOWLEDGE
- Resuscitation guidelines
- The collapsed adult
- The heart and ventricular fibrillation
- The chain of survival
- The collapsed child
- Situational life crisis
- The relatives
- The healthcare professional
- Post-traumatic stress disorder

CARE DELIVERY KNOWLEDGE
- Assessment of the collapsed infant, child and adult
- Basic life support skills required to resuscitate the infant, child and adult
- Management of a choking client
- Individual situations that require adaptation to the normal resuscitation guidelines
- Drug therapy in the resuscitation situation

PROFESSIONAL AND ETHICAL KNOWLEDGE
- The professional role of the nurse in resuscitation within hospitals and the community
- Legal and professional accountability when undertaking resuscitation
- Education and skills updating for resuscitation
- Ethical issues relating to the decision to resuscitate or not

PERSONAL AND REFLECTIVE KNOWLEDGE
- Assessment of own personal practice of resuscitation skills and identification of strengths and weaknesses
- Consolidation of knowledge through case studies

INTRODUCTION

Resuscitation encompasses more than just trying to reverse the process of a sudden death. It is a term commonly used to describe active intervention in any emergency situation.

This chapter will consider the role of the nurse in undertaking immediate and potentially life-saving care of the sick and injured patient, both in hospital and the community. The focus of this chapter is on the immediate action at an emergency and in particular, basic life support (BLS).

BLS is the initial action carried out by the rescuer on a person who has collapsed and has no effective cardiopulmonary function while awaiting help from the healthcare professionals. This action requires no extra equipment and depends on the rescuer assessing and implementing a procedure that includes mouth-to-mouth and external cardiac compression. Anyone who has undertaken first aid or resuscitation training can carry out BLS.

Advanced life support (ALS) is the second phase of emergency care and requires equipment such as airway adjuncts, drugs and a defibrillator, which are explained later in this chapter. ALS activities are usually undertaken by 'advanced practitioners', as specialized skills are required.

Immediate physical care is an issue that is often dismissed as the role of the acute hospital nurse and only really within the realm of nurses from the adult or child branches. If potential emergency situations are considered carefully it soon becomes apparent, however, that the nurses most exposed to the problems of emergency care are those working in the mental health and learning disability branches, and especially those nurses working in the community. Community nurses can have a long wait after calling for help from the emergency services and may need to be far more resourceful in their efforts to resuscitate in the emergency situation. Equally, student nurses are expected to assist in emergency situations; this may involve working alone if a situation occurs in the local supermarket, for example.

OVERVIEW

Subject knowledge

After referring to the current *Resuscitation Guidelines*, we review the most common causes of sudden collapse in children and adults, with particular reference to the altered anatomy and physiology. Under psychosocial subject knowledge, reactions to sudden trauma and death by individuals and the public are explored, with particular reference to post-traumatic stress disorder.

Care delivery knowledge

This section will present a systematic and logical approach to assessment and management of resuscitation that can be applied to any emergency situation. The 2000 *Resuscitation Guidelines* for use in the UK (Resuscitation Council UK 2000) will then be explained in more detail.

Professional and ethical knowledge

In these sections the role of the professional nurse in the emergency situation and the potential legal issues related to emergency interventions are considered. Ethical dilemmas surrounding resuscitation are also explored. The need for education and updating to maintain skills in order to be effective in the emergency situation is discussed.

Personal and reflective knowledge

Throughout this chapter, you will be able to apply theory to practice through reflective and decision making exercises and to expand your knowledge through identified research based evidence. The final section of the chapter provides case studies to consolidate your knowledge and suggests how you can assess your own practice through using specifically designed checklists.

On page 72 there are four case studies, each one relating to one of the branch programmes. You may find it helpful to read one of them before you start the chapter and use it as a focus for your reflections while reading.

SUBJECT KNOWLEDGE

BIOLOGICAL

RESUSCITATION GUIDELINES

One of the continuing dilemmas in resuscitation is the need for a consistent approach to care, that is, the same management by everyone from scouts to consultant cardiologists. An approach that is truly international has been a target of the resuscitation training bodies for many years. The European Resuscitation Council (ERC) founded in 1992 has

taken this international goal further by integrating the work of many countries. In April 1997, the International Liaison Committee on Resuscitation (ILCOR) presented advisory statements on resuscitation in order to develop a global approach (ILCOR 1997). The 2000 guidelines have further developed this process to include North America.

The reason for the term 'guidelines' is to allow for adaptations according to individual circumstances; describing them as 'rules' might discourage 'necessary' variations. Despite differences in the branches of nursing there are only two main approaches to resuscitation and these are based upon the physiological development of individuals across the lifespan (i.e. the adult and the infant). The fact that the individual has a mental health problem or a learning disability makes no difference to the general approach, as the guidelines for resuscitation remain the same. However, there may need to be slight variations from the guidelines if for example there is a specific reason for the collapse. Examples would be differences in resuscitation techniques for an infant who has stopped breathing, as opposed to an adult who has had a heart attack. It is therefore important to be able to make decisions and to have knowledge of the differences in resuscitation techniques for an infant as opposed to an adult.

> ### Reflection and portfolio exercise
>
> The easiest place to check for updates to the resuscitation guidelines is online at: http:www.resus.org.uk. Review how the guidelines have changed and the rationale for those changes. Decide whether you need any special training to be able to follow these new guidelines.
>
> The cardiac muscle is supplied with blood from the coronary arteries and it is changes such as narrowing of these vessels which may result in coronary heart disease (CHD).
>
> 1. Review how blood vessels become narrower and the potential causes for this phenomenon occurring.
> 2. How might you use the knowledge of potential causes of CHD to promote a healthy lifestyle?

The early detection of impending collapse

Survival from the pulseless collapse remains poor despite advances in the science of resuscitation and hence there is increasing interest in preventing cardiac arrest and the determination of risk factors. Hodgetts et al (2002) point out the potential advantages of a designated emergency team to attend to deteriorating patients prior to a cardiac arrest. Often it is fairly difficult to quantify events such as 'nurse concern' which occur prior to the eventual collapse; perhaps the most import observation for nurses is the routine measurement of respiratory effort and rate.

THE COLLAPSED ADULT

Before considering the practicalities of resuscitation, it is important to have an understanding of the potential mechanism of sudden collapse so that a more logical approach can be made. The Resuscitation Council guidelines have a basic assumption, which is worth mentioning: that is, the most common cause of non-traumatic sudden pulseless collapse in adults is cardiac in origin, and more specifically ventricular fibrillation (VF), which will be described further in the next section. 'Collapse' can be defined as 'a potentially reversible, sudden and unexpected loss of normal consciousness'. In infants and children, as we will see later, the situation is usually different, hence the different set of guidelines. The primary cause of infant non-traumatic collapse is classically of respiratory origin.

The aim of the BLS guidelines is to produce an accurate and rapid diagnosis, ensure appropriate help is summoned and limit the effects of hypoxia (lack of oxygen).

THE HEART AND VENTRICULAR FIBRILLATION

The heart is a four-chambered organ situated centrally and slightly to the left in the chest behind the sternum (Figs 3.1 and 3.2).

One of the characteristics of cardiac muscle is its ability to contract in the absence of any external stimulation. This independent mechanism is co-ordinated by a unique electrical system within the heart, which results in a co-ordinated contraction of the heart muscle. This is **sinus rhythm** (Fig. 3.3), a regular, co-ordinated cardiac rhythm producing a palpable pulse.

Reflection and portfolio exercise

Figure 3.3 is a representation of the normal electrical activity of the heart as measured by skin electrodes and a cardiac monitor. This is an electrocardiograph or ECG.

Referring to a physiology textbook, explain the pattern in relation to the way the electrical activity co-ordinates cardiac muscle contraction. Remember that this is only an indication of electrical activity and it does not necessarily relate directly to mechanical function.

When the normal electric conduction system in the heart fails because of ischaemic heart disease (IHD), instead of stopping 'dead' (known as asystole; Fig. 3.4), each muscle fibre independently contracts and relaxes giving the heart a shivering appearance: this is ventricular fibrillation (VF) (Fig. 3.5). Although the heart is active there is no effective pumping action, therefore the collapsed individual will have no pulse and will quickly lose consciousness.

The significance of VF is the relative simplicity of treatment – passing an electric discharge over the heart, known as defibrillation, will result in a co-ordinated muscular

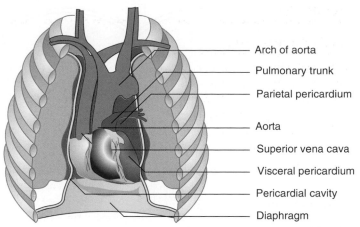

Figure 3.1   Location of the heart. (From Hinchliff et al 1996.)

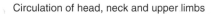

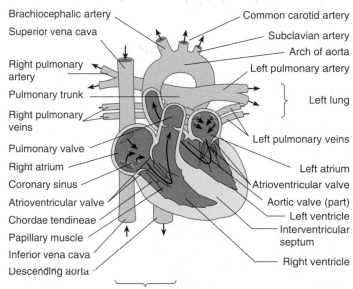

Figure 3.2   Structure of the heart and the direction of the blood flow. (From Hinchliff et al 1996.)

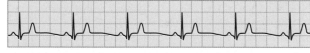

Figure 3.3   Normal sinus rhythm. (From Hinchliff et al 1996.)

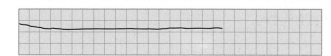

Figure 3.4   Asystole. (From Hinchliff et al 1996.)

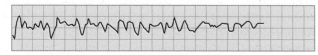

Figure 3.5   Ventricular fibrillation. (From Hinchliff et al 1996.)

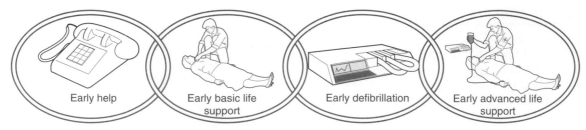

Figure 3.6   The chain of survival concept.

contraction and (hopefully) a return to a spontaneous rhythm. The key factor in the success of the process of defibrillation is time. The longer the delay between the onset of VF and treatment by defibrillation, the worse the outcome. While the patient is in VF there is no coronary circulation and therefore no myocardial oxygenation, so the patient deteriorates rapidly. It is unlikely that BLS resuscitation is very efficient in maintaining an effective coronary circulation. It does, however, buy the patient time until further help is available.

During VF the lack of oxygen supply to the cardiac muscle results in the VF activity becoming less 'strong' or 'coarse' with time and eventually decaying to asystole.

Asystole (Fig. 3.4) is the classic 'straight line' on the cardiac monitor that is frequently used in films and TV 'soaps'. The straight line indicates no apparent cardiac electrical activity and commonly occurs as a result of prolonged hypoxia or another significant illness. In practice, apparently well patients do not usually suddenly collapse into asystole as presented by the media.

The third rhythm (and the second requiring defibrillation) is pulseless ventricular tachycardia (with an emphasis on the word 'pulseless'). Within normal limits, as the heart rate increases, so does the cardiac output (rate × stroke volume); however, at very high pulse rates stroke volume will drop due to inadequate time for the heart to refill. As the heart rate increases a patient will initially become dizzy (cerebral hypoxia) and will show progressive symptoms of collapse as the blood pressure falls. Ultimately the patient will present as a cardiac arrest even though a connected electrocardiograph (ECG) will show a very rapid ventricular rate.

Pulseless electrical activity (PEA) is the fourth and least common rhythm associated with cardiac arrest. In this situation, the nurse will see a rhythm on the cardiac monitor that is similar to normal sinus rhythm, but will find no palpable carotid pulse on examining the patient. Essentially, the electrical conduction system within the cardiac muscle is functioning, but there is no associated cardiac output (hence PEA). In the simplest situation, when a patient has lost most of the circulating blood volume, the heart will continue to work while it is still oxygenated, but no significant amount of blood will be circulated. There are several causes of PEA including hypovolaemia (blood loss), pneumothorax (collapsed lung), hypothermia (low body temperature) and electrolyte imbalance in the blood and intracellular fluids. All these situations occur in adults and children so both groups can present with PEA.

THE CHAIN OF SURVIVAL

The ideal survival scenario from ventricular fibrillation is described in 'the chain of survival' (Cummins et al 1991), which indicates the links required (Fig. 3.6). Following these stages can help guide you through the emergency situation. However you will need further skills training to become competent in all aspects.

- early help ensures that defibrillation time is as short as possible
- early BLS slows deterioration
- early defibrillation is the key to reversing the situation
- finally the provision of advanced cardiac life support to stabilize the patient and ALS, which includes improving airway management and the use of drugs.

As the VF scenario is potentially so treatable, this is the target of the adult resuscitation guidelines. Conveniently, all other medical emergencies are also reasonably managed by these guidelines.

Defibrillation

Currently, the teaching and practice of defibrillation is not widespread within the preregistration education of nurses; however, the need for this role is now clearly identified.

Firstly the *National Service Framework for Coronary Heart Disease* (NHS 2000) is clear about the need for early defibrillation to be available both within and outside hospital.

Secondly the Chief Nursing Officer states within her 10 key roles for nurses that they should: 'Carry out a wide range of resuscitation procedures including defibrillation' (Mullally 2001).

Even though the statements above make the situation very clear, there still appears to be some reluctance by nurses to take on this role. Current opinion varies, from nurses being worried about the potential legal implications of nurse defibrillation and hence resistance to carrying it out, to widespread implementation across Health Trusts. It is worth pointing out to hesitant nurses that the government used the example of defibrillation by nurses as normal practice for adult branch nurses in their 1997 recruitment campaign advertisement. In order to reduce the mortality from IHD the time from VF cardiac arrest to defibrillation needs to be constantly monitored and audited. Wardrope & Morris (1993) in their review of the resuscitation guidelines stated 'defibrillate

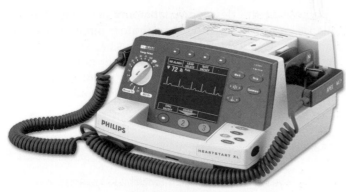

Figure 3.7   Manual defibrillator. (Philips Medical Systems.)

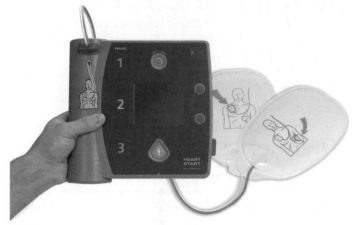

Figure 3.8   Advisory external defibrillator (AED). (Philips Medical Systems.)

as early and as often as possible'. To this end, a manual defibrillator (Fig. 3.7) is a most useful piece of equipment.

In the hospital setting, nurses are in an ideal position to carry out early defibrillation and make a significant contribution to reducing the death rate from IHD. Nurses should be able to defibrillate in all clinical environments, especially as with improving technology the process is not difficult to learn. In the pre-hospital environment, The American Heart Association argues that early bystander cardiopulmonary resuscitation (CPR) along with rapid defibrillation makes a major contribution to the survival of adults following a sudden cardiac arrest and recommend that we should move towards 'public access defibrillation' as a way of increasing survival rates (Weisfeldt et al 1995).

One of the most significant recent developments in defibrillator technology is the semi-automatic or advisory external defibrillator (AED) (Fig. 3.8). The AED system will analyse a patient's cardiac rhythm and indicate if the patient requires defibrillation or not. In use, it is simply a matter of connecting two large electrodes to the patient and following a '1, 2, 3' approach in terms of operation where '1' is on, 2 is 'analyse' (determine the rhythm) and 3 is 'fire' (defibrillate).

Since the mid-1990s, in the UK, the national news has reported on various schemes to promote the use of AEDs such as defibrillation by transport police and the fire service.

In Nottinghamshire alone there are now in the region of 60 community placed AEDs in such places as shopping centres, railway stations and leisure centres.

Experience with the use of AEDs on children is limited and the subject of current research. It is considered that it is safe to defibrillate a child from the age of 8 years old, with a standard AED using attenuated leads (Atkins et al 2001). Luckily it is rare that defibrillating an infant is required, especially outside paediatric critical care areas.

Reflection and portfolio exercise

During your practice placements review the availability of resuscitation equipment. This is usually a significant part of your orientation to any new practice setting.

1. Check whether there is a defibrillator available and how it is operated.
2. Review the local policies about when, how often and by whom resuscitation equipment is checked.
3. Discuss with your practice supervisor which members of the multidisciplinary team are allowed to perform ALS after the initial resuscitation phase (BLS).
4. How is resuscitation dealt with in primary health care settings and by individual community nurses? The documents *The Health of the Nation* (Department of Health 1991) and *Targeting Practice, The Contribution of Nurses, Midwives and Health Visitors* (Department of Health 1993) clearly identify national targets to reduce the death rates from CHD.
5. Debate the role of the nurse in helping to meet *The Health of the Nation* targets for CHD.
6. Consider the impact of training sufficient numbers of the public to instigate BLS on the adult mortality figures. How could the specialist nurse become involved in training members of the public?

THE COLLAPSED CHILD

The causes of collapse in infants (under 1 year old) and children (1–8 years old) are usually respiratory problems and resulting hypoxia rather than the cardiac problems found in adults, as degenerative heart disease is not common in children (Nadkarni et al 1997). Innes et al (1993) reviewed 45 resuscitation attempts in hospitalized children, and 21 (47%) were of respiratory origin. Cardiac failure in children and infants rarely occurs as an initial problem and is usually linked to congenital cardiac abnormalities.

The greatest mortality during childhood occurs in the first years of life. Causes include congenital problems, prematurity and infection due to the immature immune system. Sudden infant death syndrome (SIDS) remains the main cause of death in infants aged between 1 month and 1 year, although the guidelines on positioning infants have reduced this number considerably (Coyne 1996, Department of Health

1992, SIDS 2004). Over 1 year of age, trauma is the most frequent cause of death (Child Accident Prevention Trust 2002).

Those children having had an out-of-hospital cardiac arrest who arrive in accident and emergency departments not breathing and pulseless have a poor outcome due to the brain damage resulting from lack of oxygen. There are three potential outcomes of child arrest: survival, survival with neurological insult or death (Advanced Life Support Group 2001).

The respiratory system (Fig. 3.9) in children continues to develop until approximately 8 years of age. Therefore the following points need to be considered in emergency care:

- Infants tend to breathe only through their nose until the age of 3 months, which adds to the problems of resuscitation, as the nasal passages are small.
- The tongue is very large and collapses into the oropharynx easily, thus blocking the airway.
- The lower mandible is small in comparison to the large tongue, which further exacerbates the problem of airway obstruction.
- The diameter of the trachea increases threefold by puberty – the trachea is approximately the same size as the child or infant's little finger, therefore increasing the resistance to air entering and leaving the lungs.
- The epiglottis is floppy and will easily occlude the airway.

The following additional anatomical characteristics should also be borne in mind:

- The cartilaginous rings of the trachea are soft and easily compressed.
- Respiration depends upon movement of the diaphragm as the intercostal muscles are not fully developed and therefore abdominal respirations are observed until at least 6 years of age.
- The left ventricle of the heart does not develop its characteristic thick muscular wall until about 6 months of age, and this affects how well blood circulates around the body because of the limited power of each contraction.
- The basal metabolic rate and oxygen consumption in infants are much higher than in adults resulting in increased heart and respiratory rates, and therefore they are much more prone to hypoxia and resulting neurological damage.

Because of the developing anatomy and physiology a collapse is more likely to be of respiratory rather than of cardiac origin. The BLS guidelines are thus based on maintaining oxygenation rather than restoring normal cardiac rhythm. However, without oxygen an infant or child will soon become bradycardic (i.e. have a slow pulse rate) and this will quickly progress to pulselessness.

Reflection and portfolio exercise

1. How you would assess an infant/child's respiratory rate? List the key observations of respiration that you should make.
2. Recall how the pulse is taken in infants/children. Try to find out the different rates according to age and what effect illness, anxiety and pain may have on the normal values (see Ch. 6 on homeostasis).
3. If you can, observe a child and make notes on the above.

PSYCHOSOCIAL

SITUATIONAL LIFE CRISIS

The main focus in this section is on the impact of sudden collapse and death on individual family members and on society as a whole, particularly in the case of major disasters. The effects of failure to achieve a successful resuscitation on members of the healthcare team are also considered. Further study in this area of care and decision making is provided in Chapter 12 on death and dying and Chapter 8 on stress, relaxation and rest.

The term situational life crisis used by Wright (1996) defines how intensive periods of psychological, behavioural and physical disarray through loss and grief can challenge a person's existing coping mechanisms. If not addressed through crisis intervention (Caplan 1964), mental health problems may arise later.

Parkes (1975 cited by Wright 1996) identified six different determinants or predictors of grief (see below), the most significant being the mode of death (Table 3.1). Sudden death through trauma creates images of suffering and injustice for

---

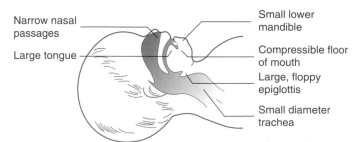

Narrow nasal passages

Large tongue

Small lower mandible

Compressible floor of mouth

Large, floppy epiglottis

Small diameter trachea

Figure 3.9 The upper airway in the infant. (Reproduced by kind permission of British Medical Journal from Advanced Life Support Group 1993.)

Table 3.1 The six determinants of grief (Parkes 1975)

Determinant
Mode of death
Nature of the attachment
Who was the person?
Historical antecedents
Personality variables
Social variables

the grieving relatives producing feelings of anger and guilt. These feeling may be directed towards the relatives themselves by thoughts of 'I should have been there' to blaming others: 'The emergency services were just not quick enough.' Anger may be compounded if monetary compensation becomes an issue at a later stage as the deceased is often seen as devalued (Wright 1996).

THE RELATIVES

The most difficult issue for relatives to grasp is the fact their loved one, who may have recently been fit and healthy, is now dead. This can be distressing when a child is involved and parents' emotions can increase if one or both parents were not present at the time of death (Rennie 1991). Reactions of relatives can vary from denial, guilt, blame to anger. Wright (1996) found relatives identified two emotions when a loved one has died suddenly:

- loss of control over their lives
- powerlessness and helplessness to support, prevent or intervene.

The needs of relatives at this time have been identified by many authors on this subject (Cook 1999, Wright 1996) and Jurkovich et al (2000) found similar results in their study where they asked what the bereaved relatives required supported these needs (Table 3.2).

Witnessing the resuscitation of a loved one is fraught with uncertainty exacerbated by lack of understanding. Rattrie (2000) and Meyers et al (2000) found health professionals were supportive to the relatives needing to be present during a resuscitation attempt, nurses more so than doctors. However, this also had more implications for further staff development and the need for a specialist clinician to support the relatives. Other issues include consent by the victim and harm of witnessing the resuscitation by the relatives. Consent is covered by the fact that resuscitation is usually an emergency event and there is evidence of increasing use of living wills. The involvement of relatives by being in the resuscitation room, seeing that everything is being done and not being separated from their loved one should offset the reaction of anger and decrease the legal risks of harm of the relatives due to the situation. The Royal College of Nursing has issued guidelines to support staff involved with relatives who find themselves in such a situation (Royal College of Nursing 2002).

Evidence based practice

Wright (1996) in his book on sudden death cites a study undertaken by Hanson & Strawser (1992) in which they survey the feelings of 47 family members who were present during the resuscitation of their relatives. Adjustment to the death was found to be easier than if they had not been with the patient according to 76% of respondents, and 64% felt that their presence was valuable to the dying person. Most respondents felt that the dying person had heard them express their love and say their goodbyes.

It has been noted that presence at resuscitation aids the grieving process and it should be an option in as many situations as possible, bearing in mind that it can cause difficulties for the healthcare professionals who may be undertaking invasive procedures in order to save the patient (Zoltie et al 1994).

Decision making exercise

John O'Neill, a 14-year-old boy with a mild learning disability, sustained a head injury in a fall from a tree at the day centre he attended. He was rushed to hospital by ambulance and his mother was called at her workplace. There was difficulty in getting information to his father as he was a long-distance lorry driver. John's mother arrived at the Accident and Emergency (A and E) department just as John began to show difficulty in breathing. The A and E team were beginning the process of intubation and ventilation. John's mother wished to be present and became increasingly agitated and aggressive when denied entrance to the emergency room.

1. Debate what the particular issues are for each person in the situation including John and what might be the long-term effects on the family.
2. What strategies could be developed by the staff of the A and E department to cope with a similar situation should it arise in the future?

Table 3.2   Needs of relatives in the event of a sudden death

Perceived needs (Cook 1999, Wright 1996)	Relatives' stated needs (Jurkovich 2000)
For information	Caring attitude
Time – with their relative, for questions, to talk, to express fears and feelings	Clarity of message
	Privacy
	Abilities to answer questions
Siblings – to be honest and involve them	Sympathy
	Time for questions
Health professionals – for support, listening, sharing and time	Autopsy information
	Clergy available
Social support – from family and friends	Direction after death
	Location of conversation
Spiritual support – minister/ hospital chaplain, carry out rites such as baptism, blessing and anointing	Timing of conversation
	Rank/seniority of news-breaker
	Follow-up contact
Physical support – food, drink, rest – caring and anxiety are exhausting	Attire of news-giver

THE HEALTHCARE PROFESSIONAL

Wright (1996) states that the cost of caring in crisis situations can physically and emotionally drain staff and suggests several different ways in which staff can support each other. These include debriefing and mutual support, re-education, activities outside work and a change of situation (see also Ch. 8 for further discussion on coping with stress).

Debriefing

Feelings of stress and anxiety can easily arise after a 'failed' resuscitation attempt. As long as the attempt has been conducted reasonably, 'failure', as it is often perceived, is more often due to the underlying pathology in the patient than the inadequacies of an effective resuscitation attempt. Debriefing after traumatic events such as a resuscitation are important not just to improve the efficiency of the next attempt, but also to ensure that staff are not left with feelings of self-blame. This can be done through a critical incident technique. The important rule to remember for debriefing is that you are there to support each other and that it should be confidential. A traumatic resuscitation attempt is not something you can just walk away from without any follow-up.

Re-education

We all become used to our own ways and it is necessary to address our knowledge to develop our skills further. Attending teaching sessions, seminars or conferences can lead to new ways of tackling this stressful situation.

Life outside work

Maintaining leisure time away from the area allows the thought processes to rest and the person to look at life differently. It is also important for the workforce as a team to socialize away from the stressful situations in the clinical areas.

Change of environment

Many professionals find that a change from a clinical area, even if only a temporary one, not only relieves the stress, but also allows a development and improvement in skills in other areas.

POST-TRAUMATIC STRESS DISORDER

Post-traumatic stress disorder (PTSD) was first described in the USA by Durham et al (1985) and involves the long-term distressing emotions that have been experienced by ancillary medical and rescue workers such as the police and firemen in response to a major disaster event. This disorder has been highlighted in recent years after major disasters such as the Hillsborough football stadium disaster, the mass shooting of children in Dunblane in Scotland in 1996 and 11 September 2001.

According to Wright (1996) sufferers of PTSD may:

- during an initial phase experience denial with a lack of awareness of the severity of the event
- during an intermediate stage seen as a phase of confrontation and disorder start to experience signs of stress such as sleeplessness, nightmares and hypersensitivity to noise and become more easily angry and irritable
- during the final phase, readjust and recover and regain control of their life, becoming more hopeful and less dependent on others.

Early recognition of the possibility of PTSD now leads to the provision of support in the form of counselling in a major disaster situation in an attempt to prevent the syndrome, while debriefing continues to play an important role for many years after the event. The ongoing difficulties for the victims of the Hillsborough disaster demonstrates this.

Reflection and portfolio exercise

Gibson (1991) in her book *Order from Chaos: Responding to Traumatic Events* has produced a helpful guide to the topic based on her experiences in Belfast, Northern Ireland. Much has been written about the complex process of helping individuals after traumatic and stressful events. If you undertake a literature search in this area, look under 'post-traumatic stress reaction'.

1. Reflect on how you would react if the rescuers in a traumatic event received more monetary compensation for PTSD than the actual relatives of the victims of the disaster. Decide how this crisis situation should be sensitively handled immediately.
2. Along with your peer group debate the legal and moral issues involved in the above dilemma.

CARE DELIVERY KNOWLEDGE

In a chapter devoted to the subject of resuscitation this section gives detailed information on how to manage an emergency situation. After initially providing general guidelines on the First Aid Process, the broad framework advocated by the Resuscitation Council is presented. However, as these will need regular updating it is important that you use this text in conjunction with a copy of the most up-to-date guidelines available. Nicol & Glen (1999) give some suggestions regarding methods to acquire and develop clinical skills.

GENERAL CONSIDERATIONS IN ANY EMERGENCY SITUATION

In any emergency situation the first aid process may be used to establish the nature of the problem you face. This is a linear process dependent upon assessment, diagnosis and action; it requires frequent assessment and reassessment. A systematic approach is also helpful as it is easy to get distracted and start to perform 'trivial' tasks before the life-saving considerations have been completed (see below).

An experienced qualified nurse is often asked by newly qualified nurses how to deal with new emergency situations. The usual answer is 'First aid and symptomatic care first, specific care for conditions is always well down the priority list.' This particular approach can be consolidated on courses such as the Advanced Trauma Nursing Course (ATNC), which has been imported into the UK over the last few years from the American College of Surgeons. Each of the phases in the first aid process will now be considered in more detail.

ASSESSMENT

Initial assessment involves assessing the situation rather than the individual (Fig. 3.10). In assessing the situation we need to:

- consider safety
- consider help required
- establish priorities.

Personal safety of the first-aider

The personal safety of the first-aider is an obvious priority so it is important to always look carefully at any situation before 'diving in'.

There is never a situation when to consider personal safety first is wrong. Potential hazards may include electricity, gas, fire, water and a casualty holding a double-barrel shotgun! Whilst a concern may relate to the time this might 'waste', in fact it only takes about the same time as putting on a pair of disposable gloves, which is probably a good thing to be doing whilst thinking (if they are available). Another health and safety consideration includes infection control. Although there is much concern in this area regarding first-aider safety, there is little current evidence that this is a great problem as long as the usual Universal Precautions

are followed, for example wearing gloves when handling body fluids (see Ch. 4 on infection control for more information).

As far as resuscitation is concerned, there are obvious risks with the spread of airborne organisms. Much concern has been raised about the potential of a rescuer catching the human immunodeficiency virus (HIV) while carrying out mouth-to-mouth resuscitation. At the time of writing, these authors have heard of no such cases. However, there are other infections that pose a potentially greater risk. Barrier devices (simple protective devices which can be placed on the patient's face) for use with mouth-to-mouth resuscitation need to be considered by the individual rescuer. Barrier devices are easily obtainable. The Ambu Company produce a 'LifeKey', which is a shield on a key ring, while the Laerdal Company produce both a shield and a pocket mask. However, in order to make use of such devices it is essential to be well practised with their use on a mannikin first as there is little point in having an emergency device that is unfamiliar. The pocket mask is especially useful as an oxygen supply can be added to the mask, increasing the percentage of oxygen delivered to the casualty from less than 20% to up to 50%, so making the whole process much more efficient.

Reflection and portfolio exercise

Refer to Chapter 4 and other literature on HIV and its mode of spread.

1. List the potential airborne infections that might be a risk to rescuers.
2. Review the effectiveness of any methods at present available to reduce risk to the first-aider.
3. Review the potential for preventive immunizations from those organisms of high risk.

Assessing help required and establishing priorities

Another consideration at the early stage is to ask whether the situation can be realistically managed or whether help is needed now, soon or not at all? In the most extreme situation, that of a multiple casualty disaster, there are two basic choices: either jump in and save a few lives while others are dying or choose to obtain a general overview of the situation and then call 999 to ensure the most appropriate

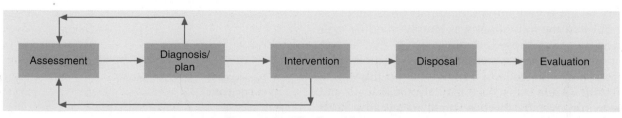

Figure 3.10   The first aid process.

response by the emergency services. Evidence from previous disasters shows that this initial stage is crucial to the overall organization of the incident. Reports of any of the British disasters usually discuss this area of management of the situation (further information regarding emergency planning can be found at the website of the Department of Health (see section on websites at the end of the chapter).

A call for help must include sufficient information to allow the emergency services co-ordinator to produce a full and adequate response (i.e. it is important to know the number and nature of the casualties). If this information is not accurately provided it will be up to the first emergency services vehicle to fulfil this role, resulting in a further delay. Clearly if a bystander is available this role can be delegated, but confirmation that the 'message passed' is passed back must be ensured.

Most acute hospitals have an emergency team who provide internal emergency support, for example the cardiac arrest team. Some smaller hospitals with limited emergency support may use the UK 999 system.

Decision making exercise

You are the first person to arrive at the scene of a road traffic accident where two cars have hit each other. In the first car the elderly male driver has severe chest pain and a minor head injury. On the back seat of the car is a 30-year-old female with profound learning disabilities who is screaming loudly. In the second car the female driver is bleeding badly from an arm laceration. In the passenger seat of the second car lies an unconscious baby.

1. How might you initially deal with the situation, assuming no help is available?
2. What information will it be necessary to give the emergency services when you make your 999 call or direct a passer-by to do so?

Diagnosis

A major consideration in the assessment process is making the diagnosis. This activity can be divided into three parts:

- history taking
- signs and symptoms
- examination.

History taking is very important; it may be as simple as finding out that the individual was simply minding their own business and collapsed, or alternatively that he was run over by a bus. Even apparently obvious situations must not be assumed – the collapsed individual on the way to hospital with a knife in his back may also be diabetic and the person run over by the bus might have had a heart attack. It is therefore never wise to make premature and potentially unfounded conclusions at any stage of an individual's care.

If the situation is not critical, time spent listening to the casualty explaining his story, and seeking clarification as necessary, is beneficial. This is both in the early stage when determining what the problems are, and later when identifying causative and exacerbating factors in order to try to prevent a recurrence.

Signs and symptoms are what the first-aider can see and what the patient says is the problem, for example apparent unresponsiveness, shortness of breath and pain. If a diagnosis has not already been reached, these signs and symptoms offer a general understanding of the situation.

There are two approaches to the examination: one for the unconscious and obviously seriously ill individual, and one for the non-life-threatening situation. For the unconscious patient, the general approach is described well in the BLS guidelines which follow. The emphasis is on:

- assessing response
- opening the airway (A)
- checking breathing (B)
- confirming the presence of a circulation (C).

This is usually known as the ABC approach, which is described in more detail in the next section. After this initial assessment, a more comprehensive assessment can be undertaken.

For the non-life-threatening emergency situation, a systematic top-to-toe approach is probably most useful (Fig. 3.11). Once it has been determined that the casualty is conscious and not bleeding, the first-aider should start at the casualty's head and work down the body (this is a skill that requires practice on a colleague) and is indicated in the Reflection and portfolio exercises.

The first-aider should take care not to be distracted in their assessment unless the situation requires immediate remedial action because something quite important may yet

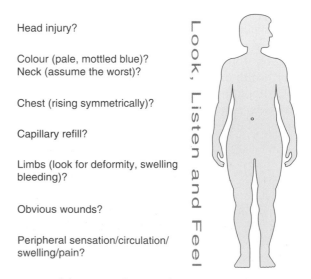

Head injury?

Colour (pale, mottled blue)?
Neck (assume the worst)?

Chest (rising symmetrically)?

Capillary refill?

Limbs (look for deformity, swelling bleeding)?

Obvious wounds?

Peripheral sensation/circulation/swelling/pain?

Look, Listen and Feel

Figure 3.11   A 'top-to-toe' approach to assessment.

Practice assessing a colleague systematically from top to toe using the following criteria. Reflect over your actions. How could you develop your skills next time?

- Starting at the head look and feel for any signs of injury, remembering that if you detect a head injury, especially if the casualty is unconscious, you must assume that there is a significant cervical spine injury until proven otherwise by a radiograph, so find a way to immobilize the neck now. (Some first aid books suggest that you examine the neck of an injured person to detect if the spinal column is in alignment or not. Although alignment of the cervical spine is interesting, its absence does not actually help you assess the significance of a spinal injury. If the history says there might be a spinal injury, you will need to treat it as such.)
- Look at the colour of the skin, the movement of the eyes and listen to the respiratory effort.
- Now assess the chest. Once you have excluded wounds (and do not forget the back) respiratory movement should be observed. Is the chest fully inflating and is movement equal on the left and right, as only one lung may be damaged?
- Checking the back (assuming the patient is on their back) involves turning the casualty and is a risky procedure, especially if you have limited or untrained staff, although on the other hand you do not want to miss anything. Ideally you need a minimum of four people to turn the casualty while you have a look. In practice this may not be possible, so you need to weigh up the possible risks with what you may gain in terms of a more comprehensive assessment.
- When looking at limbs a helpful suggestion is to look at the uninjured limb first. Although it sounds a strange idea, a good understanding of the unaffected limb makes it easier to recognize abnormality. The distressed patient might require some reassurance that you know what you are doing, but they will appreciate the reduction in touching and handling of the injured limb that will result.
- Observe for open wounds, fractures and alterations in sensation or circulation to the limb. If you are concerned about a reduction in circulation, sometimes the capillary refill test can be easier than finding a formal pulse. Light pressure on the nail bed (fingers or toes) will result in a white blanch because you have emptied the blood vessels by the external pressure. On releasing the pressure the capillary bed should refill in 2–3 seconds; if it does not refill, be concerned about the circulation.

be discovered. If there is a need to stop, the examination should be continued as soon as possible.

For further information regarding suggested interventions for wounds, etc. see: Lee et al (2002) or Caroline (1995).

INTERVENTION

General issues will be considered first, and then variations to this process for specific situations.

When assessing responsiveness, regardless of the age of the victim, there should be a response whether it is eye opening, a vocal response or movement. The unresponsive casualty may not breathe unless he or she has a patent airway (Fig. 3.12). Although it is not possible to swallow the tongue, this phrase is often used to describe the relaxed tongue dropping into and blocking the posterior oropharynx. The manoeuvres described in the guidelines aim to relieve this obstruction. When opening the airway, the position of the lower jaw is at least as important as the head tilt (Fig. 3.13), especially the need to realign it into its normal functional position with the upper and lower teeth on the same plane. (NB remember the specific needs of infants are discussed in the section of physiology earlier.)

An additional manoeuvre is the jaw thrust (see Fig. 3.14). The idea for this is to bring the lower jaw forwards – along with the jaw will come the attached tongue, hence clearing it from the airway. This is an especially important manoeuvre if the casualty has a potential neck injury, in which case it can be used alone without the head tilt manoeuvre (Fig. 3.13), which could cause further damage.

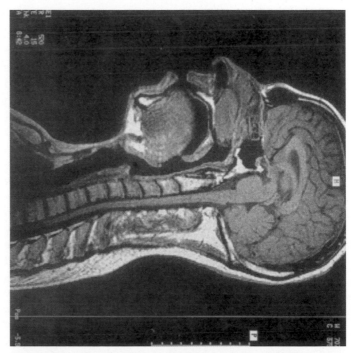

Figure 3.12   Normal anatomy of the upper airway. Nuclear magnetic image (NMI) of individual, conscious. (From the University of Nottingham.)

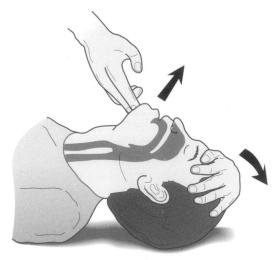

Figure 3.13   Head tilt.

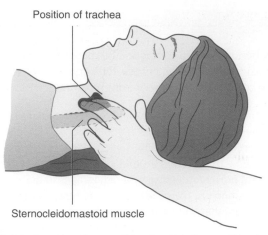

Position of trachea

Sternocleidomastoid muscle

Figure 3.15   Locating the carotid pulse. List the possible signs of a circulation, other than a pulse check.

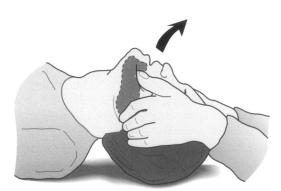

Figure 3.14   Jaw thrust.

Checking the circulation

When checking the circulation, the only appropriate pulse to check is either the carotid or the femoral pulse, as the peripheral pulses are unreliable indicators in the collapsed patient. The femoral pulse is more difficult to find even if the casualty is suitably dressed (or undressed). In order to prevent uncertainty when the rescuer is anxious and adrenaline levels are high, the carotid pulse is best felt via anatomical landmarks rather than by guesswork. On the casualty's neck the trachea and the sternomastoid muscle should be palpated. The fingers should be placed in the trough between these two structures in the midneck region and pressure exerted by the tips of the fingers until they reach the bottom of the trough (Fig. 3.15). This should be performed on the side nearest the first-aider to avoid occluding the trachea. When practising this exercise, it is essential to press on one side only, or fainting may be caused as a result of reducing blood flow to the brain. Handley et al (1997) comment that the practice of the pulse check may be a less than reliable technique, especially by lay first-aiders, and perhaps the expression 'look for signs of a circulation', which includes a more general assessment of circulation as well as a pulse check, is more appropriate.

Evidence based practice

Lack of oxygen (hypoxia) caused by a static circulation to vital organs takes various lengths of time to take effect. Lungs can withstand long periods of hypoxia: the liver 1–2 hours, the heart and kidney 30 minutes, and the brain 4–6 minutes (Newbold 1987). Therefore the effect and efficiency of compressions is very important.

The blood flow that occurs as a result of chest compressions is only about 25% of normal, and cerebral blood flow only 15% of normal, and this is assuming good quality chest compressions (Jackson 1984, Mackenzie 1964). Therefore delaying cardiac chest compressions for up to 5 minutes can result in no cerebral blood flow because of the pathological changes such as stasis of deoxygenated blood in the large veins (Lee 1984).

Mouth–to–mouth ventilation

Once the first-aider is ready to ventilate the casualty's lungs, one of the key words is 'slowly'. In the unconscious casualty, the oesophagus is relatively flat because it is not held open by cartilaginous rings as is the trachea, so slow (and low pressure) ventilations will tend to go into the lungs rather than the stomach. The harder and faster you blow, the more air will enter the stomach and the process becomes less efficient.

Unconscious people are unable to vomit. However, they can passively regurgitate their stomach contents into the upper airway, so ventilating too hard is also to the detriment of the rescuers! As far as ventilation volumes are concerned, judgement of these is a subjective art based on chest movement. According to Baskett et al (1996) 400–600 mL is needed for adults, and one-tenth of this volume (i.e. 40–60 mL) is needed for infants. Note that some adult resuscitation training mannikins may be calibrated to a larger volume.

Chest compressions

The two major theories regarding chest compressions are the cardiac theory and the thoracic pump theory. Robertson & Holmberg (1992) consider that neither of these is actually proven. It is likely that chest compression moves blood by a combination of:

- directly squeezing the heart between the sternum and the spine (cardiac pump theory)
- generally increasing the intrathoracic pressure (thoracic pump theory).

This forces blood out of the heart and chest, with the venous valve system ensuring a unidirectional flow.

As with ventilations, efficiency is related to rate and timing. Theoretically the faster the rate the greater the output, assuming a constant stroke volume (the volume of blood filling the ventricles). In practice, as the compression rate increases the stroke volume may be falling because the venous return to the chest and heart is reduced, so that the actual rate is a compromise between these factors. To make the best use of the rate remember that the relaxation phase is at least as important as the compression phase, so leave adequate time between compressions to allow thoracic and ventricular refilling before the next compression.

Combining ventilations and compressions

Debate continues regarding the most effective combination. In an adult a ratio of 15 compressions to 2 ventilations is used, as it appears to take a number of compressions to 'build up' a circulatory pressure before blood actually flows. This is only changed to continuous compressions once the patient has been intubated, when higher airway pressure can be used. In paediatrics this ratio would result in inadequate oxygenation; hence a ratio of 5 to 1 is used.

Even with the most competent rescuer, survival is not good without advanced help arriving rapidly.

Decision making exercise

John, the community psychiatric nurse, has been visiting 50-year-old Mohan Khan in his home weekly for the past 3 months. Mohan had become very depressed after he had been forced to take an early retirement offer when the company he was working for cut staff costs. Mohan's wife and two children and the local Sikh community had given him as much support as possible, but despite this and medication and counselling, Mohan has become steadily more withdrawn. On his regular Monday visit John could not get into the house and had to call Mohan's wife at the factory where she worked. On gaining entry as advised by Mohan's wife, John found Mohan collapsed in the bathroom with obvious signs of having slashed his wrists.

1. Decide on the immediate steps that John should take to provide BLS.
2. When Mohan's wife arrives, how should John direct her activities?
3. How might this family react to the immediate situation?
4. Decide what strategies John may have to use to support Mohan and his family if he survives this suicide attempt (see also Ch. 8).

Reflection and portfolio exercise

You will need access to an infant and junior resuscitation mannikin for this exercise. Using the marking grids in the chapter test your skills in BLS for infants and children following the guidelines. Ideally, ask another student to assess your skills, and remember the real situation may last a long time, so demonstrate your skills over at least 5 minutes.

A potential controversy is the issue of priorities. Pause, and reviewing information given previously in this chapter, decide which of the following is more important: the patent airway or immobilization of a potential fracture of the cervical spine? Think for a few moments about how you might open the airway of a patient who has suffered a neck injury.

Evidence based practice

McKee et al (1994) undertook an exercise training student nurses to defibrillate using automatic external defibrillators and found that they could potentially deliver the first shock within 60 seconds in the simulated situation. Considering the above factors, that is, the relative inefficiency of BLS and the need for very early defibrillation, it looks as if more widespread use of early defibrillation is the most sensible way forwards for patients with ischaemic heart disease in VF.

VARIATIONS TO THE RESUSCITATION SITUATION

So far the assumption has been that the collapse has been due to a single and relatively simple cause. Obviously in reality other factors may need to be considered in the management. In general terms, the same principles apply to adult, child, mental health or learning disability nursing. The key to success is the systematic assessment of 'the case at hand' using the simple ABC system, which has already been described. Other specific factors that need to be considered include:

- collapse due to trauma
- collapse during pregnancy
- collapse of an individual with altered anatomical airways
- collapse due to choking in the adult
- collapse due to choking in the infant or child.

Each of these situations will be dealt with briefly.

Collapse due to trauma

Remember that it is not possible to find out definitively about any spinal injury in a casualty with an obstructed airway but it must be assumed to be present if the history indicates its potential existence. However, professional nurses are expected to give a higher standard of care than that

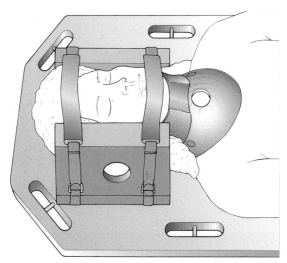

Figure 3.16   Cervical spine immobilization.

given by the general public: if the casualty has a possible cervical spine injury great care should be taken while dealing with the airway. Ideally the neck should be properly immobilized (Fig. 3.16); that is a hard collar, sandbags or equivalent should be used to increase lateral stabilization, with tape over the forehead and upper chest to hold the whole thing together. The whole procedure can be combined with the jaw thrust to maintain an open airway (see Fig. 3.14). However, this is not always realistic. It is to be hoped that any court of law would take into consideration the reality of the situation because of the difficulties with such complex interventions in an emergency.

Collapse during pregnancy

The additional requirements of the woman in late pregnancy have some significance, but are not widely highlighted. Cardiac arrest in late pregnancy is relatively rare, but potentially treatable. Physiologically the pregnant woman has higher oxygen requirements, an increased risk of regurgitation of stomach contents, and increased pressure on the diaphragm due to the pregnant uterus. Probably the most significant factor that needs to be remembered is the effect of the pregnant uterus on the unconscious casualty lying on her back (Fig. 3.17). A pregnant uterus can easily weigh 5 kg, and when it lies directly over and pressing down on the inferior vena cava there are significant sequelae. The first few chest compressions have the same effect as usual, but there will be no venous return from the legs and pelvis due to the compression on the abdominal blood vessels, so the cardiac output will quickly fall to zero.

The management of this situation is relatively simple: either the uterus is manually displaced to the left by an assistant, or the casualty's pelvis is inclined in the same direction at an angle of approximately 30 degrees, either by

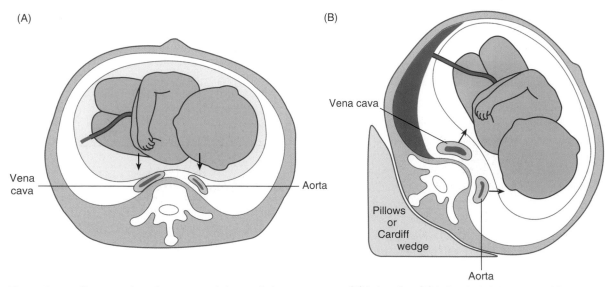

Figure 3.17   Cross-section of pregnant abdomen in late pregnancy. (A) Lying flat. (B) Lying in left lateral position (i.e. inclined to the left using a Cardiff resuscitation wedge), demonstrating relief of compression of vena cava and aorta.

pillows or by a device known as the Cardiff wedge, found in most labour suites. Either of these techniques will remove the compression from the vena cava and allow normal venous return to the chest from the lower body.

Collapse of an individual with altered anatomical airways

This is currently a relatively uncommon situation, but is on the increase as a result of reconstructive surgery following treatment for neoplasms (cancers) in the region of the throat. It is therefore probably good practice to make sure to inspect the casualty's throat down to the suprasternal notch, and definitely if any difficulty is experienced in ventilating the casualty. The management of the situation is exceptionally easy: ventilation should take place using the alternative orifice (Fig. 3.18).

Choking (foreign body airway obstruction, FBAO)

Airway obstruction is a situation which a nurse may face in almost any area of practice. It is essential that nurses can perform choking procedures quickly and efficiently to reduce the risk of respiratory and cardiac arrest.

A typical situation might arise at meal times and play times with children; it is probably the context which will alert a nurse to the potential of FBAO as it is unlikely that the obstruction will be visible during a brief airway check. Typical signs of complete obstruction are:

- hand held to the throat
- 'silent' attempts at coughing

- salivating
- distress
- rapid onset of cyanosis.

With partial obstruction stridor (a snoring sound usually on inspiration), hoarseness, 'whispering' voice and coughing may be observed.

Management of choking in the adult

If the individual still has some respiratory effort, just helping the casualty empty the mouth may prevent the situation deteriorating further. This may be especially important for individuals with swallowing difficulties such as the elderly stroke patient or the young physically disabled. Figure 3.19 shows the current recommendations for the management of choking in the adult (European Resuscitation Council 2000).

Recent evidence has demonstrated that the most effective technique in increasing airway pressure and hence 'blowing out' obstructions is the 'chest thrust' (as per chest compression) (Langhelle et al 2000). This has been implemented in the management of the unconscious patient and also makes the management procedure easier to remember.

The Heimlich manoeuvre or abdominal thrust (Fig. 3.20) aims to push the diaphragm upwards to increase the pressure in the chest cavity and so push or squeeze the object out of the trachea. If successful, the object will be ejected with some force.

Management of choking in the infant or child

The risk of choking is higher in infants and children than in adults because the upper airway is narrower and the

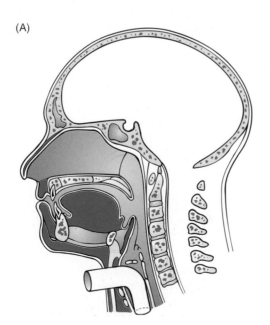 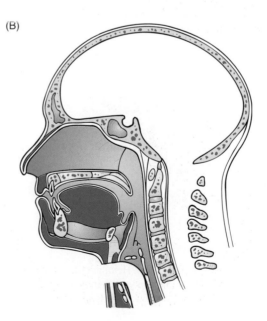

Figure 3.18   Altered anatomical upper airway. (A) Temporary artificial airway. (B) Permanent artificial airway (laryngostomy).

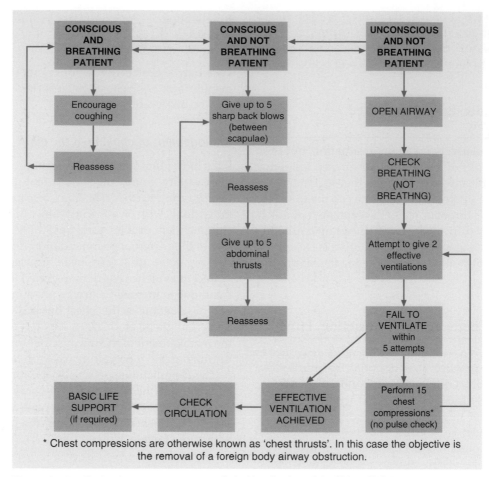

Figure 3.19   Basic airway management of choking in the adult. (After ERC Airway Management Guidelines 2000.)

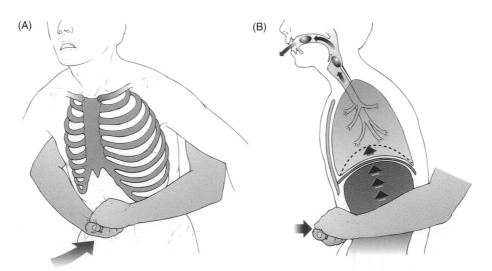

Figure 3.20   The Heimlich manoeuvre used if a patient is choking. (A) Stand behind the patient and clasp your hands over their mid–abdomen. (B) Apply a sharp movement to compress the abdomen. Repeat as necessary. (Nottingham Health Authority.)

swallowing reflex is not as well co-ordinated. The upper airway should be observed carefully during the initial assessment. Obstruction of the airway is not anticipated until the chest will not inflate. Only then is the choking procedure commenced. However, if choking is witnessed initially, the choking procedure should be started immediately.

The Resuscitation Council (UK) (2000) has produced guidelines for the management of choking in infants and

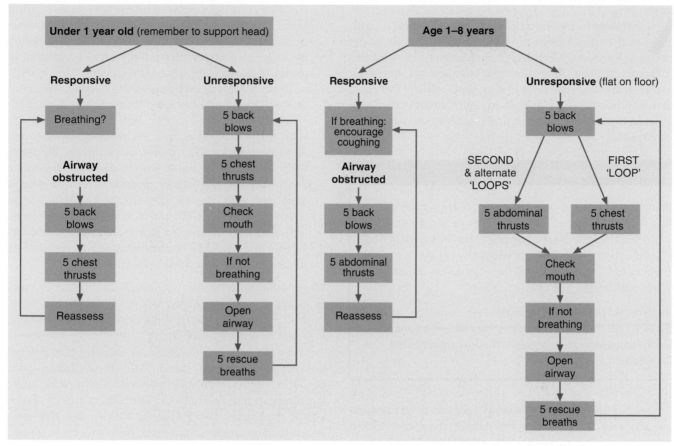

Figure 3.21   Dealing with choking in the infant or child. (From Resuscitation Council (UK) 2000.)

Table 3.3   European Resuscitation Council BLS guidelines for infants and children (based on ILCOR guidelines 2000)

Action	Rationale
Assess response by gentle shake and speak loudly	Voice and physical stimulation may cause a response in a deeply asleep infant or child
Call for help	Someone may be nearby
Open airway	Place hand on forehead and lift chin; do not overextend the head as this can close the airway
A 'sniffing' or neutral position for infants	This action may also stimulate breathing
Look, listen and feel for breathing	Allow 10 seconds, and watch the abdomen as infants and children depend on their diaphragm as the main respiratory muscle
Give two to five expired air respirations if not breathing. If no chest expansion, commence obstructed airway procedure	Watch the chest rise and fall between breaths to assess how deep you, the rescuer, need to exhale. Breaths should be delivered over 1 to 1.5 seconds to reduce abdominal distension
Palpate the pulse – the brachial in infants, the carotid in children – and look for movement	Allow 10 seconds to ensure the pulse is 60 beats or less in an infant or absent in a child
Commence chest compressions if the pulse is less than 60 in infants or absent in children	Position of chest compressions for infants and children differs because of size: • in infants, draw a line from nipple to nipple, place one finger below this line, and two fingers on the sternum, and aim for a third of the diameter of the chest at a rate of 100/minute • in children, find the point where the bottom rib joins the sternum, place two fingers above this point, then place the heel of one hand on the sternum and aim for a third of the diameter of the chest at a rate of 100/minute
Continue at a ratio of one breath to five compressions until help arrives or 15:2 if a larger child/adolescent	Always use a ratio of 1:5 on the principle of maintaining some oxygenation with some circulation

children (Fig. 3.21). The differences between the two age groups is linked to the immaturity of the liver and disconnection of the spleen from the back of the abdomen in the younger age group when the Heimlich manoeuvre (abdominal thrust) is used. Therefore this manoeuvre should be avoided at all costs in babies and replaced by the chest thrust as indicated. Chest thrusts are performed in the same manner and place as chest compressions but are carried out more rapidly.

Decision making exercise

Your friend and her 6-year-old daughter are visiting you. You and your friend go into the kitchen to prepare coffee and leave the child playing happily in the sitting room. The child is eating sweets recently bought by her mother on the way to visit you. Suddenly the child rushes into the kitchen, distressed and unable to speak.

1. What will be your first action?
2. What health promotion advice may be given to your friend to prevent an accident occuring again in the future?

There are currently some inconsistencies between resuscitation advisory bodies due to the lack of absolute evidence regarding best practice. We have therefore based the diagram on the guidance of the Resuscitation Council (UK) (2000).

FURTHER RESUSCITATION SKILLS FOR NURSES

Although the relative efficiency of BLS is not good (somewhere in the region of 15% of 'normal'), it is a significant part of the chain of survival; it buys time and must not be forgotten, especially in high-technology settings. We have already identified the significance of defibrillation in adults and airway care in children – so what are the other interventions of resuscitation?

With a patent airway, one of the early considerations is the addition of supplementary oxygen. All suddenly collapsed patients will benefit from the administration of additional oxygen. It is likely that either the patient's respiratory or cardiac function will be reduced, therefore increasing the oxygen saturation of the available circulation will be in the best interests of the patient. There are, however, two commonly expressed concerns by nurses regarding oxygen delivery.

1. Oxygen is a prescription medication and therefore a physician's signature is required before administration. Local oxygen administration policies should be read carefully and especially clauses that relate to emergency administration. When a patient is suffering from acute hypoxia, as in sudden chest pain, shortness of breath and blood loss, they will always benefit from high-flow oxygen administration during the acute phase.

2. Another concern expressed by nurses relates to administering oxygen to patients with chronic obstructive pulmonary disease (COPD). Very rarely a patient with hypoxic respiratory drive will stop breathing when given high concentrations of oxygen. All acutely ill patients on emergency oxygen are closely observed and this will therefore be noticed immediately. Even patients who are normally hypoxic will suffer adverse effects with further hypoxia. Nancy Caroline, a well-respected American paramedic trainer, summarizes the situation well: 'Never, never, never withhold oxygen therapy from any patient in respiratory distress, even (or especially) a patient with chronic obstructive pulmonary disease' (Caroline 1995: 459). The care and management of patients with COPD is a complex issue which you should study further and it should be remembered that the above only relates to acute emergency situations.

Many different types of oxygen administration devices are available, e.g. Venturi-based face masks, nasal cannulae and trauma masks. Investigate what is available in your clinical area and how they function.

Many devices are available to increase the patency of the patient's airway during the resuscitation process. Baskett (1993a) identifies the various airway adjuncts (equipment) that can help to maintain an airway. The most useful for nurses is the Guedal airway, but this requires accurate measurements to ensure the correct size is selected. These are obtained by measuring the Guedal airway alongside the jaw, the flange of the airway level with the incisor teeth and the distal part of the airway level with the corner of the jaw. In children over 5 years of age and in older age groups, the airway is inserted upside down and turned over in the mouth to hook over the back of the tongue. If the child is under 5 years of age, the tongue should be pushed down with a tongue depressor and the airway is then inserted the correct way up, preventing trauma to the soft palate.

Administration of oxygen when an airway is being used can be by a self-inflating bag. These bags are available in differing sizes according to whether the victim is an infant, child or adult. This piece of equipment has useful features such as a pop-off valve to prevent overinflation, and it can be used without a continual gas flow. It is important to select a face mask that covers the nose and mouth comfortably and creates a good seal so that the victim can receive adequate ventilation. It is also important that the user ensures patient chest movement occurs when the bag is squeezed and additional oxygen is added as soon as possible.

ADVANCED CARDIAC LIFE SUPPORT

The procedures for Advanced Cardiac Life Support (ACLS) in adults and children are shown as separate flow charts and these charts act as guidelines for a team approach to resuscitation (Figs 3.22 and 3.23). Additionally, the guidelines from the European Resuscitation Council (2000) give checklists for the appropriate actions in the case of single and two-handed rescue (Figs 3.24–3.27).

Reflection and portfolio exercise

Study Figures 3.22 and 3.23 which explain advanced cardiac life support (ACLS) in the adult and child.

1. Note the differences between the two flow charts.

2. During your practice placements, if you witness a situation where a patient (whether adult or child) has collapsed and needs resuscitation by a cardiac arrest team reflect afterwards on how the situation was managed.

3. Review the guidelines and compare your experience with the recommendations.

Discuss any differences that occur between the theory and the practice with an experienced nurse who was present at the resuscitation in order to understand the reasons behind them.

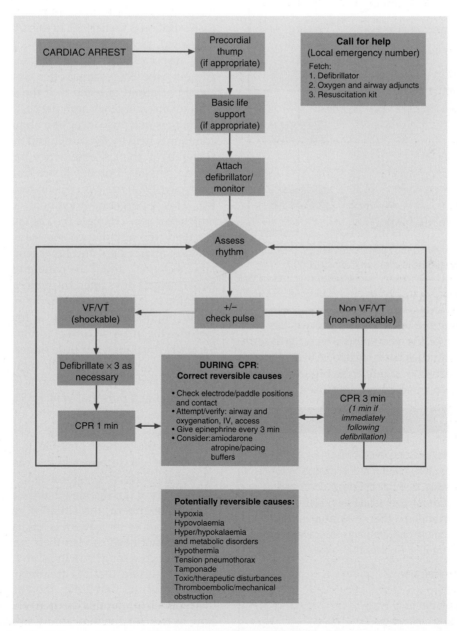

Figure 3.22 Core flow chart from the adult advanced life support guidelines. (Reproduced by kind permission of European Resuscitation Council 2000.)

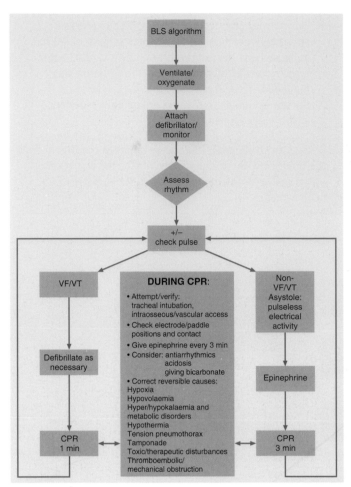

Figure 3.23 Paediatric advanced life support guidelines. (Reproduced by kind permission of European Resuscitation Council 2000.)

DRUGS AND RESUSCITATION

The use of drugs during the resuscitation process has been a controversial topic over the years and it is only recently that objective research studies have started. Although there are potentially many drugs that might be required during a cardiac arrest, the two most commonly used drugs are

---

Evidence based practice

Adrenaline (epinephrine) has become the drug of choice in resuscitation due to research conducted by Goetting & Paradis (1991). They found through animal studies and retrospective examination of adrenaline administration during cardiac arrest in children that restoration of the circulation and neurological outcome was improved. For both adrenaline and atropine identify the following:

1. The indications for their use.
2. Their actions.
3. Their potential side effects.
4. The normal adult and child doses.
5. The potential routes of administration.

---

adrenaline (epinephrine) and atropine. Adrenaline appears to improve BLS by increasing oxygen delivery to the cardiac muscle. Atropine is used in the bradycardiac (or asystolic) patient to block the inhibitory affect of the parasympathic nervous system (via the vagus nerve). For further information read any up-to-date drug handbook.

HANDING OVER RESPONSIBILITY FOR CARE

The final stage in the resuscitation process is the handing over of responsibility for care from the first-aider to healthcare professionals, who will then become responsible for the collapsed individual's welfare. This final 'disposal' of the casualty is as fraught with legal risk as any part of nursing. The same consideration should be applied when discharging the casualty into the hands of professional health carers. The easiest option is to dial 999. In this situation, continuity of care is assured, as long as handover is performed effectively, so that responsibility for subsequent care is minimized. Although the 999 system is often abused by the public, no one should be afraid of using it. If the situation is considered to warrant an emergency ambulance, then one should be called.

There is one misconception about the ambulance service commonly held by the public and that is the issue of charges. Generally in the UK emergency treatment is free and there are no charges, but the Road Traffic Act (Department of Transport 1972) has a provision for an emergency treatment fee. This emergency treatment fee will be claimed by whichever service treats the casualty first. If an ambulance is called, the ambulance service claims it; if the casualty walks to an Accident and Emergency department the hospital will claim it, and if the patient visits their general practitioner several days later, the general practitioner is allowed to claim it. Any accident involving a motor vehicle on a public highway constitutes a road traffic accident and includes the full spectrum of trauma from being run over by a lorry to breaking your little fingernail in a parked car door if the car is parked on a public highway.

The second 'disposal' option is to take the injured person to hospital in a personal vehicle. This should be considered carefully, as there may be a risk of the casualty collapsing or even just fainting in the vehicle while travelling. It is worthwhile where possible to ensure someone else is also in the car to assist if the casualty deteriorates. This allows the driver to concentrate on driving rather than the casualty. If it is decided that the casualty does not require hospital treatment, the situation must be considered very carefully before the patient is left. Is it certain that this casualty does not need to visit their general practitioner? What else could go wrong? Are there any possible complications?

If it is certain that the treatment is within the realm of expertise of the first-aider, the patient must be given full instructions (preferably written) about what to look out for, how to care for the injury now, and when to seek help. As when discharging a patient, a help option should also be left and the patient should know where to go if they are

Checklist for single rescuer basic life support for adults

Assumptions

The patient is adult and has suddenly collapsed without apparent reason.
    You are alone as the rescuer and a health care professional (or trainee)

Replies for the 'tester' are in **bold** letters,

Criteria		Correct	Incorrect sequence	Omitted
Assess safety	**SAFE**			
Assess response (shout and gentle shake)	**UNRESPONSIVE**			
Shout for help	**NONE ARRIVES**			
Brief airway check	**CLEAR**			
Open airway (head tilt, chin lift, two fingers holding jaw)				
Assess breathing (for up to 10 sec)	**ABSENT or INADEQUATE**			
Phone for ambulance/cardiac arrest team				
Brief reassess on return (as appropriate)				
Maintain open airway				
Perform two effective rescue breaths (2 sec inflation time each)				
Check for signs of circulation including carotid pulse.	**ABSENT**			
Give 15 chest compressions				
– correct position (two finger widths above base sternum, where rib margins meet centrally)				
– correct depth (4–5 cm)				
– correct rate (100/min)				
Continue cardiopulmonary resuscitation at ratio of 2 ventilations to 15 compressions				
Ensure each ventilation causes the chest to rise				
Count the compressions out aloud (1, 2, 3, …, 14, 15)				
Testing standard: Continue for 5 min at minimum of three cycles/min				

Candidate's name: ....   Date: ....
Tested by: ....   Pass/Requires further practice.

Figure 3.24 Checklist for single rescuer: basic life support for adults. (From European Resuscitation Council 2000.)

concerned. This is not only of benefit to the patient, but is also a useful defensive tactic for the nurse.

Decision making exercise

While listening to a lecture, a fellow student nurse faints and when falling, hits her head on a chair. After lying down for a few minutes, she recovers and feels better.

1. What factors should you consider when deciding if she needs to go home or to the nearest A and E department?
2. Review and decide on what your legal responsibilities might be as a first-aider if you are a student nurse.

PROFESSIONAL AND ETHICAL KNOWLEDGE

Within this section, the nurse's professional accountability is examined by focusing on:

- the role of the nurse in both BLS and ALS situations
- the nurse's responsibility to maintain his/her resuscitation skills
- the importance of the nurse evaluating his/her own level of competence.

The expectations of society will be reviewed and the ethico-legal issues surrounding resuscitation will be discussed.

Checklist for two rescuers: basic life support for adults

Assumptions

The patient is adult and has suddenly collapsed without apparent reason.
    You have assistance and you are both healthcare professionals (or trainees)

Replies for the 'tester' are in **bold** letters,

Criteria		Correct	Incorrect sequence	Omitted
First Rescuer Assess safety	**SAFE**			
Assess response (shout and gentle shake)	**UNRESPONSIVE**			
Shout for help	**SECOND RESCUER ARRIVES**			
Brief airway check	**CLEAR**			
Open airway (head tilt, chin lift, two fingers holding jaw)				
Assess breathing (for up to 10 sec)	**ABSENT or INADEQUATE**			
Send Second Rescuer to Phone for ambulance/cardiac arrest team				
First Rescuer Maintain open airway				
Perform two rescue breaths (2 sec inflation time each)				
Check for signs of circulation including carotid pulse **ABSENT**				
Give 15 chest compressions				
– correct position (two fingers above base of sternum)				
– correct depth (4–5 cm)				
– correct rate (100/min)				
Continue cardiopulmonary resuscitation at ratio of 2 ventilations to 15 compressions until return of second rescuer				
Second Rescuer returns – direct second rescuer to take over chest compressions, positioned OPPOSITE to the first rescuer				
Second Rescuer gives 15 correct chest compressions (counts compressions out loud)				
First Rescuer – gives two effective ventilations				
Continue at 2 ventilations to 15 compressions				
Testing standard: Continue for 5 min at a minimum of three cycles/min				

Candidate's name: ....   Date: ....

Tested by: ....   Pass/Requires further practice.

Figure 3.25   Checklist for two rescuers: basic life support for adults. (From European Resuscitation Council 2000.)

THE PUBLIC'S EXPECTATIONS OF THE NURSE AS A FIRST-AIDER

The public expects nurses to help in emergency situations.

When the new student nurse is first identified as 'a nurse' by their home community, everyone appears to make a mental note of this fact, so that when an emergency occurs friends and relatives know where to turn for help. This general principle appears to apply equally to nurses who have specialized in diverse areas of practice, as many members of the public only recognize the 'traditional' general nurse, and all nurses are expected to fill this role. How 'the nurse' fulfils their role in the emergency situation when called to help as 'a nurse' has many implications.

The 'duty of care' to a neighbour as a member of the public

In the UK there is no legal duty of care to a 'neighbour', which may be anyone and not just a physical neighbour.

Checklist for single rescuer: basic life support for infants (babies)

Assumptions

The patient is an infant (defined as being below 1 year of age) and has collapsed after a period of deterioration or an 'incident'

You are alone as the rescuer and a healthcare professional (or trainee)

Replies for the 'tester' are in **bold** letters,

Criteria		Correct	Incorrect sequence	Omitted
Assess safety	**SAFE**			
Assess response (shout and stimulate)	**UNRESPONSIVE**			
Shout for help				
Ensure/place or supporting surface				
Airway check	**CLEAR**			
Open airway (face parallel with chest, chin lift, two fingers holding jaw)				
Assess breathing (look, listen and feel for up to 10 sec)	**INADEQUATE or ABSENT**			
Maintain open airway				
Perform two gentle rescue breaths (from up to five attempts)				
Look for potential airway obstruction if no chest rise after five attempts				
Check for signs of circulation (including brachial pulse)	**LESS THAN 60 beats/min or ABSENT**			
Give five chest compressions				
correct position (one finger width below nipple line, on sternum) (*or encircle chest method, if two rescuers)				
– correct depth (1/3 of chest diameter)				
– correct rate (100/min)				
Continue at 1 ventilation to 5 compressions				
After 1 min phone for definitive help (if not already contacted)				
Reassess on return				
Continue at 1 ventilation to 5 compressions				
Continue for 5 min at a minimum of 15 cycles/min				

Candidate's name: .... Date: ....

Tested by: .... Pass/Requires further practice.

Figure 3.26 Checklist for single rescuer: basic life support for babies. (From European Resuscitation Council 2000.)

In practice, this means anyone can walk past an accident or step over a collapsed person in the street. Although a legal duty of care does not exist, there is, however, a moral duty towards fellow human beings that must be considered.

In the British legal system, the two major divisions are criminal and civil law. Entering a patient's house without consent may be trespass, which is a civil offence, though it may in some cases be a criminal offence. Touching a patient without consent might be considered to be assault and inappropriate treatment of a patient might result in accusations of actual bodily harm. It is no wonder that nurses worry about being sued.

One of the major considerations in criminal law is the 'intent' and 'motive' that is associated with the act. Both 'intent' and 'motive' are very complex legal issues and it would be advisable to consult a legal text to investigate these further. The courts will consider a situation where the intent when aiding an individual is to do harm in a very different light to a situation where the rescuer is trying to help. It appears more likely that the first-aider would be involved

Checklist for single rescuer: basic life support for children

Assumptions

The patient is a child (defined as between 1 and 8 years of age) and has collapsed after a period of deterioration or an 'incident'

You are alone as the rescuer and a health care professional (or trainee)

Replies for the 'tester' are in **bold** letters,

Criteria		Correct	Incorrect sequence	Omitted
Assess safety	**SAFE**			
Assess response (shout and stimulate)	**UNRESPONSIVE**			
Shout for help				
Brieft airway check	**CLEAR**			
Open airway (limited head tilt, chin lift, two fingers holding jaw)				
Assess breathing (look, listen and feel for up to 10 sec)	**ABSENT or INADEQUATE**			
Maintain open airway				
Perform two gentle rescue breaths (up to five attempts)				
Look for potential airway obstruction if no chest rise after five attempts				
Check for signs of circulation (including carotid pulse)	**ABSENT or LESS THAN 60 beats/min**			
Give five chest compressions				
correct position (one finger width above base of sternum, on sternum)				
– correct depth (1/3 of chest diameter)				
– correct rate (100/min solidus)				
Continue at 1 ventilation to 5 compressions				
After 1 min phone for definitive help (if not previously called)				
Reassess on return				
Continue at 1 ventilation to 5 compressions				
Continue for 5 min at a minimum of 15 cycles/min				

Candidate's name: .... Date: ....

Tested by: .... Pass/Requires further practice.

Figure 3.27 Checklist for single rescuer: basic life support for children. (From European Resuscitation Council 2000.)

in a case related to civil law, and most probably that of negligence where the patient has suffered additional harm due to the actions of a first-aider.

John Tingle (1991) undertook a review of the situation regarding first aid and the law. One of his major considerations was that 'legal action against Good Samaritan acts is a remote possibility'. The Good Samaritan act is simply that as described in the Bible (Luke 10: 25–37), where a stranger comes to the assistance of a fellow human being to relieve suffering. In our opinion, the principle of the Good Samaritan is one which our culture needs to encourage and support. Tingle (1991) considers this to be of significance in British

courts. If 'resuscitation' cases were brought to court and first-aiders found guilty, it might lead to the same state that is now found in the USA where members of the public and professionals are becoming hesitant to assist their neighbours. Because of these legal considerations some American states have introduced so-called 'Good Samaritan' acts to promote first aid and to some extent protect the rescuer from the nightmare of litigation.

Caroline (1995) cites one of these laws from Florida State:

Any person, including those licensed to practice medicine, who gratuitously and in good faith renders emergency care or treatment at the scene of an emergency outside of a hospital, doctor's office or other place having proper medical equipment, without objection of the injured victim or victims thereof, shall not be held liable for any civil damages as a result of any act or failure to act in providing or arranging further medical treatment where the person acts as an ordinary reasonable prudent man would have acted under the same circumstances. (Caroline 1995: 23)

The statement of particular significance is 'ordinary reasonable prudent man'. This level is difficult to determine and really left to the judgement of the court; however, the word 'man' would be replaced by 'nurse' if one were involved and an expert witness would be called in an attempt to determine what this level is. Although the current situation in the UK is not one that yet really requires this legislation, such an act might be reassuring and encourage the act of first aid by professional carers.

The 'duty of care' to a neighbour as a professional nurse

It is important to remember that although there is no duty to care for everyone, if an injured person is already 'under the care' of the potential first-aider's employer, the first-aider then has a duty to care for them. As Tingle (1991) says 'a nurse could not leave a fallen patient but could leave a witnessed accident'. Although there is no immediate legal duty of care to the witnessed accident, once the nurse has presented herself as a nurse to help, 'a duty of care' exists.

If a case were to be taken to court it would probably be in the area of negligence. The crucial factor in negligence cases is the issue of 'reasonable care' where the standard of care is expected to be that of the reasonable and ordinary nurse or first-aider considering the individual circumstances in question. In the opinion of the authors of this chapter, as long as a first-aider continually asks themself why he or she is doing each action and ensuring that their actions are always for the benefit of the injured person, litigation is considered to be unlikely. However, this is no guarantee. Barber (1993) applies a more cautionary approach to first aid and points out that 'a nurse acting on her own initiative, under no instruction from an employer and other than in the course of her own duties, is clearly responsible and liable for her own acts and omissions'.

When undertaking emergency care for individuals 'in the care' of an employer, for example a National Health Service Trust, if anything goes wrong it is more likely that the individual will sue the employer than the employee. This is likely to be the case for a nurse who is the 'designated' first-aider as described in the first aid regulations of the Health and Safety at Work Act (Health and Safety Commission 1991). Outside this situation the first-aider is 'on their own' and it seems reasonable that every nurse should have some personal indemnity insurance to cover them in such circumstances. Personal indemnity insurance is often part of a 'package' a nurse receives if they join a union or professional organization. Such an option appears to be sensible.

Barber (1993) also points out the importance of obtaining consent for all interventions and only undertaking those interventions that are 'necessary' to save life and prevent further deterioration. For nurses there is a significant additional consideration in this debate. This is the professional consideration.

It can be concluded, then, that as a member of the public there is no legal duty to help a stranger. However the Nursing and Midwifery Council (2002) puts this responsibility on all nurses in its *Code of Professional Conduct*. The code states: '(8.5) In an emergency, in or outside the work setting, you have a professional duty to provide care.'

The wording of the *Code of Professional Conduct* provides a clear mandate for all nurses that goes beyond the legal responsibilities and indicates that nurses must always act in the manner of the Good Samaritan.

Castledine (1993) cites a case from the professional conduct hearings of the UK Central Council (predecessor of the Nursing and Midwifery Council) where a district nurse passed by a road traffic accident because she feared that she did not know what to do. A member of the public reported this action and the nurse was found guilty of misconduct. Although the nurse was not removed from the register, this is a clear signal from the professional body that nurses must help in all emergency situations, even if the situation lies outside their direct realm of responsibility. The extent of this 'required' help is unclear. We would expect the minimum would be no more then ensuring competent help is on its way (i.e. someone has summoned the emergency services) and undertaking simple supportive action.

THE ROLE OF THE NURSE IN BLS AND ALS

Within the community environment, the nurse acts as a first-aider when undertaking BLS resuscitation. However, the nurse is not expected to be an expert, but should ensure a call for competent help has been made. The UK Central Council (1996) stated in reference to an off-duty nurse coming across a road traffic accident that 'in this situation it could be reasonable to expect the nurse to do no more than comfort and support the injured person'. The word 'support' still leaves the discussion fairly open as it may mean anything from holding the injured person's hand, to undertaking ALS.

Within the hospital setting, the role of the nurse in resuscitation changes in the sense that he or she is an integral part of the healthcare team. Initially, the nurse is often the locater of the incident, having found the collapsed individual. At this point, after the assessment, the nurse raises the alarm and commences BLS. A colleague will summon the arrest team and begin to collect equipment for ALS, such as a defibrillator. When the team arrives, the nurse will still have a role as they:

- have knowledge of the event
- know the ward
- know the individual and their relatives.

It is not unusual for the cardiac arrest team to be led by a nurse, either from the ward or in the role of resuscitation officer or clinical nurse manager for a 'floor' or a clinical unit. Within the trauma resuscitation protocols described by the American College of Surgeons, the nurse has a significant role. Hadfield-Law & Kent (1996) describe this role and how the resuscitation event may be managed.

EDUCATION AND TRAINING FOR RESUSCITATION

As developing resuscitation skills 'on the job' is inappropriate, a number of nationally recognized courses have been developed to provide these skills. St John Ambulance and the British Red Cross undertake excellent first aid training that develops individual skills in BLS. For more advanced training in adult cardiac collapse there is the ACLS course and for dealing with children there is the Paediatric Advanced Life Support (PALS) course. Finally, for those more interested in the trauma approach, there is the Advanced Trauma Nursing Course (ATNC). All of these courses are usually residential as they last 2–4 days and are regularly advertised in the nursing press.

All first aid and resuscitation skills require regular practice. Under local regulations, yearly updates may be mandatory in your areas of practice. Simulations set up in the work area can either be practical or 'talk through' and can be completed on a regular basis to keep skills fresh and up to date. Working as a team is especially important, so these exercises should be undertaken with as many members of the regular team as possible.

Evidence based practice

Training and maintenance of competence levels for resuscitation skills is poor among hospital personnel (Crouch 1993). Poor skill retention is linked to a lack of competence, and skills can deteriorate after 6 weeks without practice (Cavanagh 1990, Wynne et al 1990). A survey of hospital resuscitation statistics found that only 14.6% of collapsed patients survived resuscitation, but where hospital personnel are trained and competent in CPR skills 50% of collapsed patients survived (Casey 1984, Wynne et al 1990).

Crouch (1993) surveyed nurses' theoretical knowledge of resuscitation and found that less than half the sample group (62 in total) had heard of the Resuscitation Council UK. Many respondents answered questions poorly regarding the drug of choice and when the precordial thump was indicated. However, he also found that 24% had received a CPR update in the previous year, while 6.5% had never received a CPR update. Regular updating is recommended, including role play and team practice for the resuscitation team.

Decision making exercise

A crowd gathers around a motorcyclist who has fallen off his motorbike as it skidded on ice.

1. Consider what factors you need to take into consideration when you as a member of the public decide whether or not to assist at an incident.
2. How would these factors change if it became known that you were a nurse or stated you were a nurse before you started to help this motocyclist?

Review the Code of Professional Conduct (Nursing and Midwifery Council 2002).

Reflection and portfolio exercise

Review the situation of the motorcyclist in the previous exercise and decide, based on your own knowledge and skills and the requirements of the Code of Professional Conduct, how you would act in that particular scenario.

1. Identify which of the specific clauses need to be considered in the emergency situation.

ETHICAL ISSUES SURROUNDING RESUSCITATION

Much has been written about the ethics of resuscitation, the definitive document being Decisions Relating to Cardiopulmonary Resuscitation by the Royal College of Nursing and the British Medical Association (2001).

The issue of whether to actively resuscitate an individual or not is a difficult one to address. However, it must be remembered that the final decision should be in the patient's interest, respect the individual's desires as far as possible, and consider the value of human life.

Baskett (1993b) states:

In the absence of a patient's precise previous instructions to the contrary, consent to attempt CPR [cardiopulmonary resuscitation], as with other emergency procedures, is presumed since the patient is incapable of communicating his or her wishes at the moment of arrest and failure to render care immediately is certain to result in death.

'Do not resuscitate' orders are at times appropriate. It is, however, important that in this situation appropriate discussions take place between the patient, the patient's relatives and friends, and healthcare professionals. Discussion is important especially for those who are regarded as vulnerable, that is children, the mentally handicapped and those debilitated by mental illness. When resuscitation would have no effect on the process of dying or the patient does not wish to have their life extended then the decision not to resuscitate should be formally documented. These authors do not think there is a place for 'blanket orders', for example in elderly care units, where it is decided without individual consents not to resuscitate simply because all the residents are old.

'Living wills' or 'advanced directives' are sometimes used by patients to identify their wishes, with respect to end-of-life decisions. For further details see the Royal College of Nursing and the British Medical Association (2001).

Decision making exercise

You have been involved in the resuscitation of Mr James, who is 55 years old, after a severe myocardial infarction (heart attack). This gentleman was very ill before the arrest. The resuscitation continued for 30 minutes with no cardiac activity as a result. Mrs James was present when Mr James collapsed and has requested that her husband is allowed to die. The medical staff want to insert an artificial pacing device, which they feel will save Mr James's life.

1. Decide on what the legal issues are for all those involved in Mr James's care.
2. Using a model for ethical decision making (Curtin & Flaherty 1989, Seedhouse 1988) review the possible decisions that could be made that might take into consideration Mrs James's request that her husband be allowed to die.
3. What should the role of the nurse be as part of the team involved in the resuscitation process?

Reflection and portfolio exercise

Specifically in relation to emergency care investigate the issue of informed consent for:

1. Children.
2. The unconscious adult.
3. The individual with learning difficulties.
4. Those with mental health problems.

Cross-refer to Chapter 12 on death and dying and your ethico-legal textbooks.

Age of consent and incompetency

Although the above discussions have just been addressing the issue of emergency care it is important to remember the concept of consent. All nursing interventions require informed consent by the patient. In an emergency situation when the patient is unconscious it is generally accepted that the nurse may undertake what intervention is 'necessary' to save life and prevent further deterioration. Patients who are conscious need to be informed of what is going on and what treatment is proposed so that they have the opportunity to accept or refuse the treatment, unless mental incapacity is indicated. A witness can be very helpful, especially in the emergency situation, in case of any difficulties at a later date. The same rules apply for those under the age of consent (i.e. 16 years) and a parent or legal guardian must be sought for their permission if at all possible. There is currently considerable discussion about the role of the child in the process of consent, which requires further study (Department of Health 2004). The same considerations also apply for those with significant mental health problems and learning disabilities.

PERSONAL AND REFLECTIVE KNOWLEDGE

The public appears to expect nurses to help in emergency situations and therefore nurses should be able to deal with the initial management of any physical emergency until more specialist staff are available. The practice of first aid and resuscitation carries legal risks. A basic understanding of the legal and professional basis of nursing practice helps to decide how to practice safely. Nurses should not be over worried when helping out at the scene of an emergency as long as they proceed with caution according to a well-tested plan and only undertake those interventions that are 'necessary'. It also appears to be reasonable that nurses have some form of personal indemnity insurance cover.

Resuscitation is primarily a practical skill that requires a fairly wide knowledge base. As a practical skill the ability to

use it decays with lack of use. Simulation exercises need to be a common feature of the updating process. Nurses are obliged to become involved in emergency care, if not by law then by the Nursing and Midwifery Council. It is necessary that all nurses receive instruction and updating in emergency care to fulfil this role.

Overall a cautious intervention by nurses in emergency situations is to encouraged. The well-tested plan of action at any emergency is that described in the *First Aid Manual* of the voluntary first aid organizations by Webb et al (2002). The Resuscitation Council (UK) reviews and updates its guidelines based on evidence gathered from the increasing number of research studies in the field of resuscitation. These should be adhered to by all healthcare personnel in any team involved in the resuscitation process.

LEARNING TO LEARN FROM CRITICAL EVENTS

Throughout this chapter there are some reflective exercises for your portfolio. In the practice setting, it is important to learn from critical events such as those described in this chapter. Get into the habit of thinking about your actions and identifying both the positive points and those that you could improve next time.

During healthcare education and training programmes, students will receive practical BLS training. The checklists earlier in the chapter can be used for updating and revising such skills. These are specially designed for adult, infant and child resuscitation situations

CASE STUDIES IN EMERGENCY CARE

The following case histories use the content of the chapter to reflect over situations you may need to address in your particular field of nursing in the future. Completing them will help you consolidate your learning so far.

Case study: Learning disabilities

Remember the 30-year-old woman (Linda) with profound learning disabilities who was a passenger in one of the two cars involved in a crash (see p. 55). Linda was the back seat passenger in one of the cars and when you came on the scene she was screaming loudly. This lady needs to come to terms with such a traumatic event and coping strategies need to be developed to help her in the future. Obviously, Linda needs to understand how the events happened and, in some ways, most importantly of all, realize that it was an accident and no one's fault.

- Reflect on and identify some of the feelings Linda may have experienced immediately following and subsequent to the accident.
- Review again how you would have prioritized her particular care within the life-threatening scenario of the car crash.
- Linda's father recovered from his chest and head injuries, but is concerned that his daughter's needs were ignored by the rescuers. He intends to sue for negligence. Decide on the type of defence you will have in law should there be a civil case for damages.

Case study: Child

You are on a practice placement in a local school for children with special needs. Jennifer, a 4-year-old child with cerebral palsy, is found collapsed by the dinner table at school. As the only 'nurse' present you are immediately called upon by the teacher in charge to help.

- What is your first action?
- Your attempts at expired air respiration fail. What should you assume?
- After several cycles of the choking procedure a piece of meat is retrieved from Jennifer's mouth, but she is still not breathing. What should you do now?

- Rehearse practically what you have decided to do using a mannikin and self-assess your performance using the checklist for resuscitation of children.

Case study: Mental health

James is a 17-year-old client who has been admitted to an acute mental health ward with manic depression. He tells you that he has taken 50 of his lithium carbonate and haloperidol tablets over the last 10 minutes and states that he wants to die. He makes it very clear that he does not want to be treated.

- Consider whether you would undertake active resuscitation should he collapse in your presence.
- What immediate actions would you take if he did collapse?
- Reflect on and debate with your peers the ethical and legal issues involved in this particular situation.

Case study: Adult

You are having an evening out with a friend. While walking home you have come across a middle-aged man slumped against a wall, who has been vomiting profusely. He smells strongly of alcohol and is barely rousable.

- Consider how you might approach this situation.
- Should his condition deteriorate, how would you carry out mouth-to-mouth ventilations and still protect your own safety?
- It is later discovered that this patient has hepatitis B. What additional actions might you now have to take to protect yourself in the long term?

Summary

This chapter has drawn together theoretical concepts relating to resuscitation and emergency care. It has applied knowledge in relation to the practice of caring for individuals in emergency situations. It has included:

1. The causes of cardiopulmonary arrest and the physiology of care giving in relation to airway management and chest compression.
2. Knowledge for the assessment and care of individuals in situations of collapse, choking or resuscitation.
3. The professional and ethical considerations which must be taken into account in life-threatening situations.
4. The legal considerations facing nurses in relation to resuscitation and emergency care.

Annotated further reading and websites

Caroline N 1995 Emergency care in the streets, 5th edn. Little, Brown, Boston
This book was written for paramedics in the USA. It offers good insight into the skills and knowledge required of the paramedic with clear explanations and pictorial evidence. It is a text commonly used in UK paramedic training schemes.

Resuscitation Council (UK) 2002
Guidance on resuscitation. Available: http://www.resus.org.uk 7 Aug 2003

Tingle J 1991 First aid law. Nursing Times 87(35):48–49
A common sense review of British law as it relates to the nurse as a first-aider.

Webb M, Scott R, Beale P 2002 First aid manual, 8th edn. Dorling Kindersley, London
The authorized manual of the voluntary aid societies.

Wright B 1996 Sudden death: a research base for practice, 2nd edn. Churchill Livingstone, Edinburgh
This is an excellent book on the psychological impact of sudden death of a loved one (adult or child) on families, based on the research and experience of its author as a clinical nurse specialist in crisis care. The book also deals with the effects of crisis managment on healthcare staff and makes very useful suggestions for staff support and training.

Guidelines

http://www.erc.edu
European Resuscitation Council. Contains the overall European Guidelines and supporting information.

http://www.resus.org.uk
Resuscitation Council (UK). UK specific Guidelines and discussion of the implementation in the UK.

http://www.hse.gov.uk/
Health and Safety Executive. Contains UK accident figures and information regarding accident prevention.

Emergency planning

http://www.doh.gov.uk/epcu/index.htm
Emergency planning guidance for the National Health Service.

Training/Further information

http://www.bbc.co.uk/health/firstaid.shtml
Interactive First Aid training from the BBC.

http://www.child-resuscitation.org.uk
Information regarding further training for children's resuscitation.

http://www.acls.net/
Supporting information for Cardiac Life Support (USA, includes quizzes).

http://depts.washington.edu/learncpr/
Resuscitation training support information (USA).

http://www.sophusmedical.dk
Supplier of CD based training materials, downloadable sample on line.

http://www.rospa.co.uk/cms
Royal Society for the Prevention of Accidents. Statistics and information regarding Accident Prevention.

Patient support information

http://www.bfh.org.uk
British Heart Foundation. Health promotion regarding the prevention of heart disease.

http://www.bcpa.co.uk
British Cardiac Patients Association. Support site for patients suffering from heart disease.

http://www.trauma.org
Information supporting the management of trauma patients. See also the 'moulage' section for interactive exercise.

Defibrillation

http://www.medical.philips.com/
A supplier of resuscitation equipment, contains many useful educational resources.

http://www.defib.net
Defibrillation support information.

http://www.padl.org/
Public access defibrillation information.

References

Advanced Life Support Group 2001 Advanced paediatric life support. British Medical Journal, London

American Heart Association 2000 Adult basic life support. Resuscitation 46(1–3):29–71

Atkins D L, Bossaert L L, Hazinski M F et al 2001 Automated external defibrillation/public accesss defibrillation. Annals of Internal Medicine 37:S60–S67

Barber J 1993 Legal aspects of first aid and emergency care. British Journal of Nursing 2(12):641–642

Basic Life Support Working Party of the European Resuscitation Council 1992 Guidelines for basic life support. Resuscitation 24(2):103–110

Baskett P 1993a Resuscitation handbook, 2nd edn. Wolfe, London

Baskett P 1993b Ethics in cardiopulmonary resuscitation. Resuscitation 25(1):1–8

Baskett P, Nolan J, Parr M 1996 Tidal volumes which are perceived to be adequate for resuscitation. Resuscitation 31(3):231–234

Caplan G 1964 Principles of preventative psychiatry. Basic Books, New York

Caroline N 1995 Emergency care in the streets, 5th edn. Little, Brown, Boston

Casey W F 1984 Cardiopulmonary resuscitation: a survey of standards among junior hospital doctors. Journal of the Royal Society of Medicine 7(11):921–924

Castledine G 1993 Ethical implications of first aid. British Journal of Nursing 2(4):239–241

Cavanagh S J 1990 Educational aspects of cardiopulmonary training. Intensive Care Nursing 6(1):38–44

Chalk A 1995 Should relatives be present in the resuscitation room. Journal of Accident and Emergency Nursing 3(2):58–61

Child Accident Prevention Trust 2002 Safe Kids Report 2000. Available: http://www.capt.org.uk

Children Act 1989 HMSO, London

Cook P 1999 Supporting sick children and their families. Baillière Tindall, London

Coyne I 1996 Sudden infant death syndrome and baby care practices. Paediatric Nursing 8(10):16–18

Crouch R 1993 Nurses' skills in basic life support: a survey. Nursing Standard 7(20):28–31

Cummins R O, Eisenberg M S, Horwood B T et al 1990 Cardiac arrest and resuscitation: a tale of 29 cities. Annals of Emergency Medicine 19(2):179–186

Cummins R O, Ornato J P, Thies W H et al 1991 Improving survival from sudden cardiac arrest: the 'chain of survival' concept. Circulation 83(5):1832–1847

Curtin L, Flaherty M J 1989 Nursing ethics: theories and pragmatics, 2nd edn. Brady, Bowie

Department of Health 1991 The health of the nation. HMSO, London

Department of Health 1992 Back to sleep: reducing the risk of cot death. HMSO, London

Department of Health 1993 Targeting practice: the contribution of nurses, midwives and health visitors. HMSO, London

Department of Health 2004 The role of the child in the process of consent. Online. Available: http://doh.gov.uk/consent

Department of Transport 1972 Road Traffic Act. HMSO, London

Durham T W, McCammon S L, Allison E J 1985 The psychological impact of disaster on personnel. Annals of Emergency Medicine 14:7

European Resuscitation Council 2000 Basic life support: guidelines 2000. Online. Available: http://resus.org.uk

Fisher J M, Handley A J 1995 Basic life support. In: Colquhoun M C, Handley A J, Evans T R (eds) ABC of resuscitation. British Medical Journal, London, pp 1–5

Fraser S, Atkins J 1990 Survivors' recollections of helpful and unhelpful emergency nurses activities surrounding the sudden death of a loved one. Journal of Emergency Nursing 16(1):13–16

Gibson M 1991 Order from chaos: responding to traumatic events. Venture Press, Birmingham

Goetting M G, Paradis N A 1991 High dose epinephrine improves outcome from paediatric cardiac arrest. Annals of Emergency Medicine 20(1):22–26

Hadfield-Law L, Kent A 1996 Role of the trauma nurse. In: Skinner D, Driscoll P, Earlam R (eds) ABC of major trauma, 2nd edn. British Medical Journal, London, pp 80–82

Handley A J, Becker L B, Allen M et al 1997 Single rescuer adult basic life support. An advisory statement from the Basic Life Support Working Group of the International Liaison Committee on Resuscitation (ILCOR) Resuscitation 34(2):101–108

Hanson C, Strawser D 1992 Family presence during cardio-pulmonary resuscitation: Foote Hospital's 9 year perspective. Journal of Emergency Nursing 18(2):104–106

Health and Safety Commission 1991 First aid at work: approved code of practice. HMSO, London

Hinchliff S, Montague S, Watson S 1996 Physiology for nursing practice, 2nd edn. Baillière Tindall, London

Hodgetts T, Kenward G, Vlachonikolis I, Payne S, Castle N 2002 The identification of risk factors for cardiac arrest and formulation of activation criteria to alert a medical emergency team. Resuscitation 54(2):125–131

ILCOR 1997 The ILCOR advisory statements. Resuscitation 34(2):97–149

Innes P A, Summers C A, Boyd I M et al 1993 Audit of paediatric cardiopulmonary resuscitation. Archives of Disease in Childhood 68:487–491

Jackson R J 1984 Blood flow in the cerebral cortex during CPR with dogs. Annals of Emergency Medicine 13:657–659

Jurkovich G J, Pierce B, Pananem L et al 2000 Giving bad news: the family perspective. Journal of Trauma, Injury, Infection and Critical Care 48(5): 865–873

Langhelle A, Sunde K, Wik L et al 2000 Airway pressure with chest compressions versus Heimlich manoeuvre in recently dead adults with complete airway obstruction. Resuscitation 44(2):105–108

Lee S K 1984 Effect of cardiac arrest time on the cortical cerebral blood flow generated by subsequent standard CPR in rabbits. Resuscitation 17(2):105–117

Lee T, Newman L, Crawford R, Paterson J G et al 2002 First aid manual, 8th edn. Dorling Kindersley, London

McKee D R, Wynne G, Evans T R 1994 Student nurses can defibrillate within 90 seconds. Resuscitation 27(1):35–37

Mackenzie G 1964 Haemodynamic effects of external cardiac compression. Lancet i:1342

Meyers T A, Eichorn D J, Guzzetta C E et al 2000 Family presence during invasive procedures and resuscitation: the experience of family members, nurses and physicians. American Journal of Nursing 100(2):32–43

Mullally S 2001 The NHS plan: a guide for nurses, midwives and health visitors. Department of Health, London. Available: http://www.doh.gov.uk/agnmhv/agnmhv.pdf

Nadkarni V, Hazinski M F, Zideman D et al 1997 Paediatric life support. Resuscitation 34(2):115–127

Newbold D 1987 Critical care: the physiology of cardiac massage. Nursing Times 83(25):59–62

Nicol M, Glen S 1999 Clinical skills in nursing: the return of the practical room. MacMillian Press, London

Nursing and Midwifery Council 2002 Code of professional conduct. Nursing and Midwifery Council, London

Parkes C M 1975 Bereavement: studies of grief in adult life, 2nd edn. Penguin, Harmondsworth

Rattrie E 2000 Witnessed resuscitation: good practice or not? Nursing Standard 14(24):32–35

Resuscitation Council (UK) 1997 CPR '97: annual scientific symposium, Brighton, England, April 1997. Resuscitation Council (UK), London

Resuscitation Council (UK) (2000) The 2000 resuscitation guidelines for use in the United Kingdom. Resuscitation Council (UK), London Available: http://www.resus.org.uk

Royal College of Nursing 2002 Witnessing resuscitation. Royal College of Nursing, London

Royal College of Nursing and the British Medical Association 2001 Decisions relating to cardiopulmonary resuscitation. Royal College of Nursing, London

Rennie S 1991 I desperately needed to see my son. British Medical Journal 302:356

Robertson C, Holmberg S 1992 Compression techniques and blood flow during cardiopulmonary resuscitation. Resuscitation 24(2):123–132

Seedhouse D 1988 Ethics: the heart of health care. John Wiley, Chichester

SIDS 2004 Guidelines. Available: http://www.sids.org.uk

Tingle J 1991 First aid law. Nursing Times 87(35):48–49

Tingle J, Cribb A (eds) 2002 Nursing law and ethics, 2nd edn. Blackwell, Oxford

Tucker K J, Idris A 1994 Clinical and laboratory investigations of active compression–decompression cardiopulmonary resuscitation. Resuscitation 28(1):1–7

UK Central Council 1992 Code of professional conduct. UK Central Council, London

UK Central Council 1996 Guidelines for professional practice. UK Central Council, London

Wardrope J, Morris F 1993 European guidelines on resuscitation. British Medical Journal 306:1555–1556

Weisfeldt M L, Kerber R E, McGoldrick R P et al 1995 Public access defibrillation: American Heart Association medical/scientific statement. Circulation 92:2763. Available: http://www.amhrt.org:80/pubs/scipub/statements/1995/21952222html

Wright B 1996 Sudden death: a research base for practice, 2nd edn. Churchill Livingstone, Edinburgh

Wynne G, Kirby S, Cordingly A 1990 No breathing … no pulse. What shall we do? Professional Nurse 5(10):510–513

Zoltie N, Sloan J, Wright B 1994 Observed resuscitation may affect a doctor's performance. British Medical Journal 309:404

Chapter 4

Infection control

Rachel Peto

KEY ISSUES

SUBJECT KNOWLEDGE
- Main groups of microorganisms
- Routes of spread of infection
- Physical and physiological aspects related to infection control
- Infection control in relation to risk
- The influence of behaviour, attitude and culture on the prevention and control of infection
- Epidemiology related to identification and control of infection
- Health promotion

CARE DELIVERY KNOWLEDGE
- Using a problem solving approach to infection control to include assessment, planning, implementation and evaluation
- Universal precautions
- Principles of managing the control of infection to include:
  - handwashing
  - safe management of linen
  - waste and sharps
  - wearing of personal protective equipment
  - aseptic technique
  - personal care

PROFESSIONAL AND ETHICAL KNOWLEDGE
- Professional, ethical and political issues
- The role of the infection control team in hospital and the environmental health team in the community

PERSONAL AND REFLECTIVE KNOWLEDGE
- Four case studies related to the four branches of nursing with decision making exercises to apply subject matter

INTRODUCTION

Infection control, the prevention of spread of disease caused by infection, is fundamental to all nursing care. It is one of the most challenging aspects of care, as it demands both an understanding of the causes, and self-discipline to apply the theoretical knowledge to a variety of practice settings (Gould 1987).

Infectious diseases have been a threat to health and well-being since human life began, with outbreaks of infection over the centuries often generating great fear in people. Although diseases are no longer believed to be a supernatural visit as a punishment for sin, still the fear of infection is deeply rooted in the human mind (Meers et al 1997).

It is only just over a hundred years ago that the science of microbiology was born when the relationship between disease and microorganisms was discovered by Pasteur. But today at the beginning of the 21st century, despite great technological advances such as antibiotics and vaccines, infectious diseases remain a massive global threat accounting for 41% of diseases worldwide (Department of Health 2002), and the chief cause of death (Meers et al 1997).

For the Western world a particular challenge of this century is the increasing numbers of microorganisms becoming resistant to antibiotics. Much media attention has centred on methicillin resistant *Staphylococcus aureus* (MRSA), sometimes described as a 'superbug'. But of equal concern to infection control staff are the increasing cases of antibiotic resistant tuberculosis, as well as outbreaks of hospital and community wide gastrointestinal infections (Lowe 2002).

In Britain major infectious diseases kill only a small number of people compared to the past (70 000 per annum according to the Department of Health 2002). But across the world the diseases of HIV/AIDS, tuberculosis and malaria account for millions of deaths each year (Department of Health 2002).

Central to the concept of infection control is the frequently quoted statement 'Hospitals should do the sick no harm' (Nightingale 1854). One hundred and fifty years on, despite nurses and doctors still being recognized as leading authorities on infection control, one of the major challenges facing health care in Britain today is 'hospital acquired infections' (HAIs). The Second National Prevalence study of infection in hospital (Emmerson et al 1996) showed that between 9% and 10% of patients in hospital will acquire an HAI, a figure very similar to that in the first study (Meers et al 1981).

Conversely, the control of communicable diseases has traditionally been the prerogative of community staff (Worsley et al 1994) and environmental health teams. However, increasing attention needs to be paid to the care and control of infections in the community. This is due to a number of reasons and includes patients being discharged into the community with an HAI, inpatient stays following surgery being shorter, increasing numbers of ill people being cared for in their own homes, and invasive procedures such as minor operations increasingly being performed in health centres and GP surgeries (Mercier 1997, Worsley et al 1994).

Infection control must be a priority for all nurses and should underpin quality clinical practice across all areas of health care (May 2000). With the current challenge to both hospital and community staff of increasing antimicrobial resistance, no longer can healthcare staff rely on treating organisms with antibiotics; instead staff need to concentrate again on the basics – proven infection control procedures.

Therefore nurses of all branches (adult, children's, mental health and learning disabilities) have a role to play with their specific patient or client groups. Whether nursing in an institution (hospital or nursing home) or in the community (individual homes, health centres or shared housing), nurses must recognize the sources and modes of spread of infectious microorganisms and understand how to apply evidence based practice to control infection.

OVERVIEW

This chapter aims to provide you with an understanding of what infection and infection control mean for individual patients and clients (sick or well) and their carers (health professional or informal family and friends), whether this care is in a home or community setting or in a hospital or institution.

Subject knowledge

This section introduces you to the biological aspects of infection through presenting information on the four main groups of microorganisms: bacteria, viruses, fungi, protozoa. Routes, modes of spread and sources of physiological and physical control are discussed.

The complex psychosocial issues related to the control of infection are also considered, with particular reference to the influence of personal and group behaviour, attitude and culture. This section also considers epidemiology and its importance in the identification and control of infection, with particular reference to health promotion.

Care delivery knowledge

A range of nursing practices are explored using a problem solving approach of assessment, planning, implementation and evaluation. Both Universal Precautions and specific practices to prevent and control infection are considered with the aim of enabling you to apply them in practice in whatever branch of nursing you are studying and in a range of practice placements.

Professional and ethical knowledge

Professional accountability is highlighted with specific sections on ethical and political issues. The roles of the infection control team in the hospital and the environmental health team in the community are considered.

Personal and reflective knowledge

The care of individuals who may have an infection or who are particularly susceptible to an infection has important decision making implications for the nurse providing that care. Throughout the chapter there are decision making exercises and suggestions for reflection and portfolio evidence. They are provided to allow you to reflect upon practices you have observed or been involved with while in a clinical placement.

SUBJECT KNOWLEDGE

BIOLOGICAL

CLASSIFICATION OF INFECTIVE AGENTS

An infection is caused by the invasion of a person's immunological defences by the deposition of infective agents called microorganisms within the body tissues. Microorganisms are responsible for approximately half of all known human diseases (Gould 1987). Bacteria, viruses, fungi and protozoa are the four main groups of organisms capable of causing disease (Table 4.1) commonly encountered in the healthcare environment today (Wilson 2001).

Bacteria are the most common cause of HAIs (Ayliffe et al 1999, Meers et al 1997) with viruses considered to be the

---

Evidence based practice

The decline in the death rate from infectious diseases during the 20th century was dramatic (from 369 per 100 000 in 1901 to 9 per 100 000 in 2000). But infectious disease will always remain a major concern to human health – today at the beginning of the 21st century the risks posed by infectious diseases include global travel, climate change, microbial adaptation, human behaviour and impaired immune diseases (Department of Health 2002).

Table 4.1 Common organisms and infections and diseases they cause

Organism	Infections and diseases
Bacteria	
Gram positive	
Staphylococcus aureus	Wound infections, pneumonia, osteomyelitis, food poisoning
Staphylococcus epidermidis	Wound infection, associated with invasive plastic and metal devices, e.g. IV cannulas
Streptococci (group A)	Streptococcal throat, impetigo, rheumatic fever, scarlet fever
Streptococci (group B)	Urinary tract infection, wound infection, meningitis
Streptococcus pneumoniae	Pneumonia, bronchitis, meningitis, otitis media
Enterococci	Urinary tract infection, wound infection
Mycobacterium tuberculosis	Tuberculosis
Clostridium tetani	Tetanus
Clostridium difficile	Diarrhoea, hospital acquired gastrointestinal infections
Listeria	Premature delivery, septicaemia and meningitis in neonates
Gram negative	
Neisseria gonorrhoea	Gonorrhoea, pelvic inflammatory disease, conjunctivitis, infective arthritis
Neisseria meningococcus	Meningococcal septicaemia
Pseudomonas	Wound infections, chest infections
Legionella	Chest infection, legionnaires' disease
Escherichia coli	Wound infections, urinary tract infection, pelvic inflammatory disease
Salmonella	Food poisoning
Acinetobacter	Urinary tract infection, wound infections, respiratory infections
Campylobacter	Diarrhoea, gastroenteritis
Helicobacter pylori	Gastritis, gastric ulcers
Chlamydia	Trachoma, non-specific urethritis in males
Viruses	
Hepatitis A	Infectious hepatitis
Hepatitis B	Serum hepatitis
Hepatitis C	If chronic – liver disease and cirrhosis
Herpes (type 1)	Cold sores, sexually transmitted disease
Herpes (type 2)	Genital lesions
Human immunodeficiency	Acquired immunodeficiency syndrome (AIDS)
Enterovirus	Poliomyelitis
Epstein–Barr	Glandular fever
Virus-like prions	Creutzfeldt–Jakob disease (CJD)
Fungi	
Candida albicans	Vaginal thrush, urinary tract infection
Tinea	Athlete's foot, ringworm
Protozoa	
Trichomonas vaginalis	Sexually transmitted disease in women
Plasmodium falciparum	Malaria
Entamoeba	Amoebic dysentery

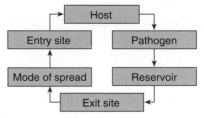

Figure 4.1 Chain of infection.

most common condition in the community, e.g. influenza, common cold (Gould 1987). However, not all microorganisms cause infection or disease. Many live quite harmlessly in soil, water and the air; in cake, alcohol and cheesemaking (yeasts). Some bacteria are vital in the production of antibiotics.

Microorganisms capable of causing disease are called pathogens, but the presence of a pathogen does not necessarily mean that an infection will ensue. The surface of the body is densely populated by a wide variety of microorganisms and every day the intestinal system excretes millions of microorganisms. These pathogens that live on their host in a specific body site without causing harm are called commensals and are often described as the normal flora of the body. They only become pathogenic and cause an infection when transferred to an abnormal body site. For example, *Escherichia coli* lives harmlessly in the gut and aids digestion, but if transferred to an abnormal body site such as a wound or the urinary tract it becomes pathogenic and causes infection and disease. For disease to ensue pathogens need to be able to multiply and to do this a chain or series of events has to take place (Fig. 4.1). Infection control principles are based on disrupting or breaking this chain.

SOURCES OF INFECTION

Bacteria

Bacteria are unicellular organisms that evolved millions of years ago. They are visible under the high magnification of an ordinary light microscope using an appropriate stain. Surrounding the bacterial cell is a membrane made up of proteins and phospholipids and surrounding the membrane is a hard cell wall, which gives the organism its shape.

Bacteria are most commonly classified by their shape (Fig. 4.2), and their response to a laboratory reaction when treated with a dye called Gram's stain. The response is determined by a chemical present in the bacteria's cell wall. Bacteria are termed *gram positive* if they stain blue/purple, and *gram negative* if they fail to take up the stain and remain the red colour of the counterstain.

Wilson (2001) states there are four main groups of bacteria: gram positive cocci and bacilli, and gram negative cocci and bacilli with other important groups including acid-fast bacilli, spirochaetes and atypical bacteria (Table 4.1).

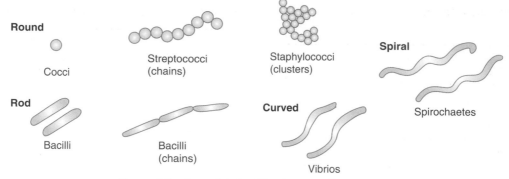

Figure 4.2   Bacterial classification according to shape.

Bacteria can cause a whole range of infections including those of the lungs, wounds, urinary tract and gastrointestinal tract. More detail regarding specific bacteria, including the increasing problem of antibiotic resistance and methods used to prevent the spread of infection are included in the Care Delivery section of this chapter.

Viruses

Viruses are not cells but are minute particles consisting of genetic material and protein. Each virus is a piece of nucleic acid that is protected by a protein coat or lipid membrane. Viruses are not usually defined as a living organism, and instead of growing and dividing like cells, they infect cells. For example the human immunodeficiency virus (HIV) infects human T cells of the immune system, while viruses that cause the common cold attach themselves to the epithelial cell membrane and invade the cell, releasing new virus particles and destroying the host cell. Viruses are extremely small and can only be seen with a high-powered electron microscope. Unlike bacteria, most viruses are very fragile and cannot survive outside a living cell for very long. Viruses are fairly resistant to disinfectants, such as chlorhexadine, which are unable to penetrate the protein coat or lipid membrane.

There are many viruses (Table 4.1), of which a number, primarily those transmitted by blood and body fluid, are of particular importance for nurses and other healthcare workers. They are referred to in some detail within the Care Delivery section of this chapter.

Prions

Prions, virus-like agents, are abnormal proteins that contain no nucleic acid. They are unique among microbes and appear to cause disease by replacing normal proteins on the surface of host cells, and then gradually compromising their function. The main prion disease in humans in the UK is Creutzfeldt–Jakob disease (CJD), although scrapie, a prion disease in sheep, has been known for centuries. CJD is associated with the destruction of brain tissue. Since 1994 there have been cases amongst young people under the age of 30 who have shown unusual neurological symptoms. Latest studies indicate that this is a variant form of CJD (vCJD) which has been linked to exposure to bovine spongioform encephalitis (BSE). Prion proteins are highly resistant to conventional methods of decontamination including heat and many chemical disinfectants.

Fungi

Fungi have a more complicated structure than bacteria and contain a nucleus. They are either branch shaped (e.g. mushrooms) or form buds (e.g. yeasts). There are over 700 000 species but few are pathogenic (Table 4.1).

Candida, the yeast that is responsible for causing thrush, destroys the normal bacteria of the area it infects, namely the mouth, large bowel and vagina. The most common, *C. albicans*, causes vaginal thrush. *Tinea* is a fungus that produces a superficial infection. It is responsible for athlete's foot and causes a painful and irritant rash in the folds of skin, most commonly between the toes. Deeper fungal infections are more common in hot climates.

Protozoa

Protozoa are microscopic single-celled animals (Table 4.1). Although unusual in the UK protozoa are very common in other parts of the world. *Trichomonas vaginalis*, a sexually transmitted infection, causes a foul-smelling, green–yellow vaginal discharge. Malaria, caused by the protozoan *Plasmodium falciparum*, remains an endemic disease in many parts of the African, Indian and Asian continents. Although malaria does not occur in the UK, around 2000 cases a year are seen in people returning from abroad (Wilson 2001). This is partly due to resistance to antimalarial drugs so physical protection is essential, e.g. insect repellents. Neither *Trichomonas* nor malaria pose any risk of cross-infection in hospitals. A third protozoan, *Toxoplasma gondii*, is a parasite that lives in the intestine of cats, cysts of which are released in their faeces. These parasites can remain alive in soil and it is possible for humans to become infected by either handling cat faeces or with contaminated soil. People at particular risk are women in early pregnancy when the infection can cause foetal death or brain damage.

Table 4.2 Environmental requirements to support the growth of organisms

Water	Most organisms require water Bacteria require a moist external environment to thrive and multiply. Spore-forming bacteria can live without water Some organisms die rapidly on drying (e.g. *Candida*, *E. coli*)
Oxygen	Aerobic bacteria require oxygen Anaerobic bacteria require no oxygen to survive, e.g. *Clostridium* Others require it when available, e.g. *Streptococcus*, *Staphylococcus*
Food	All organisms require food, e.g. organic matter – *Clostridium*, undigested food stuffs – *E. coli* Food can include inorganic matter, e.g. bed linen, work surfaces soiled with body secretions
Temperature	Organisms require a certain range of temperature Some can survive in extremes, e.g. some viruses are resistant to boiling water Cold temperature prevents bacterial growth
Light	Organisms can thrive in dark environments, e.g. in body cavities. Ultraviolet light kills some types of bacteria
pH	Acidity determines the viability of organisms Most prefer a slightly alkaline environment with pH 5–8 Some thrive in a high pH, e.g. bacteria in alkaline urine Most organisms cannot tolerate the acid environment of the stomach

GROWTH REQUIREMENTS OF LIVING ORGANISMS

All living organisms require nutrients, water, oxygen, light, temperature and a suitable pH to grow and thrive (Table 4.2). It is necessary to understand the growth requirements of organisms so that infection control measures can be based on scientific principles, not on rituals. For example, most bacteria that cause HAIs are not demanding and will readily multiply in any warm moist environment. Others require no oxygen, such as anaerobic bacteria, and are able to flourish deep in the body with little or no oxygen. Viruses, unlike bacteria, depend on living cells for their replication, and therefore need an environment that will maintain them.

ROUTES OF SPREAD OF INFECTION

All microorganisms have a reservoir where they live and multiply which may be in the environment, a person or an animal. To cause an infection, microorganisms need to find a way to enter the human body, a portal of entry, and in order to spread to another person, then require a way to leave the body, a portal of exit (Table 4.3). Once the microorganisms have left they may spread by a number of different routes.

These routes are categorized into airborne, direct contact and indirect contact (Table 4.4). Some diseases spread by a

Table 4.3 Portals of entry and portals of exit of pathogens

Respiratory tract	Inhalation and exhalation
Gastrointestinal system	Ingestion and excretion
Skin and mucous membranes	Inoculation
Reproductive system	Sexually transmitted
Urinary tract	Sexually transmitted and excretion
Blood	Congenital and trauma

Table 4.4 Routes of spread of infection

Route of spread	Source	Examples
Airborne	Human	Bedding, skin scales, coughing, sneezing, talking
	Aerosols	Nebulizers, humidifiers, showers, cooling towers
	Dust	Sweeping, dusting, building work
Direct contact	Human	Hands, uniform, sexual contact
	Food	Hands, equipment, uncooked food
	Fluids	Disinfectants, antiseptics, blood, body fluids, water
	Insects	Flies, mosquitoes
	Animals	Cows, pigs
Indirect contact	Inanimate objects	Bedpans, bedclothes, needles, washbowls, surgical instruments

specific route, while others might spread by more than one route. For example if you sneeze the tiny droplets from the nose will become airborne, but if you then put your hand up to your nose as you sneeze the droplets will come into contact with your hand. If you did not then wash your hands you could pass it on by indirect contact to the next object you touch. For this reason it is important that all healthcare workers have an understanding of appropriate infection control measures (see Care Delivery section).

The sources of microorganisms causing infections or diseases can be classified as either:

- endogenous (or self-infection) which refers to microorganisms that exist harmlessly in one part of a patient's body, but become pathogenic when transferred to another site

or

- exogenous (or cross-infection) which refers to microorganisms that do not originate from the patient but are transmitted from another source.

The host

The patient or host is the final link in the chain (Fig. 4.1) and is the most common reservoir or source of microorganisms in hospital wards and departments, particularly their body secretions, excretions and skin lesions. A person who acquires microorganisms does not necessarily develop an infection, they may simply act as a source, but be a risk to other susceptible patients. These patients are sometimes called carriers as they carry infections around and transfer them to other patients.

The hepatitis B virus and the meningitis bacterium (*Neisseria meningitidis*) are two examples of microorganisms present in carriers. There are approximately 10% of people who have had the hepatitis B virus in their blood but show no symptoms (Wilson 2001). Similarly many people are unknowingly carriers of *N. meningitidis* bacteria in their respiratory tract; they show no symptoms but can pass the bacteria onto other susceptible people.

Patients may also be carriers of antibiotic resistant microorganisms, such as MRSA, a gram positive coccus. This bacterium is an important cause of infection in both hospitals and the community.

Antimicrobial resistance

Prior to the introduction of antibiotics death from sepsis was common, and until recently many infections could be successfully treated despite the increasing problems of resistance to antibiotics. Whilst few microorganisms show resistance to all antibiotics, three common organisms, methicillin resistant *Staphylococcus aureus*, the tubercle bacilli and vancomycin resistant enterococci, are becoming very difficult to treat (Fielder & Emslie 2001). There are a number of factors that are considered to play a key role in the increasing resistance of antimicrobials, including the uncontrolled sale of and the unnecessary and inappropriate use of antibiotics (Wilson 2001).

Staphylococcus aureus, a gram positive coccus, is an important cause of infection in both hospital and the community. It is responsible for between 30% and 40% of all wound infections (Public Health Laboratory Service 2000). Today, due to this bacterium's remarkable ability to adapt to the presence of antibiotics, approximately 90% of hospital strains and 50% of community strains are resistant to penicillin. In the 1960s methicillin was introduced but because it could only be given parenterally, it was replaced by the oral drug flucloxacillin. Soon afterwards strains of methicillin resistant

Staphylococcus aureus (MRSA) were found. During the 1970s outbreaks of MRSA diminished, but in the early 1980s there were increased outbreaks. In the mid 1980s epidemics in London were reported and since then there have been sporadic outbreaks throughout the UK. Today MRSA occurs worldwide with strains usually resistant to two or more antibiotics.

Enterococci, a normal type of gut commensal, was not until recently a common cause of HAIs. Over the last two decades enterococci have become increasingly resistant to most antibiotics with now only the glycopeptide antibiotics being an effective treatment (Wilson 2001). The most susceptible patients are the seriously ill or immunocompromised, and enterococci are capable of causing septicaemia, endocarditis, urinary tract infections and peritonitis. Outbreaks of this infection show that patient-to-patient transmission occurs with the contaminated hands of healthcare staff being the most probable method of transmission. The environment is also thought to play a part (Weber & Rutala 1997).

Resistance to drugs used to treat tuberculosis (caused by mycobacteria) has occurred since streptomycin was first used in the 1940s. This resistance is due to mutation in single chromosomal genes which occurs spontaneously at a low rate within a population of mycobacteria. Treatment regimes were therefore devised to ensure that a second drug would destroy resistance to the first drug. Today, strains of tuberculosis that are resistance to the two most important drugs, isoniazid and rifampicin, are called multidrug-resistant tuberculosis (MDRTB). These MDRTB are now occurring worldwide due to inadequate supplies of drugs and non-adherence to prescribed therapy. A recent World Health Organization study found that 10% of cases of tuberculosis were resistant to at least one drug (World Health Organization 1997). In the UK, from a relatively low level of 1.6% of cases, there has been a gradual increase in resistant strains during the 1990s (Wilson 2001).

Of particular concern worldwide is the HIV related drug resistant tuberculosis. Here infection is much more likely to become active or a latent infection more likely to reactivate. The poor absorption of drugs and interactions with other drugs makes the treatment of tuberculosis in HIV-positive patients much more complicated.

CONTROLLING THE SPREAD OF INFECTION

Both physiological and physical systems of control can be used in the prevention of infection. For such control the chain of infection (Fig. 4.1) needs to be broken.

Physiological controls

The immune system is the body's physiological control which helps to resist the invasion of microorganisms and protects against foreign material. The first line of defence for the body is the non-specific or passive immune response. This provides anatomical and physical barriers against the

Table 4.5 Non-specific immune response

Route of spread	Source	Examples
Skin	Layers of skin	Mechanical and waterproof barrier
	Sebaceous glands	Secrete sebum – bactericidal properties
		Fatty acid kills bacteria
Eyes	Tears	Lysozyme – digests and destroys bacteria
	Eyelashes	Blinking reflex protects cornea from injury
Mouth	Mucosa	Mechanical barrier
	Saliva	White blood cells destroy bacteria
Stomach	Gastric secretions	High acidity destroys bacteria
Duodenum	Bile	Alkaline pH inhibits bacterial growth
Small intestine	Lymphatic tissue	Destroys bacteria
	Rapid peristalsis	Prevents bacteria from remaining in intestine
Nostrils	Hairs	Trap inhaled particles and microorganisms
	Turbinal bones	Trap inhaled particles and microorganisms
Pharynx and nasopharynx	Tonsils	Lymphoid tissue traps inspired particles
Respiratory tree (except alveoli)	Cilia	Beat mucus and particles away from lungs
	Mucus	Traps particles during inhalation
	Lung tissue	Isolates focus of infection
Vagina	Secretions	Acid pH inhibits bacterial growth
Urethra	Male length	Prevents migration of bacteria to bladder
Urine	Flushing action	Washes away microorganisms

invasion of pathogens with specific body systems playing unique roles (Table 4.5).

The body's specific or active immune response involves innate (non-specific) immunity and acquired immunity. Innate immunity is provided by genetic and cellular factors and can be influenced by age, nutritional status and any underlying disease. Active immunity describes immunity that results when the host develops antibodies following immunization. The active immune system is made up of two types of white blood cells:

- B lymphocytes, which produce antibodies
- T lymphocytes which attack cells invaded by microorganisms.

The lymphocytes have memory cells and if they encounter a particular antigen again they become active and respond by producing large numbers of specific lymphocytes and create an antibody to fight the invading microorganisms.

The body also acquires immunity artificially, through immunizations. Vaccines have been developed since the 19th century, after Edward Jenner demonstrated in 1796 that human beings could be protected from smallpox by inoculation with a similar virus that caused cowpox in cows. Vaccines are given to stimulate the production of antibodies; this induces a specific immune response, but without causing the actual disease.

The ability for people to resist and fight infection varies widely and can depend upon many factors, e.g. age, nutritional status and previous exposure to vaccinations. Young children with an immature immune system and the elderly with a diminished immune response are both at particular risk.

Physical stress from disease or major surgery are also recognized as important factors when assessing a patient's individual risk of acquiring an infection. Today there are increasing numbers of patients who have or are recovering from illnesses that have caused them to become immunocompromised. They are therefore at much greater risk of acquiring infections. Patients include those with HIV/AIDS, patients who have had an organ transplant, have received chemotherapy for cancer, or had large amounts of antibiotics when very young.

Physical controls

Physical sources of control, cleaning, disinfection and sterilization are very important in the prevention and control of infection. Inadequate decontamination has been cited as being responsible for outbreaks of infection in hospital (Wilson 2001).

Choice of a method of decontamination depends on the level of risk the item poses as a source of infection and whether the item will tolerate the method of decontamination (Wilson 2001). Many hospitals now have decontamination polices as part of their infection control procedures. The emergence of HIV has focused particular attention on the potential of medical equipment to transmit infection. To minimize risk, UK government and EU regulations, concerning the reuse of all medical devices (Plowes 1995), came into effect in January 1995.

CONTROL IN RELATION TO RISK

The decision as to whether an item requires cleaning, disinfection or sterilization depends upon whether it carries a low, medium or high risk of causing infection to the patient or client.

Low risk

For equipment or practices that are considered low risk, cleaning, that is the physical removal of microorganisms and organic matter on which they thrive (Ayliffe et al 1999), may be sufficient to control the microorganism population and so prevent the transfer of infection (Table 4.6). There are two methods of cleaning: dry and wet (Table 4.6). After cleaning, any article should have fewer microorganism on it. The dry method, however, might simply redistribute the microorganisms into the air, while the wet method may distribute and increase the microorganisms through the use of contaminated articles such as mop heads and cloths or contaminated water.

Table 4.6   Physical systems of infection control

Low risk Cleaning	Dry	Mechanical action to loosen and remove large particles but may increase airborne count of bacteria up to tenfold Does not remove stains Sweeping redisperses bacteria in dust and larger particles Dry mops may be specifically treated to attract and retain dust particles Vacuum cleaning should not increase airborne counts of bacteria Expelled air from machine should not blow dust from uncleaned surfaces back into the air Dry dusting increases the air count of dust and bacteria and recontaminates cleaned surfaces
	Wet	Water containing detergents or solvents to dissolve adherent dirt and dust Dispersal of microorganisms into the air is less likely Cleaning fluids may grow bacteria due to contamination Damp dusting is less likely to disperse bacteria into air Need to rinse after cleaning with detergent to prevent build-up of detergent film All surfaces need to be dry before use to prevent contamination from bacterial growth
Medium risk Disinfection	Heat	80°C for 1 minute or 65°C for 10 minutes kills vegetative organisms Steam heat is most effective, e.g. autoclave Damage relates to time and temperature Disinfection at a lower temperature for a longer time is possible for heat-sensitive equipment
	Chemical	Phenolics, e.g. Stericol, Hycolin, widely used for disinfecting inanimate objects Not active against bacterial spores or some viruses Toxic, unsuitable for living tissue until thoroughly rinsed Chemicals should not be used for food preparation or storage surfaces Hypochlorites (bleach) e.g. Milton, Sanichlor, mainly used for environmental disinfection, active against many microorganisms including viruses May corrode metals and bleach fabrics Chlorhexidine is used clinically, should not be used to disinfect inanimate objects Active against gram positive cocci (*S. aureus*), less active against bacilli and spores, little virucidal activity Inactivated in the presence of soap Alcohol (70% ethyl or 60% isopropyl) is rapidly active against vegetative bacteria, poor sporicidal Acts rapidly – useful surface disinfectant for physically clean surfaces, e.g. trolley tops, injection sites, hands Evaporates rapidly to leave a dry clean surface Peracetic acid (Nucidex) rapidly kills bacteria, fungi and viruses within 10 minutes. Has a strong smell and needs to be used in an area with exhaust ventilation Goggles and gloves should be worn No adverse health effects known
High risk Sterilization	Heat	Autoclaves sterilize using moist heat – steam at an increased pressure (134°C) for 3 minutes Suitable for most metal instruments, plastics, glass, fabrics Sterilizing ovens use dry heat, 160°C, for 45 minutes, 190°C for 60 minutes Heat distortion can occur, materials may become brittle or scorched
	Gas	Ethylene oxide is very toxic and requires careful control of temperature, humidity, gas concentration and pressure Used to sterilize manufactured goods
	Chemicals	Used when heat or other methods are not possible or reliable sterilization is difficult Grease, proteins (blood, tissue) or air will prevent fluids coming into contact with all surfaces Prolonged immersion times are required to kill bacterial spores
	Irradiation	Gamma rays are used industrially, e.g. for disposable plastics after packaging Repeated irradiation causes plastics to become brittle Is expensive and uneconomical to use in hospital

Evidence based practice

In 1847 Ignaz Semmelweiss (cited Parker 1990) scientifically proved the importance of antiseptic handwashing as a means of reducing hospital acquired infections. While working as an assistant obstetrician in Vienna he made the connection that putrid material causes infection. He collected and presented data that showed a much higher mortality rate when the women were delivered by physicians, compared to when delivered by a midwife. He observed that when the medical students carried out a postmortem and then immediately afterwards carried out a delivery in the obstetric ward that the women had a much higher incidence of puerperal fever. After introducing a chlorinated lime solution for use between the postmortem room and ward, Semmelweiss saw the death rate drop from 18% in April 1847 to just 2% in August (Parker 1990).

Wilson (2001) states that approximately 80% of microorganisms are removed during the cleaning procedure, but indicates that drying is equally important to prevent any remaining bacteria from multiplying. Whilst cleaning alone may be an adequate method of decontamination, it is also an essential preparation for items requiring disinfection or sterilization.

Medium risk

Disinfection, the destruction of vegetative microorganisms to a level unlikely to cause infection, reduces the number of viable microorganisms, but may not inactivate some bacterial spores (Ayliffe et al 1999). It is usually associated with equipment that may come in close contact with mucous membranes but not used for invasive procedures (Table 4.6). Pathogens remaining after disinfection may pose an infection risk to particularly susceptible patients, for example those receiving cytotoxic therapy.

The two main methods of disinfection are heat and chemicals (Table 4.6). Heat is the preferred method for disinfecting articles (e.g. surgical instruments) as it is more penetrative and easier to control than chemicals. Disinfection by chemicals may be required if heat is unsuitable, for example skin disinfection or for items that are heat sensitive such as fibreoptic endoscopes. The choice is therefore a complex matter and requires a working knowledge of the disinfectants available and the make-up of the article that requires disinfecting (Table 4.6).

High risk

Sterilization is the complete destruction or removal of all living microorganisms including bacterial spores (Ayliffe et al 1999). It involves the use of either heat (dry or moist),

gas, chemicals or irradiation (Table 4.6). Items requiring sterilization are described as being high risk to patients. It is recommended for all instruments and equipment used during invasive procedures (for example intravenous (IV) cannulas, surgical instruments, urinary catheters). As with disinfection the choice of method used depends upon the item being sterilized (Table 4.6).

OTHER METHODS OF INFECTION CONTROL

Other methods of control that are very important in the prevention of cross-infection between patient and healthcare worker include hand hygiene, waste disposal and personal hygiene. These will be discussed in detail in the Care Delivery section.

Decision making exercise

Identify some of the equipment you have used for moving and handling patients, e.g. sliding sheets, hoist slings.

- Do you consider these to be low, medium or high risk in terms of transmission of infection?
- How were they cleaned?
- Were they cleaned between patients?

Individual susceptibility to infection

Individual susceptibility varies enormously and can be caused when a person's immunity is impaired. Particular groups of patients are known to be at a greater risk (Table 4.7). It is now acknowledged that around one in 11 hospital patients at any one time has an infection caught in hospital (HAI) (National Audit Office 2000). These are infections that are 'neither presenting nor incubating when a patient enters hospital'. The cost to the National Health Service is approximately £1000 million per year (National Audit Office 2000). Whilst it is acknowledged that not all HAIs are preventable, it is stated that around 30% could be avoided through the better use of existing knowledge and the application of realistic infection control practices (National Audit Office 2000).

Table 4.7   Patients at greatest risk of infections

Group	Examples
Extremes of age	Very young and elderly
Critically ill	Patients in intensive care, multiple injuries
Chronically sick	Patients with heart and respiratory disease
Surgical patients	Abdominal surgery, trauma
Patients with underlying diseases	Patients with diabetes mellitus, malignancy
Immunosuppressed	Patients on steroids or chemotherapy; transplant patients

Although hospital patients are considered to be at an increased risk due to cross-infection between staff and patients, individuals in the community, for example in their own home, still remain at risk from many of the same risk factors as patients in hospital. The most common examples are wound infections and urinary infections whilst catheterized.

It is important to recognize not only the causal relationship and influence of physical sources and controls of infection and disease, but also the complex psychosocial issues that can be involved.

PSYCHOSOCIAL

BEHAVIOUR

Behaviour is influenced by personal beliefs and attitudes and is now recognized as one of the many determinants of disease (O'Boyle Williams 1995, Payne & Horn 1996). In the past disease and infections were normally perceived as being outside an individual's own control. For example, 100 years ago dirty water was associated with infections and diseases such as cholera, but was perceived to be the responsibility of the government and country (Parker 1990). Today many psychological, social and emotional factors are acknowledged as being particular influences, with the relationship between individuals and their lifestyles recognized as potential causes of infection and disease (O'Boyle Williams 1995).

Self-induced behaviour is an area of concern to infection control teams, as particular individuals or groups have an increased risk of disease and infection because of such behaviour or lifestyle. The intravenous drug user sharing needles and the prostitute having unprotected sex, both of whom have an increased risk of contracting HIV and AIDS, may be a first consideration. However, many other groups and individuals also have a particular risk of developing life-threatening diseases and are often ignorant or unaware of them, for example, people living in communal or shared accommodation.

Such individuals or groups may never become hospital patients through being exposed to infection as their bodies may be able to cope and fight the invasion of microorganisms or they may respond to treatment given in the community. Nevertheless some people need protecting and so infection control management needs to reach out to the community in a form that is relevant and appropriate to the particular at-risk groups or individuals.

An important aspect of health behaviour, for both staff and clients/patients alike, is compliance, the extent to which behaviour coincides with medical or health advice (Ogden 1996). For staff an example where compliance is known to be poor is in the practice of handwashing: despite staff knowing and understanding the importance of handwashing, they often fail to carry it out (Larson et al 1997).

Parents of babies and young children need to know and understand the importance of immunizations and to be able to attend the clinics. An area where change in health behaviour has occurred amongst parents has been over the issue of whether the combined mumps, measles and rubella (MMR) vaccination increases the risk of autism. This decrease in uptake of the triple vaccine has already shown an increase in numbers of reported measles cases. Parents also need to be listened to when social customs and religious practices conflict with the education that is being put forward by the health visitor.

People with mental health problems such as depression may not need hospitalization, but may have poor motivation and self-esteem, and little desire to care for themselves. This can result in food poisoning as a result of being unable or incapable of storing, preparing and cooking food adequately, and fungal and bacterial infections of the skin as a result of poor personal hygiene.

The carer of a person with a learning disability might need to take extra care and attention to ensure that behaviour and practices do not increase the risk of infection.

Reflection and portfolio evidence

Reflect upon a placement where you have cared for a person with a learning disability.

Observe how any basic infection control practices such as handwashing before meals and after using the toilet were encouraged and carried out.

- In what ways did staff teach and encourage the clients to undertake such practices?
- If such basic infection control practices were not carried out, how might you go about implementing them in a similar practice setting?
- Record your findings and ideas in your portfolio.

CULTURAL BEHAVIOUR

Behaviour adopted by particular ethnic, cultural and religious groups can put them at a greater risk of infection and disease. Examples include the eating of raw or undercooked foods by some Far East cultures, the prohibition of contraceptives including condoms by religious groups, and the non-seeking of treatment by men because it is considered unmanly or weak (O'Boyle Williams 1995).

Occupation might also increase the risk of infections and diseases, for example those who have worked in a coal mine or with asbestos have a greatly increased risk of developing chest infections and life-disabling and life-threatening lung diseases in later life.

Smoking as a cultural behaviour has over the years received a great deal of attention in the media regarding its effect on the smoker's health as well as on those who are in close contact with the smoker. For example, babies and children who live with parents who smoke have a greater risk of developing respiratory tract infections (Beeber 1996).

Behaviour, attitudes and practices do change, but this can only happen by influencing individuals and groups. This might be by education in the form of knowledge and understanding, by observation of people, peer groups and organizations, and from outside influences. During the 1980s, mass media education about safe sexual practices resulted in a dramatic reduction of HIV infections among homosexual men, although numbers among heterosexuals did similarly decline. The outcome of past behaviour is now known to take many years, for example the recent increase in numbers of cases of hepatitis C dates from 1960s behaviour, i.e. the sharing of needles to take drugs.

Certain customs and rituals, despite being considered infection control risks, are still widespread among particular cultural groups. Some examples are the practice of religious circumcisions on Jewish baby boys in their own homes and female circumcisions of young and teenage girls from certain African, Arabian and Far Eastern countries. Reasons for undertaking such practices include medical, economic, sexual, cultural and religious ones (Stewart 1997). Again the media have highlighted these practices as being dangerous and an infection risk. With regard to the practice of female circumcision, attitudes and behaviour are changing, with groups of women fighting for this practice to stop. Yet despite being illegal in Britain and Europe, female circumcision continues to be widely practised in many cultures (Cameron & Rawlings-Anderson 2001). The women argue that only by education and raising the awareness of the inherent dangers of such surgery among their own cultural groups will this practice be eradicated.

Evidence based practice

The lack of basic knowledge and development of complacent attitudes is said to be the cause of a re-emergence of syphilis in Manchester amongst gay men. A study showed a worrying level of co-infection with HIV, with a low level of knowledge of sexual partners' HIV status (Clark et al in Department of Health 2002).

EPIDEMIOLOGY

The term epidemiology can be defined as 'the study of things that happen to people' (Wilson 2001: 29), and is often used to describe the study of disease and ill health in human populations. Incidence and distribution of disease can be assessed to provide data for the control and eradication of disease. Epidemiological studies can be small (micro) or large (macro) scale. They involve determining an understanding of how infections and disease spread and who may be at risk or susceptible to the infection (Wilson 2001). Risk factors might be physical, for example infective organisms, or psychosocial, for example behavioural, such as smoking or eating raw food. The risk to the individual is partly determined by estimating the experience of the whole population.

In epidemiology whole populations are studied to determine the risk of disease occurring. By surveillance it is possible to gather facts and details of specific diseases. To measure the occurrence of a disease within a population two rates are commonly used: a prevalence rate, which measures the number of infections present at a particular time, and an incidence rate which measures the number of new infections that occur in a population. Within a population a disease that is always present at a static level is described as endemic, but if the disease is at significant increase above its normal endemic level, it is described as being an epidemic.

Epidemiologists provide healthcare workers with data to enable planning of the particular health needs and services of a community. A common infection associated with seasonal epidemics is influenza, which usually occurs amongst the elderly and those who have a diminished immunity. By monitoring influenza rates among the population as a whole, it is possible to discern early signs of an outbreak.

Outbreaks of infections are common in both institutional and community care. However, whereas an outbreak of an infection in a hospital ward or nursing home is usually on a micro scale, outbreaks of infections in the community are usually on a macro scale, at times involving hundreds of people. The influenza virus is a common cause of a macro scale infection. In a bid to try and control influenza epidemics, people over the age of 65 years and those considered at particular risk are offered free influenza immunizations.

Whilst major infectious disease outbreaks across the world are often linked to local water supplies, e.g. cholera in Tanzania in 1998, others are due to the increase in international travel and migration of populations, which makes spread to other countries inevitable (Department of Health 2002). For example, the outbreak of meningitis at the Mecca pilgrimage in 2000 was caused by a strain uncommon to the UK. When the pilgrims returned to their local communities in the UK, the disease spread to others with no known direct link to the pilgrimage (Department of Health 2002).

HEALTH PROMOTION

Health promotion is an important aspect of infection control. This can be on a small scale, such as teaching a group of ward staff, or large scale, involving large groups or entire communities. Specific groups and individuals have already been noted in this chapter as being at particular risk from infections due to their behaviours, attitudes and beliefs. For these people, health promotion attempts to prevent and control infection either to themselves or to others. The attitudes and behaviours of the health professionals carrying out such health promotion are important. Whether it is meeting a group of drug addicts to discuss the risk of sharing needles or talking to a particular cultural or religious group about child immunizations, health professionals need to be aware of their own personal beliefs, traditions and practices. Often health professionals who are not specifically specialized in infection control nursing are involved. For example, promoting the importance of immunizing babies to prevent and control potential life-threatening diseases is usually undertaken

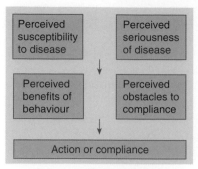

Figure 4.3   Four predictors of health belief.

by health visitors, while community psychiatric nurses usually advise drug addicts about the importance of using sterile needles and not sharing them with others.

Within health promotion there needs to be a combination of prevention, education and protection, and in the area of infection control all three aspects are influenced by personal beliefs and attitudes. The health professional needs an understanding of the influences that have an effect on a person or group's behaviour and attitude towards health education. An example referred to earlier is of a recent study which raised concerns about a potential link between the combined MMR vaccine and autism. The media seemed to grasp this topic readily and for this reason parents are confused by the conflicting advice given by different health professionals. For example, some general practitioners are readily offering the MMR by three separate injections, whilst others still give the combined vaccine.

Health behavioural models have been cited as theoretical descriptions of interactions that influence health behaviour (O'Boyle Williams 1995). There are a number of theories and models surrounding the subject of health behaviour. One model, the *health belief* model, has had major influences on health education and proposes that four predictors of health exist (O'Boyle Williams 1995) (Fig. 4.3).

Returning to the earlier example in which a community of elderly is offered an influenza immunization, the health belief model can be used in the health education and promotion of such protection. For example, the nurse assesses an elderly person's perception of the seriousness of influenza and his or her likelihood of catching it. The nurse can then help the elderly person see the benefits and constraints of the proposed immunization.

The aim of this section has been to enable you to examine and consider some the important biological and psychosocial aspects of infection control. You should by now be more aware of the relevance of the sciences surrounding infection control so that you can apply them to the more practical nursing issues examined in the next section.

CARE DELIVERY KNOWLEDGE

The prevention and control of infection is largely founded on nursing practice, which in itself must be grounded on sound research based knowledge. To help the healthcare professional there are hundreds of articles available from a broad range of journals on the subject of infection control. Many are research studies into particular infection control practices, for example handwashing (Taylor 1978a, b), the wearing of plastic aprons (Callaghan 1998), and the purchase and use of gloves (Ross 1999).

USING A PROBLEM SOLVING APPROACH TO INFECTION CONTROL

However, although there are numerous articles on specific nursing practices associated with infection control, such practices are often based on ritual rather than evidence (Ward 2000a). For over 20 years nurses have used a problem solving approach to the planning and organization of individualized nursing care (Kratz 1979), the *nursing process*, a principle still held up today by Ayliffe et al (1999). They maintain that assessing infection risk to each individual patient should be part of the overall assessment of the patient, stating that 'it is too easy to neglect infection amongst the many other priorities' (Ayliffe et al 1999: 84).

Therefore as infection control is a part of nursing practice, it seems only right that this section, Care Delivery Knowledge, uses a problem solving approach. The four stages – assessment, planning, implementation and evaluation – will be used to present the nursing knowledge and practice for infection control.

Assessment

Part of assessment is to gather information, to analyse it and to determine actual and potential problems. In the area of infection control, the two terms *clinical audit* and *surveillance* have become synonymous with assessment. Whilst visits by infection control nurses to clinical areas might be to assess the needs of specific patients or to undertake surveillance of an outbreak of a specific infection, all healthcare workers are involved with clinical audit by assessing and monitoring their patients and clinical practices.

Each individual patient needs to be assessed to determine whether they pose an infection risk to other patients or whether other patients increase the risk of infection to them (Ayliffe et al 1999). For an individual with an infection, an assessment requires an in-depth analysis of both the source of the infection and the individuals and carers at risk. Such assessments need to be routinely and systematically undertaken. By knowing the factors that increase the risk of infection to either the individual or carer, plans can be made to prevent and control the infection and appropriate nursing actions can be undertaken before an infection occurs.

The source of infection may be determined by knowing the site of infection, the organism involved and the mode or route of spread. This allows an assessment of the degree of risk and the planning and immediate initiation of preventive measures

Reflection and portfolio evidence

Consider a client with whom you have been involved in providing care. Reflecting upon this client's specific health problems:

- Assess the general and specific risk factors for infection (see Table 4.8) that you think apply. For example, an elderly patient with an infected pressure sore might have general factors such as age and malnutrition, and specific factors such as diabetes mellitus.
- Record your finding in your portfolio.

Table 4.8 General and specific risk factors for infection

General	Specific
Age of patient	Type of invasive procedure
General health	Present medication
General hygiene	Surgery
Mental state	Pressure sores
Nutrition	
Mobility	
Continence	

such as isolation of the patient or wearing protective clothing (e.g. gloves) before touching the patient or infected site. The individual and carer may both be at risk from an infection and therefore the degree of risk to both must be assessed. The risk can be considered as high, medium or low. There are general and specific risk factors that can indicate the severity of risk (Table 4.8). From these, measures can be instigated to prevent and control the infection or cross-infection.

For an institution or a particular environment an audit is carried out on a regular basis to provide a formal check to ensure that infection control measures are being routinely adhered to in areas involved in patient care. For example, during an audit of a hospital ward all areas would be inspected, both the clinical areas such as the treatment room and more indirect areas such as the ward kitchen. Both areas would be checked for general cleanliness and specific infection control measures. For example, the availability and correct use of a sharps bin would be audited in the treatment room, while the presence and correct use of a food refrigerator thermometer would be looked for in the kitchen. It is the results of such clinical audits and surveillances of HAI (Emmerson et al 1996) that have led to the development of national evidence based guidelines (Pratt et al 2001), discussed further under the section on Implementation.

Planning

Once the risks to the individual and carer have been identified, goals of care and specific nursing measures can be planned. Planning can only commence when the organism, site of infection and mode of spread have all been identified. The goals of care can be divided into those that will control, reduce and prevent self-infection (endogenous) and those that will prevent cross-infection (exogenous). This stage might also include the planning of the working environment through architectural design. For example the design of new wards and departments needs to ensure that wash-hand basins are sited in appropriate places. However, literature indicates that this planning still falls short of the mark with studies citing the lack of sinks and inappropriate and inaccessible location of wash-hand basins as one of the factors that reduce nurses' compliance with handwashing (Ward 2000b).

Planning also involves prioritizing goals of care. As the patient's condition improves or deteriorates, priorities may change. Common goals of care include prevention of exposure to an infectious organism, control of the extent of an infection, maintenance of resistance to an infection and understanding of infection control practices (Heath 1994).

Implementation

Implementation involves the use of appropriate infection control practices to reduce the risk of cross-infection and self-infection. This needs not only to be related to the requirements of each individual patient but also to include all others who might also be at risk: family, friends, and all healthcare personnel. Infection control practices will not necessarily be the same for each patient. Even when the same measures are implemented for several patients, priorities of measures may differ, but to apply unnecessary measures is considered to be a waste of time (Ayliffe et al 1999).

Safe practice should ensure that the chain of infection (Fig. 4.1) is broken, thereby preventing the transmission of pathogens to potential sites of infection. Reservoirs of infection can be eliminated, sites of entry and exit controlled, and modes of spread minimized by actions such as safe disposal of body fluids, wearing protective garments, effective handwashing and aseptic procedures.

In order to ensure that the most effective and safe practices are implemented, it is vital that all practitioners embrace the use of evidence based practice. Despite the wealth of infection control articles there has often been little or no evidence to support or refute certain infection control practices. Therefore it is imperative that nurses, due to the often close and intimate patient care given, integrate the best available evidence which must include both clinical experience and judgement.

The EPIC project (Pratt et al 2001) provides such evidence. This document, commissioned by the Department of Health, contains national evidence based principles of good practice to enable hospitals to incorporate these into their local policies and protocols. It is hoped that the implementation of evidence based guidelines will have an impact on reducing HAIs. The EPIC project includes guidelines for six specific standards:

1. Hospital environmental hygiene.
2. Hand hygiene.
3. The use of personal protective equipment.
4. The safe use of sharps.
5. Guidelines for preventing infections associated with the use of short-term indwelling urethral catheters in acute care.
6. Guidelines for preventing infections associated with the insertion and maintenance of central venous catheters.

Treatment of an infection requires elimination of infectious organisms. Although the doctor prescribes an antibiotic drug, once the causative organism has been identified, the nurse must assess the progress of infection and ensure that complications are prevented. Nursing actions include prevention of dehydration caused by a fever associated with the infection, ensuring that a drug is given aseptically, and observations for potential drug allergies.

Controlling self-infection and cross-infection is a complex task involving practices that individually or collectively control the risk of patients/carers infecting themselves by direct or indirect contact. Implementation of practices requires both adequate resources and clear communication between the patient and all those involved with their care. It is therefore important that the patient and all those who visit, either socially or professionally, are kept well informed of infection control practices being undertaken.

UNIVERSAL PRECAUTIONS

In recent years the concept of a comprehensive approach to infection control that promotes the use of safe practices to ensure protection to everyone from blood borne infections has been advocated (Wilson 2001). Called *Universal Precautions*, it embraces the notion that all blood and body fluids are potentially infectious and therefore such practices are to be used with all patients at all times, regardless of whether they are known to have a blood or body fluid infection. The impetus for the introduction of Universal Precautions began in the USA as a result of the problems of identifying individuals with HIV infection (Ayliffe et al 1999).

Reflection and portfolio evidence

In relation to the practice of Universal Precautions, reflect upon a recent placement, and some specific patients you were involved with caring for.

- Consider the rationale for when you wore gloves, a plastic apron, eye protection, or undertook the antiseptic method of handwashing.
- Decide which of these practices were undertaken to prevent you from becoming infected and which were to prevent the patient from getting an infection.
- Record your finding in your portfolio.

Universal infection control precautions have been identified as explicit policies for handwashing, skin abrasions, sharps, protective clothing, spillage and waste (Nursing Standard 1997, Royal College of Nursing 2000). These practices are applied to all patients in all healthcare settings whenever there is contact with blood and body fluids rather than only being introduced when staff consider the patient to be a high risk. One argument for implementing such precautions is that they not only protect staff from known diseases, but also protect against those that are as yet unknown.

Resistance to Universal Precautions has been both cultural and financial (Ayliffe et al 1999). In 1997 the Royal College of Nursing issued guidance regarding Universal Precautions (Nursing Standard 1997) and since then hospitals have produced their own policies to deal with blood and body fluids. Today the concept of Universal Precautions is widely accepted being used both in hospital and community (Ayliffe et al 1999).

PRINCIPLES OF INFECTION CONTROL

It is now widely acknowledged that a number of specific practices are instrumental or contribute to the control of self-infection and cross-infection and should be undertaken by all healthcare workers when caring for patients and clients in hospitals, clinics, surgeries or the home. They are:

- hand hygiene
- safe management of linen, waste and sharps
- wearing of personal protective equipment
- aseptic technique
- personal care.

Hand hygiene

The important role of handwashing in the transmission of disease was demonstrated most convincingly 150 years ago (Semmelweiss 1847, cited in Parker 1999a), and still remains today the most important technique in the prevention of cross-infection (Ayliffe et al 1999). Laboratory studies and clinical trials on handwashing have repeatedly shown that it is the most important factor in reducing HAIs (National Audit Office 2000), with many hospital infections being spread via the unwashed hands of staff (Ward 2000b). Hand hygiene is one of the six standard principles in the national evidence based guidelines (Pratt et al 2001).

The aim of handwashing is to reduce the number of bacteria to a level below that needed to establish infection when transferred to a susceptible patient. The precise number of bacteria needed is not known, but factors such as the virulence of the bacteria, the health and age of the patient, and any disruption to the body's natural defence to infection (for example from catheters, intravenous lines) affects the outcome. It has been known for over 60 years that there are two categories of bacteria on hands: transient bacteria and resident bacteria (Price 1938). Thorough handwashing with soap removes the transient bacteria, but the resident bacteria found deep in the crevices of skin and under nails persist

and are only removed after prolonged handwashing using an antiseptic (Gould 1994a). The aim of handwashing is to remove dirt and/or substantially reduce the number of organisms present on hands (Horton 1995), which are so easily transferable from hands of staff to patients (Gilmour & Hughes 1997). In particular the important role of handwashing after nappy changing and toilet use with young children and babies has been found to reduce the spread of enteric infections in day care nurseries (Worsley et al 1994).

Decision making exercise

When next out on a clinical placement watch and take note of how often you and other members of staff wash their hands.

- Note down what you had done or were about to do that made the handwashing necessary; try to determine whether the handwash was to protect yourself or to protect the patient.
- Watch the handwashing technique used – is it a quick wash or does the person take their time and ensure that they washed all the surfaces of their hands?
- What handwash solution was used and how were the hands dried?

Despite much research all highlighting the importance of handwashing and the availability of national and local guidelines, the message appears to have a limited effect (Scott 2000). Although education might seem an essential part of infection control, it is considered not enough to enhance good practice. Elliott (1996) considers that handwashing practice is strongly influenced by colleagues and role models. It is also widely accepted that there are many other factors that influence frequency of handwashing (Table 4.9). Handwashing should be carried out every time a healthcare worker moves from one patient to another, and even between performing different procedures on the same patient.

Table 4.9	Factors that influence handwashing
Products	Lack of soap
	Irritation caused by soap and towels
	Not liking soap or handrub
	Harsh products
	Hard or harsh non-absorbent towels
Facilities	Lack of handwash basins
	Inaccesible handwash basins
	Antiquated facilities
	Lack of mixer taps
	Extremes of water temperature
	Number and position of sinks and soap dispensers
Time/staff	Too busy
	Not enough time
	Not enough staff

Table 4.10   Methods of handwashing

Type	Methods	Use
Social (to remove dirt and transient organisms)	Use liquid soap and thoroughly wash with soap and water and dry with paper towel	Before: starting work, eating and drinking, feeding a patient, leaving work After: visiting the toilet, helping a patient with toiletting, handling patients and bedlinen, cleaning equipment and furniture, between each patient
Antiseptic (to remove or destroy all or most transient organisms)	Use antiseptic soap or detergent, e.g. chlorhexidine, and either thorough wash with antiseptic and water, dry with paper towel (a sterile towel may be required), or apply 5–10 mL of alcohol handrub, ensure all areas of hands and fingers in good contact with rub, and leave to dry naturally	Before: any procedure involving high-risk patients, all procedures requiring an aseptic technique, e.g. dressing, catheterization After: contact with infected patients, handling contaminated equipment and materials
Surgical (to remove or destroy transient organisms and reduce detachable resident organsims – a prolonged effect is required)	Either antiseptic soap (e.g. chlorhexidine) and water. Brush nails, wash hands and forearms for a minimum of 3 minutes, dry with a sterile towel Alternatively wash hands with soap and water and after applying minimum of 5 mL application of an alcohol handrub (as above)	Before surgery and aseptic techniques for invasive procedures.

Methods of handwashing

The method of handwashing is determined by the type of procedure to be undertaken, the handwashing agent, length of handwash and method of hand drying. Table 4.10 gives a summary of the three categories of handwashing: social, antiseptic and surgical. The procedure must include a thorough and effective technique (Fig. 4.4), ensuring that all surfaces of the hands and wrists come into contact with the washing solution (Ayliffe et al 1999).

Salisbury (1997) comments on the safe wearing of wedding rings and found that healthcare workers who wear rings had a higher bacterial count on their hands than those with no ring. Parker (1999a) recommends that the wearing of rings should be limited to wedding rings; Bernthal (1997) suggests there is insufficient evidence to conclude that wearing a ring does not put patients at risk of infections.

Length of handwash

The ideal duration of a handwash has not been determined. Times of 30 seconds (Bowell 1992) and 15–20 seconds for the whole procedure (Ayliffe et al 1999) are suggested. Gould (1994a) suggests a time of 20–30 seconds as ideal and Sprunt et al (1973, cited in Wilson 2001) suggests that even a brief wash of 10 seconds using soap and water removes the majority of transient bacteria. Ayliffe et al (1999) state that the thoroughness of application is more important than the time spent on washing or the agent used.

Handwashing agent

The type of handwashing agent is important and as Table 4.10 shows depends upon the method of handwashing being undertaken. When using soap or a medicated agent the

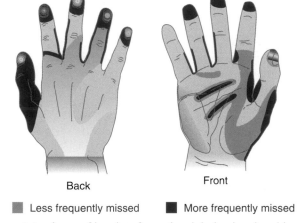

Back   Front

■ Less frequently missed   ■ More frequently missed

Figure 4.4   Areas of hand surface missed during handwashing.

mechanical action of using running water is just as important. Although the use of soap and water has been found to be sufficient for removing most transient bacteria, bar soap must not be used in clinical areas as it provides an ideal environment for the growth of microorganisms (Nursing Standard 2001). Studies have demonstrated that alcohol solutions are the most effective in reducing bacterial counts and that chlorhexadine has a residual effect in that it continues to destroy microorganisms for some time after initial application (Gilmour & Hughes 1997). Hoffman & Wilson (1994) found that one of the prime considerations to ensure handwashing took place was the selection of an acceptable handwash preparation.

Hand drying

Thorough drying after handwashing is an important part of the procedure (Wilson 2001) and plays a significant role in the control of infection (Gould 1994b). Wet hands are both

Evidence based practice

In the USA McGuckin et al (1997) developed a patient education behavioural model to increase handwashing compliance and empowering patients with responsibility for their care. This involved ongoing handwash education, and monitoring compliance of handwashing by monitoring soap/paper towel usage, additional time, staff or costs compared with potential savings of preventing HAIs. Patients in the study were asked to ask all healthcare workers carers who were to going to give direct care 'Did you wash your hands?' This study showed an increase in handwashing by at least 34% and stated that a 300-bed hospital with 10 000 admissions yearly could save over $50 000 a year. This same study was performed in one medical and one surgical ward in Oxford, with 39 patients participating. The study stated that it increased handwashing by 50% and that healthcare workers washed their hands more with surgical patients than medical (McGuckin et al 2001).

an important medium for growth and a more efficient transfer of microorganisms than dry ones (Gould 1987, 1994a). Four methods of hand-drying are commonly available:

- hand towels
- roller towels
- paper towels
- warm-air hand dryers.

Redway et al (1994) recommend the use of paper towels as being the most thorough and effective method for hand drying in clinical areas. They have a particularly important role when less effective hand decontamination agents have been used, especially following a less thorough handwash (Gould 1994b). The use of paper towels, although disliked because of their roughness, is considered to be the most effective and most appropriate method in clinical areas (Ward 2000b). Blackmore & Prisk (1984) showed cloth towels to be slightly more efficient at removing bacteria, but paper towels were found to be safer to use because they are single-use items. For cloth towels to be as safe as paper towels, they need to be used once and laundered after each use. Weiler (1965, cited in Blackmore 1987) considered warm-air dryers to be less safe than paper towels because, although they initially reduced bacteria, bacteria being fanned around in the current of warm air quickly contaminated the hands again. Two more recent studies (Knight et al 1993, Redway et al 1994) both support this, suggesting that warm-air dryers can increase the bacterial count by over 50% and increase the bacterial contamination of the local environment.

Recontamination

Hands can become recontaminated both during and following the procedure. During the procedure the dispenser containing the liquid soap can cause contamination (Bowell 1992); therefore it is recommended that soap dispensers should have disposable cartridges and be wall mounted to allow them to be elbow or foot operated (Kerr 1998). If refilling a soap dispenser is the only option, then the Infection Control Nurses Association (1998) recommends that containers are thoroughly cleaned before refilling.

Following the procedure hands can become recontaminated if a dirty surface (such as the waste bin) is touched when throwing the towel away. It is therefore important to have foot pedal-operated bins to dispose of paper towels (Ward 2000b) and healthcare workers need to be compliant in the correct use of these bins.

Alcohol handrubs

Alcohol handrubs are now recognized as a useful and effective alternative to a handwash in that they can be quickly applied without the need for either a handwash basin or hand drying equipment. However, if hands are visibly dirty then handrubs are not to be used (Pratt et al 2001). They appear to reduce skin damage and suppress regrowth of resident bacteria. Supporting the use of alcohol handrubs, a study by Bellamy et al (1993) found that alcohol preparations were more effective than both soap and water and antiseptic soap solutions in removing rotavirus from hands.

Handrubs have been found to be particularly useful where hands have to be frequently washed such as outside isolation rooms and in intensive care units (Wilson 2001) or where access to handwashing facilities may be difficult such as in a patient's own home.

SAFE MANAGEMENT OF WASTE, SHARPS AND LINEN

Clinical waste

Each year hospitals produce thousands of tons of waste (Gibbs 1990). Some, termed household rubbish, can be disposed of at a local council waste or landfill site. However, much is termed clinical waste and must be incinerated. It is imperative that all rubbish is disposed of safely and correctly to ensure that neither health carers nor clients are at risk of causing infection or becoming infected themselves. The disposal of clinical waste is an important issue wherever care is provided for clients. In the community it is becoming an increasing problem as more clients receive nursing care in their own home.

Wilson (2001) and Gibbs (1991) have defined clinical waste as including:

- blood, other body fluids, excretions
- soiled surgical dressings, swabs and instruments
- material other than linen from infectious disease cases
- all human and animal tissue
- discarded syringes, needles, broken glass
- drugs and pharmaceutical products

- waste arising from medical and nursing practice, e.g. used disposable bedpan liners, urine containers, incontinence pads, sanitary pads

In the hospital, clinical material is normally divided into three categories: rubbish (disposed into a refuse bag), sharps and soiled linen. Following the lifting of Crown Immunity in 1988, all NHS premises must comply with legislation and regulations regarding waste disposal. The Environment Protection Act 1990 requires the producers of waste to manage it safely and transfer it only to an authorized person. The Health Services Advisory Committee (1999) requires all waste to be discarded into an appropriately coloured bag with yellow for clinical waste and black for domestic (nonclinical) rubbish. From January 2002 all waste transported off a hospital site is required to be enclosed in an approved rigid container (Health Services Advisory Committee 1999).

Decision making exercise

When you are next out on a clinical placement carry out a brief audit to determine the safety of handling and disposal of sharps and clinical waste.

- Sharps – note down where sharps boxes were placed, note how full they were and find out how sharps boxes are disposed of.
- Sharps – were you aware of any special precautions taken in areas where there were particularly vulnerable patients or clients, e.g. children?
- Clinical waste – were the correct disposal bags used?
- For clinical waste – were there black bags in the kitchen and yellow bags in the clinical areas?
- If after carrying out this audit you decide that there are unsafe practices taking place, who might you speak to about it?

All blood spillages may expose healthcare workers to bloodborne viruses and other pathogens and therefore it is recommended that a hypochlorite solution containing a high concentration of chlorine releasing compounds is used, especially for large spills of blood (Wilson 2001). Chlorine releasing granules that absorb and contain the spill are preferable to a liquid that adds to the volume of spillage. In the home, thick bleaches are recommended. For large acidic spillages, such as urine, chlorine based products should not be used as they release a chlorine vapour (Department of Health 1990). Again where large spills of blood occur, for example in an operating theatre, it may be impractical to treat it using a hypochlorite, therefore it is recommended that the spill is soaked up using paper towels discarded into a yellow waste bag, and the area cleaned up with detergent and water.

Disposal of waste in the home is different with the patient or family usually being able to discard waste with their normal household waste. Healthcare workers who produce waste in the home are obliged under the Health and Safety

at Work Act 1974 to transport and dispose of clinical waste safely. Local authorities have a legal obligation to provide a collection service for infectious waste if requested.

Reflection and portfolio evidence

Think about a placement that has involved you visiting a client's home.

Identify the different types of clinical waste that were produced, e.g. wound dressings.

- Record in your portfolio the practices undertaken for disposing of clinical waste – were they disposed of by the nurse or the client?
- If by the client, were there any special arrangements made for their disposal with the council ? For example, some health authorities organize special collections of clinical waste such as colostomy bags.

Handling and disposal of sharps

Sharps are all items that may cause laceration or puncture and include needles, scalpels and broken glass (Wilson 2001). Their disposal must be into a yellow sharps container that conforms to the British Standard for sharps containers (British Standards Institute 1990). Needlestick injuries account for 16% of occupational injuries with resheathing considered to be responsible for 33% of injuries (Wilson 2001). But obtaining accurate figures for sharps injuries is difficult because many go unreported (National Audit Office 1999), therefore the actual number of injuries is considered to be far higher.

National guidelines for safe practice are included within the EPIC guidelines (Pratt et al 2001). The disposal of all sharps is the personal responsibility of the user; all sharps should be discarded into the sharps bin at the point of use (Pratt et al 2001). It is imperative that all staff, irrespective of the care setting, undertake a risk assessment and implement a clear written policy. Under the Health and Safety at Work Act 1974 all care workers have a responsibility to prevent injury to others, and this must include the safe disposal of sharps. Studies show that many of the injuries taking place could be prevented.

All sharps policies should include guidelines about:

- handling of used needles (e.g. not resheathing)
- care and handling of the sharps box (e.g. not overfilling, correct method of closure)
- disposal of the box
- what to do in the event of a needlestick injury (e.g. encouraging bleeding from the puncture site, washing the area, covering with a waterproof dressing, documenting the incident and informing the manager and occupational health).

Treatment of all sharps injuries must always be followed up properly. Although the risk of acquiring HIV following a percutaneous injury is very small (the Public Health Laboratory Service (1999) states that in the UK four healthcare workers have acquired HIV since the early 1980s), it is imperative that all staff seek guidance from their Occupational Health unit or local Accident and Emergency department as soon as possible. The role of Occupational Health units will be discussed later in this section under Personal Care.

Linen

The regulations surrounding the handling and washing of laundry in hospitals are based on Department of Health guidance (National Health Service Executive 1995) which requires hospital linen to be categorized using a national colour code for laundry bags and standards in the laundry for heat disinfection (Wilson 2001). In order to minimize the risk of cross-infection to workers who handle linen, the guidance states that infected linen should be sealed in a white water-soluble or soluble-stitched bag and placed in a red outer bag. This means that the handlers can then place the water-soluble bag directly in the washing-machine without opening it. However, not only do linen bags carry a risk of cross-contamination from pathogens, but they have also been found to contain more than just linen. Taylor (1992) reported a range of material found in linen bags, including surgical instruments, watches, patients' glasses and cutlery.

Requirements for water temperature vary between hospital and home. In hospitals the washing process must ensure that the temperature reaches 71°C for 3 minutes or 65°C for 10 minutes, whilst in the home the hot wash of a domestic washing machine is acceptable (normally 60°C) (UK Health Departments 1998).

PERSONAL PROTECTIVE EQUIPMENT

Protective equipment is used in the control and prevention of infection and should be worn by all healthcare workers when in direct contact with body fluids, to protect either the skin or mucous membranes. A risk assessment needs to be undertaken with the equipment selected depending upon the specific practice or activity and the anticipated risk of exposure (Pratt et al 2001). For example a nursing activity where there is no direct contact with blood or body fluids, such as taking a pulse or blood pressure, would not require the use of protective clothing. Conversely, an activity that may result in the contamination of hands or uniform, such as helping a patient with a commode or emptying a catheter drainage bag, would require the use of gloves and a plastic apron. It must be remembered that the use of protective equipment must not be considered in isolation to other practices, and in particular to handwashing.

Under the Personal Protective Equipment at Work Regulations (Health and Safety Commission 1992) all employers must ensure that protective clothing is available, and under the Health and Safety at Work Act 1974, such protective clothing should be worn.

Protective clothing is worn by healthcare workers to prevent:

- the user's clothing or uniform from becoming contaminated (soiled, wet or stained) with pathogenic organisms
- the transfer of pathogenic organisms to another person or inanimate object
- the user from acquiring an infection from the patient or client.

The most common items of protection include gloves, plastic aprons, masks and eye protectors, with disposable gloves and plastic aprons both the most popular and most effective items (Bowell 1993, Wilson 1990). However, if worn incorrectly (e.g. if a plastic apron is not changed between patients) they can become vehicles of infection instead of preventing infection (Bowell 1993). Other protective clothing such as shoes, hats and gowns are generally restricted to use within operating theatres and isolation units.

Although the use of protective clothing may be important, it must not be forgotten that such protection can be very alarming to the public. Therefore care needs to be taken in explaining the rationale for protective clothing to both the client and their relatives.

In examining the usefulness of the nurse's uniform as a means of protective clothing, Schwarze (1986) found that uniforms were associated with the spread of infection. Recent research found that nurses' uniforms are heavily contaminated at all times of the working day and that plastic aprons do not appear to alter the bacterial contamination of the uniform (Callaghan 1998). Previous studies had argued that personal clothing is acceptable as long as it is practical, clean and washable (Walker & Donaldson 1993).

Gloves

Gloves have been identified as being a very important barrier in two directions: in protecting the patient and in protecting staff from patient pathogens. Gloves are, however, not a substitute for handwashing, which should always be carried out following their removal (Ayliffe et al 1999). To prevent transmission of infection, gloves must be discarded after each procedure, even if procedures are on the same patient. It is therefore imperative that gloves are worn for:

- any practice that involves the handling of blood and body fluids, including procedures such as the emptying of urinary catheter bags and the handling of dirty linen, soiled dressings, colostomy bags and incontinence pads
- any aseptic invasive procedure.

The quality and effectiveness of disposable gloves vary widely. A knowledge of the different types – plastic, latex, vinyl, sterile and unsterile – is important so that the user selects the most appropriate glove according to the level of risk of the contaminant and task being performed. Gloves are provided both as sterile and unsterile, but do not need to be sterile unless for use in a sterile body site or other invasive procedure (Wilson 2001).

When wearing gloves Brookes (1994) cites the following six recommendations:

- use high-quality gloves
- choose the right glove for the job
- wash hands after removing one pair and putting on a new pair
- never reuse gloves
- change gloves when a defect is noticed
- keep fingernails short to avoid punctures.

The actual technique or procedure for putting on sterile gloves is quite complex, but very important, especially before a surgical procedure (e.g. in the operating theatre). If when putting on the gloves the wearer accidentally touches a surface that is not sterile, the outside of the gloves, which will later be in direct contact with sterile instruments and body tissues, will have become contaminated, and a vehicle of infection. The scrubbing up procedure, which lasts several minutes, would have become a futile exercise (Brookes 1994). For this reason gloves are put on in such a way that the outside of the glove never comes into contact with the hand being put inside the glove. For although the hand has been washed using an antiseptic for several minutes it will not be as sterile as the glove itself, which has undergone a very strict sterilizing procedure. In order to fully understand this quite complex procedure, watch a qualified practitioner working in an operating theatre putting on sterile gloves or a video that clearly demonstrates this practice.

Latex allergy

Since the introduction of Universal Precautions in the 1980s glove usage has increased considerably with a corresponding increase in reports of latex allergies (Clancy et al 2001). Common symptoms include itchy skin rashes, itching eyes and nose, wheezing and asthma. People with other allergies such as hay fever may be more sensitive to latex. Latex-free gloves must be available and should be used by staff who show symptoms of latex allergy. They should also attend an occupational health unit for further advice.

Aprons

Aprons have been cited as an important and effective item in the prevention of cross-infection (Curran 1991, Nursing Times 1995, Worsley et al 1994).The cotton apron, once a common feature of the nurse's uniform, fails to provide an effective barrier to organisms and offers no protection to the user against moisture and wetness (Worsley et al 1994). Disposable plastic aprons are therefore considered to be the apron of choice as they are impervious to both moisture and organisms and cheap to use. As with gloves, aprons can become a vehicle of infection if not used correctly. It is therefore recognized that the apron must be changed between patients where there is direct patient contact or contact with body fluids (Nursing Standard 2001).

Curran (1991) recommends that an apron is changed after:

- bedmaking
- total patient care
- aseptic technique
- toileting patients
- dirty tasks
- feeding patients and giving meals.

An apron should be used for only one patient and then be disposed of; the nurse's hands should then be washed and a new apron put on before attending to a new patient (Curran 1991). It is now recommended that the disposable apron worn during the serving and distributing of food should be a different colour to that worn for other purposes (Bowell 1993, Callaghan 1998).

Masks

Masks are rarely worn today outside the operating theatre with research questioning whether they need to be worn in many situations, including operating theatres (Worsley et al 1994). Previous rationale for wearing a mask was to protect the patient from getting an infection from the staff; however, there is little evidence to show that wearing a mask reduces surgical wound infection (McCluskey 1996). If a member of staff has a cold or sore throat the mask is inappropriate as the member of staff should not be on duty. Today the main rationale for wearing a mask is to protect the user from splashes of blood and body fluids onto mucous membranes of the mouth (Mangram et al 1999). Close fitting masks are recommended for use when caring for patients with open tuberculosis (Wilson 2001).

Eye protection

Eye protection should always be worn for any activity where there is a risk of blood splashing onto the face

---

Evidence based practice

Callaghan (1998) undertook a study to examine the hypothesis that wearing a plastic apron during direct patient care would significantly reduce the number of bacteria on a nurse's uniform in order to reduce the probability of the transmission of nosocomial infections. The study concluded that nurses are wearing uniforms which are heavily contaminated with a variety of bacteria and that the current use of plastic aprons does not prevent bacterial contamination of uniforms. The data did not support the commonly held perception that bacteria do not adhere to plastic. This study showed that nurses relied on the use of plastic aprons to keep their uniforms uncontaminated and consequently nurses wore their uniforms for more than one day.

(Pearson 2000). Special glasses, goggles or visors may be used in the operating theatre, and during obstetrical procedures, dentistry and endoscopy. Eye guards also offer protection against splashes of the chemicals that are used in the sterilization and disinfection of endoscopes and other surgical instruments (Worsley et al 1994).

Other protective clothing

Other items of protective clothing have traditionally involved the wearing of gowns, hats and overshoes. Studies show that hats and overshoes are of little use in the prevention of infection (Humphries et al 1991, Worsley et al 1994) and may even assist in the spread of infection.

Gowns

Gowns are mostly used in the operating theatre and delivery suite where the risk of potential contamination from blood and blood products is very high. Those made from cotton are not water repellent and when wet provide very little protection from infection (Callaghan 1998). A plastic apron worn under the gown will give protection. Increasingly, gowns made from fabrics such as Gortex are being used as they provide the necessary waterproof protection and can be laundered but have the side effect of being uncomfortably warm to wear.

Reflection and portfolio evidence

Consider any placements where you have cared for children and where they had to be nursed using protective clothing.

- Were there any strategies used to make the children less frightened? For example, were teddies and dolls dressed up in similar gowns and hats as those worn by the nurses?

Think back to the clothing the children had to wear to go to the operating theatre.

- Were the children required to wear an operating gown? If they were, were they more child-friendly perhaps by being decorated with pictures?
- If they were allowed to wear their own clothes, do you think this made an infection risk?
- Record your thoughts and answers in your portfolio.

Hats

Hats seem to be 'something of a white elephant' (Lee 1988). Nurses have traditionally worn hats, with some still considering them to be linked to hygiene and a method of keeping hair tidy (Lee 1988). The same study showed that hats are frequently touched during practice and are infrequently changed, leading Lee to believe that it is time the old ritual of wearing a hat was forgotten. However, hats are still worn in the operating theatre department where they remain an important infection control measure (Mangram et al 1999).

Overshoes

Overshoes are similarly considered unnecessary in the prevention of infection. Traditionally all visitors entering operating theatre departments and other units caring for immunocompromised patients put on a pair of paper or plastic overshoes. Whilst Humphries et al (1991) showed that there is little advantage in putting on overshoes, Weightman & Banfield (1994) concluded that disposable overshoes are unnecessary and found no evidence to suggest that the wearing of them helped decrease bacterial counts on the operating room floor. Ayliffe et al (1999) cite a study where an outbreak of *Pseudomonas* in a renal unit was linked to hands contaminated during the putting on of overshoes.

ASEPTIC TECHNIQUE

Aseptic technique aims to prevent microorganisms on hands, equipment and surfaces from being introduced to susceptible body sites (Wilson 2001). Two examples of where an aseptic procedure is required are urinary catheterization and setting up an intravenous infusion. The method and equipment for a specific procedure varies from hospital to hospital and health authority to health authority, but the principles of asepsis remain, in that the particular procedure will be undertaken in such a way that organisms will not be introduced into the treatment site.

In the past aseptic procedures have been based on much routine and ritual rather than on research or evidence based practice (Wilson 2001). For example, all wounds were strictly cared for using an aseptic procedure. Today evidence indicates that all wounds need to be assessed on an individual basis and that for some patients, wound cleansing can be a modified aseptic or 'clean' procedure using tap water (Blunt 2001, Hollinworth & Kingston 1998). There continues to be much debate and discussion over other rituals, such as whether routine cleaning of trolleys between patients is required. Thompson & Bullock (1992) argue that it serves no useful purpose. However, when an aseptic procedure is required, then certain principles must be upheld and it is then arguable whether one method or approach is any better than another.

The principles should include:

- suitable handwashing
- use of sterile packs, equipment and solutions
- the appropriate use of gloves
- maintenance of asepsis – not introducing infection
- a sterile field throughout the procedure.

Decision making exercise

Observe a practice that requires the use of an aseptic technique. Consider the principles stated in the section on aseptic technique and decide whether they were upheld.

- For example, which handwash procedure was undertaken? At the end of the observation decide whether any of the principles were breached, for example did the nurse touch something that was not sterile, such as the trolley?
- Consider the consequences in relation to infection control.

In addition to the maintenance of an aseptic technique while carrying out the procedure, it is important that the site (e.g. a surgical wound, intravenous cannula or urinary catheter) is cared for to prevent the entry or exit of infection. For example, the use of a clear film occlusive dressing over an intravenous cannula allows examination of the site without removing the dressing (Dougherty 2000), while placing a catheter bag below the level of the patient's bladder ensures there is no backflow of urine and infection that could result from this is avoided (Pratt et al 2001).

PERSONAL CARE

Attention to personal care and health is very important in the prevention of infection. Staff carrying an infection may increase the risk to specific patients. Although all patients may be at risk, the very young, the very old and the acutely ill are at particular risk. Occupational Health departments have a vital role in infection control (Mercier 1997) and liaise closely with both hospital and community infection control teams. The specific role of Occupational Health staff is focused on protecting individual staff, but all healthcare staff need to co-operate in achieving a safe and healthy working environment.

Transmission of infection between staff and patients is well recognized (Mercier 1997) with one of the main roles of Occupational Health departments being to provide staff with advice and support. One of the commonest infections frequently passed between staff and patients is gastrointestinal, usually with symptoms of diarrhoea and vomiting. A community outbreak of *E. coli* 0157 in Scotland in 1997 demonstrated this risk of cross-infection where nursing staff in the affected nursing homes became *E. coli* 0157 positive (Callaghan 1998). It is vital that staff seek advice from the Occupational Health department, as staff with symptoms of diarrhoea and vomiting must not return to work until symptom free for 48 hours.

Healthcare workers may also be symptom-free carriers of infection, e.g. MRSA, hepatitis virus B and C. In the past staff have been implicated in outbreaks of MRSA (Mercier 1997), and therefore if a healthcare worker has any suspicions that they have been infected or might be a carrier, it is imperative

that they seek advice. Occupational health staff are able to provide confidential, professional advice, specialist support and counselling. Under the *Professional Code of Conduct* (Nursing and Midwifery Council 2002), registered nurses are personally accountable for their own practice to protect and support the health of individual patients.

Personal care must also include the care of any uniform worn while caring for patients and clients. Uniforms should never be worn when off duty and ideally staff should remove their uniform before leaving their place of work and wear their own clothes to travel to and from home. Callgahan (1998) considers home laundry to be insufficient and recommends that uniforms be changed daily and washed in a hospital laundry where a temperature of 60°C should be available. This study into the bacterial contamination of nurses' uniforms confirmed that the hospital laundry could ensure that uniforms were sterile at the end of the laundry cycle, but despite staff in the study having access to the on-site laundry, only 30.6% of staff changed their uniform daily.

Care of skin, particularly that of hands, is another very important aspect of personal care for all healthcare staff. Particular attention must be paid to any breaks in the skin of hands which may be in direct contact with the patient. Waterproof dressings should always be used to cover all cuts, abrasions and lesions. Staff with dermatological conditions that cause areas of skin to become broken should assess very carefully whether they are putting themselves at risk from contamination with blood and body fluids. Such staff should seek advice from the Occupational Health department.

Bloodborne infections continue to cause much concern amongst healthcare staff, the three high risk infections being hepatitis B, hepatitis C and HIV. Under European law employers are required to offer free hepatitis B vaccinations to all clinical staff at risk from infection (Rogers et al 1999). It is vitally important that the full course of vaccinations is completed and the blood levels of immunity are checked following the course. For a few people full immunity is not achieved and again Occupational Health departments need to be involved to provide ongoing help and advice regarding increased levels of risk due to reduced immunity status.

EVALUATION

Evaluation is the final stage in a problem solving approach and involves measuring the effectiveness of nursing care. Like assessment, evaluation also involves the collection of information. However, whereas information collected during assessment is of a general nature, the data collected during the evaluation stage are more specific and often linked to a specific patient goal. Therefore data collected during evaluation can only be collected after the care has been planned and the nursing actions undertaken.

Many methods of evaluation are used to decide whether the nursing care given is assisting patients in their recovery. For example the measurement of temperature can be used to find out whether the nursing care is effective for the patient with a raised temperature caused by an infection. Measuring the overall effectiveness of infection control practices has become a very important aspect of care. Often called surveillance, research shows that data collection, analysis and feedback of results is central to detecting infections, dealing with them and ultimately reducing infection rates (National Audit Office 2000). As part of the requirements of the Controls Assurance Unit (see Ch. 2) clinical audits of infection control measures are becoming standard practice in many hospitals in the UK.

PROFESSIONAL AND ETHICAL KNOWLEDGE

PROFESSIONAL ISSUES

Professional issues are clearly stated in the *Code of Professional Conduct* (Nursing and Midwifery Council 2002) with every registered nurse, midwife and health visitor personally accountable for their own practice. When used in the context of infection control sections of the code show that nurses have several areas of direct responsibility:

- co-operate with others in the team (section 4)
- maintain professional knowledge and competence (section 6)
- act to identify and minimize the risk to patients and clients (section 8).

In the control of infection, nurses have the responsibility to educate and inform others, including both the patient and their family (Nursing Times 1995). Nurses have to demonstrate a wide range of infection control practices as well as the knowledge to enhance a patient's general or specific resistance to infection. Professional responsibility requires the nurse to remain up to date with new practices, which are often made clear through guidelines, policies and legislation. Legislation laid down in the Health and Safety at Work Act 1974 states that while the employer has responsibility to ensure protective clothing is available for use, all employees have a personal responsibility to use and wear the protective clothing provided.

Interprofessional working is important in order that all members of the team adhere to evidence based good quality practices. Policies and guidelines should be up to date and easily accessible to the team. They require regular monitoring and management to ensure that they are current and in line with new national and European legislation. The National Audit Office (2000) report into hospital acquired infections in acute NHS Trusts in England raised great concerns over this important area of practice, with the report finding a lack of infection control policies, and stated that 'written policies and procedures need to be more widely available and accessible' (National Audit Office 2000: 6). The report recommended that a national infection control manual be provided by the Department of Health (as in Scotland) with local 'add-ons'.

A further area of personal responsibility is that of self-care. All healthcare workers should ensure that they are self-protected from infections through immunizations and know where they can get advice and guidelines regarding practice. For example immunization against hepatitis B is widely available from occupational health units, thereby allowing staff who are at risk from contamination with blood to receive protection. A second area of self-care results when a member of staff has been in contact with an infection, and although not detrimental to themselves, may be detrimental to other patients who are already ill. For example, staff in contact with MRSA may be required to ensure they have not been infected themselves before moving to another ward or area of care.

Acting as an advocate, particularly for vulnerable groups, is an issue that many nurses need to uphold in the area of infection control. Some patients and clients may be particularly vulnerable to infections, but be unaware of the issue themselves. In this situation the nurse must be able to speak up on behalf of their patient or client and ensure that the care being given will not put the individual or group at risk from getting an infection. For example, a child or a person with a learning disability may not recognize the importance of washing hands after using the toilet or before eating a meal. Therefore the carer needs to ensure that this is done, thereby protecting the patient or client from a gastrointestinal infection.

ETHICAL ISSUES

Personal care by nurses to prevent infection is also an ethical issue. The declaration of personal health status by nurses and other healthcare workers is an important debatable ethical issue. On the one hand by not declaring a particular illness, a nurse could be putting a patient at risk from an infection. For example, if a nurse is known to be HIV positive and is applying for a job in a critical care unit such as the operating department, it might be argued by some that the nurse is potentially putting patients and staff at risk. Others would argue that as long as the nurse is aware of the importance of the potential causes of cross-contamination of blood and blood products and upholds good infection control practices, patients and staff would not be at risk.

Occupational Health units have the responsibility to ensure that all staff employed are free from illness and infection, and nurses have an ethical responsibility to provide an honest health declaration. However, this will inevitably mean that for a minority of staff it might be difficult to secure a job because of a specific condition.

Confidentiality is an ethical issue in infection control for staff and patients. A patient with an infection may wish to keep it confidential and not inform family and friends. However, the ethical debate over whether the patient is putting those they come into close contact with at risk requires examination. As in the previous paragraph, this is commonly seen with HIV infection or in other sexually transmitted diseases. Such a patient may demand that their condition is kept confidential, but the potential risk of infecting those they come into close contact with, such as a sexual partner or carers, needs to be assessed.

Reflection and portfolio evidence

Spend a few moments reflecting upon situations in clinical areas where you felt there was actually or could potentially have been a professional dilemma.

- For example, did you think there were any times when there was a dilemma over confidentiality, a time when a patient's diagnosis was discussed within hearing distance of other patients?
- For example, was there a situation when you felt the health and safety of a patient or staff member was at risk?
- Record your finding in your portfolio and perhaps find an opportunity to discuss them with a qualified member of staff.

Nurses have to recognize and accept that patients have the right to confidentiality over their health. Section 5 in the *Code of Professional Conduct* (Nursing and Midwifery Council 2002) states that all registered nurses, midwives and health visitors must protect confidential information and requires one 'to seek patients' and clients' wishes regarding the sharing of information with family and others'. However, this same section also states that disclosure may only be made where public interest or the law (by order of a court) is justified. This issue of confidentiality is very difficult to resolve, and in the area of infection control there will remain many areas requiring ethical and professional debate.

POLITICAL ISSUES

Infection control has become a very large and important item on the political agenda, particularly in relation to HAIs and the uncleanliness of hospital wards. Over the last 30 years within the framework of the Health and Safety at Work Act 1974 the government has legislated that healthcare professionals implement a range of policies and regulations, central to these being infection control policies.

Hospitals and other acute nursing service areas are often required to uphold local guidelines and policies to ensure that national legislation on infection control is maintained. For example, the disposal of clinical waste is required to adhere to not only national guidelines regarding the colour coding of bags for clinical waste, but also local policies dealing with the safe handling of rubbish bags and disposal to the incinerator (Health Services Advisory Committee 1999).

Despite greatly increased legislation governing working practices in hospitals and the government stressing the importance of infection control and basic hygiene, complaints about lack of hospital and ward cleanliness have increased

(Parker 1999b). Hospital cleanliness is closely associated with HAIs and new guidelines, the first for over 20 years, were published in 1999. The *Standards for Environmental Cleanliness in Hospitals* (Infection Control Nurses Association and Association of Domestic Management 1999) was the result of collaboration between several interested parties including the Department of Health, but led by the ICNA and the Association of Domestic Management.

Policies and guidelines can be considered expensive, and for this reason managers may disregard or only partially implement them. However, with the introduction in 1998 of a new framework for the NHS (Department of Health 1998), which placed a much greater emphasis on the provision of a high quality service, NHS Trusts have a much greater responsibility to ensure clinical audit and risk reduction strategies are in place, and that evidence based practice is implemented. Developing effective audit systems through the Clinical Governance framework has greatly improved compliance in the instigation and ongoing management of safe practice (see Ch. 2).

Reflection and portfolio evidence

When out in clinical practice look for the policies and guidelines appropriate to health and safety, and in particular to infection control, for example the policy on the emptying of a catheter bag.

- Select a particular policy and notice when it was last updated. If it was more than 5 years ago, carry out a brief literature search of recent studies in the same subject area.
- Try to identify whether in the light of specific research particular changes need to be made to the policy.
- If you think there should be changes, consider who you might approach about this. Consider how you might tackle this issue as a qualified nurse.
- Record your findings, thoughts and ideas in your portfolio.

Political pressure is also evident through recommendations arising from the publication of two key documents, *The Management of Hospital Acquired Infections in Acute Trusts in England* (National Audit Office 2000) and *Getting Ahead of the Curve* (Department of Health 2002). Both documents clearly identify the national and global threat and enormous financial implications of infectious diseases. The Department of Health (2002) document sets out an infectious diseases strategy for England, one of the pledges already referred to in the government White Paper *Saving Lives: Our Healthier Nation* (Department of Health 1999a).

Immunization programmes are also commonly subjected to political pressure and media coverage. On the one hand government is encouraging the uptake of this important but expensive infection control measure, both for the elderly and the very young. On the other hand, the safety of certain immunizations (e.g. the MMR triple vaccine and its alleged link with autism) has been questioned. Some parents, without clear guidelines and understanding of what constitutes safer practice, might see the government sponsored health promotion campaigns for immunizations for all babies as part of a political agenda.

The policy agenda continues to provide specific national targets for infection control. Following on from the *Health of the Nation* document (Department of Health 1992), with its targets to be met by the year 2000, the more recent White Paper, *Saving Lives: Our Healthier Nation* (Department of Health 1999a), sets similar targets to be reached by the year 2010. These include: the establishment of a new Public Health Development Fund and a Public Health Observatory in each NHS region.

Other areas of infection control are also subject to mandatory national standards to ensure the environment is safe for the total population. For example, the control of sewage, the provision of clean safe water, and the removal of household rubbish and waste are all central to a clean environment. However, the provision of these services is also determined by finance. Even though central to the control of infection for individuals and large populations, they require large financial input by local and national government. The cost of infection, if an outbreak of disease occurred due to widespread water contamination, would be enormous. It is politically and ethically correct that such environmental control on water contamination is maintained and monitored regularly for compliance.

ROLE OF THE INFECTION CONTROL TEAM

Infection control teams under the overall leadership of the Department of Health are important at national, regional and local level both in hospitals and the community. At national level there is the Public Health Laboratory Service and its Communicable Diseases Surveillance Centre which provide policy expertise and investigate outbreaks of infection and epidemics. At regional level Directors of Public Health co-ordinate health protection activities. At local level health and local authorities work together to address infections and diseases in the community with hospital based teams dealing with HAIs (Department of Health 2002).

A hospital infection control team has traditionally been made up of an infection control doctor, usually a microbiologist, an infection control nurse(s) and other members of staff with a special interest and knowledge of infection control. In 1995 the Department of Health issued guidance giving NHS Trust executives overall responsibility for ensuring the provision of effective infection control arrangements (Department of Health 1995). But although the National Audit Office (2001) report praised the work of hospital infection control staff it criticized the lack of involvement of NHS Trust chiefs, with few chief executives being members of their Hospital Infection Control Committee. It also suggested that chief executives may be unaware of the extent and cost of HAIs. The report also identified that there are currently no departmental guidelines on infection control staffing, which has led to wide variations in the ratio of infection control nurses to beds.

Interprofessional team working is a very important aspect of infection control, particularly between nurses and doctors (Greatrex 2001). To encourage team working some hospitals have ward- and department-based nurses who have a specific interest in infection control and are able to provide a very important link between the ward and infection control team in the education of staff and upholding good practice at clinical level.

A crucial aspect of infection control in both hospitals and community is that of surveillance in order to anticipate and prevent disease trends. Infection control has consistently hit the headlines over the last few years, but such political and national interest and directives have now begun to give infection control surveillance more publicity. In 1996 the Nosocomial Infection National Surveillance Scheme was launched, in response to 1995 Department of Health guidance which required infection control teams to carry out targeted, selective surveillance. The scheme aims to provide practical help and leadership for infection control teams.

Both the National Audit Office (2001) report and the Department of Health (2002) strategy recognize the important role of surveillance and the failure of the previous systems. The 2002 document stated that in the past much infection had gone unreported or undernotified so there is an incomplete picture of both the size and nature of the threat to health from infectious diseases. The 2002 strategy identified 10 key changes including a new National Infection Control and Health Protection Agency, a national expert panel to assess the threat from new and emerging infectious diseases, and stronger professional education and training programmes.

ENVIRONMENTAL HEALTH

Infection control is also concerned with environmental health, cited by the World Health Organization in 1950 as 'the control of all factors in the environment which exercise a harmful effect on human physical development, health and survival' (Worsley et al 1994: 85).

In England the mandatory enforcement of environmental health is a function of local government with qualified environmental health officers and technical support staff. Environmental health, as in the notification of communicable diseases, is a role for all healthcare professionals. While it is the doctor who is legally responsible for notifying particular communicable diseases, much of the surveillance work is undertaken by nurses, for example, the practice nurse in the health centre or a district nurse and health visitor as they visit patients and clients and their families in their own homes. Other places where informal surveillance can take place are in nursing homes, where staff may report cases of influenza or gastroenteritis so that the situation can be monitored or investigated.

Other areas of environmental health work include management of pollutants (see Ch. 2). Air pollution, noise, food hazards, health and safety and housing standards are all aspects subject to environmental control, as are control of infectious diseases, rodent and pest control, hazardous waste disposal and local authority licensing and registration to ensure the health, safety and welfare of the public. Most of the work undertaken by environmental health officers is covered by statute and enables them to have the right of entry to establishments and to prosecute offenders. Their work normally involves both surveillance through routine inspections and targeting to deal with specific issues.

Food safety is one area of specific importance, with increasing cases of food poisoning reported in recent years. Routine inspection and surveillance regarding food safety covers people, practices and premises, and is controlled under the Food Safety Act 1990. In response to concerns over food safety and in a bid to protect the public's health and consumer interests to food, a Food Standards Agency was set up. This is an independent food safety watchdog set up in 2000 by an Act of Parliament, the Food Standards Act 1999. The agency has produced a wide range of publications for the public and food industry (see section on websites).

Water used for drinking and leisure use (e.g. swimming pools) is a second important area of environmental infection control. Recent outbreaks of legionnaires' disease have been linked to natural and artificial water systems including air-conditioning systems, cooling towers and extensive plumbing of hotels and office blocks.

A third area is the licensing and registration of various activities, premises and persons to ensure that the health and welfare of the public using them is protected; for example, to ensure that safe practices of hygiene and sterilization are maintained when equipment is used for acupuncture, tattooing, ear piercing and electrolysis.

The environmental health service was introduced in the 19th century and despite better health care and improvement in the environment, the challenges facing environmental health officers are as difficult as 100 years ago. This is probably due to the fact that the need for the prevention and control of infection is increasing (Worsley et al 1994).

In conclusion, as a qualified nurse, midwife or health visitor you have a duty and personal responsibility for infection control in all its forms. It is certainly an enormous task for any one person, but by working together as a team of healthcare professionals, whether in hospital or the community, it is possible to uphold professional, ethical and legal standards that promote the prevention of infection.

PERSONAL AND REFLECTIVE KNOWLEDGE

INFECTION CONTROL AS A FUNDAMENTAL PRINCIPLE IN NURSING

This chapter has considered some of the important issues concerning infection control, a fundamental principle that must underpin all nursing practices. Although the prevention and control of infection are commonly perceived as issues that only affect the hospital patient and healthcare professionals caring for them, this chapter has demonstrated that they are increasingly important aspects of care in the community and issues that affect all, irrespective of age. Failure to prevent or control an infection may seriously affect the health of an individual or fail to ensure the health and safety of the healthcare worker.

CASE STUDIES RELATED TO INFECTION CONTROL

Case study: Adult

Ivy Brookes is 72 years old. She is married to George who is 80 years old. They live in their own two-bedroomed house. Their four children live some distance away and all are married and have children of their own. Ten years ago Ivy was diagnosed as having late onset diabetes mellitus, which is controlled by diet and oral medicine. One month ago Ivy fell and cut her left leg. The wound is healing slowly and is now infected and the district nurse has to dress the wound three times a week. Up until his retirement George was employed in a local brick making firm. He always seemed to have good health and was rarely off sick. Last winter, however, he had an episode of acute bronchitis and ever since has been troubled by a cough. Chest radiographs taken 3 months ago revealed no acute infection, and now George is being treated by his general practitioner for chronic bronchitis. On the district nurse's last visit she had suggested to Ivy and George that they have a flu vaccination before the next winter.

- What microorganisms might be involved with these two infections – one a wound infection, the second a chest infection?
- As a student nurse you are asked by the district nurse to assess Ivy and George. Which of the general and specific factors given in Table 4.8 are particularly relevant to Ivy and George?
- Whilst chatting to Ivy and George they express concern at having a flu vaccination; they tell you that a neighbour has told them that the injection can make you ill. Consider what your reply might be towards their expressed concern.

The following day you visit Ivy and George with the district nurse to change the dressing on Ivy's wound.

- What specific infection control factors would you need to consider when dressing the leg wound ?

- What type of precaution would you need to take when tending to the wound?
- How would you dispose of the dressings and dressing pack used?

Case study: Child

Emma Davis is 2 years old. She has been admitted to hospital with severe diarrhoea and vomiting. According to her mother she has been unwell for 2 days. She is complaining of abdominal pain and needs rehydration. The nurse admitting Emma decides that for the sake of other children on the ward she must be nursed in a side room. The staff nurse has asked you to be involved with Emma's care.

- How would you explain to Emma's mother the reason why she must be nursed in a side room?
- What is the risk of this infection to yourself, Emma's mother, other staff and other patients?

Basing your care on the five specific infection control practices discussed in the section Care Delivery Knowledge

- How you would go about assessing, planning and implementing your care for Emma?

Case study: Mental health

Richard Crosby is 46 years old. He was divorced 8 years ago and his wife cares for their two children aged 14 and 12 years. Over the years Richard has had several episodes of mild depression, but has managed to hold down a job. Three years ago he was made redundant from his job as an electrician and since then has only had some casual work. Until recently he has been living in a flat, but was made homeless when a fire destroyed it and all his belongings. At first Richard started to sleep rough on the streets, turning to alcohol as a way of escaping from his financial problems and homelessness. He is now living in a hostel for the homeless. One of the staff members has just discovered that Richard has started to use drugs and some used needles and syringes have been found under his mattress. You are a student on placement with a community psychiatric nurse (CPN) who has been asked to see Richard.

- Taking into account his alcohol ingestion and apparent use of intravenous drugs, what are the specific needs and actual problems Richard has in relation to his health?
- Using Table 4.3, outline the ways Richard might be putting himself and others at risk of infections.

The CPN decides that Richard needs to understand more about the particular risks of infection he and others around him face.

- Basing your health education session upon the modes of spread (airborne, direct and indirect), what are the main

infection control measures you think should be included in this talk ?

Case study: Learning disabilities

Kevin Roberts is 16 years old and was born with Down syndrome. He is able to walk with help and requires a lot of help with feeding and washing. For the last 10 years he has been attending special schools, but his mental ability has been slow to develop and he requires constant supervision. Kevin lives at home with his mother who is now in need of respite care. She has agreed reluctantly for Kevin to be admitted to a local home that cares for people with learning disabilities. You are a student nurse on placement at this home and are closely involved with Kevin's care. Outbreaks of food poisoning are not uncommon in places of communal living.

- Using the chain of infection shown in Figure 4.1 as your framework, what are the different ways in which Kevin might be put at risk of getting such an infection?

One very important way of preventing infection spreading from client to client is handwashing.

- What are the particular situations throughout the day when you would need to remember to wash your hands while caring for Kevin?

Summary

This chapter has sought to draw together all the knowledge needed to promote and maintain infection control. It has included:

1. Information on the different microorganisms capable of causing infections, their modes of transmission, the environment in which microorganisms thrive, and the body's response to infection.
2. An awareness of different behaviours, attitudes, beliefs and practices towards risk taking in relation to infection control.
3. An outline of the principle of Universal Precautions.
4. An overview of specific practices that are widely accepted as being instrumental in the control and prevention of infection: these are hand hygiene, safe management of linen, waste and sharps, wearing of personal protective equipment, aseptic technique and personal protection.
5. A presentation of the professional, ethical and political influences on the requirements for infection control.
6. An outline of the roles and responsibilities of infection control teams in hospitals and the community.

Annotated further reading and websites

Department of Health 2002 Getting ahead of the curve.
Department of Health, London
An important government document which sets out a strategy of combatting infectious diseases in England. An executive summary can be found at http://www.doh.gov.uk.

Heath H 1994 Foundations of nursing theory and practice. Mosby, London
Chapter 28 of this book gives a very good example of how to write a nursing care plan for a patient with an infection.

Pratt R, Pellowe C, Loveday H P et al 2001 The EPIC project: developing national evidence based guidelines for preventing healthcare associated infections. Journal of Hospital Infection 47 (Supplement)
This is the first phase of national evidence based guidelines for preventing healthcare associated infections and includes standard principles and specific guidelines for the care of short-term indwelling catheters and central venous catheters in acute care.

Wilson J 2001 Infection control in clinical practice, 2nd edn. Baillière Tindall, Edinburgh
An excellent book which provides a comprehensive text of the many infection control issues related to clinical practice.

Worsley M A, Ward K A, Privett S et al (eds) 1994 Infection control: a community perspective. Infection Control Nurses Association, London
This provides a very useful discussion of infection control issues in the community. In particular it gives a good overview of some of the principles of infection control, including handwashing and protective clothing.

http://www.nelh.nhs.uk/cochrane.asp
The Cochrane Library provides comprehensive research and literature reviews on a range of infection control subjects, e.g. surgical wounds, handwashing, infectious diseases.

http://www.foodstandards.gov.uk
The Food Standards Agency produces a wide range of publications of interest to the food industry, healthcare professionals and the general public.

http://www.icna.co.uk
The Infection Control Nurses Association provides lots of useful information about infection control subjects, conferences etc.

http://www.phls.co.uk
The Public Health Laboratory Service maintains an excellent site that provides a very broad range of up-to-date material about many different infection control subjects.

http://www.nhsestates.gov.uk
The website of the Standards for Hospital Cleanliness provides up-to-date information regarding the standards for hospital cleanliness, developed by the Infection Control Nurses Association and the Association of Domestic Management.

http://www.his.org.uk
The Hospital Infection Society runs an excellent site for finding out information about a wide range of topics related to infections in hospital. It is linked to the Journal of Hospital Infections.

References

Ayliffe G A J, Babb J R, Taylor L J 1999 Hospital acquired infection: principles and practice, 3rd edn. Butterworth-Heinemann, Oxford

Beeber S J 1996 Parental smoking and childhood asthma. Journal of Pediatric Healthcare 10(2):58–62

Bellamy K, Alcock R, Babb J R 1993 A test for the assessment of 'hygienic' hand disinfection using rotavirus. Journal of Hospital Infection 24:201–210

Bernthal E 1997 Wedding rings and hospital-acquired infection. Nursing Standard 11(43):44–46

Blackmore M A 1987 Hand-drying methods. Nursing Times 83(37):71–74

Blakemore M A, Prisk E M 1984 Is hot air hygienic? Home Economist 4:14–15

Blunt J 2001 Wound cleansing: ritualistic or research-based practice? Nursing Standard 16(1):33–36

Bowell B 1992 Hands up for cleanliness. Nursing Standard 6(15):24–25

Bowell B 1993 Preventing infection and its spread. Surgical Nurse 6:2, 5–12

British Standards Institute 1990 Specification for sharps containers, BS7320. British Standards Institute, London

Brookes A 1994 Surgical glove perforation. Nursing Times 90(21):60–62

Callaghan I 1998 Bacterial contamination of nurses uniforms: a study. Nursing Standard 13(1):37–42

Cameron J, Rawlings-Anderson K 2001 Cultural issues – genital mutilation: human rights and cultural imperialism. British Journal of Midwifery 9(4):231–235

Clancy J, McVicar A, Cox J 2001 Latex allergy within the perioperative area. British Journal of Perioperative Nursing 11(5):222–227

Curran E 1991 Protecting with aprons. Nursing Times 87(38):64–68

Department of Health 1990 Spills of urine: potential risk of misuse of chlorine releasing disinfecting agents. Safety Advice Bulletin 59(90):41

Department of Health 1992 The health of the nation. HMSO, London

Department of Health 1995 Hospital infection control: guidance on the control of infection in hospitals (Department of Health/Public Health Laboratory Service/Infection Working Group). HMSO, London

Department of Health 1998 A first class service in the new NHS. HMSO, London

Department of Health 1999 Saving lives: our healthier nation. HMSO, London

Department of Health 2002 Getting ahead of the curve. Department of Health, London

Dougherty L 2000 Care of a peripheral intravenous cannula. Nursing Times 96(5):51–52

Elliott P R A 1996 Handwashing practice in nurse education. Professional Nurse 11(6):357–360

Emmerson A M, Enstone J E, Griffin M 1996 The Second National Prevalence Survey in Hospitals. Journal of Hospital Infection 32(3):175–190

Environment Protection Act 1990 HMSO, London

Fielder S, Emslie A. 2001 A prescription for success. Nursing Times 97(46):62

Food Safety Act 1990 HMSO, London

Food Standards Act 1999 HMSO, London

Gibbs J 1990 Disposing of waste. Nursing Times 86(51):34–35

Gibbs J 1991 Clinical waste disposal in the community. Nursing Times 87(2):40–41

Gilmour J, Hughes R 1997 Handwashing still a neglected practice in the clinical area. British Journal of Nursing 6(22):1278–1284

Gould D 1987 Infection and patient care: a guide for nurses. Heinemann, London

Gould D 1994a Making sense of hand hygiene. Nursing Times 90(30):63–64

Gould D 1994b The significance of hand-drying in the prevention of infection. Nursing Times 90(47):30–35

Greatrex B 2001 Infection surveillance: collaborative working practices. British Journal of Nursing 10(5):310–311

Health and Safety Commission 1992 Personal protective equipment at work regulations. Health and Safety Executive, Leeds

Health and Safety at Work Act 1974 HMSO, London

Health Services Advisory Committee 1999 Safe disposal of clinical waste. Health and Safety Executive, Sudbury

Heath H 1994 Foundations of nursing theory and practice. Mosby, London

Hoffman P N, Wilson J 1994 Hands, hygiene and hospitals. Public Health Laboratory Service Microbiology Digest 11(4):211–261

Hollinworth H, Kingston J E 1998 Using a non-sterile technique in wound care. Professional Nurse 13(4):226–229

Horton R 1995 Handwashing: the fundamental infection control principle. British Journal of Nursing 4(16):926–933

Humphries H, Marshall R J, Ricketts V E et al 1991 Theatre over-shoes do not reduce operating theatre floor bacterial counts. Journal of Hospital Infection 17:117–123

Infection Control Nurses Association 1998 Guidelines for hand hygiene. Infection Control Nurses Association, West Lothian

Infection Control Nurses Association and Association of Domestic Management 1999 Standards for environmental cleanliness in hospitals. David, London

Kerr J 1998 Handwashing. Nursing Standard 12(51):35–42

Knight B, Evans C, Barrass S et al 1993 Hand drying: a survey of efficiency and hygiene. Applied Ecology Research Group, University of Westminster, London

Kratz C (ed) 1979 The nursing process. Baillière Tindall, London

Larson E, Bryan J L, Adler L M 1997 A multifaceted approach to changing handwashing behaviour. American Journal of Infection Control 23(4):251–269

Lee J 1988 Hats off! Nursing Times 84(34):59–61

Lowe S 2002 An overview of gastrointestinal infections. Nursing Standard 16(49):47–52

Mangram A J, Horan T, Pearson M L et al 1999 Guidelines for prevention of surgical site infection. American Journal of Infection Control 27(2):97–134

May D 2000 Infection control must be the priority of all nurses. British Journal of Nursing 9(3):254

McGuckin M, Waterman R, Storr J et al 2001 Evaluation of a patient empowering hand hygiene programme in the UK. Journal of Hospital Infection 48:222–227

McCluskey F 1996 Does wearing a face mask reduce bacterial wound infection? British Journal of Theatre Nursing 6(5):18–20, 29

Meers P D, Ayliffe G A J, Emmerson A M 1981 Report of the national survey of infection in hospitals. Journal of Hospital Infection 2:23–28

Meers P, McPherson M, Sedgwick J 1997 Infection control in healthcare, 2nd edn. Stanley Thornes, Cheltenham

Mercier C 1997 Infection control in hospital and community. Stanley Thornes, Cheltenham

National Audit Office 1999 The management of medical equipment in acute NHS Trusts in England. HMSO, London

National Audit Office 2000 The management and control of hospital acquired infection in acute NHS Trusts in England. HMSO, London

National Health Service Executive 1995 Hospital laundry arrangements for used and infected linen. HMSO, London

Nightingale F 1854 Notes on nursing. (Reprint) Churchill Livingstone, Edinburgh

Nursing and Midwifery Council 2002 Code of professional conduct. Nursing and Midwifery Council, London

Nursing Standard 1997 Universal precautions. Nursing Standard 11(34):32–33

Nursing Standard 2001 Prevention of cross-infection: handwashing and use of aprons. Nursing Standard 15(21):56–57

Nursing Times 1995 Infection control: the role of the nurse, Professional Development Unit no. 21, Part 2. Nursing Times 91(41)

O'Boyle Williams C 1995 The social environment. In: Soule B M, Larson E L, Preston G A (eds) Infections and nursing practice: prevention and control. Mosby, Baltimore, pp 62–79

Ogden J 1996 Health psychology. Open University Press, Milton Keynes

Parker L 1990 From pestilence to asepsis. Nursing Times 86(49):63–67

Parker L 1999a Importance of handwashing in the prevention of cross-infection. British Journal of Nursing 8(11):716–711

Parker L 1999b Managing and maintaining a safe environment. British Journal of Nursing 8(16):1053–1066

Pearson T 2000 The wearing of facial protection in high-risk environments. British Journal of Perioperative Nursing 10(3):163–166

Payne S, Horn S 1996 Psychology and health promotion. Open University Press, Milton Keynes

Plowes D 1995 Reusing or misusing? British Journal of Theatre Nursing 5(1):22

Pratt R, Pellowe C, Loveday H P et al 2001 The EPIC project: developing national evidence based guidelines for preventing healthcare associated infections. Journal of Hospital Infection 47 (Suppl.):S3–S82

Price P B 1938 The classification of transient and resident microbes. Journal of Infectious Diseases 63:301–308

Public Health Laboratory Service 1999 Occupational transmission of HIV: summary of published reports. Public Health Laboratory Service, London

Public Health Laboratory Service 2000 Surgical site infection: analysis of surveillance in English hospitals 1997–1999. Nosocomial Infection National Surveillance Scheme, London

Redway K, Knights B, Bozoky Z 1994 Hand drying: a study of bacterial types associated with different hand drying methods and with hot air dryers. University of Westminster, London

Rogers R, Salvage J, Cowell R 1999 Nurses at risk, 2nd edn. Macmillan, London

Ross S 1999 Rationalizing the purchase and use of gloves in healthcare. British Journal of Nursing 8(5):279–287

Royal College of Nursing 2000 Universal precautions for the control of infection. Royal College of Nursing, London

Sadler C 1988 Disposing of danger. Nursing Times 84(44):48–49

Salisbury D M, Hutfilz P, Treen L M et al 1997 The effect of rings on microbial load of healthcare workers hands. American Journal of Infection Control 25(1):24–27

Scott E 2000 Nurses are not washing their hands well enough. British Journal of Nursing 9(22):2264

Schwarze C 1986 The safe uniform debate. American Journal of Nursing 86:956–959

Sprunt K, Redman W, Leidy G et al 1973 Antibacterial effectiveness of routine handwashing. In: Wilson J (ed) Infection control in clinical practice, 2nd edn. Baillière Tindall, Edinburgh, pp 264–271

Stewart R 1997 Female circumcision: implications for North American nurses. Journal of Psychosocial Nursing and Mental Health Services 35(4):35–40

Taylor L 1978a An evaluation of handwashing techniques 1. Nursing Times 74(2):54–55

Taylor L 1978b An evaluation of handwashing techniques 2. Nursing Times 74(3):108–110

Taylor L 1992 Infection control policies. Surgical Nurse 5:6, 6–11

Thompson G, Bullock D 1992 To clean or not to clean? Nursing Times 88(34):66–68

UK Health Departments 1998 Guidance for clinical healthcare workers: protection against infection with bloodborne viruses, recommendation of the Expert Advisory Group on AIDS and Advisory Group on Hepatitis. Department of Health, Weatherby

Walker A, Donaldson B 1993 Dressing for protection. Nursing Times 89(2):60–62

Ward D 2000a Implementing evidence based practice in infection control. British Journal of Nursing 9(5):267–271

Ward D 2000b Handwashing facilities in the clinical area: a literature review. British Journal of Nursing 9(2):82–86

Weber D J, Rutala W A 1997 Role of environmental contamination in the transmission of vancomycin resistant enterococci. Infection Control and Hospital Epidemiology 18:306–309

Weiler E 1965 An investigation into towel hygiene. In: Blackmore A M 1987 Hand drying methods. Nursing Times 83(37):71–74

Weightman N C, Banfield K R 1994 Protective overshoes are unnecessary in a day surgery unit. Journal of Hospital Infection 28:1–3

Wilson J 1990 The price of protection. Nursing Times 86(26):67–68

Wilson J (ed) 2001 Infection control in clinical practice, 2nd edn. Baillière Tindall, Edinburgh

World Health Organization 1997 The world health report 1997. World Health Organization, Geneva

Worsley M A, Ward K A, Privett S et al (eds) 1994 Infection control: a community perspective. Daniels, Cambridge

Chapter 5

Handling and moving

Eileen Aylott

KEY ISSUES

SUBJECT KNOWLEDGE
- Relevance of spinal anatomy and physiology in relation to back care
- Concept of ergonomics and its relevance for nursing
- Factors that may contribute to back injury
- Epidemiological background to back injury in nursing
- Why individuals may participate in risk behaviours when handling clients

CARE DELIVERY KNOWLEDGE
- Four main areas for assessment in moving and handling
- Assessing handling situations
- Plans for moving a client effectively
- Equipment available to aid the moving and handling of clients
- Factors affecting the effectiveness of a handling situation
- Handling heavy patients
- Handling inanimate objects

PROFESSIONAL AND ETHICAL KNOWLEDGE
- Legal and professional guidelines for safe handling practice
- Monitoring and managing untoward incidents
- Ethical dilemmas that may occur in moving clients

PERSONAL AND REFLECTIVE KNOWLEDGE
- Personal capacity for moving and handling clients
- Strategies for personal back care
- Principles of moving and handling within scenarios set to cover all branches of nursing

INTRODUCTION

Handling situations are experienced in all aspects of life, from childhood to old age. The National Back Pain Association has identified that much adult back pain can be traced to the posture and practices of childhood (National Back Pain Association 1990). Load handling is recognized as a problem in both nursing and industry, although in nursing, however, it is important to stress that the occurrence of back injury resulting from patient handling is not a new phenomenon, with the earliest recorded back injury dating from 1500 BC (Steed et al 2000). In 1965 an article in *The Lancet* suggested that the adult human form is an awkward burden to lift or carry. Weighing up to 100 kg or more, it has no handles, it is not rigid, and it is liable to severe damage if mishandled or dropped. In bed the patient is placed inconveniently for lifting, and the placing of a load in such a situation would be tolerated by few industry workers.

It is the aim of this chapter to enable you to learn about safe principles of moving patients/clients using an ergonomic approach and to understand why, in spite of education and training, poor practice is still sometimes a problem. It is anticipated that personal recognition of the antecedents of poor practice, combined with a clear understanding of safe principles will enable you to become an effective (and uninjured!) practitioner. The development of handling techniques is a process that should continue throughout your career as part of lifelong learning. The need for safe handling should also be appreciated both inside and outside the work setting in order to be truly effective in reducing injury. Because of this, it is intended to address issues related to handling in a holistic way. This means that all areas of knowledge will be applied to encourage decision making and the questions encourage reflection and application in your personal circumstances.

It is important to realize that attending handling sessions in a classroom situation or reading and learning about safe practice is not enough to equip someone to handle effectively in practice. This chapter aims to help you develop skills in practice through assessment of handling situations, adequate planning and continuing evaluation.

OVERVIEW

Subject knowledge

You will learn about the practical aspects of back structure. The anatomy and physiology of the spine and posture is addressed and the implications of this knowledge are applied in relation to developing an ergonomically friendly work environment. The epidemiology of back pain and injury is highlighted, and psychosocial considerations are discussed.

Care delivery knowledge

This section explains the decision making approach that handling situations now require from health professionals. It includes detailed information on assessment processes and tools, outlines the importance of planning for the use of appropriate equipment and human resources and gives more detailed information on the aids available for handling and moving patients/clients.

Professional and ethical knowledge

Current legislation and professional issues are presented for discussion both in relation to ensuring safe practice and in seeking recompense for injured parties should an incident occur. Support agencies are included at this point for further reference. Finally, some of the dilemmas faced by nurses in providing individualized care related to moving and handling are presented for discussion.

Personal and reflective knowledge

The case studies within this section will enable you to develop your ability to make decisions in handling situations while encouraging reflection on practice experiences. Depending on the situation, there may be straightforward solutions to the problems encountered. However, other situations may lend themselves to a variety of options, the choice of which may depend on the individuals concerned, the environment and the client.

On pages 119–123 there are four case studies, each one relating to one of the branch programmes. You may find it helpful to read one of them before you start the chapter and use it as a focus for your reflections while reading.

SUBJECT KNOWLEDGE

BIOLOGICAL

The purpose of this section is to examine spinal anatomy and physiology and relate these to the prevention of problems caused by poor posture and poor load handling techniques. A consideration of the provision of an ergonomically friendly environment for moving and handling clients is also explored. 'Ergonomics aims to design appliances, technical systems and tasks in such a way as to improve human safety, health, comfort and performance' and 'as a consequence of its applied nature the ergonomic approach results in the adaptation of the workplace or environment to fit people, rather than the other way around' (Dul & Weerdmeester 1993).

Decision making exercise

1. Think of daily life events and tasks and compile a list of activities during which you might put your back at risk. You may be surprised at how extensive this list will be.
2. Look at your list and decide which of the actions identified in the bullet list on page 108 may be involved.
3. Many health trusts are now advocating a 'non-lifting' policy at work. However, it is important that good handling practices are pursued both in and out of work to protect your back from injury. Look at your list again and decide what alternative actions may be possible to protect your back.

THE SPINAL CORD

The spinal column is composed of 33 vertebrae. It acts as a protective cover for the spinal cord and provides attachments for ligaments, muscles and ribs (Fig. 5.1).

The spinal cord has five sections (Fig. 5.2). Note that the vertebrae change shape and size according to their type and function. For instance, the cervical vertebrae are smaller and their shape is designed to facilitate movement of the head and neck, whereas the lumbar vertebrae have larger bodies in order to sustain more weight.

From Figure 5.3 you can see that each vertebra is composed of a main body of bone and this is the anterior aspect of the vertebra. Bony projections are situated posteriorly. These provide the attachment for muscles and ligaments.

The human spine, of which the spinal column and cord are component parts, has a unique design: it is constructed to withstand tremendous pressure and to facilitate a variety of movements (Fig. 5.4). It can be seen that the spine is quite flexible. For good posture, the spine needs to be maintained in normal alignment, and forward bending, extension, side bending and rotation of the spine avoided. Persistent poor posture, not sitting correctly, standing incorrectly, slumping, twisting the back, and pulling, pushing and handling loads incorrectly will eventually damage the spine.

Intervertebral discs

Between each two vertebrae is a disc consisting of an outer fibrous elastic ring and a soft jelly-like nucleus. The function of the disc is to act as a shock absorber, and provided it is not subjected to undue persistent pressure, it will serve

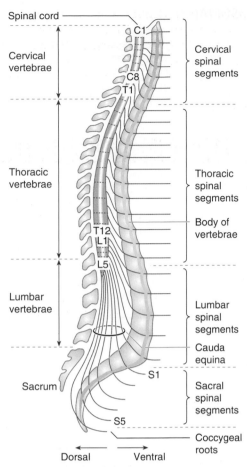

Figure 5.1 The spinal cord. (From Hinchliff & Montague 1988.)

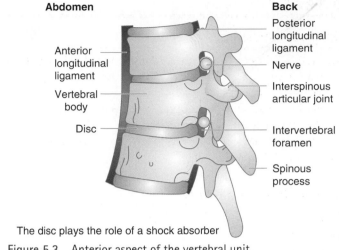

The disc plays the role of a shock absorber

Figure 5.3 Anterior aspect of the vertebral unit.

Cervical region
This consists of seven vertebrae, which are small and designed for maximum movement of the head and neck.

Thoracic region
This region consists of 12 vertebrae, which are slightly larger with a smaller range of movement. These vertebrae also provide attachment for the ribs.

Lumbar region
This region consists of five vertebrae. These are the largest vertebrae to allow maximum weight bearing. They also provide a wide range of movement.

Sacral region
This consists of five fused vertebrae and provides support for the spine.

Coccyx
This consists of four fused vertebrae and forms the base of the spine.

Figure 5.2 The five sections of the spinal cord.

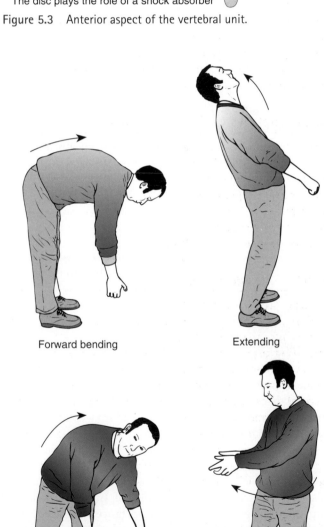

Forward bending

Extending

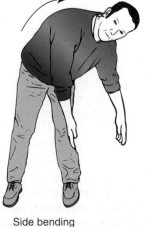

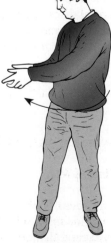

Side bending

Rotating

Figure 5.4 Movements of the spine.

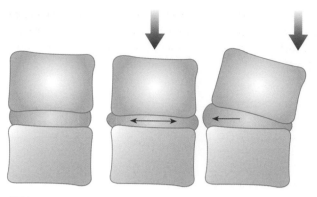

Without pressure   Under pressure

Figure 5.5   Under pressure, the disc is compressed and shapes itself to the angle and impact of pressure. When the pressure is released the disc returns to its original shape. Permanent one-sided pressure will cause wear and tear of the disc. Think of the disk as a jam doughnut – if you compress one side what happens to the jam? That can be likened to a herniation.

this function well. Figure 5.5 indicates how the disc modifies its position to take account of this pressure. Bending forwards puts a great deal of pressure on the posterior aspect of the disc and if the pressure on the disc is too great, it will herniate and acute pain may be felt if the nerves that emerge from the spinal cord become trapped by the herniation.

BACK INJURY

Injury to the back results from activities that involve:

- stooping
- twisting
- uneven loads
- forward bending
- prolonged, fixed postures.

In fact any activity that increases pressure on the intervertebral discs, particularly if the pressure is one-sided, will increase wear and tear on the discs and may ultimately contribute to disc herniation.

Cumulative strain

Walsh (1988) explores the concept of human kinetics in more detail, highlighting the importance of correct body movement. This is also important in relation to the concept of cumulative or repetitive strain, which in nursing is becoming recognized as a contributing factor to ultimate injury (Dolan & Adams 1998). Poor practice may not result in one identifiable injury but rather to ongoing gradual wear and tear, which may cause pain and disability. According to Dolan & Adams (1998) repetitive lifting tasks fatigue the back muscles and increase the bending movement on the lumbar spine.

PSYCHOSOCIAL

THE EPIDEMIOLOGY OF BACK INJURY

Although it is important to understand what may contribute to back injury, it is also essential to have some notion of the extent of the problem both in the population generally and in nursing. Information to aid your understanding and perspective of this problem includes the following:

- Back pain is the largest single cause of absence from work, the cost of which is £50 billion per year to the British economy (Back Care 2001).

- In nursing every year an estimated 80 000 nurses injure their backs (Institute for Employment Studies Report no 315: see Seccombe & Smith 1996) and approximately 5% have to take early retirement due to muscular skeletal injury (Seccombe & Smith 1996, 1999).

- The health service union Confederation of Health Service Employees (COHSE) conducted a survey among their members and found that up to one in four nurses experiences back pain either at work or at the end of the working day (Confederation of Health Service Employees 1992).

- A total of 1977 incidents of handling injuries were reported to Health Service Executive (HSE) in 2000–2001.

- Of the 134 major injuries reported (includes over 3 days injuries) 32% were due to lifting patients and 16% were due to awkward movements (Health Service Executive 2002).

- In a Royal College of Nursing case (BBC News Online 2000), a nurse was awarded over £800 000 for a back injury sustained at work.

What cannot be calculated from these figures is the personal misery, loss of independence and chronic illness that may additionally result. A knock-on effect, which is also difficult to quantify, is the cost of treatment and welfare benefit needed to support people who become injured. Although there appears to be a downward trend in the rate of both reported and unreported injury in the past 5 years, the nursing profession is deeply concerned about the above situation.

Evidence based practice

The Third European Survey on Working Conditions undertaken by the European Foundation for the Improvement of Living and Working Conditions (2001) suggested that 25.3% of UK workers reported that work had affected their health in the form of backache. This compared to 42.1% in Greece, 39.6% in Finland and 11.3% in Ireland. The overall EU average was 31.7%.

Behavioural issues

When all of the above is taken into consideration, it seems inconceivable that much of this suffering arises out of poor practice; however, nurses' attitudes are identified as being slow to change. Much evidence of routine and ritual prevails in the area of manual handling in spite of documented research to inform nursing practice (McGuire & Dewar 1995). However, more encouragingly a survey to investigate NHS Trusts compliance with the Royal College of Nursing's (1996b) *Safer Patient Handling Policy* was published in July 2002, which suggests there has been a change in the culture for the manual handling of patients within the NHS, and that practitioners are no longer manually lifting patients without questioning the practice (Crumpton et al 2002).

Decision making exercise

With time allocated to practice placement learning increasing, you will be spending more time undertaking patient care skills. Manual handling tasks are part of everyday practice and you may be required to undertake a variety of activities while working within the interprofessional team.

During a morning shift you observe a patient who has suffered a stroke, being stood with the aid of a Sarah hoist. The patient has a very dense hemiparisis on his left side and is unable to weight bear fully on that side. He is complaining of pain during the manoeuvre and appears very distressed.

Consider these questions and discuss them with your practice educator or skills laboratory tutor.

1. Is the equipment being used suitable for a patient with this condition?
2. How would you respond if asked to participate in this manoeuvre?
3. What other options may be available to the staff to transfer this patient?
4. Which clause within your code of professional conduct could be contravened and why?

Preventing back injury

Everyone needs to take care of his or her back and the logical point at which to start would be to encourage good posture from early childhood. Studies across Europe show that back pain is very common in children, around 50% experiencing back pain at some time. However, a recent study in France (Viry 1999) recorded four out of five children having back pain in the last year. In that study the weight of their school bags was one of the strongest predictors as was how they wore them (one or two straps).

The notion that 'prevention is better than cure' is well acknowledged. Organizations such as the Health Education Authority with its *Look After Yourself* project (1994) aimed to educate people into preventive measures.

Certain predisposing factors help identify those who are at greatest risk of developing low back pain. People at greatest risk are likely to have one or more of the following characteristics:

- excess weight
- extreme lordosis
- absence of regular exercise
- weak abdominal muscles
- tight hamstrings or hip flexors
- weak or tight back muscles
- general muscular tension.

CARING FOR YOURSELF

You need to know how to care for yourself and your own back both at work as a nurse and in your lifestyle generally. Keeping yourself fit using gentle exercise programmes can help. Regular walking and swimming are also to be recommended. Keeping to your desirable weight can be a preventative measure in back problems, and can also be avoided by wearing sensible footwear. Further reading on exercising to strengthen your back and keeping fit generally can be found in a wealth of publications and websites such as that of Back Care, which are regularly updated (see section on websites).

Reflection and portfolio evidence

Having just read about factors predisposing back injuries:

- Which of your clients do you consider may be at particular risk of injuring their backs?
- Design a list of health promotion tips for use with clients you perceive to be 'at risk' on return to their own homes.
- Use this work as evidence for your portfolio.

During your practice placements you should always wear flat lace-up shoes, usually outlined in a uniform policy. This type of footwear will give you maximum support for your feet and assist you to maintain correct traction

---

Evidence based practice

A study undertaken by Palmer et al (2000) which compared two prevalence surveys undertaken at 10-year intervals concluded that although more back injuries were being reported, this may be due to cultural changes leading to greater awareness of more minor back injuries and a willingness to report them. If this is correct then the solution to the growing economic burden from back pain may lie in modifying people's attitudes and behaviour rather than in the interventions aimed at reducing physical stresses on the spine.

when undertaking manual handling tasks with others. The type of footwear worn by someone who sustains a back injury would be investigated to see whether it has been a predisposing factor to the injury, and the wrong type of footwear could nullify or reduce a claim for compensation.

CARE DELIVERY KNOWLEDGE

GENERAL PRINCIPLES OF LOAD HANDLING

This section explains the decision making approach that handling situations now require from health professionals. It includes detailed information on assessment processes and tools, outlines the importance of planning for the use of appropriate equipment and human resources and gives more detailed information on the aids available for handling and moving patients/clients.

The principles of safe handling include the need to use a systematic approach to all handling situations. General principles of load handling include:

- knowledge of the patient
- deciding on the most appropriate method
- agreeing commands
- identifying a leader for the task
- explaining to the patient what is to happen
- competence in using any handling aids
- preparing the environment
- keeping your spine in normal alignment
- being relaxed with the lead foot pointing in the direction of movement
- always moving or sliding towards yourself.

ASSESSMENT OF HANDLING SITUATIONS

Maitland (1989) observes that 'In our society we are over concerned with getting things done and that not enough emphasis is placed on the way in which we do things.' This is true of many nurses in relation to handling situations. It is often argued that there is not time to assess patients, as the work needs to be done. However, thorough assessment of a situation is the key to successful handling and requires knowledge, time and a framework for a systematic approach.

So many assessment factors to take into account may seem daunting at first, but the planning and safety of any manoeuvre depends upon accurate assessment. Handling assessment skills can be likened to learning to drive a car. Initially, this requires careful thought and learner drivers may be slow because of all the things that need to be taken into account and their actions may be uncoordinated. However, as with practice, driving theory and skills become second nature, so it is to some extent with client handling. If an assessment is initially completed thoroughly, then on subsequent occasions discomfort for the client and risk of injury to the nurse can be reduced.

There are numerous assessment tools that can be used that incorporate all the elements to be considered when handling and moving a load. It is important to use the tool correctly but also to be aware that all tools have their limitations.

It must be acknowledged that assessment tools are simply an aid to healthcare workers. Knowledge and professional judgement are also needed to select the appropriate manoeuvre. Once it is established that the risk is low, medium or high, then planning the handling task will follow more easily. However, no handling situation is without risk. The risk of injury can only be minimized.

The National Back Pain Association (1991) states that the **T**ask, **I**ndividual, **L**oad, and the **E**nvironment need to be assessed as do the **R**esources available (TILER; see below). These are now considered in more detail.

Assessing the task

For each individual client there may be several tasks to take into account, and manual lifting should be avoided if at all possible. Separate assessments will be necessary for each task. For example transferring a patient from a bed to the commode, from a chair to the bathroom, or from a wheelchair into a car will probably require the use of different strategies. Depending on the manoeuvre, different numbers of handlers may be required as well as a variety of techniques and postures. It is important to take into account the weight of the load and this is as important in lifting as it is in pushing, pulling, transferring or sliding. There is a tendency to acknowledge the risk of back injury, but other injuries due to repetitive strain or excess strain such as those utilized in sliding can be as debilitating to the nurse. It has been documented that prolonged postures and repetitive movements are tiring and in the long term can lead to muscle and joint injuries (Dolan & Adams 1998). Other important factors are positions used for handling, unsatisfactory or prolonged static postures, the height at which the manoeuvre is carried out (Royal College of Nursing 1996a, 1999), or repetition rates over a period of time (National Back Pain Association 1992). All these factors can increase the cumulative stress on the body that may subsequently lead to injury.

Assessing the individual handler

In assessing any handling situation the capabilities of the individuals undertaking the handling is vital. What may be an appropriate handling plan for an experienced nurse may be beyond the capabilities and competence of the junior student. In addition, the individual may have limitations due to factors other than their nursing experience. Carers may feel discomfort adopting recommended positions or postures for particular techniques and in some instances may need referral to occupational health for assessment for such discomfort. Also many female nurses are of childbearing age and if they are or think they may be pregnant, they need advice for manual handling. Such advice is offered by the Royal College of Nursing (1995) in their guide *Hazards for Pregnant Nurses: An A–Z Guide*. In addition, the drive to recruit more mature staff into nursing may mean that some have existing back problems, which may be compounded by the practices they are undertaking.

Assessing the load or person

The weight of the load is an important consideration and lifting should be avoided if at all possible. In today's society average body weight has increased due to social and economic factors; this has enhanced the need for fuller risk assessment and an increase in the knowledge base of the professional planning the task of load handling. Some health authorities have produced guidance on handling heavy patients (these are patients weighing over 20 stone (127 kg)) and have highlighted the need to weigh patients and document this information in their notes. Ideally patients should be identified prior to admission to allow for the correct equipment to be obtained to nurse them; this information should also be made available to the community prior to discharge. It is important to note that many students will be working with district nurses in people's homes and that equipment may need to be ordered before a successful and safe discharge can occur.

Identification of any factor that makes the load difficult to handle should be taken into account, for example, the psychological state of the patient. Patients who are unpredictable in their responses will increase the risks in handling situations to both carers and themselves (Royal College of Nursing 1993). In addition, the use of certain pieces of equipment may be socially unacceptable to the patient, and this is where good communication skills as well as the rights of the nurse to protect themselves from injury can be extremely important. This can be even more crucial in a community setting where the health carer is a guest in the client's home and not able to implement changes that one may automatically be able to make in a ward setting (Hemple 1993).

Assessing the environment

The optimum working environment is one that is ergonomically sound. However, since caring for patients takes place in many different settings it may not always be possible to control the setting in this way. Additionally, it is important to note that since all individuals are different, an ergonomically friendly environment for one individual may be dangerous for another. All environments for moving and handling must therefore be assessed before a manoeuvre takes place.

Obstructions or hazards within the working area need to be assessed as well as specific environmental problems. Environmental problems can be interpreted as the wider physical environment (e.g. the room or bed area). Alternatively, they may pertain to the client's immediate environment. This may include a wide variety of such factors, from the presence of a urinary catheter to the client's painful joints that are aggravated by movement. All these aspects may require specific planning and careful assessment is perhaps especially pertinent in areas where clients have a learning disability, are young children or are unconscious and so are unable to contribute their views to the assessment.

Assessing the equipment and resources

In utilizing any equipment for a manual handling situation, the first question that must be asked is whether the equipment is appropriate for the task you wish to undertake. This may include assessing such things as whether the equipment has the capacity to cope with the weight of the client you wish to move or whether the equipment is suitable to use in that particular environment. If appropriate equipment is not available it may be pertinent to obtain this equipment either from another area or through local protocols that are in place. Checking that the equipment is in working order and that there are no apparent defects is essential. Specific checks will vary according to the type of equipment employed, for example, cracks in a plastic transfer belt, brakes that are not efficient on a hoist or clasps that are worn out on a transfer belt will mean that this equipment is unsafe and should not be used.

Reflection and portfolio evidence

Look at the documentation for manual handling, risk assessment and care planning in your clinical area.

- Talk to your mentor about the assessment process.
- Undertake an assessment of a patient using the TILER format.
- How long did it take you? Did this surprise you?
- Talk to the patient about your plan and note the responses for your reflection.
- Write up and add to your portfolio.

If appropriate, the last occasion on which the equipment was serviced (i.e. a hoist) should be noted, and the equipment should not be used if the date does not comply with local protocols. For all equipment, social cleanliness needs to be observed to prevent the risk of cross-infection between patients; if soiled, the equipment will require cleaning in accordance with local policy.

PLANNING

Once an assessment has been undertaken the information is used to form the basis of planning the moving and handling task (Fig. 5.6). A major factor to consider here is the resources available in human terms and in relation to the equipment available.

Patient's name	District nurse

Body build   Obese ☐   Above average ☐   Average ☐   Below average ☐   Tall ☐   Medium ☐   Short ☐

Weight (if known)   **Risk of falls** High ☐   Low ☐

Problems with comprehension, behaviour, cooperation (identify)

Handling constraints, e.g. disability, weakness, pain, skin lesions, infusions (identify)

Tasks (see examples)	**Methods to be used** (see examples)	**Describe any remaning problems, list any other measures needed** (see examples)

Date(s) assessed:

Assessor's signature:

Proposed review dates:

Finishing date:

Examples of tasks:
✓ sitting/standing
✓ toiletting
✓ bathing
✓ transfer to/from bed
✓ movement in bed
✓ sustained postures
✓ walking
✓ in/out of car

Examples of methods/ control measures
Organization
✓ Number of staff needed?
✓ Patient stays in bed
Equipment
✓ Variable height bed
✓ Hoists
✓ Slings/belt
✓ Bath aids
✓ Wheeled sani-chair
✓ Monkey poles
✓ Patient hand blocks
✓ Rope ladders
✓ Turntable
✓ Sliding aids
✓ Stair lift
Furniture
✓ Reposition/remove

Examples of problems/ risk factors
Task
✓ Is it necessary? Can it be avoided?
✓ Involves stretching, stooping, twisting, sustained load?
✓ Rest/recovery time?
Patient
✓ Weight, disability, ailments, etc.
Environment
✓ Space to manoeuvre, to use hoist?
✓ Access to bed, bath, WC, passageways?
✓ Steps, stairs?
✓ Flooring uneven? OK for hoist?
✓ Furniture: movable? height? condition?
✓ Bed: double? low?
Carers
✓ Fitness for the task, freshness or fatigue?
✓ Experience with patient and with handling team?
✓ Skill: handling, using equipment?
Furniture
✓ Reposition/remove

Figure 5.6   Royal College of Nursing community care plan. (Reproduced by kind permission of Royal College of Nursing 2003.)

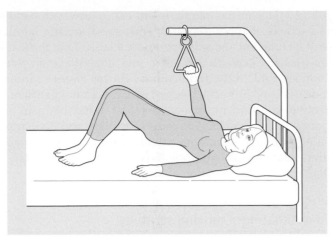

Figure 5.7   Patient lifting herself.

Often a forgotten resource is the patients themselves. If consulted and included in the care planning process, patients may often be able to move themselves with small adjustments such as a monkey pole (Fig. 5.7). Sometimes the simplest of things are overlooked like asking the patient if they could stand or roll themselves. The culture of nursing is that we should be doing things for patients rather than encouraging independence wherever possible.

Many types of handling equipment are available, some of which is sophisticated and expensive while other equipment is simple and relatively inexpensive. Some examples of handling aids are given below.

Equipment may include:

- sliding equipment
- transfer equipment
- turning equipment
- leg lifting equipment
- lifting equipment
- handling equipment

or a combination of any of the above.

These will now be considered in more depth.

Sliding equipment

When using sliding equipment it is important to think carefully about the safety of the patient and the handlers. Although the nurse is not handling the full weight of the patient, effort is required to complete the manoeuvre and therefore this task should be planned carefully and carried out in manageable stages. When a combination of sliding equipment is used, such as a slide sheet and a pat slide, extra caution should be taken to protect the patient as the effort required to move them using this method is considerably less than conventional means and could result in the patient either being turned rapidly through 180 degrees or being launched off the bed and onto the floor.

Transfer equipment

There are many types of transfer equipment. Individual capacity and the weight and co-operation of the patient will affect whether the choice of a transfer aid is appropriate. Transfer equipment may take the form of a pat slide used under a sheet or in combination with other equipment such as a sliding sheet. This equipment, such as banana boards, may also be used independently by patients (e.g. amputees), so as to maintain the patient's dignity and independence as well as ensuring that arm muscles are used.

Turning equipment

Turning equipment may include specialist beds such as Stoke beds used in the care of spinal injured patients. This type of equipment reduces the amount of manual handling that may be required as it is the bed that moves, but it is important that correct instruction is obtained before using such specialist equipment and that assessment of the patient's condition is undertaken prior to any movement. This category may also include sliding sheets and turntables.

Leg lifting equipment

This type of equipment may be powered or manually operated and is commonly used by disabled people living in the community. Manual leg lifters look like stiff dog leads which may be looped over the foot to aid the leg up into the bed. They tend to be more useful to people who only have leg impairments as good sitting balance and adequate strength in at least one arm is required to operate the manual aids. Manually lifting a patient's legs into bed without the use of equipment will usually involve the handler adopting a poor posture by side flexing and rotating the spine; the use of leg lifters may eliminate the risk to carers (Demain et al 2000). Powered leg lifters are easily operated by the use of a handset but are relatively more expensive to purchase. Both types of equipment may enable patients to maintain independence and reduce the requirements for community care. Simple devices such as these may enable older people to maintain autonomy over simple choices such as the time they go to bed or get up in the morning.

Lifting equipment

A hoist (Fig. 5.8) takes the full weight of a patient, but hoists have specified weight limits and it is still important for the nurse to adopt a safe posture when putting a sling onto a patient and while using the hoist. It is also important to assess the patient for the size of sling used and that it is compatible with the hoist. Confusion may occur in ward areas when more than one type of hoist is present and slings are taken into side wards where patients are being barrier

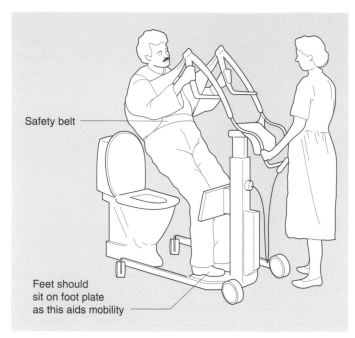

Safety belt

Feet should
sit on foot plate
as this aids mobility

Figure 5.8   Patient using a Sarah hoist. (Reproduced by kind permission of Arjo.)

nursed to control the spread of infection. Single-patient-use slings are now available for this purpose.

Lifting cushions or seats are inflatable devices used to aid fallen patients to be lifted from the floor. The unit consists of an inflatable cushion and a compressor unit; the cushion is placed under the sitting patient and inflated to a height that enables the patient to stand easily. This device requires the patient to have reasonable sitting balance to ensure safe usage and to minimize the risk to both patient and handler. Care should be taken to assess the patient fully for injury prior to the use of this device, and findings should be fully documented in the patient's notes.

Handling equipment

Usually handling equipment takes the form of material belts which may be purchased in different sizes. These belts have secure handles around their circumference and can be used to guide patients who may just need a little support during transfers or while walking. These are not lifting aids and careful consideration should be given with reference to the type of task to be undertaken and the condition and understanding of the patient with whom it is used.

In conclusion, during the planning stage, a key principle is to avoid lifting if at all possible while making a move as easy as possible for both client and handler. The solution needs to be chosen using knowledge about the patient and professional judgement. Any assistants need to agree to the manoeuvre and it must be ascertained that the handlers have the capacity and expertise to undertake the procedure. All aids such as hoists or sliding equipment can reduce the

risk of injury to the handlers, but can injure both handler and patient if the individuals concerned are not familiar with its function and safe operation. Clause 13 of the leaflet *Practitioner–Client Relationships and Prevention of Abuse* (Nursing and Midwifery Council 2002a) states: 'Physical abuse is any physical contact which harms clients or is likely to cause them unnecessary and avoidable pain and distress.' This may include rough handling and poor application of manual handling techniques and as such negotiation with the patient should be viewed as essential, as should the documentation of any outcome decision.

Co-ordinating a moving strategy

A decision needs to be made about how many people are required to undertake the chosen procedure. If more than one handler is required, a leader must be appointed to avoid confusion during the handling and so reduce the risk of injury. Any commands to be used during the procedure need to be agreed in advance. This ensures that the handling is co-ordinated and that weight will be evenly distributed between handlers, thereby reducing the risk of injury.

The checklist when planning is as follows:

- assessment information is available; use TILER (see facing page)
- avoid lifting if at all possible
- choose the appropriate method for all concerned
- ensure all staff involved are familiar with the equipment and procedure
- choose a leader if appropriate
- decide on commands to be used
- communicate with the patient
- check the environment and the equipment.

IMPLEMENTATION

Every handling situation carries a potential risk to the handler and care must be taken to reduce the risk. Assessment and forward planning will help to reduce the risk as will sound knowledge regarding handling loads or patients. Some additional points that need to be taken into consideration when implementing handling plans are: optimum height for handling; handling in confined spaces; moving inanimate objects; and handling children.

Optimum height for handling

The National Back Pain Association suggests that there is an optimum height for handling a patient in bed which should maintain the patient between the handler's knee and shoulder (National Back Pain Association 1991: 12). This is to minimize the risk of poor posture that may lead to stress on the spine. If variable-height beds are available,

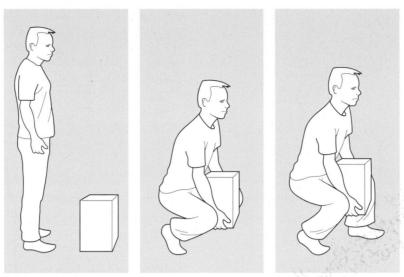

Figure 5.9   Lifting a box from the floor. (Reproduced by kind permission of Stephen Gee.)

they should be adjusted accordingly so as to avoid one-sided pressure on the vertebral column. If two handlers are working together the bed should be adjusted so that the pelvis of the shorter individual is level with the bed when moving. Fixed-height beds or specialist beds and cots can present a hazard due to the adoption of unsafe postures when handling patients. If assessment and planning have been adequate, hazards should be avoided through the choice of an appropriate handling method for the situation.

Hoists should be used when moving an adult or large child from the floor. If such equipment is not available a sliding sheet may be an alternative provided there are sufficient handlers to minimize the risk of back injury due to lifting heavy loads. A good method for handling babies who may wriggle and therefore present a hazard can be found in the guide *The Handling of Patients* (National Back Pain Association 1992: 114).

Handling in confined spaces

As it is impossible to optimize all environments completely, it may be best to identify areas that are not suitable for handling dependent patients. This will help to avoid unsafe postures and reduce the risk of injury to carers. If a patient falls in a confined space, it may be necessary to slide the patient into a more accessible area so that a safe procedure can then be planned.

Handling inanimate objects

The majority of this chapter has been dedicated to the moving and handling of patients, but it is important to remember that many handling tasks are carried out on

inanimate objects such as boxes, beds, drip stands and laundry bags. It is therefore important that these areas are also given careful consideration.

Picking up a box from the floor (Fig. 5.9) and transferring it to another location requires the same methodology as planning to move a patient – TILER:

- Task
- Individual
- Load
- Environment
- Resources/equipment.

A good base position should be adopted to ensure a stable stance is maintained by observing the handler's centre of gravity, which when standing with feet shoulder-width apart lies between the feet. To then lift a box from the floor the knees should be bent and the back kept as straight as possible. One foot may be placed in front of the other to steady the handler when descending. The box should be held as close as possible to keep the centre of gravity within the base while rising to a standing position (reverse for lowering). As for every load reassessment should be carried out even between boxes.

Handling children

The handling of children often presents dilemmas in staff who, when dealing with sick children, often feel obliged to pick them up to comfort them, or transfer them in and out of the bath, etc. Again correct handling techniques should be applied in almost the same method as the box above (Fig. 5.10). The child should be supported within the handler's centre of gravity keeping the heaviest part as close to the body as possible. Handling may be avoided or reduced by encouraging the parents to provide as much of the child's

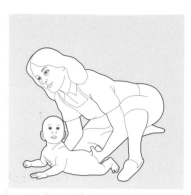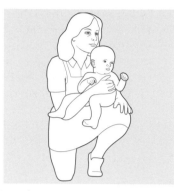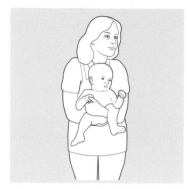

Figure 5.10   Lifting a child from the floor. (Reproduced by kind permission of Stephen Gee.)

care as is reasonable. This is beneficial to both the nurse and the child as family contact is important for the child's well-being.

EVALUATION

Once the procedure has been decided upon it is the nurse's responsibility to document and evaluate the outcome of each handling task to create a handling plan that is available for the multiprofessional healthcare team. The importance of good record keeping cannot be overemphasized, as records are an essential and integral part of care. Records should provide accurate, current, comprehensive and concise information about a patient, including a record of any problems that arise and the action taken in response to them. The quality of your record keeping is also a reflection of the standard of your professional practice. Good record keeping is a mark of the skilled and safe practitioner (Nursing and Midwifery Council 2002b). The Health Service Commissioner's annual report (National Health Service Training Directorate 1994) stated that poor record keeping continues to crop up in reported cases. For clinical risk management, comprehensive records are a vital requirement in relation to manual handling situations.

A handling plan for the patient must include the task being addressed, the weight of the patient, the type of equipment to be used, the number of staff required and the level of expertise necessary to make the procedure as safe as possible. Inexperienced handlers must take care not to act beyond their level of competence when participating in the planning of patient care. If any problems arise these must be recorded in the plan together with the actions taken to resolve problems.

Evaluation is an integral part of the systematic approach to handling situations and is necessary to identify the level of success of the handling plan that has been implemented. If problems are identified they need to be documented and acted upon. Evaluation provides the basis for reassessing, replanning or altering the methods used and assists the multiprofessional team in building up a body of knowledge that is of great value in future moving and handling situations.

PROFESSIONAL AND ETHICAL KNOWLEDGE

LEGAL GUIDELINES FOR SAFE PRACTICE

Since the Manual Handling Operations Regulations came into force in Britain on 1 January 1993 (Health and Safety Executive 1992), the need to use equipment to reduce manual handling risks has been widely recognized by health professionals (Demain et al 2000).

Today, management of load movements is not focused on lifting, and most areas are now emphasizing that 'no lifting' policies are implemented (Moore 1993). Safer handling policies have been introduced into hospitals and other healthcare settings. These state that patients 'should never be lifted manually, should be encouraged to assist in their own transfers', and that 'appropriate equipment and furniture should be used to minimize the risk of injury' (Tracy & Ruszala 1998). It is sometimes argued that equipment should not be used, as the patient may not like to be handled using a mechanical aid. However, it must be remembered that although patient preferences are important, the safety of the handlers needs to be considered.

Although there have been attempts for many years to gain legislation to protect employees including a European Community directive (Commission of the European Communities 1990) leading to the development of manual handling regulations, until recently the occurrence of back pain and injury was an accepted risk factor in being a nurse.

In spite of these changes, however, there are still back injuries occurring and many of these are as a result of poor handling practices involving the continued use of 'banned' lifts (National Back Pain Association 2002).

Risk assessment of any manual handling task should be considered using an ergonomic approach that looks at the relationship between the task, the person being moved, the environment and the worker (Lloyd 1996, Wilson 2001), but its benefits are yet to be substantiated (Hingnett 1996, Stubbs 2000). The word 'ergonomics' is Greek in origin and means natural laws ('nomo') of work ('ergo'). One of the guiding principles of the science is creating a balance between the demands of a task and the capabilities of the individual performing it. If the demands of a task, whether physical or mental, are greater than the capability of the individual doing the work, then stress (physical or psychological) and consequently strain and injury, can result (National Back Pain Association 2002).

Before January 1993, in the UK, the Health and Safety at Work Act 1974 was in place to prevent industrial accidents (see Ch. 2). This Act had some weaknesses, thereby rendering it somewhat inadequate; a major area of weakness being assessment of risk, which is now being addressed by employers through the Clinical Governance agenda.

In 1992, the UK government adopted the European Community Directive 90/269/EEC (Commission of the European Communities 1990). This requires greater attention to be given to all aspects of any handling situation and stated that assessment should be used to avoid risk of injury.

Managers of care settings are now required to establish and implement safe policies and procedures with respect to handling. They must ensure that regular training and updating are given and reinforced to all employees. Careful records should be kept of this training. Attention must be paid to the environment in which handling takes place and an ergonomic approach is recommended.

Nurses in supervisory positions (i.e. qualified nurses) are responsible for carrying out a comprehensive risk assessment of each handling situation and must ensure that the handling task is completed safely. Information related to technique, equipment and load involved must be communicated to other parties and also documented in patient/client records. Consideration must be given to the capacity of the individual handlers in every situation, as this will affect any technique selected.

PROFESSIONAL GUIDELINES FOR SAFE PRACTICE

The first Royal College of Nursing *Code of Practice for Handling of Patients* (Royal College of Nursing 1993) advocated a 50 kg (8 stone) weight limit for a patient being lifted by two nurses under ideal conditions. Further editions (Royal College of Nursing 1996a, 1999) advocate eliminating hazardous manual handling in all but exceptional or life-threatening situations such as fire, bomb, structural collapse or drowning. However, clients may still need to be handled manually and this should only be considered if it does not involve lifting all or most of the client's weight. As far as possible aids should be used to assist client handlers. Supporting or transferring a client can still pose a hazard to carers and care should be taken when selecting the appropriate method. The client should always be encouraged to assist in the manoeuvre as much as they are able. This will not only

reduce the risk of injury for the carer, but will also promote client independence and therefore increase self-esteem.

The Resuscitation Council (UK) (2001) produced guidance for safer handling during resuscitation in hospital which outlines safe practice techniques that are unique to cardiopulmonary resuscitation. The production of such guidance is a huge step towards the recognition of risk assessment in the workplace and good practice in handling patients. When a patient collapses safe handling techniques are often forgotten in order to act quickly to save life. In this way the rescuers may put themselves at risk. Emergency situations require quick thinking and good assessment skills on the part of the rescuers and good communication skills to co-ordinate the team effort.

Following resuscitation the patient may need to be lifted from the floor onto a bed or trolley. The safest method would be to hoist the patient from the floor but some situations do not allow for this method (e.g. suspected spinal injury). In extreme cases a manual lift may be required. This type of transfer is high risk and should only be considered as a last resort.

Those organizations that have introduced safer handling policies since the legislation in 1992 have recognized the improvements in handling practice and also minimized the risk of large compensation claims for back-injured employees (Royal College of Nursing 1996b).

The *Code of Professional Conduct* of the Nursing and Midwifery Council (2002c) guides both qualified and student nurses in deciding whether to participate in a handling situation if there is any uncertainty regarding professional accountability. You are personally accountable for your practice and you must not involve yourself in anything that you know to be dangerous, for example continuing to use a method of handling that is considered as 'bad' practice. The first clause of the code of conduct states that you should always act in such a manner as to promote and safeguard the interests and well-being of patients and clients. You therefore need to be knowledgeable and up to date in all aspects of current practice.

Evidence based practice

In an attempt to quantify how well NHS Trusts were complying with the 1996 Safer Patient Handling Campaign messages, the Royal College of Nursing Working Well Initiative commissioned an exploratory survey during 2001 undertaken by Crumpton et al (2002). The aim of this survey was to quantify the impact of the 1996 campaign and to assess whether or not the aims were achieved.

The conclusion made was that the RCN's Safer Patient Handling Campaign seems to have fulfilled its aims in that the majority of Trusts either have a back care advisor (BCA) in post or have access to one. Therefore safer patient handling and risk awareness are being promoted within Trusts.

MANAGING UNTOWARD INCIDENTS IN HANDLING AND MOVING

In spite of the careful provision of both legislation and professional and local guidelines and policies, incidents leading to compensation claims for back injuries are still occurring. It is estimated that the UK economy loses approximately £50 billion each year as a result of inability to work due to back injuries (Back Care 2001). Case studies show that the fight for compensation is a slow process with detrimental effects on many aspects of an individual's life.

The following list indicates the areas that are likely to be investigated should a claim for compensation be pursued through the law courts:

- staff training, updating and attendance
- hazards, loads
- footwear and clothing at the time of the incident
- written policies for handling
- written plans for handling particular loads
- equipment provided or used to assist in load handling
- incident reporting
- follow-up treatment at the time of the injury
- any history of previous injury
- current work practices, staffing and workload.

Decision making exercise

You are on placement in the orthopaedic outpatients department and note a patient who has sustained a shoulder injury while handling loads in the store room of a company. He has been unable to work for 3 months and indicates that he intends submitting a claim for compensation against the company.

- List the factors that you think would need to be considered and investigated in connection with this claim.
- Consider what advice you could give this patient at this stage.

The previous section on Care Delivery highlighted the need for careful documentation of handling plans and evaluation of practices. Documentation communicates to all effective techniques or those that have been tried and found to be unsuccessful. There can be serious implications on any claim for compensation if an employee has ignored their employer's handling plan.

Additionally there is a requirement for adverse incidents to be clearly documented and such documentation can provide essential information in the event of an incident investigation.

The Health and Safety at Work Act 1974 has defined responsibilities for both employer and employee in this respect (outlined in Ch. 2). However, it would appear that healthcare staff need to improve record keeping considerably. The National Health Service Training Directorate (2001) indicate that more than one-third of the complaints are upheld regarding patient care involving lack of or incorrect information (i.e. poor record keeping). Often the problem is not writing down the wrong thing, but not writing anything.

MONITORING ACCIDENTS

A final aspect related to safety in moving and handling is the monitoring of accidents and incidents. Monitoring and reporting accidents regarding back injury is the responsibility of Occupational Health departments, who maintain detailed records of accidents and incidents that occur including follow-up care and the outcomes of treatment. This information can then be of use should an injured party seek legal compensation.

As a nurse you are at risk of injury and an occurrence such as back pain unrelieved by a night's rest should be documented on an appropriate incident form and reported to your Occupational Health department. Follow-up advice should be obtained to protect yourself from further injury.

Monitoring also enables Occupational Health personnel to identify areas where practices should be investigated. Where staff are reporting high levels of injury and absenteeism through back injury, specific support may be beneficial. In some hospitals, ergonomists have been appointed to provide advice. In certain situations it may be appropriate for the Health and Safety Executive to investigate working practices.

Evidence based practice

A survey conducted by Palmer et al (2000) stated that almost half the adult population of the UK (49%) report low back pain lasting at least 24 hours at some time during the year. In a similar survey conducted 10 years earlier by Walsh et al (1992) the percentage was one-third of the adult population.

ETHICAL DILEMMAS IN THE PROVISION OF SAFE HANDLING

Within any handling situation that involves the movement of clients it is paramount that wherever possible their wishes are respected: however, one must recognize that at times this may have unacceptable consequences for carers (e.g. a possible injury to carers as a result of not using a hoist). This is one example of a moral and ethical dilemma with which carers may be faced when planning to move clients. There are no easy answers and careful negotiation is required to achieve an acceptable outcome for all concerned.

Decision making exercise

Mrs Townshend is an obese 65-year-old diabetic lady who has just undergone an above-knee amputation of her right leg. It is proposed that she sits out of bed in a chair for a while and the nurses propose to use a hoist to help transfer her from bed to chair. However, Mrs Townshend refuses to get out of bed saying she is worried that she will fall out of the hoist and end up on the floor.

Please discuss and debate the following questions with particular reference to the Human Rights Act 1998:

1. Does the use of handling aids such as a hoist infringe on a client's rights?
2. If a client states that he or she does not wish to be moved using a hoist, do carers have any right to insist that the aid is used?
3. What might you do in the above circumstances?

Under the Human Rights Act 1998, public authorities are now under a duty to act compatibly with the European Convention rights of disabled people, including their rights under Article 3 (not to be subjected to inhuman or degrading treatment) and Article 8 (to develop their personality in their relations with others). Indeed public authorities (which includes agencies that may be private but are carrying out a 'public function', such as providing personal assistance under contract with a local authority) may be obliged by the coming into force of the Act to revisit their interpretation of their duties under health and safety legislation. Health and safety at work regulations must be interpreted so as to be compatible with those rights. According to legal advice sought by the Disability Rights Commission, '"no lifting" policies are likely to be unlawful to the extent that they preclude consideration of the particular needs of the individual concerned' (Disability Rights Commission 2002).

Falling patients are a great concern for nurses who often attempt to catch them in an effort to prevent harm. With all good intentions this practice is extremely dangerous and is responsible for numerous back injuries to nursing staff, some of which have ended that individual's career. The guidance is that if a patient is falling backwards and someone is with them, to take a step backwards away from the patient and guide him or her to the floor. If next to a wall encourage the patient to use it to slide down as a method of breaking the fall. Never attempt to catch a falling patient. If you can prevent them from banging their head then you have done a good job but do not feel guilty if you have not stopped the fall altogether.

PERSONAL AND REFLECTIVE KNOWLEDGE

PERSONAL CAPACITY FOR MOVING AND HANDLING PATIENTS

In this chapter, the importance of accurate assessment has been emphasized, as it is the basis for effective planning and implementation of skills. Safe practice requires you to be a knowledgeable professional and to develop the appropriate skills for your particular client population. These require continual development and updating throughout your career. Moving and handling practice is no exception. A safe practitioner must keep up to date with the latest legislation, guidelines and practices in order to move clients most effectively and safely. It is also essential to participate in the ongoing evaluation and development of equipment used in moving and handling clients in their own particular setting.

You have already reflected on your personal needs in relation to caring for yourself and ensuring optimum personal performance in the light of the knowledge offered in this chapter and reflective practice requires practitioners to review their nursing actions and interventions critically.

Should you personally experience an injury in relation to manual handling, the following organizations may be able to provide advice and support:

- The National Back Pain Association is a charity specifically concerned with the back pain sufferer and their family. Its address is National Back Pain Association, 16 Elmtree Road, Teddington, Middlesex TW11 8ST. Telephone: 02089775474. Website: www.backcare.org.uk.
- Work Injured Nurses' Group (WING) is affiliated to the Royal College of Nursing. It provides advice, information and support to any RCN member affected by injury, illness or disability. The group offers guidance on NHS and social security benefits and pensions, a range of information and advice guides, study days, a network of members and local support groups throughout the UK, and the WING quarterly newsletter. Its address is: 20 Cavendish Square, London W1G ORN. Telephone: 020 7647 3465. Website: www.rcn.org.uk.

Reflection on practice can be achieved by a comprehensive consideration of the four main branches of nursing. Case studies and reflective exercises are provided for you to consider these issues. Because of the practical nature of this chapter, a worked discussion is included for each case study. It is envisaged that this will allow you to compare your thoughts with those of the authors and generate ideas for your own practice.

CASE STUDIES RELATED TO HANDLING AND MOVING

The following case study scenarios will be used in the next section so that you can explore the importance of assessing the task, load, environment and individual handler's capabilities. All names used are pseudonyms.

Case study: Learning disabilities

Martin Richards is a 15-year-old boy with learning disabilities. He weighs 8 stone (50 kg), lives at home with his parents, and attends a day centre during school periods. His mobility needs are met by transporting him in a wheelchair both at home and in the day centre, but he does need transferring from wheelchair to the toilet and vice versa on a regular basis. At the day centre he receives regular physiotherapy to prevent joint contractures. He is subject to bouts of anger, which make him unco-operative at times. Both Martin's home and the day centre have been adapted to allow access for equipment.

1. In relation to Martin:
   - List all the Tasks that require assessment.
   - Are there any additional factors relating to Individual handlers that need to be taken into account?
   - Identify factors to take into consideration regarding the 'Load' to be handled.
   - Jot down any pertinent Environmental factors that may affect Martin's handling situation.
   - Consider equipment/Resources that may be useful and why you would choose to use it.
2. Using the scenario make notes on the handling plan you might make for Martin.
3. In the middle of a bout of anger, Martin indicates that he needs to use the toilet. He is shouting at carers and making punching gestures at anyone who approaches him. How would you deal with this situation?
4. Compare your ideas with the thoughts of our authors outlined below.

Suggested management for Martin Richards

1. Assessment
   - *Tasks.* Manoeuvring the wheelchair: pivotal transfer will be necessary from wheelchair to the toilet and vice versa.
   - *Factors affecting Individual handlers.* Staff need to be aware of signs that precede Martin's bouts of anger that lead to his difficult behaviour. It has already been established that the environment is suitable for clients in wheelchairs and those who require transfer. The main focus for Martin is his unpredictability. Therefore, it is vital that staff have identified and documented both verbal and non-verbal cues that precede his bouts of anger. These warning signs must be made known to all carers so that they can avoid situations that carry a high risk of resulting in injury.
   - *Load.* Martin is unpredictable at times, although in ideal conditions his weight is acceptable for handling.
   - *Environment.* Suitable access for wheelchairs and transfers.
   - *Equipment/Resources.* A transfer belt could assist the pivotal transfer. No equipment is necessary for manoeuvring the

wheelchair but good posture needs to be taken into account here.
2. Handling plan
   - *Transfer.* Martin does not usually have to be lifted. In using a pivotal transfer the nurse uses the principles of leverage and the patient takes some weight through their legs and feet. The choice here may be for one or two nurses to transfer Martin, possibly using a transfer belt or board. It must be remembered that the individual's capabilities in relation to handling are important here. It is also often recommended by employers that two people should be present for any handling situation and it is vital that you check the local policy about this. It is usually useful to have a second person strategically placed to assist in the transfer should the need arise. Using a transfer belt or board will also assist the individual who has reduced or absent muscle tone. The joints of such patients can be damaged if the nurse's grasp is at the joints. In addition, if the patient suddenly becomes a 'dead weight' through not taking some weight through their lower limbs the nurse may be put at risk. A transfer aid enables the assistant to help take some weight from the main transfer person.
   - *Unpredictable behaviour.* Martin's bouts of anger leading to uncooperative behaviour are a key factor. Careful observation may mean that subtle signs of developing anger can alert the nurse to potentially hazardous **situations** when manual handling should be avoided until the situation has been defused or resolved. If problems are encountered during the transfer it may be appropriate to use controlled fall techniques (National Back Pain Association 1991) to lower Martin to the floor until he can be handled safely. As long as Martin is not a danger to himself or others the nurse should let him vent his anger and only attempt to handle him once the situation is over and he is co-operative again.
   - *Communication.* Nursing staff must not rely on recognizing the signs of Martin's anger intuitively: they must be recorded. This is particularly important for students who may be in placements for short periods of time and so do not know the patients as intimately as the permanent staff. Close supervision of a student by experienced staff can form the basis of a positive learning experience for the student in this sort of situation.
3. Dealing with Martin's anger and his need to use the toilet
   An occurrence like this will pose a dilemma for the carers. To maintain Martin's dignity and promote normality it is important to help him meet his physical needs. However, the carer has to balance meeting his immediate needs with the possibility that Martin or his carers may sustain injuries as handling under these circumstances would be less than ideal.

Case study: Child

Emma Newton is a 2½-year-old girl who is being treated at regular intervals in hospital for leukaemia. The treatment leaves her feeling very weak, but in spite of this she is a determined little girl who dislikes staying in her cot and becomes distressed if she cannot continue to play with her toys on the floor. She weighs 2 stone (12.7 kg). Her drugs are given intermittently through a line inserted into a major vein in the upper thorax and care needs to be taken not to dislodge this. Her mother stays with her while she is an inpatient and she is visited regularly by her twin brothers who are 5 years old. The environment is a happy cheerful setting and provides many toys and equipment for the children to play with. Friends are encouraged to visit and the ward is often full of children.

1. In relation to Emma:
   - List all the Tasks that will require assessment.
   - Are there additional factors relating to the Individual handlers that need to be taken into account?
   - Identify factors to take into consideration regarding the 'Load' to be handled.
   - Jot down any pertinent Environmental factors that may affect Emma's handling situation.
   - Consider any equipment/Resources that may be used and why you would choose to use it.
2. Using the scenario make notes on the handling plan you might make for Emma.
3. Emma's mother comments to you that she is concerned that Andrew, one of Emma's twin brothers, spends a lot of time trying to pick Emma up and cuddle her. Although she says she can understand that he wants to make her better, she is concerned about him dropping her and also about the long-term effects on his back from carrying her around. Given that spinal damage often begins in childhood (National Back Pain Association 1990), devise a programme to help educate Emma's brothers about the importance of caring for their backs.
4. Compare your ideas with the thoughts of our authors outlined below.

Suggested management for Emma Newton

1. Assessment
   - *Tasks.* Moving from cot to floor and chair, moving from floor to cot, assisting with toileting and hygiene needs.
   - *Factors affecting Individual handlers.* Fitness for task and assistance required. Although Emma's weight may make it easy for one nurse to manage her, other factors such as taking care not to displace the intravenous line mean that additional help may be required. If Emma's mother is involved in Emma's care, it is important to consider the educational needs of the mother in relation to handling. The nurse should also consider her own posture when lifting the child from the cot. Does this mean reaching forward, forward bending or rotation of the spine, or can the cot sides be lowered to allow a good posture? In addition, when lifting from the floor, the handler's knees are fully bent, which reduces the handler's lifting capacity. These factors, together with possible clutter and hazards of other children present, create a high-risk manoeuvre that requires careful thought and planning by the nurse. However, as Emma is

cared for regularly in this setting it may be pertinent for the nurse to consult previous assessments and plans that have been formulated for Emma. They could provide invaluable information about how Emma has been handled successfully in the past. Alternatively, the evaluations may provide information about which manoeuvres have been unsuccessful.
   - *Load.* Emma's weight should be acceptable for one nurse to manage under ideal conditions, but assistance may be required because of attachments.
   - *Environment.* May be cluttered with toys. Other children present may be a hazard. Cot is fixed height and has side bars to negotiate.
   - *Equipment/Resources.* Equipment may not be necessary, but wrapping Emma in a blanket may make her more secure.
2. Handling plan
   - *Movement in bed.* Moving Emma within her cot poses little risk due to her weight, but could be hazardous if the height of the cot is unsuitable as the nurse may find it difficult to adopt a safe posture. It may help to lower the cot side and put one knee on the cot to get close to Emma and to help keep the spine in normal alignment. Forward bending must be avoided.
   - *Movement from cot to floor.* This could be quite hazardous. The nurse needs to ensure that there are no obstacles in the way and may need assistance to protect the venous line. Moving from an upright position to the floor needs to be carried out with care to maintain normal spinal posture. Holding Emma close to the trunk will help reduce spinal loading on the nurse.
3. An educational strategy for Emma's brothers
   This could include making up a game or rhyme to help the children think about bending their knees and keeping the spine in alignment when reaching for items on the floor. Also, obtaining leaflets and posters that are appropriate for children would be helpful for the ward Emma is on. This type of information would also help Emma's mother handle her daughter safely.

Case study: Adult

Robert Sinclair is a 70-year-old man who has always had a problem with his weight. He weighs 20 stone (127 kg) and over the years this excess weight has caused degeneration in his joints. The net result is that he is unable to stand and take his own weight. This is the main reason why he is living in a nursing home. Robert is an articulate gentleman who pays a great deal of attention to his personal hygiene and likes to bath on a daily basis. He likes to sit in the conservatory as he has enjoyed gardening in the past. The nursing home is modern and the nurse managers have taken account for the need for access for specialized equipment in the design of the building.

1. In relation to Robert:
   - List all the Tasks that will require assessment.

- Are there additional factors relating to Individual handlers that need to be taken into account?
- Identify factors to take into consideration regarding the 'Load' to be handled.
- Jot down any pertinent Environmental factors that may affect Robert's handling situation.
- Consider equipment/Resources that may be of use and state why you would choose to use them.

2. Using the scenario make notes on the handling plan you might make for Robert.
3. While you are working on placement in the nursing home you hear that a care assistant has transferred Robert from his bed to a chair using the hoist and sling that is normally used for his transfer. After the manoeuvre Robert complains bitterly that he was extremely uncomfortable and that the sling has scraped the skin on the back of his thighs. It becomes apparent that the care assistant has only been shown once how to use the hoist by another care assistant.
   - What should the qualified nurse in charge of the shift need to do about this situation?
   - What measures could have been implemented to prevent this type of occurrence?
4. Compare your ideas with the thoughts of our authors outlined below.

Suggested management for Robert Sinclair

1. Assessment
   - *Tasks.* Moving Robert from bed to a chair, chair to the toilet and transfer to other areas in the home, moving Robert up the bed and turning him on his side.
   - *Factors affecting Individual handlers.* Staff will need education in the use of hoists and other equipment. In using equipment there may be a risk of repetitive strain injury. Because Robert is able to co-operate he will be able to participate in the assessment process. This will be helpful as the pain in his joints may vary in intensity. The ability to communicate this will enable the variations in handling techniques to be employed, i.e. the type of sling to use with the hoist for maximum patient comfort. Adequate pain relief also needs to be provided to ensure patient comfort.
   - *Load.* Robert's weight is far too great for even two nurses to handle without using aids.
   - *Environment.* The home is well adapted for the residents, but may become cluttered with the residents' personal belongings. Carpets may mean that hoists and wheelchairs will be difficult to manoeuvre.
   - *Equipment/Resources.* A hoist with sling suitable for Robert's weight would be used to move him from bed to chair, chair to toilet, and transfer within the home. A sliding sheet could be used for turning Robert and sliding him up the bed.
2. Handling plan
   - *The options to choose in most handling situations are to avoid lifting.* To promote Robert's quality of life it is necessary to make him as mobile as possible without lifting and putting the nursing staff at high risk of injury.

- *Moving in bed.* Sliding may be an option for movement up the bed or the use of the 30 degrees tilt (Preston 1988) for turning. However, Robert is rather heavy and it is unlikely that two nurses could manage these manoeuvres without risk. If enough staff are available these may be viable options.
- *Movement from bed to chair or toilet.* A hoist would be the most appropriate piece of equipment and would also be the safest way to move Robert up and down the bed. There are many hoists available and it is important to choose within any area the one that is most versatile and useful for the type of patients nursed. Other considerations are the weight limit of the hoist and the selection of slings available for use with the hoist. The noise levels produced, the way the hoist is operated, and how easy it is to manoeuvre in the environment are other important factors. In relation to the nursing staff, the postures adopted when operating the hoist and the type of operating controls can result in repetitive strain injury to the wrists, shoulders and spine. Also strain when pushing or pulling the hoist (e.g. on carpeted areas) may put the nurse at risk of injury. Some hoists may require additional force to move them. It is vital that nurses have adequate training and supervision for operating any equipment used. This prevents discomfort for the patient and reduces the risk of injury to both nurses and patients.
- *Environment.* Clearing the environment of patients' personal belongings as well as other equipment is vital to reduce potential hazards. Timing of procedures may help with this and can contribute to the safety of all involved. In addition, preparing things such as the chair the patient is to sit in will save time and minimize distress for the person being moved. It can be most undignified to be left supported in a hoist while nurses look for a suitable chair for the patient to sit in.

3. Managing Robert's 'transfer' problem
   - The nurse in charge of the shift on this occasion would have a duty to ensure that any treatment and care necessary for the skin abrasion was carried out and documented. An untoward incident form would require completion, detailing all aspects of the incident, including the outcome of interviews with the care assistant and any other witnesses to the incident. Robert's relatives would need to be informed and also the manager of the nursing home.
   - The provision of training for staff should be considered to prevent such an incident. Training is required under the Health and Safety at Work Act 1974.

Case study: Mental health

Doreen Jones is a 66-year-old lady with advanced dementia. She has extremely limited communication skills and is really only able to communicate pain by screaming at the nurses. Doreen weighs 11 stone (70 kg) and is unable to perform activities of living unaided as her body is permanently rigid with arms and legs flexed and in a fixed position. She frequently slips down the bed, but is unable to sit out in a chair because when she does she arches her back and is at risk of falling out of the chair and injuring herself. The care setting is purpose built, but to make it as homely as possible, much of the area is taken up by bedside tables, chairs and personal belongings for the residents.

1. In relation to Doreen
   - List all the Tasks that require assessment.
   - Are there additional factors relating to Individual handlers that need to be taken into account?
   - Identify factors to take into consideration regarding the 'Load' to be handled.
   - Jot down any pertinent Environmental factors that may affect Doreen's handling situation.
   - Consider equipment/Resources that may be of use and state why you would choose to use them.
2. Using the scenario make notes on the handling plan you might make for Doreen.
3. Compare your ideas with the thoughts of our authors outlined below.

Suggested management for Doreen Jones

1. Assessment
   - *Tasks*. Moving Doreen up and down the bed, turning from side to side.
   - *Factors affecting Individual handlers*. Staff need to be aware of maximizing communication with Doreen. Awareness of the signs of pain that Doreen demonstrates and analgesia available for her are important factors to take into consideration. For Doreen, continuous slipping which will result in repetitive tasks will increase the risk of injury considerably, particularly as communication is difficult. These factors, together with a cluttered environment, pose a potential hazard. Therefore, the assessment in this type of situation will need to be detailed to allow effective planning.
   - *Load*. Doreen is 11 stone (70 kg) and will require an appropriate handling plan or the use of handling aids.
   - *Environment*. The environment is cluttered and will therefore pose a hazard to staff that needs to be eliminated.
   - *Equipment/Resources*. A sliding sheet to move Doreen up the bed or a sheet for the 30 degrees tilt (Preston 1988).
2. Handling plan
   - Movement in bed. Doreen presents a high-risk handling situation. This is compounded by communication difficulties, her flexed, rigid posture, and the level of pain she suffers. The most sensible option for Doreen would be to use a sliding sheet to move her up and down the bed and the 30 degrees tilt to turn her to prevent pressure sore formation. Utilizing these manoeuvres will reduce the pain she suffers and will help to prevent joint injuries due to poor grasp of the patient by nursing staff. Use of the same techniques by nursing staff may help to reduce some of Doreen's fear about what is happening to her. Another important factor is the use of prophylactic pain relief rather

than waiting for Doreen to scream out in pain before analgesia is administered. Slipping down the bed frequently not only means that Doreen will have to be handled frequently, but can also contribute to the development of pressure sores. To help prevent slipping down the bed it is important to check that the lumbar curve of the spine is well supported. This can be done by inserting your hand between the pillows and lumbar curve. If there is a gap between the pillows and the spine, the pillows need to be rearranged to fit comfortably into the lumbar curve. If this is not done, the lack of support will give Doreen backache and make her fidget to get comfortable, and as a result she will slip further down the bed. In addition, a soft pillow support underneath her flexed legs will fulfill a similar function to the lumbar curve support. Alternatively, using a hoist with an appropriate sling may be another option. Due to difficulties in communicating with Doreen the sight of a large piece of mechanical machinery may increase her fear. Over time, though, the efficient use of the equipment with minimal discomfort to Doreen may help alleviate this. However, it is vital that nursing staff know how to use the equipment correctly as one disastrous attempt with such equipment will lead to further patient fear, distrust and lack of cooperation.

Summary

This chapter has introduced you to the knowledge required to make effective nursing decisions in moving and handling situations. It has included:

1. An outline of the applied anatomy of the spine and the effects of cumulative back strain/injury on a person's lifestyle.
2. A description of the key issues that need to be assessed along with the use of an assessment tool and a handling and moving plan.
3. Discussion on how evaluation can contribute to safer handling of patients.
4. An emphasis on the importance of accurate record keeping in relation to manual handling.
5. Focus on the importance of legislation on manual handling.
6. A brief review of potential ethical problems arising in handling situations.
7. An emphasis on the need to care for your own back.

Annotated further reading and websites

1. Books published by the Health and Safety Executive (HSE) Manual Handling Operations Regulations 1992: Guidance on Regulations, 2nd edn. HSE Books 1998

Getting to grips with manual handling: a short guide for employers. HSE Books 2000 (single copies free, multiple copies in priced packs)

Manual handling: solutions you can handle. HSE Books 1994

Five steps to risk assessment. HSE Books 1998 (single copies free, multiple copies in priced packs)

A pain in your workplace? Ergonomic problems and solutions. HSE Books 1994

Manual handling in the health services (Health Services Advisory Committee). HSE Books 1993

Guidance on manual handling of loads in the health service (Health Services Advisory Committee). HSE Books 1998

Upper limb disorders: assessing the risks. HSE Books 1999

Lighten the load: guidance for employees on musculoskeletal disorders: employer (INDG 109). HSE Books 1995

Lighten the load: guidance for employees on musculoskeletal disorders: employee (INDG 110). HSE Books 1995

HSE priced and free publications can be obtained from:
HSE Books
PO Box 1999
Sudbury
Suffolk CO10 2WA
UK
Tel: 01787 881165
Fax: 01787 313995
http://www.hsebooks.co.uk

2. Books published by the Royal College of Nursing (RCN)
RCN code of practice for patient handling (Working Well Initiative)
Introducing a safer patient handling policy (Working Well Initiative)
Manual handling assessments in hospitals and the community
The guide to the handling of patients, 4th edn

RCN publications can be obtained from:
RCN Direct
Tel: 0845 7726100 or
Royal College of Nursing
20 Cavendish Square
London W1G 0RN
UK
Tel: 0207 4093333

3. Books published by the Disabled Living Foundation (DLF)
Handling people: equipment, advice and information

Chambers R, Hawksley B, Smith G, Chambers C 2001 *Pain matters in primary care.* Radcliffe Medical Press, Oxford

DLF publications can be obtained from:
DLF
360–384 Harrow Road
London W9 2HU
UK
Tel: 0207 289 6111

4. Books published by the National Back Exchange
The interprofessional curriculum: a course for back care advisors. Published by National Back Exchange (NBE), the Chartered Society of Physiotherapists (CSP), the College of Occupational Therapists (COT), the Ergonomics Society and the Royal College of Nursing (RCN)

This publication can be obtained from:
National Back Exchange
Plantation House

The Bell Plantation
Towcester
Northamptonshire NN12 6HN
UK
Tel: 01327 358855
Fax: 01327 354476

5. Books published by UNISON
Ending back pain from lifting: a safety representative's guide to preventing injury through manual handling. UNISON 1999

Inspecting for lifting and handling hazards. UNISON 1996

UNISON publications can be obtained from:
UNISON
1 Mabledon Place
LONDON WC1H 9AJ
UK
Tel: 0207 388 2366

6. Books published by the Chartered Society of Physiotherapy
Joint Statement on Manual Handling. Chartered Society of Physiotherapy (CSP), Royal College of Nursing (RCN) and College of Occupational Therapists (COT). Information Paper no. 41 1997

Delegation of tasks to assistants: a guide for qualified members and assistants. Information Paper no. PA6 May 2002

Vocational rehabilitation: briefing document

CSP publications can be obtained from:
Chartered Society of Physiotherapy
14 Bedford Row
London WC1R 4ED
UK
Tel: 0207 306 6666
Fax: 0207 306 6611

http://www.think-back.com
Think Back is a key management programme for those with long-term back problems providing support, contact and information.

http://www.learninglink.ac.uk/moveit/moveit.htm
An Internet course that covers all aspects of basic handling, managing risk and load carrying. A simple approach to ensure safe moving and handling.

http://www.iea.cc
International Ergonomics Association. The federation of ergonomics and human factors societies provides this site. Its mission is to elaborate and advance ergonomic science and practice, and to improve the quality of life by expanding its scope of application and contribution to society.

http://www.hse.gov.uk
Site connection to The Manual Handling Operation Regulations 1998.

http://www.hmso.gov.uk/si/si1998/19982307.htm
Links with the Health and Safety Executive website offering leaflets, new publications, research and statistics.

http://www.nhs.uk/backinwork
The NHS Back in Work campaign website is aimed at everyone who works in the NHS. Offering practical

guidance for implementing local policies for dealing with back pain.

http://www.backcare.org.uk
Back Care is a charity for healthier backs. It provides education on how to avoid back injuries and support for those with back pain through education, information and publications.

http://www.nationalbackexchange.org.uk
National Back Exchange is a multidisciplinary group for those with an interest in back care and prevention of work related musculoskeletal disorders.

http://www.unison.org.uk
UNISON's site, providing news and campaigns.

References

Back Care 2001 UK charter for back care. Available: http://www.backpain.org/pages/c_pages/charter.php

BBC News Online 2000 Nurse wins £800 000 for back injury. Available: www.bbconline.com

Commission of the European Communities 1990 Council directive on the minimum health and safety requirements for the manual handling of loads where there is a risk of back injury to workers, 4th Directive 90/269/EEC. Official Journal of the European Communities 156:9–13

Confederation of Health Service Employees 1992 Backbreaking work. Confederation of Health Service Employees, Banstead

Crumpton E, Bannister C, Maw J 2002 Survey to investigate NHS trusts compliance with the RCN safer patient handling policy 1996. Royal College of Nursing, London

Demain S, Gore S, McLellan D L 2000 The use of leg lifting equipment. Nursing Standard 14(39):41–43

Disability Rights Commission 2002 Background paper on health and safety, risk management and independent living for disabled people. Disability Rights Commission Online. Available: http://www.drc-gb.org.uk

Dolan P, Adams M A 1998 Repetitive lifting tasks fatigue the back muscles and increase the bending movement on the lumbar spine. Journal of Biomechanics 31:713–721

Dul J, Weerdmeester B 1993 Ergonomics for beginners, 9th edn. Taylor and Francis, London

European Foundation for the Improvement of Living and Working Conditions 2001 Third European Survey on Working Conditions 2000. European Foundation, Dublin

Health and Safety at Work Act 1974 HMSO, London

Health and Safety Executive 1992 Manual handling operation regulations. HMSO, London

Health Education Authority 1994 Look after yourself: tutors' manual. Health Education Authority, London

Hemple S 1993 Home truths. Nursing Times 89(15):40–41

Hingnett S 1996 Work related back pain in nurses. Journal of Advanced Nursing 23:1238–1246

Hinchliff S, Montague S 1988 Physiology for nursing practice. Baillière Tindall, London

Human Rights Act 1998 HMSO, London

Lloyd P 1996 The guide to the handling of patients, 4th edn. National Back Pain Association, Teddington

Maitland J 1989 The Alexander technique. Nursing Times 85(42):55–57

McGuire T, Dewar J 1995 An assessment of moving and handling practices among Scottish nurses. Nursing Standard 9(40):35–39

Moore W 1993 Reporting back. Nursing Times 89(22):29–30

National Back Pain Association 1990 Better backs for children: a guide for teachers and parents. National Back Pain Association with British Petroleum, Teddington

National Back Pain Association 1991 Lifting and handling: an ergonomic approach. National Back Pain Association, Teddington

National Back Pain Association 1992 The handling of patients, 3rd edn. National Back Pain Association in collaboration with the Royal College of Nursing, Teddington

National Back Pain Association 2002 National Back Pain Association website. Available: http://www.backpain.org

National Health Service Training Directorate 1994 Formal investigation and legal issues: just for the record. National Health Service Training Directorate, Leeds

National Health Service Training Directorate 2001 Work related back disorder statistics information sheet. National Health Service Training Directorate, Leeds

Nursing and Midwifery Council 2002a Practitioner–client relationship and the prevention of abuse. Nursing and Midwifery Council, London

Nursing and Midwifery Council 2002b Guidelines for records and record keeping. Nursing and Midwifery Council, London

Nursing and Midwifery Council 2002c Code of professional conduct. Nursing and Midwifery Council, London

Palmer K T, Walsh K, Bendall H et al 2000 Back pain in Britian: a comparison of two prevalence surveys at an interval of ten years. British Medical Journal 320:1577–1578

Preston K W 1988 Positioning for comfort and pressure relief: the 30 degree alternative. Care, Science and Practice 6(4):116–119

Resuscitation Council (UK) 2001 Guidance for safer handling during resuscitation in hospitals. Resuscitation Council (UK), London

Royal College of Nursing 1993 Code of practice for handling of patients. Royal College of Nursing, London

Royal College of Nursing 1995 Hazards for pregnant nurses: an A–Z guide. Royal College of Nursing, London

Royal College of Nursing 1996a Code of practice for handling of patients. Royal College of Nursing, London

Royal College of Nursing 1996b Introducing a safer patient handling policy. Royal College of Nursing, London

Royal College of Nursing 1999 Code of practice for handling patients. Royal College of Nursing, London

Royal College of Nursing 2003 Manual handling assessment in hospital and community: an RCN guide, 3rd edn. Royal College of Nursing, London

Seccombe I, Smith G 1996 In the balance: registered nurse supply and demand, Institute for Employment Studies Report no. 315. Institute for Employment Studies, London

Seccombe I, Smith G 1999 The Institute of Employment Studies Report to the Royal College of Nursing on incidence of back injuries in nurses. Unpublished

Steed R, Tracey C 2000 Equipment for moving and handling: hoists and slings. British Journal of Therapy and Rehabilitation 7(10):430–435

Steed R, Wiltshire S, Cassar S et al 2000 Moving and handling: legislation and responsibilities. British Journal of Therapy and Rehabilitation 7(9):382–386

Stubbs D A 2000 Implementing and evaluating an ergonomics intervention. Conference presentation, Robens Centre for Health Ergonomics, University of Surrey.

Tracy M, Ruszala S 1998 Introducing a safer patient handling policy. In: Lloyd, P (ed) The handling of patients: a guide for nurses, 4th edn. National Back Pain Association, Teddington, pp 23–29

Viry P 1999 Non-specific back pain in children: a search for associated factors in 14 year old school children. Revue du Rheumatisme (English edn) 66:381–388

Walsh K, Cruddes M, Coggon D 1992 Low back pain in eight areas of Britain. Journal of Epidemiology Community Health 46(3):231–233

Walsh R 1988 Good movement habits. Nursing Times 84(37):59–61

Wilson C B 2001 Safer handling practice for nurses: a review of the literature. British Journal of Nursing 10(2):108–114

Chapter 6

Homeostasis

Helen Dobbins, Gary Adams and Diane Hewson

KEY ISSUES

SUBJECT KNOWLEDGE
- Behavioural, cultural and environmental factors that affect health
- Mechanism of feedback loops in maintaining homeostasis
- Biological basis of thermoregulation, blood pressure maintenance, pulse and respiratory homeostasis

CARE DELIVERY KNOWLEDGE
- Measurement and assessment of body temperature
- Measurement and assessment of blood pressure
- Measurement and assessment of respiration

PROFESSIONAL AND ETHICAL KNOWLEDGE
- Accountability
- Consent
- Health promotion

PERSONAL AND REFLECTIVE KNOWLEDGE
- Ideas for portfolio and skills laboratory learning
- Case study consolidation

INTRODUCTION

Being healthy implies a feeling of general well-being. Although originally focused primarily on physical well-being, it is now recognized that there are multiple, inter-dependent, dimensions to feeling healthy, including psychosocial, spiritual and emotional dimensions. To maintain health individuals need to constantly adapt to changes within their own internal environment and to the changing external environment. An individual becomes 'unhealthy' or 'unwell' when any of the dimensions of their health are affected by internal or external forces to which they are unable to adapt. The nurse supports the patient or client's ability to adapt through health education, assessment and therapeutic interventions.

This chapter will explore the ways in which the human establishes and maintains a stable internal environment. This balance of the system is known as homeostasis. The word homeostasis is derived from the Greek words 'homeo' (same) and 'stasis' (staying). Many mechanisms exist within the body that can rapidly respond to change in order to maintain homeostasis.

This chapter will examine the fundamental bases of homeostasis and the ways in which the body responds in an attempt to meet the specific demands placed upon it by a changing blood pressure, body temperature and respiration. The role of the nurse in monitoring temperature, blood pressure and respiration will be explored and the related professional and ethical issues. As the content of this chapter focuses on these three specific areas of homeostasis, it is expected that you will cross-reference with many other chapters for other complementary aspects of homeostasis, for example Chapter 3 on resuscitation, Chapter 14 on skin integrity, Chapter 7 on nutrition and Chapter 8 on stress, relaxation and rest.

OVERVIEW

Subject knowledge

The mechanisms of feedback loops are explored. These are essential to maintaining homeostasis. The chapter will then concentrate on how normal temperature, blood pressure and respiration are maintained and controlled by the body.

Individual behavioural, environmental, social and emotional factors also have an effect on how internal body balance is maintained. These factors are explored under psychosocial and environmental subject knowledge.

Care delivery knowledge

The knowledge needed by the nurse for making a comprehensive assessment of temperature, blood pressure and respirations is explored. The nursing management of some common problems that threaten homeostasis are also included in this section.

Professional and ethical knowledge

Professional issues that influence the role of the nurse in the assessment of homeostasis are identified. The discussion includes an exploration of how the issues of consent, professional accountability and health promotion apply to the nurse's role when undertaking observations and measurements.

Personal and reflective knowledge

Suggestions are made for portfolio development and experiential exercises in which assessment of homeostasis can be practiced in a safe environment. Consolidation of knowledge gained from the chapter and through your practice experience is facilitated through case study work.

On pages 148–149 there are four case studies, each one relating to one of the branch programmes. You may find it helpful to read one of them before you start the chapter and use it as a focus for your reflections while reading.

SUBJECT KNOWLEDGE

MECHANISMS IN HOMEOSTASIS

Before outlining specific knowledge needed for clinical decision making regarding body temperature, blood pressure and respiration, it is important to understand the internal mechanisms involved in maintaining balance in all body systems and also consider potential external influences.

Internally, most of the control systems of the body are based on the principle of negative feedback, that is, any deviation from the normal range results in the body correcting the high or low value and re-establishing a state of equilibrium. Within the process of negative feedback, there is an inhibitory component that prevents the body from becoming too cold or too hot. For example, when the body is too hot, peripheral vasodilatation occurs and heat is lost under the direction of the hypothalamus. As a consequence, body temperature drops. A further reduction in temperature is

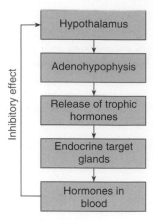

Figure 6.1 Negative feedback loop.

prevented by thermoreceptors in the skin sending messages to the hypothalamus to inhibit vasodilatation. Thus the inhibitory message 'kicks in' (Fig. 6.1).

The hypothalamus is the 'brain of the brain' and is part of the limbic system, which helps to maintain homeostasis. The hypothalamus regulates eating and drinking, sleeping and waking, body temperature, hormone balances, heart rate, sex drive and emotions. It also directs the master gland of the brain – the pituitary gland – which is responsible for regulating hormonal balance within the body. The brain is therefore the major organ of adaption and can respond to changes in the external and internal environment quickly and flexibly to maintain health. How homeostasis is specifically maintained is the major focus of this chapter, but although homeostasis is concerned with the stability and maintenance of internal physiological systems, it is also important to consider such balance as being within a context of some external influence.

EXTERNAL INFLUENCES ON HOMEOSTASIS

Psychosocial, cultural, economic and environmental factors can affect homeostasis and need to be considered. Influences on behaviour are individual to each person, but are usually associated with the family and school in childhood, peers in early adolescence, social groupings and religious beliefs, the media and multiple other sources. The beliefs of society are influential and how individuals become ill or remain healthy is affected by cultural beliefs on what is good and bad

---

Evidence based practice

Calman & Johnson (1985) examined the perceptions about health of women from middle class and working class backgrounds. The middle class women were more likely to talk about engaging in exercise, being fit and active, and eating the right food. Working class women focused on getting through the day without being ill.
Both groups felt that being healthy meant not visiting the doctor or taking time off.

'healthy' behaviour. Many sociologists have commented on the 'lay' perceptions of health as opposed to how professionals describe, label and classify 'ill-health' (Helman 1994, Kleinman 1980, Mishler 1981).

All these differences can be important in deciding how to approach individuals and groups when involved in health promotion activities. Cultural beliefs can also lead to misunderstandings and may even be a threat to health. An example would be using a hot water bottle during the shivering phase of a fever for a young child aged between 6 months and 3 years. Besides the danger of burning the skin, the child's temperature may rise rapidly, leading to an increased risk of febrile convulsion.

Environmental factors, which include political and economic factors over which individuals have limited control, have often been underestimated in the past as a source of ill-health (Blackburn 1991, Townsend & Davidson 1982). Government legislation and policy are important in controlling situations that have a detrimental affect on health (see Chapter 2 on safety and risk). The government made a commitment in the National Health Service plan (Department of Health 2000a) to reduce health inequalities. This has recently been made a key priority area and specific targets have been set for the Primary Care Trusts (PCTs) to achieve between 2003 and 2006 (Department of Health 2003). These include improving infant mortality and life expectancy across socioeconomic and geographical disadvantaged groups. It is well established that unskilled men are three times more likely to die prematurely from heart disease (Department of Health 2000b) and this pattern of inequality is reflected across a range of other diseases such as diabetes. In the context of this chapter, the most significant aspects of this policy are those in relation to smoking cessation and the prevention and treatment of coronary heart disease (CHD), in particular the early detection and management of hypertension.

Smoking is the principal avoidable cause of death in the UK. A comprehensive smoking cessation plan is now in place to help reduce disease and deaths from smoking and the effects of passive smoking, particularly in public places and at work (Department of Health 1998). This involves the provision of free advice, services and treatments to help individuals give up smoking.

The National Service Framework for CHD (Department of Health 2000b) clearly states in standards two and three the importance of screening to identify people with symptoms of CHD or those at risk of developing it. Early detection and treatment of hypertension is a very important step in reducing CHD. Nurses make a significant contribution towards achieving these standards through their role in activities such as lifestyle checks and hypertension clinics, where they can offer health advice and support, alongside monitoring blood pressure and other physical signs.

Government economic policy has also had a direct impact on individuals in society who are at risk of hypothermia. It could be argued that imposing a tax on fuel and limiting extra payments to the elderly and disabled until certain low temperatures have been reached over consecutive days has little impact overall on reducing morbidity and mortality due to hypothermia during the winter months. Research in this area is fraught with difficulties as hypothermia is often not the main recorded cause of death (Watson 1996); however, the Department of Health (2001a) suggest that there are about 80 000 cold-related deaths each year in the UK. Although health promotion may be addressed at the levels of behaviour and lifestyle, it may still be the cost factor that predominates in an individual's ability to keep warm in winter.

A more recent concern is that of the health effects of climate change in the UK (Department of Health 2001a). It is anticipated that there will be a gradual fall in cold-related deaths and an increase in heat-related deaths due to global warming over the next few decades. Surprisingly there are about 800 heat-related deaths in the UK per year; these are mainly related to the effects of heat waves on the elderly.

Health promotion is a complex and challenging activity. Both Tannahill (1985) and Tones (1993) recognize the interrelationship between individual behaviours and environmental factors in relation to health promotion and recommend a mixture of political action, creating supportive and strong community action groups, changing the approach of health services and professionals, and developing the individual's personal esteem and ability to make informed choices.

Good health is a fundamental building block of wellbeing and as stated in the Introduction, the body strives to maintain balance and adapt to changes through homeostasis. The rest of this chapter will focus upon the maintainance of homeostasis within the three key areas already identified: control of body temperature, blood pressure maintenance and respiratory regulation.

THE BALANCE OF BODY TEMPERATURE

The main organ for maintaining normal body temperature or thermoregulation is the skin. The skin has many vital functions. However, in this particular section, thermoregulation and its homeostatic control will be the main focus (see Chapter 14 for other functions of the skin).

Evidence based practice

Case & Waterhouse (1994) indicate that homeothermy is dependent upon continual thermoregulation. Environmental temperature variation studies demonstrate that these may be circadian (diurnal), circannual or geographic. Diurnal ranges of 35°C are commonly recorded in continental hot deserts. The largest circannual temperature variations occur in the centre of large land masses where winter temperatures can fall to −65°C and summers have a mean of +20°C. Geographically, individual populations live in environmental temperatures ranging from −65°C to 50°C.

Humans are homeothermic and can only maintain core temperature within a narrow range of 36–38°C despite the day-to-day fluctuations encountered as a consequence of environmental temperatures and our own metabolic activities. Homeothermy is dependent upon continual thermoregulation (Case & Waterhouse 1994) with the scales finely balanced between heat production and heat loss.

Four major physical processes are involved in the loss of heat from the skin to the environment:

- evaporation
- conduction
- radiation
- convection.

Each of these processes is important to understand when managing the care of patients and clients.

Evaporation (22% of heat loss)

By wetting the back of your hand and then blowing on the area, you can experience the process of evaporation. The body loses heat through the use of sweat glands present in the skin. Sweat is composed mainly of water and as it evaporates the energy used in the process of evaporation cools the body. Water is constantly being lost from the body; insensible water loss (i.e. too small or gradual to be perceived) is approximately 500 mL/day as a result of evaporative loss from the skin and the respiratory passages. This loss can be increased as a result of exercise or sweating.

Conduction (3% of heat loss)

In conduction, heat loss or gain is brought about by contact between the surface of the skin and some other object. For example, if the skin temperature is higher than the temperature of the clothes you wear, then heat will be lost to the clothes. This is particularly relevant when discussing heat loss and gain in the elderly and children for whom it is important to wear additional clothing in low environmental temperatures. The additional clothing provides insulation from the cold and therefore heat is lost much more slowly.

Radiation (60% of heat loss)

Radiation is a process whereby heat is transferred from one heat source to another. For example, when you are cold it is possible to gain heat by standing in the sunshine. The human body also loses heat via radiation. This factor can be life-saving as it enables the emergency services to use heat sensitive cameras to locate victims buried in building rubble or lost underground.

Convection (15% of heat loss)

As air moves over the skin heat is lost through convection. When there is little movement of air it forms an insulating

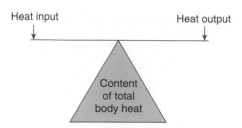

Figure 6.2   Balancing the scales of body heat.

barrier and reduces the amount of heat lost; when air movement increases heat loss also increases.

Reflection and portfolio evidence

In your practice placements you may encounter many ways of managing heat loss or gain in both children and adults. Reflect on and decide which of the four processes opposite is primarily involved in each of the following methods used in practice.

- A baby placed in an incubator
- A child wrapped in a foil blanket or 'space blanket'
- Fan therapy in the room of a person with a high temperature
- Tepid sponging of an adult with a high temperature.

Homeostatic control of body temperature

Body temperature is regulated by a feedback loop. Heat is constantly being produced by metabolic activity. In order for this heat production to become and remain homeostatically balanced, there has to be a heat loss of the same proportion. This is obtained by balancing the scales between heat input and heat output (Fig. 6.2).

Physiological response to low temperatures

Thermoreceptors located in the periphery and central nervous system respond to a lowering of temperature and transmit impulses to the preoptic area located in the hypothalamus, stimulating the heat promoting centre. As a consequence, there is sympathetic nervous system stimulation resulting in vasoconstriction, increased metabolism and shivering (Fig. 6.3).

Sympathetic stimulation resulting in the release of adrenaline and noradrenaline increases the basal metabolic rate by mobilizing the fat stores from adipose tissue and as a consequence generating heat. This process is known as chemical thermogenesis or non-shivering thermogenesis and its function is vital in the newborn because their heat loss is large due to their large surface area. This adipose tissue is called 'brown fat' and humans have only a small quantity and can therefore only raise their body heat production by 10–15%.

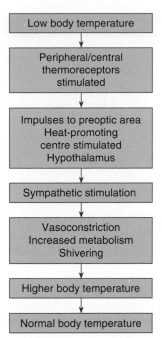

Figure 6.3 Thermoregulatory mechanism when the body temperature is low.

Physiological response to high temperatures

A rise in temperature is recognized by peripheral and central thermoreceptors, which relay this information to the preoptic area of the hypothalamus and the heat losing centre is stimulated. As a result, there is parasympathetic stimulation; cutaneous vasodilatation, diaphoresis (sweating) and decreased metabolism ensue and heat loss is increased. Shivering is inhibited.

Physical factors that affect thermoregulation

These include:

- exercise
- hormones
- drugs
- food intake
- circadian rhythms
- age.

Thermoregulation failure

Under certain conditions the normal thermoregulatory mechanisms can be compromised. These include:

- fever (pyrexia)
- heat stroke
- heat exhaustion
- hypothermia.

Fever

Fever (pyrexia) is an elevation in body temperature up to 41°C and can be caused by inflammation as a result of pyrogen/interleukin-1 release. This initiates an upward displacement of the hypothalamic 'set point' for temperature control. As the set point has been raised the body responds by increasing temperature to this new level. A rise in temperature is said to help the body's immune responses eliminate the pathogens.

Heat stroke

This is caused by a failure of the thermoregulatory system. The body becomes dangerously overheated when there has been prolonged exposure to heat (often as a result of high ambient air temperatures). The condition can develop rapidly; initially there is a loss of energy and irritability, followed by more serious neurological and mental disturbances. There is a large reduction in sweating and coma occurs as the core body temperature approaches 42°C.

any increased environmental temperature. Age-related deficits, decreased perception of changes in ambient temperature or limited mobility may all be factors precipitating heat stroke. The sweat threshold increases and sweat volume decreases with age and older people, who may be dehydrated or have cardiovascular disease, can neither sweat appropriately nor increase their cardiac output. The elderly are also more likely to be taking medication that can impair their physiological response to an increased environmental temperature.

Heat exhaustion

Heat exhaustion is caused by a loss of salt and water through excessive sweating. It usually happens to people who are unaccustomed to a hot humid environment. It can cause cramps in the legs, arms or back with associated fatigue and dizziness. Appropriate rehydration is a necessary intervention for both types of deficiency.

Reflection and portfolio evidence

During a practice placement with the school nurse you observe a health promotion session in which the issue of taking alcohol and drugs is discussed. The teenagers involved argue that the nightclub scene is the main venue for taking mood enhancing drugs and they are not involved in taking drugs regularly. The school nurse goes on to discuss the combined effects of prolonged exercise and drugs and alcohol on health.

- Review the effects of exercise on the mechanisms for controlling body temperature.
- Decide what both the physical and psychological effects of alcohol and/or a mood enhancing drug might be that would potentiate the effects of exercise on thermoregulation.
- Decide how the above knowledge will influence the advice to be given to teenagers who enjoy clubbing.
- (For information about 'ecstasy' and water intoxication see Ch. 16.)

Hypothermia

The effects of hypothermia vary with the speed of onset and how far the temperature falls. At 35°C there may be shivering, cold, pale, dry skin and apathy. A fall of body temperature to below 33°C causes mental confusion and sluggishness and further reductions result in dysfunction of the thermoregulatory system. Shivering in an attempt to gain heat ceases and loss of consciousness results. Muscle rigidity follows with associated cardiac dysrhythmias and eventual

---

Evidence based practice

Watson (1996) suggests that the 'extent to which hypothermia is responsible for death in the elderly is controversial'. Opinions vary between questioning the existence of hypothermia and it being a major cause of death. Hypothermia may contribute to or result from other illnesses, which makes the epidemiology complex and as a result it is rarely cited as the primary cause of death.

Causes of hypothermia in the elderly are usually multi-factorial and include reduced efficiency of thermoregulation mechanisms, immobility, malnutrition, falls, attitudes towards heating, poverty, poor housing, medication and alcohol consumption.

---

death. The elderly, the very young and homeless people are particularly vulnerable during the winter months in the UK. Alcohol and drugs can exacerbate hypothermia.

Children have a protective mechanism that is triggered if they fall into cold water. This response is referred to as the dive reflex, and results in a decreased heart rate and an increased cerebral and cardiac blood flow. As children are small in size they have a relatively smaller circulating blood volume, which means that the cold water in the lungs rapidly chills the blood in the pulmonary circulation which then results in brain cooling and a reduction in the brain's oxygen (O_2) requirements. Consequently, a child may survive immersion in cold water for longer periods of time than an adult.

THE BALANCE OF BLOOD PRESSURE

Blood pressure is the pressure that is exerted on the walls of the blood vessels in which blood is contained. Its level is dependent upon the interaction of three components:

- the volume of blood in the circulatory system
- the heart rate (velocity)
- the resistance offered by constricted blood vessels (peripheral resistance).

Normotension (i.e. normal blood pressure) is the pressure of the blood within the systemic circulation and the range varies according to age (Table 6.1). Systolic blood pressure (upper value) indicates the maximum pressure produced by the left ventricle during contraction or systole. Diastolic blood pressure (lower value) represents the pressure in the artery at the end of the diastole or relaxation of the left ventricle.

Factors contributing to a change in blood pressure

If the needs of the body increase then the delivery of blood to those areas will also have to increase to meet the needs.

Table 6.1 Average blood pressure values, taken from 250 000 healthy individuals (from Durkin 1979)

Age (years)	Blood pressure (mmHg) Systolic	Diastolic
Newborn	80	46
10	103	70
20	120	80
40	126	84
60	135	89

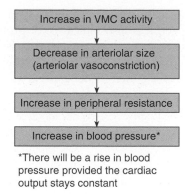

*There will be a rise in blood pressure provided the cardiac output stays constant

Figure 6.4 Increase in vasomotor activity.

The speed with which the heart contracts each minute (heart rate) multiplied by the amount of blood it expels (stroke volume) is referred to as the cardiac output (i.e. cardiac output = heart rate × stroke volume) and should this increase a corresponding increase in blood pressure will be observed.

Another factor that must be borne in mind is the degree of friction created when blood travels rapidly through the blood vessels. This is referred to as peripheral resistance. The widening (vasodilatation) or narrowing (vasoconstriction) of a blood vessel will result in either a reduction or increase in this friction of blood against the walls of the blood vessels and, as a consequence, a decrease or increase in the blood pressure. A division of the autonomic nervous system called the sympathetic nervous system regulates the size of blood vessels. The middle layer in the arteriolar wall called the tunica media is in a state of partial contraction as a result of continual activity by the sympathetic division of the autonomic nervous system. This is referred to as sympathetic tone and the tone derives from a group of cells in the vasomotor centre within the medulla oblongata in the brain. An increase or decrease in vasomotor centre (VMC) activity will lead to a corresponding increase or decrease in blood pressure (Fig. 6.4).

Reflection and portfolio evidence

Using your biological sciences textbook review the effects on the homeostatic control of blood pressure of:

- The baroreceptor control system
- The chemoreceptor control system.

Review the relative effects of each of these mechanisms when:

- You get patients up suddenly from a lying position to a standing position and they complain of feeling dizzy and faint.
- You start to get a headache in a smoke-filled room.

Reflection and portfolio evidence

Blood pressure is constantly adapting to meet the changing needs of the body. Review the list below and decide whether blood pressure will be increased or decreased and explain why in each case.

- Exercise
- Stress
- Sleep
- Digestion
- Time of day.

THE PULSE

Contraction of the left ventricle forces blood into the aorta and as a result creates distension and elongation in the arterial wall. As a consequence of this distension, the wave passing along an artery can be felt whenever it is pressed carefully against a bone in places such as the wrist (radial and ulnar pulses), ankles (posterior tibial pulse), neck (carotid pulse) and groin (femoral pulse) areas (Fig. 6.5). In babies of less than 1 year of age, heart rate is measured by listening with a stethoscope to the apex beat. This is defined as the heart beat which is heard at the apex or lower tip of the heart. The nurse listens for the characteristic 'lub-dub' sounds and counts each full cardiac cycle for 1 minute to determine the apical rate (Lewis & Timby 1993). In young children the brachial pulse is the most common site for measurement of pulse.

When trying to establish information about a patient's pulse, it is important to consider three factors:

- rate
- rhythm
- strength of the pulse wave.

Pulse rate

Pulse rate (Table 6.2) indicates the speed with which the heart is beating, and it varies with age. A rapid pulse is called a tachycardia and may be triggered by excitement, anxiety or exertion; however, it is also indicative of problems such as haemorrhage or fever. Conversely, a slow pulse is referred to as bradycardia. In health, a well-trained athlete may exhibit bradycardia because their heart muscle is very efficient. Bradycardia can be indicative of heart and neurological disease and is also caused by stimulation of the parasympathetic nervous system.

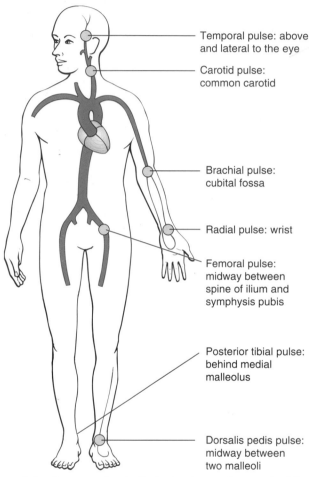

Figure 6.5   Common sites in the body where pulses can be felt. (From Hinchliff et al 1996.)

Pulse rhythm

The normal pulse is regular and the time between each beat is constant. If the normal rhythm of ventricular contraction alters, the interval between beats is interrupted. This can be due to a heart beat occurring earlier (premature) or later or a missed beat. An irregular pulse pattern is called an arrhythmia or dysrhythmia and can be either continuous or intermittent. Sinus arryhthmia is a change in rhythm more commonly found in children and is associated with an increase in heart rate on inspiration and a decrease on expiration (Hinchliff et al 1996). Other changes are often associated with cardiovascular disease and can be life-threatening if cardiac output is seriously affected (see Ch. 3 on resuscitation).

Pulse strength

Pulse strength can be separated into two important factors:

- volume
- tension.

Pulse volume is the degree of distension felt in the arterial wall in response to the pressure wave exerted on ventricular contraction. It usually relates to the amount of blood pumped out with each contraction.

An altered pulse volume is often described as being:

- weak and thready; here the pulse is difficult to feel and disappears if slight pressure is exerted
- bounding and full; here the pulse is easy to feel, it is pronounced and strong and does not disappear with moderate pressure (Lewis & Timby 1993).

Tension is specifically related to blood pressure. More force is needed when compressing the artery to feel for a pulse when the blood pressure is high. Conversely, less force is required when the blood pressure is low. When automated equipment is used to measure the pulse rate such as a pulse oximeter it is important to manually check rhythm and strength as the equipment will not detect this.

Reflection and portfolio evidence

In the practice laboratory:

- Measure and comment on the rate, rhythm and strength of the pulse rate of your peer group.
- Note any differences related to age and other factors such as recent exercise.

In your practice placements:

- Observe the different sites for taking the pulse in different client groups.
- Under supervision practice taking the pulse of individual clients and note any changes and the reason for those changes in rate, rhythm and strength.

Table 6.2   Normal pulse rates per minute at various ages

Age	Approximate range	Approximate average
Newborn	120–160	140
1 month to 12 months	80–140	120
2 years	80–130	110
2 years to 6 years	75–120	100
6 years to 12 years	75–110	95
Adolescence	60–100	80
Adulthood	60–100	80

RESPIRATORY HOMEOSTASIS

This section is concerned with the physiology of breathing and gaseous exchange, and the way that respiratory and cardiovascular systems work together to maintain homeostasis.

The balance of respiration

The primary purpose of respiration is to supply the cells of the body with oxygen (O_2) and remove carbon dioxide (CO_2). The three basic processes involved include:

- pulmonary ventilation, otherwise known as breathing, which is concerned with air passing into (inspiration) and out of (expiration) the respiratory passageways in an exchange with the atmosphere
- external respiration, which refers to the exchange of respiratory gases between the lungs and the blood
- internal respiration, which is the exchange of respiratory gases between the blood and the cells of the body.

In the processes of pulmonary ventilation, there is an exchange of respiratory gases as a result of a pressure gradient, which exists between the atmosphere and the alveoli of the lungs. Through the action of the diaphragm and the intercostal muscles the chest cavity and the lungs expand.

This creates a pressure within the alveoli lower than that of the atmosphere, leading to a movement of air from the atmosphere to the lungs during inspiration. However, on expiration when the diaphragm and the intercostal muscles return to their normal position, the pressure gradient is reversed and air moves out of the lungs.

Once the tissues of the body have used the O_2 it is essential that not only is the waste product CO_2 removed, but that O_2 concentrations are replenished. External respiration is the process whereby there is an exchange of O_2 inward and CO_2 outward between the pulmonary blood capillaries and the lung alveoli. This is achieved by the pressures exerted by the O_2 and CO_2. Figure 6.6 refers to the partial pressure of O_2 (pO_2). This is the pressure exerted in its particular location and is proportional to its concentration and can be measured in mmHg or kPa. Because the pO_2 in the alveoli is greater than in the pulmonary blood vessels, O_2 moves down the concentration gradient. The diffusion of O_2 from alveoli to blood capillaries allows deoxygenated blood to be converted to oxygenated blood. The diffusion of CO_2 from the blood capillary to the alveoli works on exactly the same principle as O_2 diffusion. Due to the relatively high partial pressure of CO_2 (pCO_2) in the pulmonary blood capillary and the low pCO_2 in the alveoli, CO_2 diffuses down its concentration gradient (see Fig. 6.6).

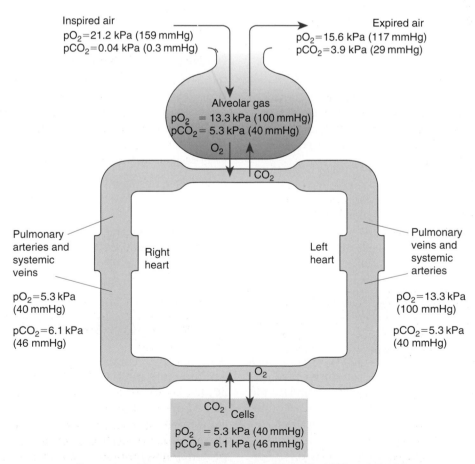

Figure 6.6   The process of respiration. (From Hinchliff et al 1996.)

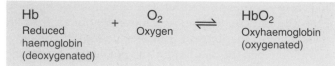

Figure 6.7   The association of oxygen with haemoglobin. This is a reversible reaction as denoted by the two-way arrow.

On completion of external respiration, oxygenated blood is transported back to the left atrium via the pulmonary veins, and thence to the circulation and tissue cells via the aorta. Exchange of gases between the blood capillaries of the tissues and the tissue cells themselves is referred to as internal respiration and works on the same principles as external respiration (see Fig. 6.6).

Oxygen transport

Because of its reduced solubility in water, the greater part of O_2 is carried in chemical combination with haemoglobin in the erythrocytes (red blood cells). Haemoglobin (Hb) is a protein in which the haem portion contains four atoms of iron, each of which is capable of attaching itself to a molecule of O_2. Therefore, four molecules of O_2 can combine with one molecule of Hb (Fig. 6.7). When the Hb is fully saturated with O_2 (oxyhaemoglobin) it is bright red, while a gradual diminution in the O_2 content results in a dark red coloration (deoxyhaemoglobin).

Reflection and portfolio evidence

Haemoglobin (Hb) is so important in the carriage of O_2 that a reduction in Hb concentration from whatever cause will be a threat to the patient or client. In maintaining or restoring homeostasis the patient or client may need to have a blood transfusion. During your practice placements:

- Find out where, how and from whom blood is obtained for transfusion.
- How soon after obtaining blood from a donor should it be transfused into the recipient and what changes can occur to donor blood during storage?
- Are there any other intravenous fluids that can be given as a replacement for blood? What are the problems with these fluids in relation to restoring O_2 homeostasis?

Control of the respiratory system

The control of the respiratory system is an interrelated one between neural and chemical stimuli, which regulate the rate of respiration in order to meet the metabolic requirements of the body. Many factors affect respiratory rate and are summarized in Figure 6.8.

Chemical control is related specifically to levels of CO_2 in the blood, the primary stimulus to breathe being the response of the respiratory centre in the brain to an increase in CO_2 concentration in the blood passing over central chemoreceptors in the medulla and peripheral chemoreceptors in the arch of the aorta. A high level of CO_2 stimulates a feedback loop through the respiratory centre that will result in an increase in the rate and depth of breathing in order to return the blood CO_2 concentration to normal and therefore maintain homeostasis.

Neural control is via areas within the respiratory centre, which have the ability to stimulate and inhibit respiration. These areas include:

- medullary rhythmicity area controls the rhythm of respiration
- pneumotaxic area controls the smooth transition between inspiration and expiration and inhibits inspiration to prevent overinflation of the lungs
- apneustic area controls the smooth transition between inspiration and expiration and inhibits expiration.

An understanding of the neural and chemical control of respiration is helpful when assessing respiration. The voluntary control of breathing is achieved through descending pathways from the cerebral cortex to the medullary respiratory centre. Voluntary control is limited in duration, it is demonstrated during hyperventilation, breath holding, singing, speech and deep breathing for relaxation. Enhancing voluntary control through teaching patients how to adapt their breathing can be useful in managing respiratory problems.

Reflection and portfolio evidence

Although most of the time we are not conscious of our breathing as we go about our daily lives, attention will be drawn to how we breathe in certain situations. Reflect on whether control of our breathing is voluntary or involuntary in each of the following situations and explain why.

- When singing in an opera
- In a panic when breathing shallowly and at a very fast rate
- When swimming
- When breathing is very shallow and slow after drinking many pints of beer.

CARE DELIVERY KNOWLEDGE

A fundamental component of a nurse's role is the thorough and accurate physiological assessment of children and adults in whatever healthcare setting. The information gained provides the foundation for nursing decisions and contributes towards the decisions of other health professionals. It is vital that changes in homeostasis are detected promptly and monitored as they can indicate serious alterations in health due to disease, injury, treatments, surgery

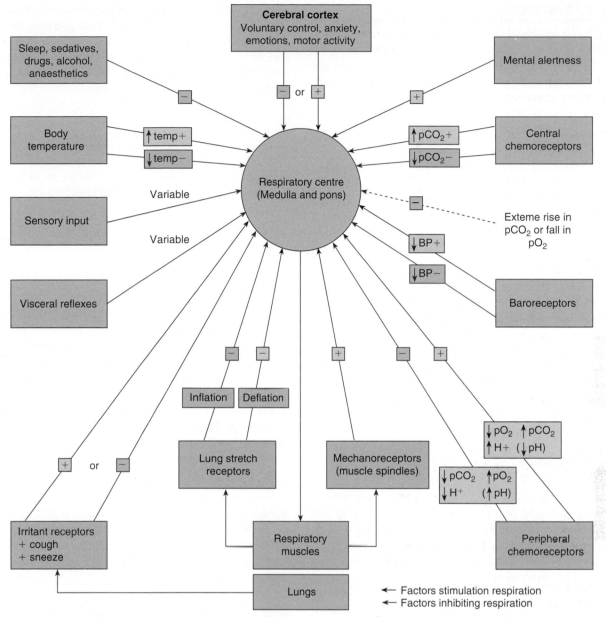

Figure 6.8 Factors that affect respiratory homeostasis. (From Hinchliff et al 1996.)

and medications. Screening for changes that occur more slowly is also important within the context of health promotion and the prevention of disease.

Physiological assessment involves the collection of both measurable and subjective information, the most common of which are:

- blood pressure
- pulse
- temperature
- respiration
- fluid balance
- skin condition and pallor.

These measurements and observations are often referred to as vital signs.

It is important to recognize that vital signs can remain within the normal range despite serious illness or injury. Compensatory mechanisms can mask an underlying problem as the body strives to maintain homeostasis. It is therefore crucial to always assess the whole patient for any change, using a range of measurements and observations and listen to how the patient reports feeling. The converse situation can also arise; you may detect a low blood pressure in a patient who appears perfectly healthy.

Single measurements are not generally acted upon in isolation as temporary changes can occur in response to emotional, physical and environmental factors such as pain and anxiety, or the measurement could be inaccurate. Monitoring for any pattern or trends emerging in the observations is a more reliable indication of a change.

GENERAL PRINCIPLES

When carrying out observations the nurse must ensure that the person's privacy, dignity, safety and comfort is maintained and that when possible verbal consent is sought before commencing the procedure (this is discussed later). The results of observations should be explained to the patient. The nurse must also ensure that:

- correct equipment is used and maintained in good working order
- correct techniques are followed and reflect local/national guidelines
- measurements taken are accurate, clearly documented and communicated to the patient's doctor and nurse if they fall outside the normal range for that person
- measurements are performed when there is a rational patient-centred reason to do so
- any problems identified and subsequent nursing interventions are recorded in the patient's nursing records
- measurements are performed by competent healthcare staff.

MEASUREMENT OF TEMPERATURE

A thorough knowledge of thermoregulation and the factors that influence it provides a valuable contribution to decision making in many aspects of nursing practice. This knowledge can be applied to health education, for example when advising an elderly person on how to prevent hypothermia. It influences decisions about the environment of care, such as minimizing an infant's heat loss during bathing by ensuring a warm, draught-free environment. Importantly, this knowledge also forms the basis for the assessment, planning, implementation and evaluation of care of those individuals who have the potential for or an actual altered body temperature. Those most at risk of thermoregulatory disturbance are the very young, the elderly and people with chronic or acute illness (Childs 1994). The effects of limited

mobility and an inadequate nutritional intake are particularly important as they limit heat-gaining mechanisms. Alterations in body temperature may indicate a physical problem, as occurs when temperature is raised due to an infection or a behavioural problem such as dressing inappropriately for the weather conditions.

ASSESSMENT OF TEMPERATURE

The assessment of temperature involves observing and touching the skin, noting any change in behaviour, and listening to how the patient reports feeling (Woollons 1996). Specific aspects to consider are:

- Is the skin excessively warm or cool, dry or moist? (Use the back of your fingers as they are more sensitive to temperature.)
- Are the extremities pale, mottled or flushed?
- Is the patient shivering? Shivering can occur when a person is cold or during the heat-gaining phase of pyrexia. It causes discomfort in the short term; however, prolonged uncontrolled shivering can lead to exhaustion, pain and helplessness (Holtzclaw 1990). It is also important to remember when caring for young infants (under 1 year of age) that they cannot shiver.
- Has the patient's behaviour changed (e.g. restlessness, lethargy, delirium)?
- Does the client's behaviour indicate that they are feeling hot or cold?

It is important both in the home and in institutional settings to assess the environment, particularly air temperature, heating and ventilation, dampness and draughts, and if appropriate to ensure that clothing and bedding are available. Nurses are responsible for providing a safe and comfortable environment of care and must report promptly any problems that arise.

Reflection and portfolio evidence

Consider what sort of actions or behaviour an adult, an infant and a child might demonstrate with decreased body temperature and raised body temperature.

- During your practice placements note any differences between expected behaviour and what you witness.
- Discuss the possible reasons for these differences with practice staff and your tutor.

Decision making exercise

During the winter when on an inner city practice placement with a community psychiatric nurse (CPN), you observe the CPN three times a week working with a group of young drug addicts who attend a drop-in centre. You notice that one of the group, Sean, does not appear to be caring for himself and is now frequently missing from the group sessions.

- What physical, social and environmental factors might threaten Sean's health?
- How might the CPN assess the present situation?
- Decide on a long-term health promotion strategy that you think might be successful in Sean's case.

ACCURATE MEASUREMENTS OF TEMPERATURE

The aim of temperature measurement is to provide an objective approximation of core body temperature. Measurements must be accurate and the method used safe and acceptable to the patient.

Safety is particularly relevant when considering the risks of broken glass and mercury toxicity associated with the use of a glass and mercury thermometer. Although used less frequently these are still available in some healthcare settings. Mercury is a highly toxic substance and is extremely hazardous. If a thermometer breaks, mercury vapour is emitted into the atmosphere and may be inhaled or absorbed through the skin, and if not correctly disposed of, mercury remains in the environment for years (Cutter 1994). The handling and disposal of mercury is controlled by the 1989 Control of Substances Hazardous to Health (COSHH) regulations (Health and Safety Commission 1988). The Medical Devices Agency (2002) recommends the use of safer alternatives. The clinical thermometer has been largely replaced by the use of electronic/digital probes, disposable and infrared tympanic thermometers. These devices are quicker and safer to use and generally considered to be accurate (Carroll 2000).

The nurse needs to consider the three main variables that influence the accuracy of temperature measurement (Woollons 1996). These are:

- the site
- the measuring device
- the technique.

Choosing a site

The best sites for core temperature measurement are those that are in close proximity to major arteries and organs in the central core of the body and are well insulated from external factors. The pulmonary artery is considered the optimal core site, but this measurement requires the insertion of a pulmonary artery catheter and thermistor, which are only suitable for use in high-dependency or critical care areas (Fulbrook 1993). Key factors to consider when choosing a site are:

- the individual's age and health status
- the degree of accuracy required
- accessibility and acceptability
- the degree of co-operation (Erickson and Yount 1991).

Evidence based practice

Research available that compares the accuracy of different sites includes the following:

- Erickson & Yount (1991) compared measurements of the tympanic and oral sites and their findings suggest that either site can be used for adults having major surgery.
- Fulbrook (1993) provides a thorough review of the available literature comparing sites and suggests that contrary to popular belief it is possible to achieve an accurate axilla temperature if the correct recording time is used.
- Nyholm et al (1994) investigated the accuracy of oral and rectal electronic thermometry and found oral measurements were unacceptably inaccurate for routine daily measurement. They advocate the use of rectal thermometry on a routine basis. The doctors performing this research did not consider other factors that influence a nurse's choice of site such as acceptability to the patient or clearly identify possible reasons for the variances they found.
- Board (1995) compares the use of disposable and glass thermometers in a health care of the elderly environment. Her findings in this small study indicate a good correlation between oral and axillary temperature and suggest that disposable thermometers are an accurate, efficient and cost-effective method for obtaining oral and axillary temperatures.

Decision making exercise

Woollons (1996) provides a good overview of some of the products currently available in the UK. Find out which devices are used in your area and ask why they have been chosen. Decide which devices and sites would be suitable when measuring the temperature of:

- An infant with an ear infection.
- A drunken young adult in the Accident and Emergency department.
- An adult with a mild learning disability who is a planned admission to an acute unit for routine surgery that afternoon.
- A hypothermic elderly confused adult in the community.

The most commonly used sites are the mouth, tympanic membrane, axilla and less frequently the rectum. All have relative advantages and disadvantages that require consideration. Table 6.3 lists these and the devices suggested to take the measurement.

Tympanic thermometry is now frequently encountered in practice. A probe is inserted into the ear canal and this measures the infrared emissions from the surface of the tympanic membrane, which is in close proximity to the hypothalamus and cerebral arteries. A number of studies report a good correlation between pulmonary artery temperature and tympanic membrane measurements (Edge & Morgan 1993, Ferra-Love 1991); however, there is debate about its accuracy if the thermometer is not used correctly (Casey 2000).

Choice of thermometer

The devices available are:

- glass and mercury thermometer
- electronic (probe and digital display) thermometers (Fig. 6.9)

Table 6.3   Advantages and disadvantages of different thermometry sites

Site	Advantages	Disadvantages	Thermometer
Oral	• Good correlation with core temperature due to close proximity of the lingual and sublingual arteries and thermo receptors • Suitable for most older children and adults • Easily accessible and usually acceptable to patients	• Needs accurate positioning of the thermometer in the sublingual pocket • Prior eating, drinking and smoking or mouth breathing, poor lip seal and talking during the measurement can influence accuracy • Not suitable for infants, young children and confused or restless adults • Cross-infection is a potential risk with any shared thermometer	• Glass and mercury • Electronic/digital • Tempadot
Typanic	• Good correlation with core temperature due to close proximity of the eardrum to the carotid artery and hypothalamus • Suitable for most children and adults • Ease of access and very rapid reading time	• Poor positioning, use of incorrect probe size and poor operating technique can influence accuracy	• Tympanic infrared
Axilla	• Useful for patients when you can't use the oral or tympanic site, e.g. following surgery or trauma • Provides a good approximation of temperature, as long as site is documented	• Peripheral measurement, therefore not to be used in hypothermia or shock • Site not well insulated from the environment; position difficult to maintain • Need to disrupt bedding and clothing	• Glass and mercury • Electronic/digital • Tempadot
Rectal	• Good correlation with core temperature • Useful for patients with hypothermia or who are unconscious. Although very accurate in young children, its use is in decline and questioned	• Potential discomfort, trauma/rectal perforation and embarrassment • Site not easily accessible • Unsuitable for a restless child or adult • Accuracy affected by presence of stool	• Glass and mercury • Electronic/digital

• liquid crystal thermometer (disposable forehead strip)
• tempadot (a disposable strip impregnated with heat-sensitive chemicals, which change colour as temperature alters)
• tympanic membrane thermometers (Fig. 6.10).

The criteria for choosing a device include accuracy, reliability, adaptability across age groups and sites, safety, ease of use, low risk of cross-infection, cost-effectiveness, full range of temperature measurements, durability, maintainability and anti-theft properties. Careful consideration needs to be taken in choosing an appropriate site and device for children; a recent study identified that children preferred the tympanic thermometer because it was fast and comfortable (Pickersgill 2003).

Technique

Using the correct technique should ensure a safe and accurate temperature measurement. This involves having knowledge of both the site and the device being used and minimizing extraneous variables such as drinking before an oral measurement. Manufacturer's guidelines must be followed and electronic equipment will need regular servicing to ensure accuracy. Minimizing the risk of cross-infection with any device is paramount and disposable covers must be used with all probes.

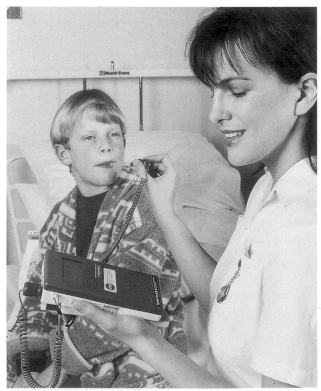

Figure 6.9   An electronic thermometer. (Reproduced with kind permission of IVAC Medical Systems.)

There are inconsistencies in practice and in the literature regarding the time required to record temperatures at all sites when using a glass and mercury thermometer (Closs 1987, Cutter 1994). It is generally accepted that in most situations a clinically significant measurement can be achieved by taking the oral temperature for 3 minutes (Pugh Davies et al 1986).

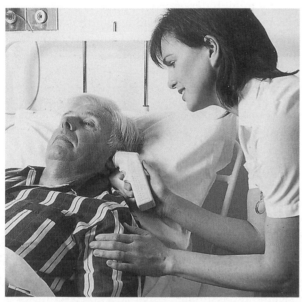

Figure 6.10   A tympanic thermometer. (Reproduced with kind permission of IVAC Medical Systems.)

Pyrexia

Pyrexia is defined as a core temperature above 38°C; this commonly occurs in response to an infection or tissue damage. Decisions about nursing care are determined by the stage of the pyrexia (Table 6.4). If the rise in temperature is slight, symptoms may not be observable.

If the temperature rises above 40°C it can affect cerebral function and cause restlessness and delirium due to nerve cell irritability. Febrile convulsions are a particular risk in infants and young children because their thermoregulation mechanisms are immature.

Hypothermia

Hypothermia is defined as a core temperature below 35°C (Roper et al 1993). It can develop gradually over a period of time or have a sudden acute onset. The main aims of care are to reduce further loss of heat and to promote the return

Table 6.4   Stages in pyrexia with nursing management

Stage	Features	Nursing management
Stage 1: heat gaining	- Patient complains of feeling cold and shivery - If a child, looks pale and feels cold to the touch peripherally	- Promote rest and comfort in a warm draught-free environment and adjust bedding to maintain comfort - Administer antipyretics prescribed
Stage 2: heat dissipation	- Patient looks flushed and complains of feeling hot - Diaphoresis (sweating) - Thirst and dry mouth - Headache - Reduced appetite - Disorientation - Lethargy - Aching - Weakness - Pulse and respiratory rate increase	- Promote rest - Adjust environment and bedding to increase the circulation of cool air – use a fan, but do not direct at the patient as this causes vasoconstriction - Encourage fluids - Reassure and explain what is happening - Administer prescribed antipyretics
Stage 3	- Return to normal	

of a normal body temperature with the minimum of complications, if possible by natural warming. The temperature should return to normal at a rate of no more than 0.5°C/hour. Rapid uncontrolled rewarming will lead to peripheral vasodilation; this causes a fall in blood pressure and the return of cold acidotic peripheral blood to the heart. This may precipitate a cardiac arrest.

Early signs of hypothermia (i.e. when the core temperature is between 35°C and 33°C) are:

- patient looks and feels cold
- puffy face and husky voice
- pale, cool and waxy skin
- shivering (the ability to shiver decreases as temperature falls below 34°C)
- fatigue and impaired cognitive function
- drowsiness.

Later signs of hypothermia (i.e. when the core temperature is lower than 32°C) are:

- reduced heart and respiratory rate and blood pressure
- cyanosis and mottled peripheries
- cardiac arrhythmias
- reduced responsiveness leading to loss of consciousness.

Prevention is central to caring for individuals who are at risk of hypothermia and this is best achieved by educating such individuals and their family and friends about their personal vulnerability and how to minimize their risk (Webster 1995).

Slow, natural rewarming can be achieved by caring for the patient in bed, with lightweight blankets and maintaining a warm environment (26–29°C). Warm drinks and food can commence as the patient's condition improves. Active strategies are usually decided upon by the medical staff and may include the use of a warming mattress and administering warm intravenous (IV) fluids.

MEASUREMENT OF BLOOD PRESSURE

Blood pressure is a frequently undertaken assessment procedure in adults. It is completed less frequently in children, in whom abnormal blood pressure is usually secondary to an underlying disease (Goonasekera & Dillon 2000).

Assessment

Blood pressure can only be recorded by a physical procedure, unlike some other observations. However, common physical symptoms are associated with abnormal blood pressures. These are listed in Table 6.5. An absence of symptoms does not exclude a problem. People can adapt to an abnormal blood pressure, and have no symptoms at all.

There are several ways in which blood pressure can be measured.

Direct/invasive

This method is infrequently used as it requires insertion of a catheter into an artery, which can be attached to a monitoring system via a pressure transducer. It is a technique used frequently in high dependency and intensive care settings, and provides a continuous reading which is very accurate.

However it is impractical and invasive, and therefore unsuitable for most practice situations.

Indirect/non-invasive

Non-invasive methods are the most frequently used. This can be done using automated machines or manual equipment.

- Automated machines
  Automated blood pressure equipment is now the most common method of measuring blood pressure in most clinical settings. It is often the preferred method in children who can become distressed or impatient with manual measurement and as such can make detecting the sounds required (see below) very difficult.

  These machines usually use the oscillometric method (detect vibrations). A compressive cuff is attached to a machine and is inflated either on a timed setting or by the user. The machine then detects oscillations in pressure due to arterial wall movement beneath the cuff. Most machines detect the mean blood pressure reading, the machine then uses empirically derived algorithms to determine the systolic and diastolic values.

  Research is being undertaken to determine the accuracy of these machines, and the British Hypertension Society has made equipment recommendations as a result (O'Brien et al 2001).

Table 6.5 Symptoms associated with abnormal blood pressure

Hypertension	Hypotension
Pounding headache	Dizziness
Nose bleeds	Fainting
Visual disturbances	Confusion
Chest pain	Palpitations

It is still important, despite the accuracy of the recommended machines, that healthcare workers have the skill to perform manual blood pressure measurements. Mechanical errors/failures can occur and readings may need verification before treatment is commenced.

Evidence based practice

Webster et al (1984) found a mean difference of 11–12 mmHg between the arm in a dependent position and the arm held at heart level. Croft & Cruikshank (1990) found that for most adults using the large-size adult cuff provided a satisfactory degree of accuracy in blood pressure measurement.

- Manual

This technique requires a measuring device with means of manually inflating the compressive cuff. It also requires some means of detecting the reading, usually by auscultation (listening).

The measuring device used is called a sphygmomanometer, of which the most common is the mercury device. As identified in temperature measurement, mercury use is controversial. The Medical Devices Agency (2002) recommends using an alternative whenever possible.

Aneroid sphygmomanometers can be used, and are safer. However they need regular calibration as they lose accuracy over time. It is for this reason that mercury sphygmomanometers are often still used (O'Brien et al 2001).

A stethoscope is the most common means of listening to the Korotkoff sounds that enable the pressures to be identified (Fig. 6.11). However in small children it can be difficult to hear and therefore a Doppler flow detector

may be used. This device uses ultrasound technology to amplify the sound. Only systolic recordings can be detected with the Doppler.

It is important to note that in some patients there is an auscultatory gap in the Korotkoff sounds. After the systolic pressure appears it can briefly disappear again and this can be mistaken for the systolic pressure reading.

Palpation is a means of estimating the location of the systolic pressure. This is done by feeling for the pulse disappearing when inflating the cuff. The cuff can then be inflated to 30 mmHg above this value for auscultation to increase accuracy.

Some very skilled health professionals can accurately palpate the systolic pressure and do not use an auscultatory method at all.

Procedure

Blood pressure measurement is a skilled procedure that requires practice and consistency. The British Hypertension Society has made recommendations that enable uniform practice when adhered to (O'Brien et al 1997):

- Patients should sit for 3 minutes before measurement takes place.
- Full explanations are needed regardless of age to gain consent and reduce anxiety.
- Equipment should be checked for condition and maintenance before use.
- Cuff selection is very important. Guidelines state that the bladder in the cuff should circle at least 80% of the limb. A selection of cuffs should always be available, particularly in areas attended by children.
- The cuff should be inflated to 30 mmHg above estimated systolic pressure and deflated by 2–3 mmHg/per second. This ensures accurate visualization of reading.
- The limb should be at heart level during measurement.
- Pressure should be recorded to the nearest 2 mmHg. Rounding off to the nearest 5–10 mmHg creates inaccuracies.
- The diastolic reading should be recorded as phase 5 during auscultation (this is when the sounds disappear). In some patient groups the sound may still be present at 0 on the device. If this occurs phase 4, when muffling occurs, should be used. This should be clearly recorded.
- Clinical decisions should never be made on a single reading; the reading should be repeated and other factors disregarded first. For example, patients with coarctation of the aorta will have a high reading on one arm but not the other.

Documentation

Accurate documentation is very important. Measurement of blood pressure is most useful when considering trends. Therefore each recording needs to be comparable.

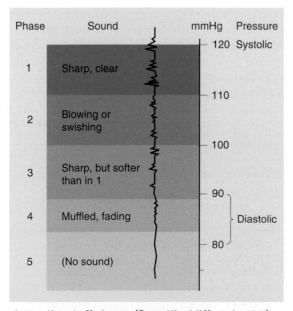

Phase	Sound		mmHg	Pressure
			120	Systolic
1	Sharp, clear			
			110	
2	Blowing or swishing			
			100	
3	Sharp, but softer than in 1			
			90	
4	Muffled, fading			Diastolic
			80	
5	(No sound)			

Figure 6.11 Korotkoff phases. (From Hinchliff et al 1996.)

The following information should be recorded, and subsequent readings performed in the same way:

- the limb used
- the size of cuff
- equipment used
- position of patient
- status of patient (any other important observations such as anxiety).

Hypertension

Hypertension (high blood pressure) is the chronic elevation of blood pressure above a normal value which is acceptable for the patient's age. This is usually accepted as 100 plus the chronological age of the patient for systolic pressure, and for the diastolic pressure it is usually above 90 mmHg. Hypertension may be mainly systolic, or a combination of systolic and diastolic (Thomas et al 1992). Hypertension can be separated into two categories:

- primary hypertension
- secondary hypertension.

Evidence based practice

McGee et al (1992) state that the distribution of blood pressure in human populations is unimodal, suggesting a polygenic inheritance (i.e. a combined action of a number of genes). This fact has been confirmed by twin studies and comparing the blood pressures of adopted and natural children with the same parents. With regards to race, hypertensive black Afro-Caribbean men have a death rate about six times that of hypertensive white men. Essential hypertension is more common and has a better prognosis in women.

The prevalence of hypertension in a population correlates with salt intake. Cigarette smoking increases the risk of malignant hypertension (i.e. blood pressure rises very rapidly causing serious damage to organs) and urban populations have higher blood pressures than rural ones.

Primary hypertension

This is commonly referred to as essential hypertension and usually occurs in people who are 35–45 years of age. It is not caused by any specific disease but is associated with a combination of factors. The effects are insidious and develop over many years. Hypertension is frequently discovered by chance at routine health checks. Factors known to predispose individuals to primary hypertension include:

- genetic factors
- racial factors

- age and sex
- diet
- smoking
- environmental factors
- stress.

Secondary hypertension

This develops as a consequence of an underlying disease, and occurs in approximately 5–10% of patients with hypertension and is more common in young patients. The primary causes for secondary hypertension are:

- renal in origin
- stenosis of the aorta, commonly called coarctation
- arteriosclerosis, which causes a narrowing of the lumen of blood vessels leading to increased peripheral resistance.

White coat hypertension

This is a well-documented phenomenon. Patients, particularly children, can become very anxious during procedures involving health professionals. This can cause a rise blood pressure, which could be misdiagnosed as hypertension (Sorof & Portman 2000). Ambulatory blood pressure measurement (ABPM) is now being used to detect this group of patients in whom treatment is not necessary. A compact automated device is worn at home continuously for 24 hours, and is preset to take regular readings. The data are then downloaded once the equipment is collected, when a trace can be analysed. Other individual/biological factors that should be considered when assessing blood pressure are listed in Table 6.6.

National Service Framework for coronary heart disease

Hypertension is just one risk factor in heart disease, and is closely linked to myocardial infarction and stroke (Beevers

Table 6.6 Factors that may alter blood pressure

Increased blood pressure	Decreased blood pressure
Environmental/physiological factors which alter blood pressure	
Exercise	Sleep
Environmental factors	
Full bladder	
Alcohol	
Smoking	
Procedural errors which alter blood pressure	
Limb below heart level	Limb above heart level
Cuff too small	Cuff too large
Limb unsupported during measurement	

et al 2001). Over 110 000 people die from heart problems each year and 300 000 have heart attacks.

This is a very serious issue, and as a result it has become the target for one of the National Service Frameworks. Prevention is a major focus, identifying people who are at high risk. Monitoring of people with hypertension is an area that is identified, and national strategies are being developed as a result.

Hypotension

Hypotension is usually a condition in which the systolic blood pressure falls below 100 mmHg in the adult. Remember that a child's normal blood pressure is age related (see Table 6.1). A hypotensive state can be precipitated by either a loss of blood or a fluid shift from one physiological fluid compartment to another. Children are particularly vulnerable as they have a relatively low circulating blood volume and can develop hypovolaemic shock very rapidly. A fall in blood pressure initiates a cyclical chain of events, which initially brings about hypoxia (i.e. a reduction of O_2 to the tissues). Hypoxia leads to cell and tissue damage, resulting in the release of vasodilator substances and a further fall in blood pressure.

MEASUREMENT OF RESPIRATION

Nurses require a sound knowledge of normal respiration together with an understanding of how and why respiratory homeostasis can be disrupted. The factors that influence respiration are complex, often interrelate and can be broadly described as being physical, psychological, social and environmental. In fact very few health problems do not affect respiration in some way.

Knowledge of factors affecting respiration can be effectively used by nurses to:

- promote health and provide health education
- detect respiratory problems through screening
- assess and monitor respiratory status
- provide competent care for individuals with respiratory problems.

Many of the frequently encountered respiratory diseases such as asthma, chronic obstructive pulmonary disease and

---

Reflection and portfolio evidence

With reference to *The Health of the Nation* (Department of Health 1997):

- Review the targets the government has set that relate to respiratory disease.
- Make a list of the possible opportunities nurses have to promote healthier living that could reduce the incidence and symptoms of respiratory disease.

---

lung cancer have been closely linked to environmental factors and individual lifestyle and are considered by health professionals to be largely preventable.

Assessing respirations

It is relatively simple for a nurse to assess breathing directly by observing the rate, depth and rhythm of respiration (Table 6.7). These observations provide a good basic indicator of respiratory function. Impaired gas exchange during external and internal respiration is more difficult to assess. If more detailed information is required additional assessment methods can be used such as:

- an oximeter, which measures the O_2 saturation level in the blood
- laboratory equipment to measure arterial blood gases
- apnoea monitors, which alarm if an infant has an episode of apnoea.

The use of technology supplements the information gained through observation and measurement and allows the nurse to note both subtle and rapid change in a patient's condition. In children there can be a rapid deterioration in condition with diseases such as asthma and bronchiolitis. The oximeter and apnoea monitors are essential.

Observation of breathing

At rest, normal respiration is passive and quiet, and the chest wall and abdomen gently rise and fall with each breath. In more active breathing (e.g. following exercise) there is an increase in the use of the intercostal and accessory muscles, which allows greater lung expansion. This increase in depth of respirations can be observed by the rise and fall of the shoulders, increased movement of the ribcage and the contraction of the accessory muscles in the neck during inspiration. It is important to assess the symmetry of chest

---

Table 6.7   Respiratory rates and volumes for infant, child and adult (from Wong 1993)

Age	Rate (breaths/min)
Newborn	35
1 to 11 months	30
2 years	25
4 years	23
6 years	21
8 years	20
10 years	19
12 years	19
14 years	18
16 years	17
18 years	16–18

movement and the type of breath, while noting the amount of effort required to breathe at rest and during activity. Prolonged, laboured breathing at rest and use of the accessory muscles is a cause for concern and indicates serious respiratory dysfunction. Nasal flaring, rib recession and head bobbing in the infant and young child indicate problems that lead to a rapid deterioration in the child's condition (see Ch. 3 on resuscitation).

It can be difficult to assess breathing during sleep, especially with children; placing a hand gently on the upper abdominal area allows respiratory movement to be felt.

Respiratory rate

The respiratory rate is simply assessed by counting each full breath over 1 minute. Extraneous variables such as talking and the effects of activity need to be considered. An awareness of being observed may alter respiratory rate and depth; counting respirations while appearing to take the patient's pulse can minimize this. The rate of pulse and breathing tends to maintain a ratio of approximately 5:1 (Faulkner 1985). Table 6.7 indicates normal respiratory rates.

Tachypnoea is a respiratory rate above age-adjusted normal values. Tachypnoea is a normal response to increased activity, but can also be an indication of hypoxia (low O_2), hypercarbia (high CO_2), acidosis, raised temperature, pain, stress and anxiety.

Bradypnoea is a respiratory rate lower than the normal age-adjusted values. It is less commonly seen than tachypnoea and can be an indication of severe hypothermia, opiate drug overdose, acid–base imbalance and neurological dysfunction.

Apnoea is the absence of breathing for at least 10 seconds. It can be transitory as in 'sleep apnoea', which is associated with a brief obstruction of the upper airway and causes snoring or it may be life-threatening as in sudden infant death syndrome.

Respiratory depth

The depth of respiration is dependent upon the amount of air inhaled, which is known as the tidal volume. For an average adult at rest it is about 500 mL of expired air. Depth is assessed by observing the degree of movement of the chest wall during inspiration. A more objective way is to measure the amount of air exhaled with a spirometer or peak flow meter (Fig. 6.12). This method is particularly beneficial when caring for individuals with respiratory problems such as asthma and chronic obstructive pulmonary disease.

Posture can affect the depth of respiration; supine, lateral and slumped positions can limit chest expansion. Orthopnoea is the term used to describe difficulty in breathing when lying down. Depth is also reduced when the movement of the diaphragm is restricted by obesity, pregnancy and ascites. Patients with respiratory disease tend to

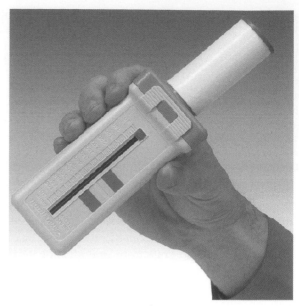

Figure 6.12 Peak flow monitor. (Reproduced with kind permission of Vitalograph Ltd.)

feel more comfortable sitting well up and leaning slightly forward or standing as gravity enhances lung expansion. Before making decisions it may be valuable to assess which position if any provides relief from symptoms.

Respiratory rhythm

Normal breathing in adults is regular and uninterrupted except for the occasional sigh, but infants and young children can have a less regular pattern. The rhythm is maintained by the carefully controlled timing of the respiratory cycle. Many of the abnormal patterns in breathing occur as the result of brain injury or disease that affects the respiratory centres in the brain such as the apneustic or pneumotaxic centres mentioned above.

Cheyne–Stokes respiration may occur as death approaches and is characterized by a gradual increase in the rate and depth of respiration followed by a gradual decrease over 30–45 seconds in the depth and rate of respiration. This cycle may be followed by a period of apnoea for up to 20 seconds (Faulkner 1985). It can be distressing to observe and families need an explanation and reassurance.

Breath sounds

Further information can be gained by assessing the sounds of breathing. Normal respiration is almost silent, therefore any respiratory sound requires investigation. Noisy respiration is referred to as stertorous breathing and can be caused by:

● secretions in the trachea and bronchi, which make a gurgling type of noise

- obstruction to air flow, which sounds like a wheeze or a harsh crowing sound (e.g. stridor in children).

Observation of skin colour

Cyanosis occurs when the blood is not carrying sufficient O_2 to the tissues and deoxygenated haemoglobin accumulates in the tissues. A grey, blue or mauve discoloration of the skin occurs. Peripheral cyanosis is usually seen in the hands and feet and occurs when the circulation is restricted. Central cyanosis is more serious and indicates a lack of arterial blood from the lungs. It is most clearly seen in the tissues of the face and trunk, but it can be difficult to assess in dark-skinned people. Cyanosis is an unreliable and late sign of hypoxia so you should be alert to alterations in the rate and depth of breathing and any behavioural changes in the individual. The use of an oximeter to monitor oxygen saturation levels is strongly indicated in the assessment and monitoring of patients who are at risk of hypoxia.

Behavioural changes

Common responses to inadequate respiratory function include restlessness, confusion, anxiety, fatigue, agitation and loss of concentration. There can be an altered level of consciousness, which will depend upon the degree of cerebral hypoxia and acidosis.

Cough, sneeze and sputum

Coughing and sneezing are the respiratory system's protective mechanism against irritants and obstructions. However, if the nature and frequency of a cough change there may be a respiratory problem. Sputum coughed up from the lungs provides valuable information, and the amount, consistency, colour and odour need to be assessed. Blood-stained sputum is referred to as haemoptysis.

Pain and dyspnoea

Pain on breathing needs to be assessed to determine its cause and can indicate infection, inflammation or trauma. Dyspnoea describes the feelings experienced by a patient of difficult and laboured breathing. Gift (1990) describes dyspnoea as a subjective sensation that is often associated with chronic lung disease and stresses that the intensity of the dyspnoea is not always reflected in the findings when respiratory function is assessed. Gift also provides a useful model based upon three dimensions of dyspnoea: physical, psychological and social. This model is very important for nurses to consider as it reminds us of the holistic needs of our patients and focuses our attention on the effects of living with dyspnoea.

PROFESSIONAL AND ETHICAL KNOWLEDGE

ACCOUNTABILITY

Clinical decision making is an area that is reliant upon professional judgement and knowledge. This is especially important in an age where the use of technology is increasing, and it can be very easy to become dependent upon its use. As identified earlier in this chapter, there are other means of assessing homeostasis, which should also be used, such as visual observation. Equipment can produce inaccuracies, and means of verifying abnormal results are needed.

Equally nurses need to be aware of their own limitations in practice. If they are not confident in the results they are obtaining they should seek clarification and guidance. This can be difficult to acknowledge; however, ritualistic practices and inaccurate documentation of observations are not acceptable. The Nursing and Midwifery Council *Code of Professional Conduct* states this very clearly (Nursing and Midwifery Council 2002).

CONSENT

Consent is another area that is covered in the *Code of Professional Conduct*. In 2001 the Department of Health published revised good practice guidelines for consent. Within this it states that: 'Patients have a fundamental ethical and legal right to determine what happens to their own bodies' (Department of Health 2001b: 9). Observations such as measuring blood pressure, pulse and temperature that involve physically touching patients need to be considered within these guidelines.

Informed consent is fundamental to this, but can become very complex in situations where a patient's health status (physical or mental) is compromised. Although in most situations it is unnecessary to document consent for observation, it may be important to do so in these circumstances.

Ultimately, 'You have a duty of care to your clients, who are entitled to receive safe and competent care' (Nursing and Midwifery Council 2002: 3).

HEALTH PROMOTION

An important aspect of the nurse's role in health promotion is to empower the patient through sharing information so that they can take an active role in their care and contribute to their own well being. Explaining why observations are made and the results will often provide the opportunity to answer the patient's questions and discuss related health issues. This may lead to increased insight into their health and promote healthier choices.

Evidence based practice

McBride (1994) studied the attitudes, beliefs and health promotion practices of hospital nurses in acute adult wards and found that the nurses in general had a positive attitude to health promotion activities and that other health professionals acknowledged that nurses had an important role to play in this domain of practice.

Wilson-Barnett & Latter (1993) found that the health promotion activities of nurses in acute hospital wards were focused on giving health advice and information to patients and was seen as a separate activity rather than integrated with other nursing activities. Lack of time and knowledge were recognized as major constraints in carrying out the health promotion role effectively.

PERSONAL AND REFLECTIVE KNOWLEDGE

IDEAS FOR PORTFOLIO AND SKILLS LABORATORY LEARNING

Undertaking the assessment of patients involves understanding a considerable amount of theoretical knowledge as well as mastering a wide range of skills and being able to use your professional judgement. This chapter has alerted you broadly to the scope of knowledge and skills needed, but this knowledge should be supplemented by other more specialized texts and consolidated through reflection and discussion of learning in your practice placements. Many of the exercises throughout the chapter will have encouraged you to reflect on your practice experiences. Keeping a record and reviewing these experiences will help you to develop your portfolio.

It is recommended that you take the opportunity to practice your skills in a learning laboratory before commencing your placements. This will help develop your confidence and is important in terms of the quality of care being delivered to clients. When learning how to assess temperature, pulse, respirations and blood pressure on your peers take note of any differences you observe. Experiential exercises could include testing the effects of factors such as exercise, rest, noise, time of day on 'vital signs'.

CASE STUDIES RELATING TO HOMEOSTASIS

The following case studies are included so that you can consolidate knowledge gained from this chapter and your practice experience. In addition to your reflective writing it is useful to collect relevant policies, procedures and literature for your portfolio.

Case study: Adult

Pauline Scott is 56 years old and has had progressive multiple sclerosis for 30 years. She is unable to mobilize and is confined to a wheelchair for most of her day. She lives with her husband, John, who is a retired farmer and her main carer. They live in a rural area in an old farmhouse. The living area is comfortable and warm, but Pauline finds the bathroom and bedroom very cold in the winter and as a result is now washing and dressing in the kitchen, which she finds unsatisfactory.

- What factors would you need to consider when assessing Pauline's ability to maintain her body temperature?
- What advice would you give to Pauline and John about minimizing the risk of hypothermia?
- Find out what other agencies or members of the primary care team could help with this problem.

Case study: Learning disabilities

Malvika Singh is an 8-year-old girl with mild learning disability and profound physical disability. She attends a special needs school in a wheelchair which has been made to accommodate her needs. Malvika's posture is severely affected by scoliosis of her spine and her trunk deviates to the right; she is unable to sit upright. Over the last year she has had repeated chest infections, which have required antibiotic therapy.

- What are the factors that make Malvika at risk of recurrent chest infections?
- Decide on what observations you should take when Malvika has a chest infection and why?
- What could you do to minimize her risk of developing a chest infection?

Case study: Mental health

Paul Grey is a 47-year-old recently divorced man with three school-aged children who live with his wife. Paul has become increasingly anxious and unable to deal with his daily workload. The head of his department, who is aware of the stresses in Paul's personal life, has asked him to seek help through the occupational health unit. The occupational health nurse finds that Paul's blood pressure is elevated at 160/105 mmHg and he is 5 kg overweight. Paul and the nurse discuss his lifestyle and personal problems.

- Review the factors that might have led to the increase in Paul's blood pressure.
- Explore how lifestyle and life events can lead to hypertension (see also Ch. 8 on stress, relaxation and rest).
- Decide on what ongoing monitoring and health promotion would be appropriate for Paul.

Case study: Child

Jade, a 9-month-old infant, has been admitted to the children's ward accompanied by her 18-year-old mother, Mandy, who lives at home with her mother and father. Jade looks flushed and has a pyrexia of 38°C; she has been crying and irritable and is not taking her feeds. Mandy is very tearful and worried about her baby.

- Decide on which 'vital signs' you need to assess and how often.
- What would you need to consider when assessing these 'vital signs' in Jade?
- Review possible nursing interventions that could be implemented to control Jade's temperature.

Summary

This chapter has drawn together theoretical concepts relating to homeostasis and applied this knowledge in relation to the practice of caring for individuals. It has included:

1. The biological theoretical basis of thermoregulation, blood pressure maintenance, pulse and respiratory homeostasis, and the maintenance of feedback loops in maintaining homeostasis.
2. Behavioural, cultural and environmental influences that may affect an individual's ability to maintain homeostasis.
3. Consideration of factors influencing nurse decision making in monitoring and aiding maintenance of homeostasis for patients. These factors relate to the measurement, assessment and nursing management of body temperature, blood pressure and respiration.
4. Professional and ethical dimensions of patient consent, and nursing accountability in relation to the provision of nursing care.
5. Considerations relating to the use of medical technology in assessment.

Knowledge illuminated within this chapter has been combined with evidence from other referenced sources and applied within a range of situations. Suggestions have been made for portfolio development in relation to management of homeostasis.

Annotated further reading and websites

Blows W 2001 The biological basis of nursing: clinical observations. Routledge, London

Childs C 1994 Temperature control. In: Alexander M, Fawcett J, Runciman P (eds) Nursing practice: hospital and home, the adult. Churchill Livingstone, Edinburgh, pp 679–695
A very good overview of thermoregulation in adults with the biological basis covered in more detail.

Fulbrook P 1993 Core temperature measurement in adults: a literature review. Journal of Advanced Nursing 18:1451–1460
A good summary of the literature on temperature measurement up to the early 1990s. A critical appraisal and summary of research completed. Again the focus is on the adult.

Helman C G 1994 Culture, health and illness, 3rd edn. Butterworth-Heinemann, Oxford
This is a good comprehensive text on cultural influences on health. Although only referred to briefly in this chapter there is much information that is useful to support other chapters in this textbook. See especially Chapter 2 on cultural definitions of anatomy and physiology.

Hinchliff S, Montague S, Watson R 1996 Physiology for nursing practice. Baillière Tindall, London
This excellent physiology textbook, and particularly the chapters outlined below, provides good back-up information in relation to the biological basis of the elements of homeostasis covered in this chapter. There are also useful sections that relate theory to the practice of nursing. See Chapter 6.1 on temperature regulation Chapter 4.2 on cardiovascular function and Chapter 5.3 on respiration.

Mallett J, Doughty L 2000 The Royal Marsden NHS Trust manual of clinical nursing procedures, 5th edn. Blackwell Science, Oxford
A good reference book about how to carry out the skills of measuring homeostasis. The rationale for each of the activities is provided.

Torrance C, Serginson E 1996 An observational study of student nurses' measurement of arterial blood pressure by sphygmomanometry and auscultation. Nurse Education Today 16:282–286
This is a very instructive piece of research because of the use of observation of accuracy in the application of skills in blood pressure measurement. It highlights the need for students to be taught and supervised in skills acquisition in nursing.

Wong D L, Hockenberry M J, Wilson D et al 2003 Whaley and Wong's Nursing care of infants and children, 7th edn. Mosby, St Louis
For students who wish to specialize in children's nursing, this book is a very comprehensive resource book for all aspects of infant, child and teenage care. Maintaining homeostasis in infants and children differs from that in adults and requires specialist knowledge and skills. See Chapter 1 on assessment of the child.

http://www.doh.gov.uk
From the Department of Health's web page you can access numerous useful web pages on public health policy and health education, national service frameworks and screening and environmental issues and health.

http://www.abdn.ac.uk/BHS/
Website of the British Hypertension Society. This is a good website with guidelines on measuring blood pressure.

References

Beevers G, Lip G H, O'Brien E 2001 ABC of hypertension, 4th edn. British Medical Journal, London

Blackburn C 1991 Poverty and health: working with families. Open University Press, Milton Keynes

Board M 1995 Comparison of disposable and glass mercury thermometers. Nursing Times 91(33):36–37

Calman M, Johnson B 1985 Health, health risks and inequalities: an exploratory study of women's perceptions. Sociology of Health and Illness 14(2):233–254

Carroll M 2000 An evaluation of temperature measurement. Nursing Standard 14(44):39–43

Case R M, Waterhouse J M (eds) 1994 Human physiology: age, stress and the environment, 2nd edn. Oxford Science Publications, Oxford

Casey G 2000 Fever management in children. Nursing Standard 14(40):36–40

Childs C 1994 Temperature control. In: Alexander M, Fawcett J, Runciman P (eds) Nursing practice: hospital and home – the adult. Churchill Livingstone, Edinburgh, pp 679–695

Closs J 1987 Oral temperature measurement. Nursing Times 83(1):36–39

Croft J, Cruikshank J 1990 Blood pressure measurement in adults: large cuffs for all. Journal of Epidemiology and Community Health 44:107–173

Cutter J 1994 Recording patient temperature: are we getting it right? Professional Nurse 9(9):608–616

Department of Health 1997 The health of the nation, 2nd edn. HMSO, London

Department of Health 1998 Smoking kills: a White Paper on tobacco. HMSO, London

Department of Health 2000a The NHS plan. HMSO, London

Department of Health 2000b National Service Framework for coronary heart disease: modern standards and service models. HMSO, London

Department of Health 2001a Health effects of climate change. HMSO, London

Department of Health 2001b Good practice in consent: achieving the NHS plan commitment to patient-centred consent practice. HMSO, London

Department of Health 2002 Tackling health inequalities: summary of cross cutting review. HMSO, London

Department of Health 2003 Priorities and planning framework (PPF) for 2003–06 Improvement, expansion and reform: the next three years. HMSO, London

Durkin N 1979 An introduction to medical science: comprehensive guide to anatomy, biochemistry and physiology. MTP Press, Lancaster

Edge G, Morgan M 1993 The Genius infrared tympanic thermometer. Anaesthesia 48(7):604–607

Erickson R, Yount S 1991 Comparison of tympanic and oral temperatures in surgical patients. Nursing Research 40(2):90–93

Faulkner A 1985 Nursing: a creative approach. Baillière Tindall, London

Faulkner A (ed) 1990 Oncology. Scutari Press, London

Ferra-Love R 1991 A comparison of tympanic and pulmonary artery measures of core temperature. Journal of Post Anaesthetic Nursing 6(3):161–164

Fulbrook P 1993 Core temperature measurement in adults: a literature review. Journal of Advanced Nursing 18:1451–1460

Gift A 1990 Dyspnoea. Nursing Clinics of North America 25(4):955–965

Goldman M B, Nash M, Petkovic M S 1994 Do electrolyte-containing beverages improve water balance in hyponatraemic schizophrenics? Journal of Clinical Psychiatry 55(4):151–153

Goonasekera C D A, Dillon M J 2000 Measurement and interpretation of blood pressure. Archives of Disease in Childhood 82:261–265

Halle A, Repasy A 1987 Classic heatstroke: a serious challenge for the elderly. Hospital Practice 22(5):26

Health and Safety Commission 1988 The control of substances hazardous to health, regulations. HMSO, London

Helman C G 1994 Culture, health and illness, 3rd edn. Butterworth Heinemann, Oxford

Hinchliff S, Montague S, Watson R 1996 Physiology for nursing practice. Baillière Tindall, London

Holtzclaw B 1990 Shivering: a clinical nursing problem. Nursing Clinics of North America 25(4):977–985

Kleinman A 1980 Patients and healers in the context of culture. University of California Press, Berkeley

Lewis L W, Timby B 1993 Fundamental skills and concepts in patient care. Chapman & Hall, London

McBride A 1994 Health promotion in hospitals: the attitudes, beliefs and practices of hospital nurses. Journal of Advanced Nursing 20:92–100

McGee J, Isaacson P G, Wright N A 1992 Oxford textbook of pathology: principles of pathology. Oxford Medical Publications, Oxford

Medical Devices Agency 2002 Medical devices containing mercury: current position in the UK and Europe. Online. Available: http:/www.medical-devices.gov.uk/mda/mdawebsitev2.nsf/ 3 Feb 2003

Mishler J 1981 Social contexts of health, illness and patient care. Cambridge University Press, Cambridge

National Heart, Lung and Blood Institute 1987 Report of the second task force on blood pressure control in children: 1987. Paediatrics 79(1):1–11

Nursing and Midwifery Council 2002 Code of professional conduct. Nursing and Midwifery Council, London

Nyholm B, Jeppensen L, Mortensen B et al 1994 The superiority of rectal thermometry to oral thermometry with regard to accuracy. Journal of Advanced Nursing 20:660–665

O'Brien E T, Petrie J C, Littler W A et al 1997 Blood pressure measurement: recommendations of the British Hypertension Society. British Medical Journal, London

O'Brien E, Waeber B, Parati G et al 2001 Blood pressure measuring devices: recommendations of the European Society of Hypertension. British Medical Journal 322:531–536

Orstein R, Sobel D 1988 Bodyguards. In: Orstein R, Sobel D (eds) The healing brain. Touchstone, New York, pp 35–54

Pickersgill J 2003 Temperature taking: children's preferences. Paediatric Nursing 15(2):21–25

Pugh Davies S, Kassab J, Thrush A et al 1986 A comparison of mercury and digital thermometers. Journal of Advanced Nursing 11:535–543

Roper N, Logan W, Tierney A 1993 The elements of nursing, 3rd edn. Longman, Edinburgh

Sorof J M, Portman R J 2000 Ambulatory blood pressure monitoring in the pediatric patient. Journal of Pediatrics 136(5):578–586

Tannahill A 1985 What is health promotion? Health Education Journal 44(4):167–168

Thomas C, Gebert G, Hambach V 1992 Textbook and colour atlas of the cardiovascular system. Chapman & Hall, London

Timms-Hagen J 1984 Thermogenesis in brown adipose tissue as an energy buffer. New England Journal of Medicine 311:1549

Tones K 1993 The theory of health promotion: implications for nursing. In: Wilson-Barnett J, Macleod Clark J (eds) Research in health promotion and nursing. Macmillan, London

Torrance C, Serginson E 1996 Student nurses' knowledge in relation to blood pressure measurement by sphygmomanometry and auscultation. Nurse Education Today 16(6):397–402

Townsend P, Davidson N 1982 Inequalities in health: the Black report. Penguin, Harmondsworth

Watson R 1996 Hypothermia. Elderly Care 8(6):25–28

Webster C 1995 Health and physical assessment. In: Heath H (ed) Foundations in nursing practice. Mosby, London, pp 71–102

Webster J, Newnham D, Petrie J et al 1984 Influence of arm position on measurement of blood pressure. British Medical Journal 288:1574–1575

Woollons S 1996 Temperature measurement devices. Professional Nurse 11(8):541–547

Wilson-Barnett J, Latter S 1993 Factors influencing health education and health promotion practice in acute ward settings. In: Wilson-Barnett J, Macleod Clark J (eds) Research in health promotion and nursing. Macmillan, London

Wong D L 1993 Whaley and Wong's Essentials of pediatric nursing. Mosby, St Louis

Wong D L, Hockenberry M J, Wilson D et al 2003 Whaley and Wong's Essentials of pediatric nursing, 7th edn. Mosby, St Louis

Chapter 7

Nutrition

Lindsey Bellringer

KEY ISSUES

SUBJECT KNOWLEDGE

- Energy producing and non energy producing food, what it is and why it is needed in the body
- The chemical structure of the different food groups
- Storage and use of food in the body
- How metabolism extracts energy from food
- Social and psychological influences on nutrition

CARE DELIVERY KNOWLEDGE

- Assessing nutritional status
- Calculation of body mass index and the healthy range
- Identification of different nutritional needs related to age
- Feeding patients
- Identification of appropriate alternative and supplementary methods of feeding when patients are unable to eat normally
- A review of common disorders of nutrition

PROFESSIONAL AND ETHICAL KNOWLEDGE

- Legal aspects of food safety
- Professional accountability
- Ethical dilemmas in feeding
- Patients' rights

PERSONAL AND REFLECTIVE KNOWLEDGE

- Review of main points
- Explore your personal beliefs about nutrition
- Apply your knowledge to professional practice

INTRODUCTION

Food is essential for life; it provides the nutrients we need to maintain our bodies. It also is an integral part of our social and cultural life. In the UK there is a greater range of affordable foods available than ever before and it should be possible to ensure the population, as a whole, does not suffer from diseases caused by lack of essential nutrients. More and more a healthy diet is implicated in the prevention of diseases such as coronary artery disease, bowel cancer and diabetes and there is no lack of information available to the general public about these facts. Why then are health professionals still dealing with impaired health and disease due to poor nutrition? Nurses may well be called upon to explain the vast amount of occasionally conflicting information about diet to patients. They must give informed, up-to-date advice and ensure that patients are not left feeling guilty because they have not eaten all the right foods or that they have been unable to provide a healthy diet for their families.

Reflection and portfolio evidence

Identify some of the information you have encountered about food, diet or nutrition in the past week. Sources of such information may include television, radio, newspapers books and magazines, as well as friends.

- How do you think this information has affected your attitudes or behaviour?
- Discuss your reflections with your peer group of learners.
- Debate how your findings will influence your decisions in offering health promotion advice to your patients/clients.

The provision of nutritional care is a challenge to nurses, particularly in the institutional setting, as demonstrated in the report *Hungry in Hospital* (Community Health Council 1997). Much has been published about nutritional assessment tools, how to monitor patients' risk of malnutrition and recommendations for changing practice (Collier 2002, Devlin 2000, Ledsham & Gough 2000). In 2001 the Department of Health produced the resource pack *Essence of Care* (Department of Health 2001) aimed at improving standards of care in England by using benchmarks of good practice. The food and nutrition benchmark requires that 'Patients/ clients are enabled to consume food (orally) which meets their individual need'. Nurses are encouraged to compare practice in their clinical area to the benchmark of good practice and formulate action plans on how to improve the standard of care from initial assessment through to health promotion.

This chapter aims to provide you with core knowledge on good nutritional care as well as exploring with you the many ways of providing food. It also provides information on the professional, ethical and legal responsibilities of the nurse in ensuring that their patients meet their nutritional needs.

Subject knowledge

This section deals with functions of food as a source of energy, growth and repair. It outlines the physiological processes that allow the body to use nutritional components and throughout this section you are asked to consider the physiological evidence against the common contemporary dietary myths. Social and psychological factors and their influence on nutrition are discussed.

Care delivery knowledge

This section concentrates on the assessment of the patient's nutritional status. Nutritional needs vary according to age, gender and lifestyle. Pregnant and breastfeeding women have particular needs to ensure their own health and that of their babies. Strategies for planning, implementing and evaluating nutritional care are discussed. Alternative methods of feeding when patients are unable to eat normally are explored.

Professional and ethical knowledge

This section outlines legislation surrounding the provision of food and the nurse's responsibility to the client related to the code of professional conduct. It also touches on the ethical issues surrounding food and drink, for instance when caring for the terminally ill or those in a persistent vegetative state.

Personal and reflective knowledge

The final part of the chapter asks you to reflect on what you have read and consider how you can put it to practice and produce evidence for your learning portfolio.

Four case studies are presented at the end of the chapter, each one relating to one of the branch programmes.

SUBJECT KNOWLEDGE

BIOLOGICAL

ENERGY PRODUCING FOODS

All of the activities we undertake involve the expenditure of energy. Even when we are asleep or unconscious the muscles of our heart and respiration need energy. Heat energy is needed to maintain body temperature and cells are constantly being replaced as they wear out and die. All of the energy for these processes is derived from food in the form of carbohydrates, fats or proteins.

The amount of food we need is controlled by our energy expenditure; this is called the energy balance. If we take in less energy than we are using we are said to be in a negative energy balance and will lose weight. On the other hand taking in excess energy, regardless of the type of food eaten, will result in weight gain. Many people maintain the same weight for many years, which indicates a very accurate control of energy balance, although how this regulating mechanism works is uncertain.

The amount of food we eat is determined to a large extent by appetite. The main control of appetite is physiological, involving two centres within the hypothalmus – the feeding (hunger) centre and the satiety (full) centre – which work in opposition to each other. The satiety centre is mainly controlled by the blood glucose concentration and functions to suppress the hunger centre. As the blood glucose level decreases the power of the satiety centre is lowered and the hunger centre becomes active giving rise to the feeling of hunger and the desire to eat. This explains why something sweet at the end of a meal (consequently containing a large amount of simple sugars that are rapidly absorbed to raise the blood sugar level) leaves an individual feeling satisfied and in need of no further food. Other physiological influences on appetite are the body fat deposits and the distension of the gut. Pychosocial influences are also important as will be discussed later in this chapter. How the body uses energy producing foods, i.e. carbohydrate, proteins and fats, is discussed below.

Carbohydrates

Carbohydrates should account for more than half the energy intake in the diet. They have a general formula $(CH_2O)_n$ and are manufactured by plants from carbon dioxide, water and energy from sunlight through the process of photosynthesis. By this means the energy of the sun is trapped and made available to animals when they eat the plant.

The most simple carbohydrates, such as glucose, fructose and galactose, contain six carbon molecules and are called monosaccharides. These three monosaccharides all have the formula $C_6H_{12}O_6$ but the positions of the carbon atoms in relation to the oxygen atoms differ. These monosaccharides can combine to form pairs of molecules called disaccharides.

This is achieved by the removal of a water molecule and is known as a condensation reaction. Depending on the combination of monosaccharides, different disaccharides are produced. For example:

- the disaccharide we are most familiar with is sucrose – table sugar – and this is simply one glucose molecule joined to one fructose molecule
- two molecules of glucose form maltose, which is a disaccharide
- one molecule of glucose and one molecule of galactose form lactose.

Because of their relatively uncomplicated molecular structure, monosaccharides and disaccharides are quickly absorbed and utilized. They are also referred to as simple sugars. Many glucose molecules joined together form a polysaccharide called starch, which plants use as an energy store, for example the starch in potatoes and cereals. Foods containing these will therefore be high in complex carbohydrate.

Plants use another carbohydrate called cellulose to form their structure. Humans are unable to digest this structural carbohydrate, but ruminants such as cows or sheep are able to break it down and use it for energy.

Many people believe that some forms of simple carbohydrate are more natural and therefore healthier than others and these myths are exploited by the food industry who try to convince us that their products are more healthy than those of their competitors. It is worth remembering that from a nutritional viewpoint there is no difference between glucose, fructose and sucrose and certainly no advantage to cane sugar over beet sugar. Pure carbohydrate from whatever source releases 4.1 kcal/g when metabolized, although foods containing a higher proportion of water and cellulose will have a lower energy density.

Digestion, transport and storage of carbohydrates

All complex carbohydrates must be broken down by the digestive system into monosaccharides before they can be absorbed. The process begins with the action of salivary amylase, which converts starch into the disaccharide, maltose. Other starches are split into disaccharides by the pancreatic amylase. The final step is for a series of enzymes in the small intestine to break down the disaccharides into monosaccharides. There is a specific enzyme for each disaccharide, but the names are easy to remember:

- maltose is split by maltase
- sucrose is split by sucrase
- lactose is split by lactase.

Splitting disaccharides also involves putting the water back, a process known as hydrolysis (from the Greek words 'hydro' meaning water, and 'lysis' meaning breaking down).

This is the opposite process to the condensation reaction, which removes water to join the two monosaccharide molecules. Once broken down to monosaccharides in the digestive system, carbohydrates are absorbed in the small intestine and transported via the portal vein to the liver. This raises the concentration of the plasma glucose and stimulates the secretion of insulin by the beta cells of the pancreas. This in turn increases the rate which the large glucose molecules are able to pass through the cell walls into the cells where they will be broken down to provide energy.

Excessive plasma glucose can be converted into an insoluble carbohydrate, glycogen, which is similar to starch in plants, through the process of glycogenesis. Glycogen is stored mainly in the liver and the muscles and can be converted back to glucose (glycogenolysis) when the plasma glucose concentration falls. When glycogen stores are full any remaining glucose may be converted into fat and stored until it is needed. As the glucose in the blood is used up, insulin secretion decreases and glucagon secretion from the alpha cells of the pancreas increases. Glucagon converts glycogen back into glucose to restore the blood glucose concentration and mobilize the stored fat.

Decision making exercise

The hormone glucagon is secreted by the alpha cells of the pancreas when the blood glucose concentration falls. This causes a reduction in glycogenesis and an increase in glycogenolysis, which leads to an increase in blood glucose concentration. Glucagon can also be manufactured synthetically and administered by injection.

- What are the indications for the use of synthetic glucagon?
- What is the usual dosage?
- What are the limitations of using synthetic glucagon?

Utilization of carbohydrate: respiration

Carbohydrates are made in the chloroplasts of plant cells through the action of photosynthesis as follows:

$$6H_2O + 6CO_2 + energy \rightarrow C_6H_{12}O_6 + 6O_2$$

When the equation is moving in this direction, energy from the sun is used to form carbohydrate. However, in the mitochondria of animal cells this action is reversed, in the process of respiration, as follows:

$$C_6H_{12}O_6 + 6O_2 \rightarrow 6H_2O + 6CO_2 + energy$$

The energy produced in respiration takes two forms, heat and chemical energy. The heat energy maintains the body temperature. This explains why we get hot when we exercise, as an increase in the metabolism of food in the muscles generates more heat. The chemical energy is used to join phosphate to another molecule to store energy for future use. The commonest example of this action is phosphate (P) joining adenosine diphosphate (ADP) to form adenosine triphoshate (ATP). When energy is required the phosphate bond is broken to revert back to ADP and P so releasing the stored energy.

The process of obtaining energy from glucose occurs in three stages:

1. The first stage, glycolysis, takes place in the cytoplasm of the cell. Here the six-carbon glucose molecule is split into two three-carbon pyruvate molecules. Glycolysis releases eight ATP molecules.
2. If there is no oxygen present (i.e. anaerobic conditions) pyruvate is converted to lactate, which will be reconverted to pyruvate when oxygen becomes available. This costs six ATP molecules. Therefore in the absence of adequate oxygen, the energy yield from glycolysis drops two molecules of ATP. In the presence of oxygen, however, the pyruvate is transported to the mitochondria where it is converted to carbon dioxide and acetyl coenzyme A (acetyl CoA). The acetyl CoA enters the Krebs cycle where the hydrogen is removed and carbon dioxide is released (aerobic metabolism).
3. In the third stage of the process, called the electron transport chain, the energy is once more used to combine phosphate with ADP to produce ATP. The hydrogen is then combined with oxygen to form water.

The three stages of this glucose metabolism will release sufficient energy from one molecule of glucose to produce 38 molecules of ATP.

The more mitochondria there are in a cell the more reactions can take place and the greater the amount of energy available. The mitochondria increase in response to the energy demand made upon a cell. Consequently this increases the individual's basal metabolic rate. When there is less demand the number of mitochondria decrease. You may notice this effect if you decide to increase your fitness by regular exercise. You will notice that as you continue a programme of training the length of time you are able to engage in activity increases. You see yourself becoming fit. Cells are able to engage in more activity as the number of mitochondria increase in response to the demand made on them during training.

Fats

Fats are solid and oils are liquid, and they are referred to collectively as lipids. They are insoluble in water and have the general formula $CH_3(CH_2)_nCOOH$, which looks complicated but like carbohydrate they only contain carbon, hydrogen and oxygen. Most lipids in the diet are in the form of triglycerides. These are made up of three fatty acids, each attached to a glycerol molecule to form a structure like a letter E, with the glycerol being the vertical stroke. Fatty acids are a line of carbon atoms with hydrogen atoms attached. There are three different forms of fatty acids known as:

- saturated fatty acids, which contain the maximum possible number of hydrogen atoms

- monounsaturated fatty acids, which have two hydrogen atoms missing from each molecule
- polyunsaturated fatty acids, which have more than two hydrogen atoms missing from each molecule.

Saturated fats are solid at room temperature whereas mono- and polyunsaturated fats are liquid oils. Generally animal fats are saturated and those from vegetables and fish are unsaturated (two exceptions to this rule are palm and coconut oil). Saturated fat in the diet tends to raise the concentration of the blood cholesterol level whereas monounsaturated fats such as olive oil tend to lower it. Because a high blood cholesterol concentration is linked to arterial disease, the current recommendation is to reduce the total amount of fat in the diet and to limit the intake of saturated fat so that it constitutes not more than 10% of the energy intake. Examples of fatty foods include butter, margarine, lard, cooking oil and the fat on meat.

Reflection and portfolio evidence

Read the Cochrane review 'Reduced or modified dietary fat for preventing cardiovascular disease' by Hooper et al (2003). Based on the reviewers' conclusion:

- Reflect on your personal dietary habits and review whether there is a need for you to change your habits to maintain your health.
- Make notes on how you would advise a patient with a high risk of cardiac disease about dietary fat consumption.
- Write a short information sheet explaining the differences between saturated fatty acids, monounsaturated fatty acids and polyunsaturated fatty acids.
- How would you explain the difference between high density and low density lipoprotein cholesterol?

Under supervision provide the above information to a patient/client at risk and complete for your portfolio of evidence.

Fats are often thought of as being bad but a certain amount is essential for our health and well-being. Fats are needed to make cell membranes, steroid hormones, prostaglandins and bile, and to store energy. They are a very efficient way of storing energy as they contain 9.3 kcal/g, which is more than double the energy content of carbohydrates and proteins. However, because fats pack many calories into a small volume it is easy to take too many calories in a high fat diet.

Digestion, utilization, transport and storage of lipids

Lipids are insoluble and form large globules in water; therefore they need to be emulsified. This is achieved in the body by the action of bile (Fig. 7.1). Once emulsified the triglycerides are split by the enzyme lipase into fatty acids

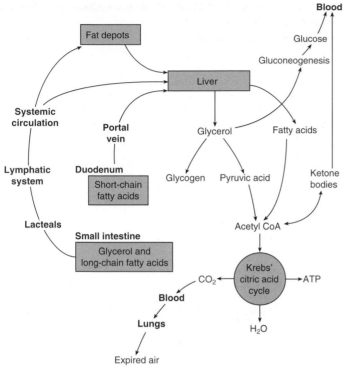

Figure 7.1   Diagram of fat metabolism. (From Hinchliff et al 1996.)

and monoglycerides. Short chain fatty acids are absorbed into the blood directly at this point. Most fatty acids are long chain (i.e. they have more than 12 carbon atoms) and these and the monoglycerides take a different pathway to the blood. By combining with bile salts, long chain fatty acids and the monoglycerides form micelles and in this form are then able to enter the epithelial cells of the villi. Once in the epithelial cells lipase acts on the monoglycerides to reduce them to glycerol and fatty acids. Here they are combined with cholesterol and phospholipids to form chylomicrons. These in turn are absorbed into the lacteals of the small intestine and transported through the lymphatic system to enter the blood at the subclavian vein.

As fats are insoluble, absorbed fats are either transported in the blood as chylomicrons or as free fatty acids attached to albumin. These transport molecules are also known as lipoproteins. Because fat is lighter than water the higher the percentage of fat in a lipoprotein the lower the density. Low density lipoproteins (LDLs) carry a high percentage of cholesterol and are therefore associated with a risk to health. The high density lipoproteins (HDLs) on the other hand transport fat from the tissues to the liver to be excreted.

Lipids are either stored on adipose tissue as triglcerides or metabolized by the liver in a process called beta oxidation. The liver cells split pairs of carbon atoms from the fatty acids to form acetyl CoA, which can then enter the Krebs cycle. Excess acetyl CoA is converted into ketones and circulated to other tissues in the body where it is converted back to acetyl CoA and used for energy.

Proteins

Chemical structure

Proteins share the same properties of fats and carbohydrates. They contain the same three chemicals – carbon, hydrogen and oxygen – but additionally all proteins contain nitrogen. Complex proteins are made up of amino acids linked together by a peptide bond. There is no general formula, but all amino acids have an amine group (NH_2) and an acidic carboxyl group (COOH) in common, with the remainder of the molecule varying depending on which amino acid it is. Although there are only 20 amino acids, the number of possible combinations to form proteins is almost infinite. One very important characteristic of proteins is that each one tends to fold itself into a particular shape which will determine its function. For example if the haemoglobin molecule does not assume its correct shape sickle cell anaemia results. The action of enzymes, which are proteins, also relies on their shape and if this is altered by heat or pH they will not function.

Sources

Many amino acids can be synthesized in the body; those that cannot are known as essential amino acids and must be taken in the diet. Many plants are deficient in one or more of the essential amino acids but a mixture of plant proteins is capable of supplying all the amino acids needed. Meat, fish, eggs and milk have a high protein content. Plant sources rich in protein are seeds, with peas, beans and nuts particularly valuable. Cereals and potatoes have a comparatively low percentage of protein but because of the large amount in most diets they can make a significant contribution to total intake.

Decision making exercise

A colleague has spent the weekend demonstrating against the export of live farm animals. She has decided to become a strict vegan. Of the 20 amino acids in the body it is only possible to synthesize 10 in adequate amounts and it is not possible to synthesize eight at all nor is it possible to store protein in the body. Therefore if amino acids are to be synthesized it is only possible if combinations of foods containing the elements of amino acids are consumed together.

- What are the implications of protein synthesis for your colleague?
- Which foods contain essential amino acids?
- Which foods contain no essential amino acids?
- Using this knowledge, how would you help your colleague to devise a dietary plan to ensure she receives enough protein?

Utilization, transport and storage

Protein is unique in containing nitrogen so intake and the loss of protein from the body is termed nitrogen balance. Digestive enzymes split the proteins into individual amino acids which can then be absorbed. Once absorbed, the amino acids are used for repair and replacement of cells, and the manufacture of enzymes and hormones; any excess will be deaminated by the liver. This process involves splitting off the nitrogen and converting it into urea, which can then be excreted by the kidneys. The deaminated amino acid remnants can be used to form glucose (glucogenesis), stored as fats, or metabolized to provide energy.

NON ENERGY PRODUCING DIETARY COMPONENTS

The remaining components of the diet do not provide energy but are essential for health. These are vitamins, minerals and fibre.

Vitamins

Vitamins are a series of unrelated organic substances that are needed in very small amounts for normal body metabolism. They are divided into those that are fat soluble and those that are water soluble: see Tables 7.1 and 7.2.

Minerals

These inorganic salts are an essential part of the diet and are required for many processes. They include sodium, potassium, chlorine, iron, iodine, chloride, copper, cobalt, zinc, calcium and selenium. The most common minerals are shown in Table 7.3.

Fibre

Fibre is the indigestible part of the diet that comes from plants; it consists of bran, cellulose and other polysaccharides. Although fibre is not essential for life, deficiency is associated with a variety of diseases. Fibre passes unchanged into the colon adding bulk to the faeces, stimulating peristalsis which prevents constipation. Fibre may reduce the risk of bowel cancer by diluting any toxins and carcinogens in the faeces and reducing the length of time they are in contact with the colon.

PSYCHOSOCIAL

PSYCHOLOGICAL AND SOCIOCULTURAL ASPECTS OF NUTRITION

So far the physiology of nutrition has been considered. This assumes that people are rational dispassionate consumers who will choose to eat the quantity and type of foods best suited to maintaining their energy balance and supplying all the essential nutrients when they feel hungry. Nutritional value is only one of many things taken into account by the majority of people when faced with a choice of food. There are a host of influencing factors such as what sorts of food have been eaten in the past, for example a particular food may be associated with an enjoyable evening out with friends or the bad experience of being made to 'eat your greens'. Sweet things may be associated with being given rewards or treats as a child and in buying them we may be

Table 7.1   Fat soluble vitamins

Vitamin and chemical name	Source	Functions	Recommended daily intake (adult)	Effects of deficiency
A *Retinol* (*provitamin carotene in plants*)	Milk, butter, cheese, egg yolk, fish liver, oils, yellow and green vegetables	Maintains healthy epithelial tissue, cornea and is required for the synthesis of visual purple	600–700 micrograms	Night blindness; atrophy and keratinization of the epithelium; increased infections of ear, sinuses, urinary and alimentary tracts; drying and ulceration of the cornea
D *Calciferol*	Can be synthesized by the action of ultraviolet light on 7-dehydrocholesterol in the skin; milk, butter, cheese, eggs, fish liver	Aids the absorption and utilization of calcium and phosphorus to promote healthy bones and teeth	10 micrograms	Ricketts (in children), osteomalacia in adults
E *Tocopherol*	Egg yolk, nuts, seeds, olive and other vegetable oils, green vegetables	Prevents catabolism of polyunsaturated fats, needed for the structure of cell membranes	3–4 milligrams	Anaemia; ataxia; cystic fibrosis
K *Phylloquinone*	Dark green leafy vegetables, liver, fish	Needed for the formation of prothrombin and factors VII, IX and X	60–70 micrograms	Easy bruising and prolonged blood clotting time

Table 7.2   Water soluble vitamins

Vitamin and chemical name	Source	Functions	Recommended daily intake (adult)[8]	Effects of deficiency
B₁ *Thiamine*	Yeast, liver, germ of cereals, nuts, pulses, egg yolk, legumes	Metabolism of carbohydrate and nutrition of nerve cells	0.8–1 milligram	Fatigue; neuropathy; loss of memory; beriberi
B₂ *Riboflavin*	Liver, yeast, milk, eggs, green vegetables, kidney and fish roe	Carbohydrate metabolism; maintains healthy skin and eyes	1–1.3 milligrams	Angular stomatitis; dermatitis; blurred vision
B₆ *Pyridoxine*	Meat, liver, fish, vegetables, bran of cereals	Protein metabolism; production of antibodies	1.2–1.4 milligrams	(Rare)
B₁₂ *Cyanocobalamin*	Liver, milk, poultry, fish; not found in plants	Maturation of the red blood cells, DNA synthesis	1.5 micrograms	Pernicious anaemia
B *Folic acid/folacin*	Synthesized in the colon; dark green vegetables, liver, kidney, eggs	Formation of red blood cells; DNA synthesis	200 micrograms	Anaemia; N.B. pregnant women need to take a supplement
B *Nicotinic acid/niacin*	Synthesized in the body from tryptophan; yeast, offal, fish, pulses, wholemeal cereals, potatoes	Inhibits production of cholesterol; needed for cell respiration	12–17 milligrams	Prolonged deficiency causes pellagra
B *Pantothenic acid*	Meat, liver, yeast, fresh vegetables, egg yolk, grains	Amino acid metabolism	3–7 milligrams	Vague – loss of appetite, abdominal and limb pains; associated with alcoholic neuropathy
B *Biotin*	Yeasts, liver, kidney, pulses, nuts	Carbohydrate and fat metabolism (essential for Krebs cycle)	10–200 micrograms	Scaly skin; anorexia; elevated blood cholesterol levels
C *Ascorbic acid*	Citrus fruits, currants, berries, green vegetables, potatoes	Formation of collagen; absorption of iron from the gut; required to convert folic acid to its active form	40 milligrams	Slow wound healing; anaemia; scurvy

rewarding ourselves for a job well done or comforting ourselves when feeling rejected.

Food plays a part in religion and culture; not only the type of food consumed but in the preparation and timing of meals. The taste and texture of food also influence the choice of foods. Fat, salt and sugar have a very widespread appeal as evidenced by the popularity of chips and crisps and chocolate.

Food advertising encourages us to eat the manufacturer's product whether we are hungry or not. This huge industry is very versatile and can respond to current fashion by targeting the consumer for example with low fat, low calorie foods. Food cookery programmes appear on the television every day; few of these are aimed at low income groups though some demonstrate that interesting meals can be made quite cheaply. Much has changed in family life; often both parents are working and families may eat at different times of day with snacks in between. Ready meals that can be microwaved are often preferred to home made meals, which take time and planning, despite being cheaper and usually tastier.

With all the above factors it is hardly surprising that nutritional values are low on the list of priorities when it comes to food. Current government guidelines recommend five portions of fruit and vegetables daily, which can be difficult to achieve for the less well off or for those working in areas that have restricted food available, for example out of town industrial estates. Schools throughout the country have been looking at ways of improving the diet of children (Turner et al 2000). Many innovative schemes are being tried, for example offering free fruit at infant schools, breakfast clubs, tokens issued for choosing healthy options to enable cheap access to sports centres and inviting celebrity chefs to host cookery classes.

We live in a multicultural society and nurses need to have an awareness of dietary restrictions that may be part of a patient's culture or religion. For example the Islamic religion requires all healthy adults to fast, i.e. to take no food, drink or medication from dawn to sunset during the month of Ramadan. People with diabetes would be able to refrain from fasting, as exceptions are made for those who are ill, but many people are reluctant to accept this concession (Pinar

Table 7.3   Minerals

Mineral (chemical symbol)	Source	Importance in the body	Problems	
			Excess	Deficit
Sodium (Na)	Fish, table salt, cured meats, most other foods	The most common cation found in the extracellular fluid; principal electrolyte in maintaining osmotic pressure and water balance; essential for normal neuromuscular function	Implicated as a cause of hypertension	Nausea; abdominal and muscle cramps; convulsions
Potassium (K)	Most foods, especially fruit and vegetables	Helps maintain intracellular osmotic pressure; essential for normal nerve impulse conduction, muscle contraction, protein synthesis and glycogenesis	Cardiac arrhythmia; paraesthesia; muscular weakness	Cardiac arrhythmia; heart failure; muscular weakness; paralysis; nausea and vomiting
Calcium (Ca)	Milk, cheese, eggs, vegetables and shellfish	Required for the hardening of bones and teeth, blood clotting, transmission of nerve impulses and muscle contraction, normal heart rhythm	Impaired neural function; lethargy and confusion; muscle pain and weakness; calcium deposits in soft tissue; renal stones	Muscle tetany; osteoporosis; retarded growth and rickets in children
Chlorine (Cl)	Table salts	With sodium, helps maintain osmotic pressure and pH of extracellular fluid; required for the formation of hydrochloric acid in the stomach	Vomiting	Alkalosis; muscle cramps; apathy
Iron (Fe)	Red meat, liver, green vegetables, whole meal bread, egg yolk	Essential for the formation of haemoglobin in the red blood cells and the oxidization of carbohydrate	Damage to heart, liver and pancreas	Iron deficiency anaemia; pallor, lethargy, anorexia
Iodine (I)	Salt water fish, cod liver oil, vegetables grown in iodine rich soil, iodized table salt.	Required to form thyroid hormones T_3 and T_4 which help to regulate metabolic rate	Depressed synthesis of thyroid hormones	Myxoedema; impaired learning and motivation in children
Magnesium (Mg)	Nuts, fruit, leafy green vegetables, whole grains	Needed for normal neural function; lactation; oxidization of carbohydrates and protein hydrolysis	Appears to be linked to obsessive behaviour, hallucinations and violent behaviour	Not known
Zinc (Zn)	Seafood, meat, cereals, nuts, wheat germ, yeast	Required for normal growth, wound healing, taste, smell and sperm production	Ataxia, slurred speech, tremors	Loss of taste and smell; depressed immunity

2002). Nurses must be able to advise on how best to avoid or minimize the problems observing the fast might cause, while respecting the individual's right to observe his/her faith.

CARE DELIVERY KNOWLEDGE

All the components of a healthy diet are required by everyone at all stages in the life cycle in both health and illness. However, nutritional needs change throughout the various stages of our lives. By carrying out a nutritional assessment on patients nurses can help individuals by educating them

about diet and the part it plays in health and well-being. The following section gives a brief overview of special requirements at different stages in the life cycle.

NUTRITIONAL REQUIREMENTS THROUGH THE LIFE CYCLE

Pregnancy

Energy requirements increase during pregnancy to provide for the increase in tissue mass of the fetus, and the mother. The energy requirement varies according to the trimester but overall an increase in intake of 71–120 kcal per day is adequate for most well-nourished women (Coutts 2000a). A well-balanced diet provides most of the nutrients to maintain a healthy pregnancy, but evidence suggests that some supplements are advisable.

Lack of essential micronutrients (vitamins and minerals) is thought to be a cause of some birth defects and possible susceptibility to diseases later in life. Folic acid is particularly important as its deficiency is implicated in neural tube defects of the newborn. Most literature suggests that women should take a supplement of folic acid as it is difficult to achieve the recommended daily intake in pregnancy by diet alone. It is also recommended that women who are planning to have a baby supplement their folate intake. The current advice from the Department of Health (2000) is that all women of child-bearing age who may become pregnant or who are planning a pregnancy should take a supplement that provides 400 micrograms of folic acid per day. As preplanned pregnancies are not always the norm, there has been discussion on the need to fortify staple foods such as bread with folate for the total population. Other supplements that may be required by some pregnant women include vitamin D and iron.

Pregnant women are also advised not to eat dishes containing raw or partially cooked eggs, soft or mould ripened cheeses as these foods are possible sources of the bacteria *Salmonella* and *Listeria monocytogenes*. Current opinion is that liver and liver paté should be avoided during pregnancy as they contain high concentrations of vitamin A which may be teratogenic in high doses in early gestation (Goldberg 2003).

Lactation

During lactation the extra energy required by a breastfeeding mother is approximately 450 kcal per day rising slightly as the baby gets older. To achieve these extra requirements only a small amount of extra food is needed as the mother can use energy from stores laid down during pregnancy.

Babies

In the first few months babies receive all their energy requirements of life from breast or formula milk. The required energy intake for a baby is much higher than that of an adult: 110 kcal/kg of expected weight per day which approximately equates to between 100 and 250 mL of breastmilk per kg body weight per day (British Nutrition Foundation 1998a). After about 4 months, milk no longer fulfils all the baby's nutritional needs and other foods should be introduced. It is currently recommended that this process, known as weaning, does not commence before the age of 4 months (Coutts 2000b) as the infant's gut is limited in the type of foods it can digest and absorb. The infant should also be able to sit only slightly supported and turn his head away to indicate food refusal (British Nutrition Foundation 1998a). Infant diets need to be high in lipid for energy and for essential long chain fatty acids and fat soluble vitamins. Infants are also at

risk of iron and zinc deficiency so it is important to ensure the diet has sufficient micronutrients. There is much evidence and continued research into the effects of weaning diet on long-term health and health professionals need to be well informed about this aspect of child care (Coutts 2000b).

Schoolchildren

A varied diet containing adequate energy and nutrients is essential for normal growth and development of children. They have a high energy requirement for their size. To achieve this energy intake, foods that are high in energy and also rich in nutrients should be eaten as part of small frequent meals. A good supply of protein, calcium, iron and vitamins A and D are also necessary as childhood is an important time for tooth and bone development (British Nutrition Foundation 1998b). Concern is growing over the increase in obesity among schoolchildren. The combined effect of an increased intake of high-fat snacks and sugary fizzy drinks with less physical activity has been cited in several papers (Dietz 2001, Ludwig et al 2001). There is evidence that overweight children and adolescents are being diagnosed with Type 2 diabetes, a condition that is normally associated with adults over 40 (Perry 2001).

Evidence based practice

Obesity in adults and children: a call for action (Holm et al 2001). This report examines obesity as a worldwide health problem associated with substantial economic burden. Obese people experience more hypertension, elevated cholesterol, Type 2 diabetes and joint and mobility problems. This trend is becoming more prevalent amongst children. Data from a nationally representative sample of English children showed that the frequency of overweight ranged from 22% at age 6 to 31% at age 15. Childhood obesity is associated with elevated serum lipids, hypertension and abnormal glucose tolerance. Often these children have psychosocial problems that persist into adolescence and adulthood. Obese children are often sedentary and prefer fast food to a healthy diet, encouraged by the attitudes of countries with improved living standards. Holm et al suggest that a call for action is needed for all modernized societies, to alter environments and attitudes to support rather than hinder healthy dietary intake and being physically active.

Teenagers

Teenagers are particularly susceptible to media images which portray thinness as desirable. They are also at a stage where mood swings may be compensated for by comfort foods. As a result they can be prone to eating disorders which leave them short of nutrients and threaten their physical as well as mental health. Teenagers are the most common age group to suffer the disorders of anorexia nervosa and bulimia nervosa (these conditions are covered more fully further on in this chapter).

Adults

Adults need to eat a well-balanced diet to maintain their optimum weight. The recommendation of foods as a percentage of the daily intake is a simple way of planning a varied and healthy diet. Recommendations (Donellan 2001) are as follows:

- Bread, other cereals and potatoes 34%
- Fruit and vegetables 33%
- Milk and dairy foods 15%
- Meat, fish and alternatives 12%
- Fatty and sugary food 7%.

Often activity decreases with age; if a middle aged person consumes the same amount of food as when an active teenager, weight gain will occur. The government's recommendation of eating five portions of fruit and vegetables daily and reducing intake of saturated fats has been linked with improved health benefits, especially in the prevention of heart disease and some cancers (Coutts 2001).

Older people

Older people are particularly at risk of poor nutrition and its consequences. Between 10% and 40% of older people admitted to hospital are already malnourished (Bond 1997). There are a variety of causes of poor nutrition in the older person, such as loss of appetite due to decreased sense of taste and smell, poor dentition, lack of agility and mobility, social isolation and depression. Medical conditions or the side effects of drugs can interfere with nutrient absorption and metabolism as well as suppressing appetite (Devlin 2000). Particularly at risk are patients with dementia as this group of patients often refuse food and exhibit choking behaviour when attempts to spoon-feed are made; this causes stress and poses ethical problems for the carers (Biernacki & Barratt 2001). Tube feeding may be used if tolerated but issues surrounding consent need to explored.

Whether in their own home, nursing or residential home or hospital elderly people need to have a thorough nutritional assessment if presenting with an illness, as undernutrition has been demonstrated to increase morbidity and mortality especially during the winter months.

When planning food intake for older people the decline in basal metabolic rate (BMR) with age should be taken into account as should the reduction of physical activity. The Committee on Medical Aspects of Food Policy recommend that a standard value of 1.5 times the BMR should be used to calculate the minimum energy requirement for all people over 60 (Department of Health 1992). Nurses have the

responsibility that following the assessment and planning of energy intake, sufficient help and supervision are provided to the individual to enable meals to be eaten.

> ### Evidence based practice
>
> Protein and energy supplementation in elderly people at risk from malnutrition: Cochrane review (Milne et al 2003). The review examines the evidence from trials for improvement in nutritional status and clinical outcomes when sip feeds providing extra protein and energy are provided. Thirty-one trials with 2464 participants have been included in the review. The conclusion was that supplementation appears to produce a small but consistent weight gain. There was a statistically significant beneficial effect on mortality and a shorter length of inpatient stay. However, more data are needed to provide conclusive evidence. Few trials addressed practical or organizational difficulties faced by practitioners trying to meet the individuals needs and preferences of those at risk of malnutrition.

PATIENT/CLIENT ASSESSMENT

The extent of the nursing assessment will vary depending upon the client. A variety of assessment tools can be accessed from the literature and used in clinical practice to ensure that sufficient information is gathered to formulate a plan based on the risk of malnutrition for each individual client. The tool may incorporate recommendations for actions such as keeping food charts or offering nutritional supplements, and should indicate when to refer to a dietitian (Fig. 7.2).

Information required includes:

- an estimation of the basal metabolic rate (BMR)
- a calculation of body mass index (BMI)
- an assessment of physical conditions affecting the client's ability to eat
- a history
- socioeconomic information
- cultural and religious beliefs.

> ### Reflection and portfolio evidence
>
> Conduct a literature search and identify four tools used for nutritional assessment. If your clinical area has an assessment tool in use include it. To help you choose criteria for reviewing tools see Malnutrition Advisory Group (2000) and Bond (1997).
>
> - Critically review each tool using the same criteria.
> - Identify one that you feel is most appropriate for your current clinical area.
> - Record the results of your findings in your portfolio.

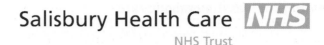

NUTRITIONAL RISK ASSESSMENT

Surname:	Forename: ....
Hospital No ☐ ☐ ☐ ☐ ☐	Age (in years): ☐ Height: ☐
Date of Admission: ☐ ☐ ☐	Consultant: ....

RISK FACTORS

1. AGE	Score	2. REASON FOR ADMISSION	Score	3. DIET	Score	4. APPETITE	Score
< 40 years	1	No planned surgery	1	Normal	1	Good (manages 3 meals a day)	1
40 – 60 years	2	Minor surgery	2	Restricted (e.g. special diet)	2	Poor (eating ½ meals or less)	2
60 – 80 years	3	Chronic medical conditions	4	Fluids only	3	Refuses, or is unable to drink or eat	3
> 80 years	4	• Major surgery • Trauma • Infection associated with pyrexia • Acute medical conditions • Existing pressure sore • Post-op complication • Substance abuse	8	Nil by mouth	4	Vomiting and diarrhoea	4

5. WEIGHT	Score	Risk Score		6. ABILITY TO EAT	Score
No weight loss	1	**< 10 LOW RISK**	• *No action necessary*	Able to eat without help	1
Recent weight loss Up to 10%	2	**11 – 17 MODERATE RISK**	• *Needs Monitoring* • Check weight weekly • Encourage eating and drinking, Observe and record intake • Replace missed meals with supplements • Review weekly, if no improvement refer to dieticians	Requires some help	2
Recent weight loss >10% or BMI 16 – 18	3			Needs to be fed	3
Skeletal BMI < 16	4	**>18 HIGH RISK**	• *Needs Action* • Refer to Dietician • Consider NUTRITIONAL SUPPORT • Review twice weekly	Unable to swallow	4

Date	Clinician	Weight	BMI	Risk Score

Figure 7.2   Nutritional risk assessment tool. (Reproduced with kind permission of Salisbury Health Care NHS Trust.)

Estimating the basal metabolic rate

The BMR of an individual varies according to surface area as this determines the rate of heat loss. Tall thin people lose heat faster than short fat people because they have a larger surface area in relation to their volume. Babies have a large surface area in relation to their volume and also have comparatively large heads with little hair so they can lose heat very quickly. The BMR declines with age. The physical activity of an individual will affect their calorie requirements so a nursing assessment must take this into account.

Calculating the body mass index

Many clinical areas now have BMI charts in prominent positions to allow for a quick estimation of BMI. However, when dealing with patients in the community it is necessary to be able to calculate the BMI and to know the normal range and what risk deviations outside this range may have for the client.

To calculate the BMI you will need to measure the height of the patient/client in metres (m) and their weight in kilograms (kg).

The formula for calculating BMI is: weight divided by height^2.

For example, if a man weighs 70 kg and is 1.75 m tall the calculation is:

$$70/(1.75 \times 1.75) = 70/3.0625 = 22.8$$

Therefore this man's BMI = 22.8.

Table 7.4 gives the normal range for BMI and the meaning of BMI values outside the normal range. Figure 7.3 shows a ready reckoner for calculating BMI.

Assessment of physical conditions affecting the patient's ability to eat

Difficulties in eating may result from physical conditions such as arthritis, hemiplegia or dysphagia following a stroke, hand or arm injuries, lack of motor skills in for example those with learning difficulties or very young children. Poor teeth, ill-fitting dentures or no dentures will all cause difficulty and may mean certain foods are avoided or need special preparation.

History

Taking a history from the client can reveal many conditions that affect their nutritional status.

- Medical conditions which may be related to diet.
- Medication that may affect nutritional status (e.g. thiazide and loop diuretics can cause potassium deficiency, corticosteroids can cause sodium and water retention and excessive vitamin and mineral intake can lead to toxicity).
- A history of constipation or self-medication with laxatives may indicate dietary fibre deficiency.

Table 7.4	Range of BMI
Less than 20	Underweight
20–24.9	Normal
25–29.9	Overweight
30 and over	Obese

- A history of a high alcohol intake which can cause vitamin deficiencies, particularly B$_{12}$, and lead to medical problems such as peripheral neuropathy.
- Unexplained weight loss in the recent past can indicate underlying disease.

Socioeconomic information

It is important to take into account the client's living circumstances:

- Does the client live alone?
- Are they recently bereaved?
- Can they afford a balanced diet?
- Do they have adequate cooking facilities?
- Are there any agencies already involved, e.g. Meals on Wheels?

Cultural and religious beliefs about food and its preparation

Specific dietary requirements must be noted. It is best to ask the client or relatives and not make assumptions; for instance, not all members of the Jewish faith follow the same strict dietary code (Collins 2002).

PLANNING

The nursing assessment will indicate what particular dietary requirements and conditions the patient requires. In the institutional setting planning will ensure that the client is provided with a diet that meets these requirements and is able to eat it. Alternatively, if the client is in the community it may be necessary to plan information giving sessions to enable them to select and prepare appropriate foods within their financial means and own preferences. The role of the nurse is not to tell the patient what he should eat: planning diet must be patient centered as enjoyment of food is a very individual thing.

If on the other hand the client wishes to change his or her dietary pattern, for example to lose weight or because of fear of arterial disease, then a detailed planning procedure should be instituted. Firstly, the client should be encouraged to identify benefits and difficulties of the proposed course of action. It is very easy for the client to make a decision to lose weight without thinking of the fact that the

BODY MASS READY RECKONER

Salisbury Health Care NHS
NHS Trust

HEIGHT (Feet and Inches)

WEIGHT → (Kilograms)

← WEIGHT (Stones & pounds)

WEIGHT (Kilograms)	4'6"	7"	8"		9"	10"	11"	5'		1"	2"	3"		4"	5"	6"		7"	8"	9"	10"		11"	6'	1"	2"	3"		4"	5"		6"	7"	WEIGHT (Stones & pounds)
110	59	58	56	56	53	52	50	49	48	46	45	44	43	42	41	40	39	38	37	36	36	35	34	33	32	32	31	30	30	29	29	28	27	
109	59	57	56	54	53	51	50	48	47	46	45	44	43	42	41	40	39	38	37	36	35	34	34	33	32	32	31	30	30	29	28	28	27	7lbs
108	58	57	55	54	52	51	49	48	47	46	44	43	42	41	40	39	38	37	37	36	35	34	33	33	32	31	31	30	29	29	28	28	27	
107	58	56	55	53	52	50	49	48	46	45	44	43	42	41	40	39	38	37	36	35	35	34	33	32	32	31	30	30	29	28	28	27	27	
106	57	56	54	53	51	50	47	47	46	45	44	42	41	40	39	38	38	37	36	35	34	33	33	32	31	31	30	29	29	28	27	26	26	17st
105	57	56	54	52	51	49	47	47	45	44	43	42	41	40	39	38	37	36	35	35	34	33	32	32	31	30	30	29	28	28	27	27	26	
104	56	55	53	52	50	49	47	46	45	43	43	42	41	40	39	38	37	36	35	34	34	33	32	31	31	30	29	29	28	28	27	27	26	
103	56	55	53	51	50	48	46	46	45	43	42	41	40	39	38	37	36	36	35	34	33	33	32	31	30	30	29	28	28	27	27	26	26	7lbs
102	55	54	52	51	49	48	46	45	44	43	42	41	40	39	38	37	36	35	34	34	33	32	31	31	30	29	29	28	28	27	27	26	25	
101	55	54	52	50	49	47	45	45	44	42	42	40	39	38	38	37	36	35	34	33	33	32	31	30	30	29	29	28	27	27	26	26	25	
100	54	53	51	50	48	47	45	44	43	42	41	40	39	38	37	36	35	35	34	33	32	32	31	30	30	29	28	27	27	27	26	26	25	16st
99	54	53	51	49	48	46	44	44	43	41	41	40	39	38	37	36	35	34	33	33	32	31	31	30	29	29	28	27	27	26	26	25	25	
98	53	52	50	49	47	46	44	44	42	41	40	39	38	37	36	36	35	34	33	32	32	31	30	30	29	28	28	27	27	26	26	25	24	
97	52	51	50	48	47	46	43	43	42	42	40	40	39	38	37	36	35	34	34	33	32	31	31	30	29	29	28	27	27	26	25	25	24	7lbs
96	52	51	49	48	46	45	43	43	42	40	39	38	37	37	36	35	34	33	32	32	31	30	30	29	28	28	27	26	26	26	25	24	24	
95	51	50	49	47	46	45	42	42	41	40	39	38	37	36	35	34	34	33	32	31	31	30	29	29	28	27	27	26	26	25	25	24	24	
94	51	49	48	47	45	44	43	42	41	40	39	38	37	36	35	34	33	33	32	31	30	30	29	28	28	27	27	26	25	25	24	24	23	15st
93	50	49	47	46	45	44	42	41	40	39	38	37	36	35	35	34	33	32	31	31	30	29	29	28	27	27	26	26	25	25	24	24	23	
92	50	48	47	46	44	43	42	41	40	39	38	37	36	36	34	33	33	32	31	30	30	29	28	28	27	27	26	25	25	24	24	23	23	
91	49	48	46	45	44	43	42	40	39	38	37	36	36	35	34	33	32	31	31	30	29	29	28	27	27	26	26	25	25	24	24	23	23	7lbs
90	49	47	46	45	43	42	41	40	39	38	37	36	35	34	33	33	32	31	30	30	29	28	28	27	27	26	25	25	24	24	23	23	22	
89	48	47	45	44	43	42	41	40	39	38	37	36	35	34	33	32	32	31	30	29	29	28	27	27	26	26	25	25	24	24	23	23	22	
88	48	46	45	44	42	41	40	39	38	37	36	35	34	34	32	32	31	30	30	29	28	28	27	27	26	25	25	24	24	23	23	22	22	14st
87	47	46	44	43	42	41	40	39	38	37	36	35	34	33	32	32	31	30	29	29	28	27	27	26	26	25	25	24	24	23	23	22	22	
86	45	45	44	43	41	40	39	38	37	36	35	34	34	33	32	31	30	30	29	28	28	27	27	26	25	25	24	24	23	23	22	22	21	
85	46	45	43	42	41	40	39	38	37	36	35	34	33	32	32	31	30	29	29	28	27	27	26	26	25	25	24	24	23	23	22	22	21	7lbs
84	45	44	43	42	41	39	38	37	36	35	35	34	33	32	31	30	30	29	28	28	27	27	26	25	25	24	24	23	23	22	22	21	21	
83	45	44	42	41	40	39	38	37	36	35	34	33	32	32	31	30	29	29	28	27	27	26	26	25	25	24	23	23	23	22	22	21	21	
82	44	43	42	41	40	38	37	36	35	35	34	33	32	31	30	30	29	28	28	27	26	26	25	25	24	24	23	23	22	22	21	21	20	13st
81	44	43	41	40	39	38	37	36	35	34	33	32	32	31	30	29	29	28	27	27	26	26	25	24	24	23	23	22	22	22	21	21	20	
80	43	42	41	40	39	38	37	36	35	34	33	32	31	30	30	29	28	28	27	26	26	25	25	24	24	23	23	22	22	21	21	20	20	
79	43	41	40	39	38	37	36	35	34	33	32	32	31	30	29	29	28	27	27	26	26	25	24	24	23	23	22	22	21	21	21	20	20	7lbs
78	42	41	40	39	38	37	36	35	34	33	32	31	30	30	29	28	28	27	26	26	25	25	24	24	23	23	22	22	21	21	20	20	19	
77	42	40	39	38	37	36	35	34	33	32	32	31	30	29	29	28	27	27	26	25	25	24	24	23	23	22	22	21	21	20	20	20	19	
76	41	40	39	38	37	36	35	34	33	32	31	30	30	29	28	28	27	26	26	25	25	24	23	23	22	22	22	21	21	20	20	19	19	12st
75	41	39	38	27	36	35	34	33	32	32	31	30	29	29	28	27	27	26	25	25	24	24	23	23	22	22	21	21	20	20	20	19	19	
74	40	39	38	37	36	35	34	33	32	31	30	30	29	28	28	27	26	26	25	24	24	23	23	22	22	21	21	20	20	20	19	19	18	
73	39	38	37	36	35	34	33	32	32	31	30	29	29	28	27	26	26	25	25	24	24	23	23	22	22	21	21	20	20	19	19	19	18	7lbs
72	39	38	37	36	35	34	33	32	31	30	30	29	28	27	27	26	26	25	24	24	23	23	22	22	21	21	20	20	20	19	19	18	18	
71	38	37	36	35	34	33	32	32	31	30	29	28	28	27	26	26	25	25	24	23	23	22	22	21	21	21	20	20	19	19	18	18	18	
70	38	37	36	35	34	33	32	31	30	30	29	28	27	27	26	25	25	24	24	23	23	22	22	21	21	20	20	20	19	19	18	18	17	11st
69	37	36	35	34	33	33	32	31	30	29	28	28	27	26	26	25	24	24	23	23	22	21	21	21	20	20	20	19	19	18	18	18	17	
68	37	36	35	34	33	32	31	30	29	29	28	27	27	26	25	25	24	24	23	22	22	21	21	21	20	20	19	19	18	18	18	17	17	
67	36	35	34	33	32	31	31	30	29	28	28	27	26	26	25	24	24	23	23	22	22	21	21	20	20	19	19	19	18	18	18	17	17	7lbs
66	36	35	34	33	32	31	30	29	29	28	27	26	26	25	25	24	23	23	22	22	21	21	20	20	19	19	18	18	18	18	17	17	16	
65	35	34	33	32	31	30	30	29	28	27	27	26	25	25	24	24	23	22	22	21	21	21	20	20	19	19	18	18	18	17	17	17	16	
64	35	34	33	32	31	30	29	28	28	27	26	26	25	24	24	23	23	22	22	21	21	20	20	19	19	18	18	18	17	17	17	16	16	10st
63	34	33	32	31	30	30	29	28	27	27	26	25	25	24	23	23	22	22	21	21	20	20	19	19	19	18	18	17	17	17	17	16	16	
62	34	33	32	31	30	29	28	28	27	26	25	25	24	24	23	22	22	21	21	20	20	20	19	19	18	18	18	17	17	16	16	16	15	
61	33	32	31	30	29	29	28	27	26	26	25	24	24	23	23	22	22	21	21	20	20	19	19	18	18	18	17	17	17	16	16	16	15	7lbs
60	32	32	31	30	29	28	27	27	26	25	25	24	23	23	22	22	21	21	20	20	19	19	19	18	18	17	17	17	16	16	16	15	15	
59	32	31	30	29	28	28	27	26	26	25	24	24	23	22	22	21	21	20	20	19	19	19	18	18	17	17	17	16	16	16	16	15	15	
58	31	30	30	29	28	27	26	26	25	24	24	23	23	22	22	21	21	20	20	19	19	18	18	18	17	17	16	16	16	15	15	15	14	9st
57	31	30	29	28	27	27	26	25	25	24	23	23	22	22	21	21	20	20	19	19	18	18	18	17	17	16	16	16	15	15	15	15	14	
56	30	29	29	28	27	26	26	25	24	24	23	23	22	21	21	20	20	19	19	18	18	18	17	17	17	16	16	16	15	15	15	14	14	
55	30	29	28	27	27	26	25	24	24	23	23	22	21	21	20	20	19	19	18	18	18	17	17	17	16	16	16	15	15	15	14	14	14	7lbs
54	29	28	28	27	26	25	25	24	23	23	22	22	21	21	20	20	19	19	18	18	17	17	17	16	16	16	15	15	15	14	14	14	13	
53	29	28	27	26	26	25	24	24	23	22	22	21	21	20	20	19	19	18	18	18	17	17	16	16	16	15	15	15	14	14	14	14	13	
52	28	27	27	26	25	24	24	23	23	22	21	21	20	20	19	19	18	18	18	17	17	16	16	16	15	15	15	14	14	14	14	13	13	8st
51	28	27	26	25	25	24	23	23	22	22	21	20	20	19	19	19	18	18	17	17	16	16	16	15	15	15	14	14	14	14	13	13	13	
50	27	26	26	25	24	23	23	22	22	21	21	20	20	19	19	18	18	17	17	17	16	16	15	15	15	14	14	14	14	13	13	13	12	
49	26	26	25	24	24	23	22	22	21	21	20	20	19	19	18	18	17	17	17	16	16	15	15	15	14	14	14	14	13	13	13	12	12	7lbs
48	26	25	24	24	23	23	22	21	21	20	20	19	19	18	18	17	17	17	16	16	15	15	15	14	14	14	14	13	13	13	12	12	12	
47	25	25	24	23	23	22	21	21	20	20	19	19	18	18	17	17	17	16	16	16	15	15	15	14	14	14	13	13	13	12	12	12	12	
46	25	24	23	23	22	22	21	20	20	19	19	18	18	18	17	17	16	16	16	15	15	15	14	14	14	13	13	13	12	12	12	12	11	7st
45	24	24	23	22	22	21	21	20	19	19	18	18	18	17	17	16	16	16	15	15	15	14	14	14	13	13	13	12	12	12	12	11	11	
44	24	23	22	22	21	21	20	20	19	19	18	18	17	17	16	16	16	15	15	15	14	14	14	13	13	13	12	12	12	12	11	11	11	
HEIGHT (Metres)	1.36		1.4		1.44		1.48		1.52		1.56		1.6		1.64		1.68		1.72		1.76		1.8		1.84		1.88		1.92		1.96		2	

HEIGHT (Metres)

- Very Obese.
- Obese
- Overweight
- Healthy
- Underweight. At risk during hospital admission

Figure 7.3 BMI ready reckoner. (Reproduced with kind permission of Salisbury Health Care NHS Trust.)

change will affect their social life and will require a permanent change in lifestyle. Once the decision has been made the client should be involved in the planning. Giving a patient a diet sheet and telling him to stick to it is not helpful, client centered or individualized. A useful strategy is for the client to keep a food diary making a note of what food is consumed and when. The nurse can then identify how difficult it would be for the client to omit or increase items in the diet. The aim should be to make the least possible change consistent with achieving the outcome. To be successful and to avoid the client being on a permanent 'diet' or experiencing a 'yo-yo' pattern of weight loss a gradual loss of 1 kg per week should be the target (British Nutrition Foundation 1998c). It is useful to plan with patients how they will deal with problems such as dinner parties with friends and in restaurants. This enables patients to be prepared rather than having to make a snap decision to refuse or accept a particular item.

INTERVENTION

In the institutional setting, nursing intervention may involve ensuring that patients are provided with food, can reach it, can cut it up and transfer it to their mouths, and can chew, swallow and digest it. The nurse must ensure that the food is accessible, and the patients are sitting up and able to feed themselves. Patients that have difficulty transferring the food to their mouths should be assessed by an occupational therapist who may be able to provide eating utensils that will make this easier.

The patient may not be able to take food in the normal way due to his medical condition and this may necessitate feeding in a different way. Tube feeding using the functioning gut is known as enteral feeding. When the gut does not work, patients can be fed intravenously, i.e. directly into a large vein; this is known as parenteral feeding. Enteral and parenteral feeding will be discussed later in the chapter.

In the community setting, the client may need help with shopping or cooking and the nurse may be involved with the social services in organizing the support services to do this. Many large supermarkets now provide an ordering and delivery service using the internet which may be appropriate for some patients.

Mealtimes are a social event; in the institutional setting this is especially important as the day is usually structured around mealtimes. Mealtimes break the monotony, provide structure and are an opportunity to socialize. Food is often a common topic of conversation within hospital wards and in the busy setting it is easy to undervalue its social importance as well as its contribution to recovery and wellbeing. Ward staff should attempt to ensure that meal times are not interrupted by doctors' rounds, dressings or other routine tasks. Unpleasant sounds, sights and smells need to be minimized as they can destroy patients' appetite; ideally a separate dining area should be provided for those able to mobilize.

FEEDING A CLIENT

Prior to feeding the patient it should be noted whether the patient has any condition that may compromise swallowing. A full swallowing assessment by a speech therapist may be needed for some patients (e.g. following a stroke or severe head injury) and the care plan may need to include special instructions of how to position and feed the individual to ensure safety.

If patients require feeding they should be sat up in position where they can see the food and the method of feeding should be as normal as possible. The nurse should sit in a comfortable and relaxed manner to avoid any suggestion of hurry, be at the same eye level as the patient and in a position to make eye contact. Every effort should be made to maintain the dignity of the patient. Being unable to feed oneself is associated with early childhood and it is very easy to treat such patients as if they are children. The use of plastic bibs reinforces this image and they should be avoided. The use of a large napkin is preferable when there is a need to protect the patient's clothing. Whenever possible the food should be cut up and given in the same way as the patients would eat it if they were able to feed themselves. The practice of cutting up all the food at once and then feeding the patient with a spoon should be avoided. Although feeding a patient is often left to the most junior staff it requires considerable skill and knowledge as well as sensitivity if it is to be done well (Weetch 2001).

Enteral feeding

Patients may not be able to take sufficient food orally to ensure adequate nourishment or they may be unable to swallow because of surgery, trauma or stroke. This may be a relatively short-term problem or it may be for life. As long as the digestive system is working normally, enteral feeding is a simple and, when managed correctly, safe method of providing nourishment.

Enteral feeding involves passing a feeding tube via the nose into the stomach or jejunum or directly into the stomach or jejunum, by an X-ray guided or surgical procedure forming a gastrostomy or jejunostomy. If enteral feeding is only going to be short term a size 12 french gauge nasogastric tube can be used for adults. A tube of this size has the advantage of being easily aspirated to check absorption and position and is less likely to block than a finer tube. However this type of tube is uncomfortable for the patient and needs to be changed after a week (Arrowsmith 1993, Lord 1997, Riley 2002a).

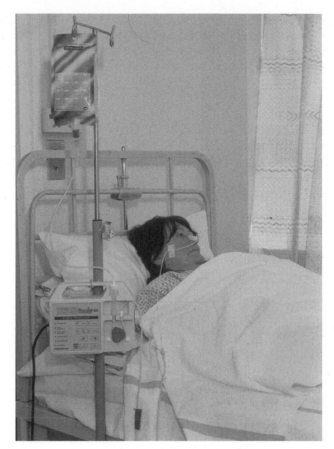

Figure 7.4   A 'patient' (the author) with fine-bore feeding tube and delivery pump. (Reproduced with kind permission of Salisbury Health Care NHS Trust.)

Evidence based practice

Bedside methods of determining nasogastric tube placement: a literature review (Christensen 2001). This article selected 50 articles out the 68 identified in a search covering 1982–2000.The article reviewed the three traditional methods of determining enteral tube placement: auscultation of insufflated air, aspiration of gastrointestinal fluid and pH measurement of gastrointestinal fluid. The author concludes that little progress has been made to establish any new technique to determine enteral tube placement at the bedside and that there is a need for rigorous nursing research. Based on the evidence available he concludes that the most reliable bedside method is testing the pH of the aspirated fluid.

If feeding is to be continued for a longer period of time a fine-bore tube size 8 french gauge for adults should be used as these are better tolerated by patients and less likely to cause damage to the nasal passages or oesophagus (Fig. 7.4). Fine-bore tubes do have some disadvantages: it is not as easy to check the correct position by testing gastric contents as aspiration of the tube can be difficult and an X-ray may be needed. The narrow lumen of the tube can block quite easily especially if used for administering medication; however, when managed correctly they can be used for long-term feeding in hospital and in the community.

If enteral feeding is going to be necessary for a long time or permanently, a gastrostomy can be formed which allows food to be administered directly into the stomach. This has the advantage of being easier to manage and interferes less with body image. If overnight feeding or bolus feeding is used patients can get out and about in the day without others being aware of the tube. Jejunal feeding is used when there is a danger of the patient aspirating stomach contents, for example a spinally injured or ventilated patient.

It is generally thought to be more beneficial to administer the feed continuously using a volumetric pump, rather than have bolus feeds, as there is evidence to suggest that bolus feeds are more likely to cause stomach cramps and diarrhoea. Enteral feeding regimes are tailored to the individual using complete ready made feeds and include 'flushes' of additional water to maintain hydration and to keep the tube patent. A rest period is usually included in a gastric feeding regime to allow the pH of the stomach contents to return to a more acidic level and kill bacteria (Riley 2002b). When feeding via the jejunum it is usual to maintain continuous feeding as stopping and starting can reduce tolerance; discreet lightweight pumps are available for home use.

Parenteral feeding

If the digestive system is not functioning or not available, intravenous feeding or parenteral nutrition (PN) should be considered. The solution is concentrated and usually needs to be delivered through a catheter fed into a large central vein, e.g. the subclavian vein. Short-term peripheral vein feeding can be achieved but it is labour intensive requiring frequent changes of cannula and careful monitoring to prevent thrombophlebitis (Manning & Wilkinson 1996).

Inserting a central venous catheter needs to be undertaken by an experienced practitioner in an appropriate clinical area to minimize the risks associated with the procedure for example infection, air embolus, pneumothorax. It can also be uncomfortable for the patient and nursing support should be provided throughout the procedure. The benefit of providing the patient's complete nutritional needs and the risks need to be considered by the multidisciplinary team, patient and relatives before commencing PN (for more detailed information about the insertion of central lines and management of PN please see a specialist text and refer to your own local policies and guidelines).

Parenteral nutrition solutions are prepared in a sterile environment and should always be administered using a volumetric pump by nurses trained in their use. The patient will need to be carefully monitored in the early stages of establishing parenteral nutrition, requiring frequent blood tests and fluid balance monitoring. However once feeding is established and as long as the underlying medical condition permits, parenteral nutrition can also be managed in the community with back-up from specialist nurses, community nurses and day centres.

DISORDERS OF NUTRITION

In everyday practice nurses, regardless of the specialist branch they undertake, are likely to be involved with children or adults with common dietary disorders. They are also likely to be exposed to malnutrition in the elderly both on admission to hospital or during their community placements and need to use their assessment skills and knowledge to promote an improved diet and outcome for these patients.

All nurses should have a working knowledge of the following three chronic conditions

- diabetes mellitus
- obesity
- anorexia nervosa.

Diabetes mellitus

This common condition is characterized by an inability to control plasma glucose concentration. In Type 1 or insulin dependent diabetes mellitus (IDDM) no insulin is produced, and glucose spills over into the urine (glycosuria) causing osmotic diuresis and dehydration. In addition the body metabolizes excessive amounts of fat, resulting in a rise in plasma ketone concentration which may be sufficient to cause acidosis and coma. Type 2 non insulin dependent diabetes mellitus is when there is not enough insulin produced by the pancreas or when the insulin produced is ineffective; it usually results in hyperglycaemia, glycosuria and dehydration.

Both are serious medical conditions that require careful management to prevent long-term health problems. Diabetes mellitus of both types can be treated with medication but dietary management remains important. Patients will have an individual regime based on their basal metabolic requirements and level of physical activity. The principles of the diet are similar to those for any normal healthy diet but the amount, type and frequency of carbohydrate is controlled to allow a constant blood glucose concentration to be maintained. The objectives of the diet are:

- to maintain or achieve desirable weight (i.e. BMI of 20–25)
- to eat regular meals based on starchy foods such as bread, pasta and rice choosing those containing high fibre when possible
- to maintain a low fat intake of 30–35% of calories choosing monounsaturated fats, e.g. olive oil and rapeseed oil; use less butter, cheese and fatty meats; choose low fat dairy foods
- eat more fruit and vegetables – aim for five portions a day
- cut down on sugar and sugary foods; use sugar-free drinks and squashes.
- drink alcohol in moderation only and never on a empty stomach.

When planning the type of carbohydrate to include in the diet, the glycaemic index can be used. The index measures how blood glucose concentration is affected by eating a particular carbohydrate. Glucose itself has an index of 100 whereas the same amount of pasta will be absorbed more slowly and cause a smaller increase in the blood glucose concentration. This would consequently give a lower score on the glycaemic scale. Combinations of high and low glycaemic index foods eaten together will cause a lower increase in blood glucose concentration than when a high index food is eaten alone.

One of the key factors in controlling diabetes mellitus is client education and the development of a partnership between the patients and those responsible for their care. Patients who do not understand their condition are less likely to comply with the diet and treatment thus risking the long term complications of diabetes. Diabetic Nurse Specialists have made a valuable contribution to patient care by demonstrating that it is possible to tailor the diet and medication to suit the individual's lifestyle rather than the other way round.

Obesity

Overweight is defined as a body mass index of 25–29.9 and obesity by a body mass index of 30 or above. Being overweight is not considered to constitute a serious risk to health but may bring with it some restriction of mobility and social activities. However, being obese carries significant health risks such as heart disease, stroke, diabetes, high blood pressure, some cancers, osteoarthritis of weight bearing joints, gallstones, reproductive disorders and complications during and after pregnancy.

Obesity also affects the quality of life of children and adults in many ways. The UK has the fastest growing rates of obesity in Europe. Unless effective action is taken 20% of men and 25% of women could be obese by the year 2005 (National Audit Office 2001). This would have significant cost implications for the National Health Service. The increase in obesity is not just restricted to adults; children are becoming obese and thus experiencing diseases that are normally associated with adults (Perry 2001).

Why obesity is increasing so rapidly is by no means clear, although a correlation with an increase in dietary fat has been demonstrated. There has been a steady increase in the amount of fat in our diets over the last 50 years. One of the problems seems to be that fat does not increase the blood glucose concentration to give feedback to the satiety centre to stop eating, whereas carbohydrate does (Lissner & Heitmann 1995). In addition, if the intake of complex carbohydrates is increased there is an increase in carbohydrate oxidation to compensate. In fat metabolism there is no comparable mechanism. It would therefore be reasonable to assume that the increased fat intake in the diet of developing countries is an important factor in the rise of obesity.

In developed countries much of the energy expended by people at work and in the home has decreased with the introduction of machines and labour saving devices. As many jobs become more sedentary increased activity at home could compensate. However, many homes now have personal computers, and playing complicated and exciting games on the computer or getting information from the internet uses much less energy than playing football or walking to a library and carrying books back home. The individual doing light work (4 kcal/min) for 7 or 8 hours will use far more energy than someone doing half an hour of vigorous exercise (12 kcal/min) two or three times a week.

Obesity not only has recognized physical health risks, but also has stigmas attached to it, associated with laziness and gluttony which can significantly disadvantage individuals who may then seek help. A walk round a bookshop reveals a plethora of self-help books to overcome obesity; some will be based on science and up-to-date nutritional principles, others claim novel and bizarre ways to lose weight. Most glossy magazines and many home web pages have celebrity diets and supermarkets have low fat, low calorie healthy option foods to be used as part of a calorie controlled diet. Targeting the overweight and obese is big business and yet the incidence of obesity in the population continues to rise.

For every kilogram that someone is overweight he or she has stored 7000 kcal of energy and the only way to get rid of it, excluding surgery, is to metabolize it. This can only be achieved by decreasing energy intake or increasing energy output by the requisite amount. The amount of energy used during exercise is very little; for example using an exercise bicycle at a pedal load sustainable for any length of time by an unfit individual will use approximately 5 kcal/min. In other words it would take about 24 hours of cycling to lose 1 kg of weight. Exercise on its own is not an effective way of losing weight though it does have its own benefits, for example an individual who becomes fitter as a result of exercise is likely to be more active, benefiting heart, lungs, muscle and bones. To reduce weight effectively means cutting down on energy intake by altering the diet.

Fad diets will achieve weight loss, for instance a grapefruit or banana diet, but are difficult to sustain and over time produce shortages in essential macro and micronutrients. Success depends on finding the diet that contains less energy than the individual is metabolizing and that she or he is happy with. Slimming clubs tend to help individuals to choose foods from a variety of categories to suit the individual's lifestyle and offer education and support. As a result the more reputable ones have notable successes; however, their services are not free and clubs do not appeal to everyone.

For a nurse planning a reducing diet, permanent weight loss is more likely to be achieved if the points below are followed.

1. Establish a realistic rate of weight loss. It may have taken years to gain the weight and it unrealistic to expect to lose it within weeks. A target of 0.5–1 kg per week is reasonable, but the client may have seen diets advertised saying 'Lose 10 lb in a week' and be disappointed that you suggest so little. Point out that much of this loss would be water rather than fat and that even not eating anything at all would only result in the loss of 1.5–2 kg per week.
2. Calorific intake should be reduced by 500–1000 kcal per day. A smaller reduction will mean weight loss is very slow, a greater reduction may risk a loss of lean body mass and vitamin and mineral deficiencies. Moderate exercise will help, but it should be something the individual enjoys doing otherwise they are unlikely to keep it up.
3. Fats can be restricted quite drastically without essential fatty acid deficiency developing, and because of their high calorie content this can account for much of the reduction of calories in the diet.
4. Some increase in fibre may help the client to feel satisfied after a meal.
5. Several small meals will increase metabolic rate (postprandial thermogenesis) and reduce the chance of overeating, which can occur with one meal a day.
6. A change in eating habits that results in slow weight loss is more likely to result in a permanent weight loss.

Overall the advice is to maintain a healthy diet with plenty of fruit and vegetables and starchy foods with fat kept to minimum. It is far better not to ban specific foods but allow the client to plan for the odd treat without increasing their calorific intake for the day.

Anorexia nervosa and bulimia nervosa

Eating disorders are common amongst adolescents and although more prevalent in females they can also affect males. Anorexia is not always easy to diagnose, as when does dieting to lose weight become anorexia? The generally accepted diagnostic criteria for anorexia are

- refusal to maintain body weight at or above a minimally normal weight for height and age (or failure to make expected weight gain during a period of growth)
- intense fear of gaining weight or becoming fat, even when underweight
- disturbance in the way in which one's body weight or shape is experienced
- amenorrhoea in females.

The disease can be further divided into two specific types:

1. Restricted, i.e. no binge-eating or purging behaviour (anorexia nervosa).
2. Binge-eating and purging type (bulimia nervosa).

Patients with anorexia believe they are fat even when obviously emaciated. The desire to be thin is largely determined by culture. In affluent countries where food is easily available and affordable by the majority of society, being overweight becomes synonymous with sloth, self-indulgence and greed. Thinness conversely is associated with discipline and self-control; this tends to be reinforced by the media and advertising (Killen 2001).

Many sufferers of eating disorders may have family problems, for instance, being described as model children by parents may be associated with non-assertive behaviour and the eating disorder is a way of gaining control. This aspect of the disease can make it very difficult to treat as many patients see the disorder as part of their identity and may deny they have a problem or feign compliance.

Many patients with anorexia are treated as outpatients but admission to hospital will be necessary for the severely underweight who need intervention to ensure their survival. Treatment is aimed at correcting the physiological problems that are life threatening and feeding by enteral or parenteral routes may be necessary (Royal College of Physicians 2002). Once the patient is out of immediate physical danger, psychotherapy with or without drugs is commenced. Inpatient treatment is often based on behavioural interventions that use a combination of non-punitive reinforcement. The aim is to gain weight and restore normal eating patterns and body functions, aiming for a BMI of at least 18 in most individuals (Muscari 2002). Treatment is also aimed at teaching the client to understand and change dysfunctional behaviours and attitudes and to improve personal self-esteem; this may require family involvement and therapy but each plan of care will be unique to the individual.

PROFESSIONAL AND ETHICAL KNOWLEDGE

FOOD SAFETY

The nurse should be aware of legislation regarding food, in particular the work of the Food Standards Agency, the Food Safety Act 1990 and the Food Standards Act 1999. The Food Safety Act is a wide ranging law that covers the food safety and consumer protection throughout the UK. It affects everyone working in the production, processing, storage and distribution and sale of food. Hospitals are subject to the same rigorous rules as restaurants for storing, preparing and serving food. The Act also states that people handling food will need appropriate training in hygiene.

The Food Standards Act includes regulation on accurate labelling of foodstuffs. This is particularly important when buying processed food as many individuals are sensitive or allergic to certain food products. For example many products contain peanuts or peanut oil and can produce fatal anaphylaxis if ingested by individuals allergic to them (Stewart-Truswell 1999).

Food poisoning may be defined as 'an illness caused by food or drink contaminated by pathogenic microorganisms or their toxins, or by chemicals' (Microbiological Safety of Food Committee 1990: 6). In the UK all clinicians have a statutory duty to notify the local authority of cases of food poisoning. The incidence of food poisoning is increasing at an alarming rate, although a true picture of the risk to health is difficult to obtain because many cases probably go unreported by individuals and clinicians. This increase could be due changing behaviour, as more and more people in developed countries eat out, eat more convenience foods and buy food in bulk to store.

Reflection and portfolio evidence

Look at the evidence on one of the following topics: new variant Creutzfeldt–Jakob disease; *Campylobacter* contamination of food; genetically modified food.

- How is this reported in newspapers, professional journals and in government reports?
- How easy was it to find the information?
- How accurate was the information from each source?
- How might a nurse working in a school use this information when advising an anxious mother on the safety of food?

A general outbreak of food poisoning is defined as one that affects members of more than one household or residents of an institution (Department of Health 1994). Hospital catering departments have a duty to provide safe food for patients and their employees must adhere to strict codes of hygiene. When food arrives in ward areas it should be stored correctly and served at the correct temperature. Ward kitchens need to be inspected regularly and food kept in refrigerators should be dated and labelled. All members of staff, volunteers or relatives must wash their hands effectively before handling food for patients. Patients should be enabled to wash their hands prior to mealtimes. Nursing staff and housekeeping assistants should be trained in food hygiene and should be monitored by the charge nurse or ward sister.

Any outbreak of diarrhoea and vomiting within a hospital needs to be immediately managed by the infection control team. Isolating and barrier nursing the patients affected should be instigated immediately without waiting for confirmation from laboratory specimens. Any staff affected will need to stay off work and monitoring by the Occupational Health department may be necessary (See Ch. 4 and consult your own Trust's infection control policies for more detailed information).

Institutions and businesses are controlled by strict laws relating to food production and consumption; however, many incidences of food poisoning are the result of poor personal and domestic hygiene. The principles of the advice given to the food industry are just as relevant to the domestic setting. Poor hygiene, the misuse of refrigerators, poor storage and inadequately heated food pose a risk to individuals in their own homes.

PROFESSIONAL ACCOUNTABILITY

Following the report *Hungry in Hospital* (National Association of Community Health Councils 1997), the UK Central Council Registrar wrote to every hospital in the UK to remind nurses that: 'Nursing has a clear responsibility for ensuring that the nutritional needs of patients are met.'

Within the *Code of Professional Conduct* (Nursing and Midwifery Council 2002) there are a number of clauses that should be kept in mind when considering nursing responsibility and nutrition, for example:

Clause 4 As a registered nurse or midwife, you must cooperate with others in the team.

4.1 *The team includes the patient, the patient's or client's family, informal carers and health and social care professionals in the National Health Service, independent and voluntary sectors.*

4.2 *You are expected to work cooperatively within teams and to respect the skills, expertise and contributions of your colleagues. You must treat them fairly and without discrimination.*

4.3 *You must communicate effectively and share your knowledge, skill and expertise with the other members of the team as required for the benefit of patients and patients.*

Involving the patients and their relatives in planning nutritional care will make it more likely that compliance and cooperation are achieved. Communicating with all the agencies will help ensure that your patients receive any help available to assist with the provision of nutritional needs, e.g. dietary advice information, Meals on Wheels, help with shopping. Maintaining good and collegiate relationships with dieticians, the catering department, ward housekeepers and kitchen porters benefits the patient by making the best use of all the team has to offer.

Evidence based practice

The importance of patients' nutritional status in wound healing (Russel 2001). This article demonstrates the need for adequate levels of calories, protein, vitamins and minerals to support wound healing. Alteration in nutritional status preceeding or during injury may alter the wound healing response. Protein deficiency has been demonstrated to cause poor healing rates with reduced collagen formation and wound dehiscence. Russel identifies the roles of glucose, fatty acids, vitamins and trace elements whilst recognizing that more research is needed to establish the key micronutrients involved in the complex process of wound healing. Russel states that the nurse is the ideal person to carry out nutritional assessment and monitor wound healing and then decide on appropriate nutritional care.

Clause 6 As a registered nurse or midwife, you must maintain your professional knowledge and competence.

6.2 *To practise competently you must possess the knowledge, skills and abilities required for lawful, safe and effective practice without direct supervision. You must acknowledge the limits of your professional competence and only undertake practice and accept responsibilities for those activities in which you are competent.*

6.3 *If an aspect of practice is beyond your level of competence or outside your level of registration you must obtain help and supervision from a competent practitioner ….*

Consider a patient with specific dietary needs, for example renal failure; if you have insufficient knowledge to give dietary advice to this patient or client you must consult or refer to a dietician or other suitably qualified practitioner.

When offering advice to patients care must be taken not to endorse particular products, for instance recommending a brand of slimming product or a particular slimming club or gym (Nursing and Midwifery Council 2002: Clause 7).

Nurses able to use their knowledge of nutrition and their skills in assessing and detecting patients at risk will devise and deliver an individual nutritional plan aimed at improving the outcome for their patient. They must retain the responsibility for the supervision of meals and nutrition of their patients even when skill mix and resources make this difficult.

ETHICAL CONCERNS

Although nurses and all members of the multiprofessional team need to ensure that their patients' nutritional needs are met, there are ethical issues surrounding food and drink. Should nurses, as part of the multiprofessional team, be encouraging the use of invasive techniques like enteral feeding to ensure nutrition for the patients at all times? Consider the patient in a persistent vegetative state, a patient dying from incurable illness, or the patient with advanced dementia or anorexia.

Vegetative state is defined as a complete unawareness of self or the environment and an inability to interact with others (Lennard-Jones 1999). It can be transient but recovery is unusual when it persists for longer than 12 months after trauma or 3–6 months after an anoxic episode and a prognostic description of persistent vegetative state (PVS) is made. Tony Bland was a victim of the 1989 Hillsborough Stadium disaster whose cerebral cortex was destroyed as a result of prolonged oxygen deprivation (Thompson et al 2000). In 1993 the Law Lords allowed the tube feeding of Tony Bland to be discontinued. Tube feeding is now regarded in law as a medical treatment. The judgement in the Tony Bland case was not that the tube should be withdrawn but that it was not in his best interest for it to be continued. The proposed action by the doctor to remove the tube was therefore ruled in a declaratory judgement not to be illegal, but it was still his decision whether or not to do so (Airedale NHS Trust *v.* Bland 1993).

Towards the end of life patients may refuse food and many of the ethical considerations in palliative care settings are concerned with feeding and providing adequate hydration to patients, elderly or otherwise, who have not long to live. These issues must be discussed with the multidisciplinary team, relatives and patients if they are able. The aim of palliative care is to provide comfort, support and relief of symptoms; persisting with diet and fluids or commencing a tube feed may not be appropriate. Local measures such as sips of fluid or ice to suck for comfort may be all the patient wants and enforcing fluids and nutrition is intrusive (see Ch. 12).

Patients with advanced dementia often refuse food and drink and exhibit dysphagia and choking symptoms; this makes it difficult and frightening for their carers when attempting to feed them. The role of tube feeding for these patients is controversial as the tube may be poorly tolerated and feeding has not been shown to reduce mortality significantly (Sanders et al 2000). However, there is not enough evidence to justify refusing a trial of tube feeding for patients with dementia and more research may be needed into providing alternative methods of nutrition for these patients (Biernacki & Barratt 2001, Gillick 2000).

Anorexic patients as discussed earlier can occasionally starve themselves so severely that their lives become at risk. As anorexia nervosa is a recognized mental illness compulsory admission to hospital can be arranged under the Mental Health Act 1983. There is provision in this act to treat the illness without consent and enforced tube feeding as part of the treatment is legal, but each individual case needs to be considered carefully. Advice and further information is available to the multiprofessional team from the Mental Health Act Commission.

Decision making exercise

Based on observations in practice and/or on debates with your peers, review how you would justify the decisions you might make in circumstances where there are obvious ethical dilemmas related to food and nutrition:

- In what circumstances should patients be able to refuse food?
- Does your decision alter according to the medical diagnosis?
- How does this integrate with the responsibilities of the nurse stated in the *Code of Professional Conduct* (Nursing and Midwifery Council 2002)?
- Should food ever be withheld from patients?

PERSONAL AND REFLECTIVE KNOWLEDGE

THE NURSE AS ROLE MODEL

In reflecting on your practice and in the knowledge gained from this chapter it is important that you manage your own personal nutritional needs, not only to maintain your health but also to provide a role model for your patients and clients. Meeting the nutritional needs of patients is a core function of nursing and there are many opportunities available to learn through your practice experience and the collection of evidence for your portfolio. For example, find out if there is any audit or benchmarking taking place in your clinical area and ask to be involved. Outbreaks of food poisoning, food scares and new ways to lose weight will always cause interest in the public domain and nurses must be prepared to offer sensible advice based on the evidence available.

CASE STUDIES IN NUTRITION

To consolidate your learning from this chapter work through the following case studies.

Case study: Adult

Peter Dawson is a 58-year-old man who lives at home with his wife. He is very overweight, being 1.8 m tall and weighing 100 kg. He admits to drinking and smoking 'quite a bit' most evenings and says he has no time to exercise. He has recently been diagnosed as having non insulin dependent diabetes mellitus, for which he has been prescribed a diabetic diet and a hypoglycaemic drug.

- Calculate Peter's BMI. What grade of being overweight does this represent?
- Apart from reduced insulin sensitivity, why might his diabetes be made worse by his obesity, smoking and drinking of alcohol?
- What help and advice could Peter be given to improve his lifestyle?

Case study: Mental health

Sally, aged 17 years, lives at home with her mother, who is divorced. Sally start dieting 2 years ago, but continued to diet after reaching her target weight. She is now 20 kg underweight but says she still feels fat. Sally's mother has always believed that her place was in the home looking after Sally and her younger brother, and is very worried because Sally looks so thin.

- Apart from lacking energy intake what other factors may be missing from Sally's diet?
- What sort of social pressures are there on young girls to account for the high incidence of eating disorders?
- Consider how Sally's schoolfriends and her parents may have unwittingly contributed to her problems.

Case study: Child

Marcus and Yvonne are strict vegans. They have fed their son, Jason, of 4 months with soya milk and are now considering weaning to solids.

- What are the ramifications of Marcus' and Yvonne's dietary preferences on Jason's dietary needs?
- Plan a diet that is compatible with Marcus' and Yvonne's beliefs and Jason's nutritional needs.
- How could the nurse later assess that the diet is meeting all Jason's nutritional requirements?

Case study: Learning disabilities

Andrew is 38 years of age and suffers from a moderate learning disability. He attends a social centre on a daily basis but otherwise lives with his parents. Andrew is 1.76 m tall and weighs 98 kg. He enjoys his food and has a hearty appetite, eating a cooked breakfast every morning and a full dinner at night. This is supplemented by a cooked snack at the social centre every day and bars of chocolate. Andrew's parents feel that although he's a little overweight he is otherwise happy. They have no time for special diets or 'rabbit food'.

- Calculate Andrew's BMI.
- What are the long-term physiological consequences for Andrew should this situation continue?
- How might the nurse help Andrew lose weight but continue to eat the food he and his family enjoy?

Summary

This chapter has outlined knowledge needed for decision making in promoting health and providing good nutrition for patients or clients. It has included:

1. Information on the various components of a balanced diet, the common sources from which they may be obtained, and the way various foods are digested and used within the body.
2. An awareness of cultural differences and how food plays such an important part in psychological and social aspects of life.
3. Knowledge on the key components of a nutritional assessment and the application of a variety of nutritional assessment tools.
4. The promotion of a healthy diet, ensuring that myths are dispelled and there is a balanced approach to media advertising.
5. Acknowledgement that people with common nutritional problems are encountered in all branches of nursing practice, and provided information that is essential to give good quality advice and support.

6. Information on research to audit standards for evidenced based nutritional care for patients.
7. Legal aspects of food safety that need to be adhered to in order to prevent outbreaks of food poisoning at home or in healthcare institutions.
8. Ethical issues related to feeding which should be debated and decisions made based on patient, family and healthcare team participation.

Annotated further reading and web sites

Benyon S 1998 Metabolism and nutrition. Mosby, London
Written for medical students but well laid out and easy to follow with short modules and good clearly drawn diagrams. Recommended for getting to grips with the chemistry of metabolism and nutrition. It also has a section on history taking and clinical nutrition disorders.

Bond S 1997 Eating matters. Newcastle University, Newcastle upon Tyne
An excellent practical workbook for improving nutritional standards in hospital wards. It recognizes the need for multiprofessional team work throughout departments and suggests novel ways to educate staff. Try the quiz with colleagues.

Draper H 2000 Anorexia nervosa and respecting a refusal of life prolonging therapy: a limited justification. Bioethics 14(2):120–133
Read and discuss this paper with a group of colleagues. A thought-provoking insight into the arguments for and against respecting a patient's right to refuse treatment.

Marieb E 1998 Human anatomy and physiology, 4th edn. Benjamin/Cummings, Menlo Park
This has very detailed chapters about the digestive system and nutrition, metabolism and body temperature regulation. It is easy to read with a very clear diagram of the Krebs cycle. You need to bear in mind the difference in recommended daily intake of vitamins and minerals between the USA and the UK.

http://www.nutrition.org.uk
The British Nutrition Foundation (BNF) is an independent charity which provides reliable information on nutrition and related health matters to the public, press and health professionals. It produces leaflets and briefing papers and some books.

http://www.bapen.org.uk
The British Association for Parenteral and Enteral Nutrition is registered charity whose aim is to improve the nutritional treatment of all sufferers from illness who have become or are likely to become malnourished. The association provides in depth reports and information for healthcare professionals and patients.

http://www.diabetes.org.uk
Diabetes UK runs this site which gives sensible and reliable information to diabetics, their carers and health professionals. It uses plain language in its advice sheets.

http://www.foodstandards.gov.uk
The Food Standards Agency has been created to protect public health from risks that may arise in connection with the consumption of food. This is useful site for information on food poisoning, genetically modified food, etc.

References

Airedale NHS Trust v. Bland 1993 Judgements of Family Division, Court of Appeal (Civil Division) and House of Lords. In: Fennel P, Harpwood V, Harpwood H et al (eds) Medico-Legal Reports: 12. Butterworth, London

Arrowsmith H 1993 Nursing management of patients receiving a nasogastric feed. British Journal of Nursing 2(7):1053–1058

Biernacki C, Barratt J 2001 Improving the nutritional status of people with dementia. British Journal of Nursing 10(17):1105–1114

Bond S 1997 Eating matters. Newcastle University, Newcastle upon Tyne

British Nutrition Foundation 1998a Pregnancy. Online. Available: http://www.nutrition.org.uk/information/dietthrulife/pregnancy.html 12 Sept 2002

British Nutrition Foundation 1998b School children. Online. Available: http://www.nutrition.org.uk/information/dietthrulife/children.html 12 Sept 2002

British Nutrition Foundation 1998c Yo-yo dieting. Online. Available: http://www.nutrition.org.uk/medianews/pressinformation/yoyodiet.html 26 Sept 2002

Christensen M 2001 Bedside methods of determining nasogastric tube placement: a literature review. Nursing in Critical Care 6(4):192–199

Collier J 2002 Using a nutritional risk screening tool in the hospital setting. Nurse 2 Nurse 2(6):32–33

Collins A 2002 Nursing with dignity. Part 1: Judaism. Nursing Times 98(9):34–35

Community Health Council 1997 Hungry in hospital. Association of Community Health Councils for England and Wales, London

Co-operative Group 2001 The plate of the nation. In: Donellan C (ed) Healthy eating. Independence, Cambridge, pp 4–5

Coutts A 2000a Nutrition and the life cycle. Part 1: Maternal nutrition and pregnancy. British Journal of Nursing 9(17):1133–1138

Coutts A 2000b Nutrition and the life cycle. Part 2: Infancy and weaning. British Journal of Nursing 9(21):2205–2216

Coutts A 2001 Nutrition and the life cycle. Part 4: The healthy diet for the adult. British Journal of Nursing 10(6):362–369

Department of Health 1992 Dietary reference values for food energy and nutrients for the United Kingdom. HMSO, London

Department of Health 1994 Management of outbreaks of foodborne illness. Department of Health, London

Department of Health 2000 Folic acid and the prevention of disease. HMSO, London

Department of Health 2001 Essence of care: patient focused benchmarking for health practitioners. HMSO, London

Devlin M 2000 The nutritional needs of the older person. Professional Nurse 16(3):951–955

Dietz W H 2001 The obesity epidemic in young children. British Medical Journal 322:313–314

Donellan C (ed) 2001 Healthy eating. Independence, Cambridge

Food Safety Act 1990 HMSO, London

Food Standards Act 1999 HMSO, London

Gillick M R 2000 Rethinking the role of tube feeding in patients with advanced dementia. New England Journal of Medicine 342:206–210

Goldberg G 2003 Nutrition in pregnancy: the facts and the fallacies. Nursing Standard 17(19):39–42

Hinchliff S, Montague S, Watson R 1996 Physiology for nursing practice. Baillière Tindall, London

Holm K, Li S, Spector N et al 2001 Obesity in adults and children: a call for action. Journal of Advanced Nursing 36(2):266–269

Hooper L, Summerbell C D, Higgins J P T et al 2003 Reduced or modified dietary fat for preventing cardiovascular disease.

Cochrane review. In: The Cochrane Library, Issue 1. Update Software, Oxford

Killen M 2001 The rich get thin, the poor get fat. In: Donellan C (ed) Healthy eating. Independence, Cambridge, pp 11–12

Ledsham J, Gough A 2000 Screening and monitoring patients for malnutrition. Professional Nurse 15(11):695–698

Lennard-Jones J 1999 Ethical and legal aspects of fluid and nutrients in clinical practice. Emap, London

Lissner L, Heitmann B L 1995 Dietary fat and obesity: evidence from epidemiology. European Journal of Clinical Nutrition 49:79–90

Lord L 1997 Enteral access devices. Nursing Clinics of North America 32(4):685–703

Ludwig D, Peterson K, Gortmaker S 2001 Relationship between consumption of sugar sweetened drinks and childhood obesity: a prospective, observational analysis. Lancet 357:505–508

Malnutrition Advisory Group 2000 Source of evidence and information for screening tool guidelines In: Guidelines for the detection and management of malnutrition. British Association for Parenteral and Enteral Nutrition, Maidenhead, pp 19–27

Manning E, Wilkinson D 1996 Peripheral parenteral nutrition techniques: the way forward. Oxford Clinical Communications, Oxford

Microbiological Safety of Food 1990 Report of the Committee on the Microbiological Safety of Food: Part 1. HMSO, London

Milne A C, Potter J, Avenell A 2003 Protein and energy supplements in elderly people at risk from malnutrition. Cochrane review. In: The Cochrane Library, Issue 1, Update Software, Oxford

Muscari M 2002 Effective management of adolescents with anorexia and bulimia. Journal of Psychosocial Nursing and Mental Health Services 40(2):23–31

National Audit Office 2001 Tackling obesity in England. HMSO, London

Nursing and Midwifery Council 2002 Code of professional conduct. Nursing and Midwifery Council, London

Perry M 2001 The problem of obesity and the onset of Type 2 diabetes in children. Professional Nurse 17(6):376–378

Pinar R 2002 Management of people with diabetes during Ramadan. British Journal of Nursing 11(20):1300–1303

Riley M 2002a Establishing nutritional guidelines for critically ill patients: Part 1. Professional Nurse 17(10):580–583

Riley M 2002b Establishing nutritional guidelines for critically ill patients: Part 2. Professional Nurse 17(11):655–658

Royal College of Physicians 2002 Nutrition and patients: a doctor's responsibility. Report of a working party. Royal College of Physicians, London

Russel L 2001 The importance of patients' nutritional status in wound healing. British Journal of Nursing (supplement) 10(6):S42–S49

Sanders D S, Carter M J, D'Silva J et al 2000 Survival analysis in percutaneous endoscopic gastrostomy feeding: a worse outcome in patients with dementia. American Journal of Gastroenterology 95: 1472–1475

Stewart-Truswell A 1999 ABC of nutrition, 3rd edn. British Medical Journal, London

Thompson I, Melia K, Boyd K 2000 Nursing ethics, 4th edn. Churchill Livingstone, Edinburgh

Turner S, Levinson R, McLellan-Arnold B et al 2000 Healthy eating in primary schools: an educational perspective from a socially deprived area. Health Education Journal 59(3):196–210

Weetch R 2001 Feeding problems in elderly patients. Nursing Times Plus 97(16):60–61

Chapter 8

Stress, relaxation and rest

David Howard

KEY ISSUES

SUBJECT KNOWLEDGE
- The concept of stress
- Short-term and long-term physiological changes in stress
- Psychological and emotional changes associated with stress
- Life events and stress
- Personality types susceptible to the negative effects of stress
- Burnout
- Post-traumatic stress disorder
- Relaxation, rest and sleep
- Circadian rhythm and patterns of sleep

CARE DELIVERY KNOWLEDGE
- Assessing stress, relaxation and sleep
- The management of stress
- Promoting sleep

PROFESSIONAL AND ETHICAL KNOWLEDGE
- The context of care in the UK and some stress-related implications for clients and carers
- Stress in the workplace

PERSONAL AND REFLECTIVE KNOWLEDGE
- Become aware of your own response to stress
- Become aware of how others respond to stress
- Using stress management in professional practice

INTRODUCTION

Although stress, relaxation and rest are separate concepts there is a high degree of interdependence. Underpinning each concept, however, is the influence of psychological stress and associated stressors. Consequently, emphasis has been placed on developing awareness of managing stress, in the self, in others and within an organization, as it is from this foundation that understanding relaxation and rest can develop.

OVERVIEW

Subject knowledge

This section addresses the nature of stress, its effects on individuals and the role stress plays in everyone's lives, together with the physiological, psychological and social changes that occur in response to stress. At the end of this section the consequences of exposure to very stressful events and prolonged exposure to stress are addressed by burnout and post-traumatic stress disorder. Finally, the concepts of relaxation, rest and sleep are examined and their relationship to stress explored.

Care delivery knowledge

Here, the assessment of stress and sleep and strategies for planning stress management are explored. First stress in clients is addressed. The reasons why clients may suffer from stress and what should be assessed and why are examined. Nurses will also encounter clients' relatives who may be suffering from stress. Reasons why, and the signs that indicate this are explored. The workplace is potentially a very stressful environment and this is given attention where signs of stress in colleagues and stress in the self are identified. Then, in the final part of assessment, consideration is made of methods of assessing sleep. Following assessment, strategies for stress management, for clients, carers and in the workplace, are discussed and the section concludes by examining ways that sleep can be promoted.

Professional and ethical knowledge

This section examines the context within which stress arises. Emphasis is placed on the ability of the individual to control stress from the following perspectives: stress resulting from illness, stress resulting from caring, and the relationship between stress and employment.

As controlling stressors is a fundamental component of stress management, and with so many stressors outside individuals' control in health and social care, the ethical issues here focus on the policy agenda and its implementation.

Personal and reflective knowledge

This chapter has been designed to enhance learning through developing self-awareness. In the final part of the chapter, there are exercises that will enhance awareness of personal stressors, personal coping mechanisms, and opportunities to consider alternative methods of promoting relaxation and rest, based on the knowledge gained in the preceding sections.

On pages 195–196 are four case studies, each one relating to one of the branch programmes. You may find it helpful to read one of them before you start the chapter and use it as a focus for your reflections while reading.

SUBJECT KNOWLEDGE

Think about being stressed. Then think about being relaxed. Are they opposite ends of the same scale, or are they more difficult to define? Is being relaxed the same as resting and sleep? Or can you relax and be active at the same time? Is stress always bad, or can it be helpful sometimes? The answers to these questions are not as simple as they originally seem. So, to begin this chapter the concepts of stress, relaxation and rest will be examined in greater detail.

STRESS

Seyle (1984: 74) defined stress as 'the non-specific response of the body to any demand'. Generally it is associated with negative effects on health; however, a certain amount is necessary for survival. If the degree of stress becomes too great, however, performance, and ultimately health, will deteriorate. This reflects the arousal curve (Hebb 1954) where the individual's performance increases in proportion with the level of arousal. Once the individual's maximum capacity for arousal is exceeded though, their performance falls and negative consequences on health occur (Fig. 8.1). Consequently, all individuals require a certain amount of stress to achieve optimal functioning. Once this is reached, however, any increase results in negative effects. This explains why people in very demanding, high-pressure jobs are at risk of developing stress-related disease.

If this singular explanation of the pathology of stress is true then why do people who have low stimulating repetitive jobs also suffer from stress-related diseases? This question

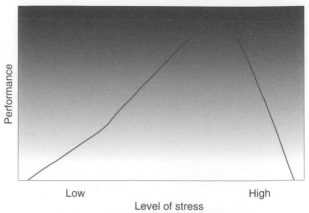

Figure 8.1 The arousal curve. (From Hebb 1954.)

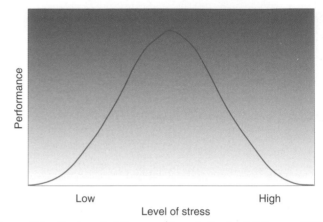

Figure 8.2 The inverted U curve. (From Sutherland & Cooper 1990.)

was pondered by Sutherland & Cooper (1990). While they agreed that overstimulation caused stress, they also argued that stress could be caused by understimulation. In response, they developed the arousal curve into an inverted U which identified an optimal level of performance in the centre of excessive levels of stress characterized by understimulation and overstimulation (Fig. 8.2). This shows that boredom is just as stressful as overstimulation, and the effects on individuals just as damaging.

On the definition of stress, Seyle (1984) felt a single term was inadequate, arguing that stress could be positive or negative. Positive stress he called eustress (from the Greek word 'eu', good), which was likened to excitement or euphoric feelings. Negative stress was called distress (from the Latin word 'dis', bad). Although the body undergoes similar physiological changes on exposure to both types of stress, it is the long-term effects of distress that are damaging. This definition integrates well with the inverted U hypothesis in that individuals require a certain amount of arousal to perform optimally (whether this occurs when working or relaxing, such as when reading a book). This occurs in eustress stimulation. If the arousal becomes too great or too little, however, then eustress is replaced by distress.

Often, whether stress is positive or negative can be related to whether or not the individual has control of the stressor (the object triggering the stress). Stress that occurs where the individual retains control is positive and exhilarating. On the other hand, where the individual has little control of the threat then the experience is negative and damaging.

RELAXATION AND REST

The concepts of relaxation and rest are linked strongly with those of stress. Sometimes relaxing is doing something different from work or normal pursuits. Thus, relaxation can be active or recreational, for example cycling or gardening (eustressful activities). At other times relaxing means reducing physical activity (such as sunbathing).

Relaxation is generally the precursor to rest. Rest is the period where the body engages in minimal activities to allow restorative processes to occur and, following which, the individual feels refreshed, or rested. Often this coincides with sleep.

There is a close relationship between stress and relaxation, but they are not opposite ends of a scale. It depends on context and the amount of control the individual has over the situation. Sitting down and doing nothing may be relaxing; however, being forced to sit and do nothing in an airport because your flight has been delayed is far from restful! Consequently, people interpret relaxation in a variety of ways. For clarity within this chapter, each concept will be examined independently which, in turn, will provide the rationale for the interventions discussed in the Care Delivery Knowledge section.

PHYSIOLOGICAL RESPONSES TO STRESS

The General Adaptation Syndrome

Seyle (1984) described the physiological changes that occur in response to stress in the General Adaptation Syndrome (Fig. 8.3).

On exposure to the stressor the limbic system sets in motion the physiological response. Initially the hypothalamus is stimulated and this invokes the general adaptation syndrome which occurs over three consecutive stages.

1.   Alarm reaction

This is the very rapid immediate physiological response activated by the sympathetic nervous system and adrenal medulla, and its function is to prepare the body for defensive action to counter the stressor. It causes an increase in the secretion of adrenaline (epinephrine) and noradrenaline (norepinephrine) and invokes the fight or flight response, causing the major physiological changes summarized in Table 8.1, which prepare the body for intense physical action to either confront and fight, or to escape quickly, from the object of stress.

2.   Resistance reaction

The alarm reaction is followed by the resistance reaction. This is a long-term reaction brought about by hormones secreted by the hypothalamus and both provides the energy to sustain the stress response and protects the body by counteracting the effects of physical damage. The hormone pathway (Fig. 8.3) begins with the release of corticotrophin releasing hormone. This stimulates the anterior pituitary gland to secrete adrenocorticotrophic hormone which in turn stimulates the adrenal cortex to increase the secretion of cortisol. The action of cortisol increases glycogenesis and catabolism of body proteins leading to hyperglycaemia, providing copious energy to sustain the response. Cortisol also suppresses the inflammation response, enabling the body to continue action if it is damaged, and it increases the constriction of peripheral blood vessels to maintain blood pressure should blood loss occur though damage to the body surface. Cortisol also suppresses reconstruction of connective tissue and the immune system, however, which can have serious adverse consequences in the long term. In practice, this is likely to be of particular significance during recovery from illness or surgery.

3.   Exhaustion

This is the final stage of the General Adaptation Syndrome (Seyle 1984). It occurs following prolonged excessive distress and, if continued, leads to illness and, eventually, death. Thus, repeated use of the general adaptation syndrome, as occurs in stressful environments where there is no escape, has adverse consequences on the health of individuals.

Continued exposure to stressful events

One of the most obvious effects of continued exposure to stress is on the circulatory system. Within the General Adaptation Syndrome, the heart rate increases and blood pressure rises. In turn, continued exposure to stressful events can damage the circulatory system as it tries to compensate. Friedman & Rosenman (1974) Legault et al (1995), Levi & Lunde-Jensen (1996) and Bosma et al (1997) demonstrated this phenomenon, all reporting associations of high levels of psychological distress with coronary heart disease.

In Figure 8.3 it is shown that the action of cortisol suppresses the immune response. A suppressed immune

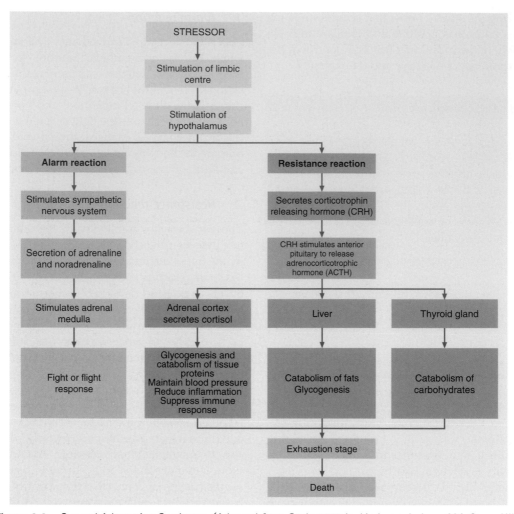

Figure 8.3 General Adaptation Syndrome. (Adapted from Seyle 1984 by kind permission of McGraw-Hill.)

Table 8.1 Major physiological changes associated with the flight or fight response

System	Effect	Outcome
Circulatory system	Increased heart rate and force of contraction Peripheral vasoconstriction	Concentrates blood in the body core, increases blood pressure and increases the flow of blood to the large skeletal muscles that will be used either in fighting or running away
Respiratory system	Increase in respiration rate Dilation of bronchi	Increases oxygenation of the blood, providing the muscles with vast amounts of oxygen in anticipation of the increased aerobic respiration involved in major exertion
Eyes	Pupil dilation	Allows more light into the eyes, resulting in better vision
Skeletal muscles	Increased tension	Quicker response
Excretory system	Increased micturition	Removes excess fluid to reduce body weight and allow a quicker response
Digestive system	Diarrhoea Vomiting Dry mouth	Reduces weight Reduces weight Prevents eating and adding to weight
Skin	Sweat gland activation	Increases cooling in anticipation of muscle activity

response leaves the individual less able to fight off disease. People often find that when they are tired, such as when they have been working for a long time without a holiday break, they become more susceptible to minor infections such as colds and that once they contract an infection it takes longer than usual to recover. Indeed, the incidence of sickness in the workplace is an indicator of employee stress.

The immune system also protects the body against more sinister disease. However, following major life events it has been observed that people have an increased susceptibility

Table 8.2   Mental defence mechanisms (Freud 1934)

Mechanism	Definition	Example
Denial	When reality is too unpleasant or painful to face then individuals may deny that it really exists. In some circumstances this is a healthy process as it allows the individual time to come to terms with the problem. Indeed it is the first stage of the grieving process (Kubler-Ross 1975) (see Ch. 12). In other situations denial may be more serious (see example)	A woman may deny that she could have a serious illness and may delay seeking medical help for a lump she has recently found in her breast
Displacement	When it is impossible to address the cause of stress then anger may be redirected on another, innocent but reachable object	You may have been given a hard time by your boss to whom you are unable to retaliate. When you return home you immediately have a blazing argument with your partner
Intellectualization	To use intellectual powers of thinking, analysis and reasoning to detach oneself from emotional issues	For people working in life or death situations, such as in high dependency units, this defence mechanism may be necessary for survival. If the emotional bluntness extends into other areas of the individuals' lives, however, then the mechanism becomes problematic
Projection	Blaming someone else for how you feel	The ward manager who is unable to manage the ward effectively may blame the situation on incompetent staff
Rationalization	To find an acceptable explanation for an act that you find unacceptable	'It's in the overall best interest' 'You have to be cruel to be kind' 'I don't really care that I lost the interview. I didn't really want the job anyway'
Reaction formation	To conceal what you really feel by thinking and acting in the opposite way	Some people who have an issue in their life about which they feel uncomfortable may campaign against the issue For example, individuals who have led promiscuous lives may campaign strongly for the sanctity of family values
Regression	Individuals engage in behaviours from an earlier, more secure, life stage	Losing your temper and engaging in tantrums when things go wrong Eating when feeling stressed
Repression	Painful thoughts are forced into the unconscious. Although they are out of the conscious they may resurface in dreams	An accident victim may utilize repression to have no recollection of the events surrounding the accident
Sublimation	To redirect the energy from unacceptable sexual or aggressive drives into another socially acceptable activity	Unacceptable aggressive energy focused into a sporting activity This may not always be a positive mechanism. For example, an ambitious manager may utilize sublimation to secure promotions at the expense of family and social commitments

to cancers (Totman 1990). This effect was also reported by Fawzy et al (1993) who examined the survival of individuals with malignant melanomas to find that those who received early psychological interventions to reduce stress had an improved survival rate.

PSYCHOLOGICAL CHANGES IN RESPONSE TO STRESS

Psychological responses to stress vary according to the level of threat. A mild level of stimulation, where the individual remains in control, is accompanied by positive feelings. As the level of stress increases, however, the pleasure changes to a feeling of being overwhelmed. The ability to function effectively decreases and although individuals may be aware of what is happening, they find it difficult to engage in problem solving thinking. Consequently, individuals find they have ever-increasing demands that they are

unable to meet, which in turn perpetuates their feelings of distress. Interpersonal relationships may deteriorate as they become short tempered, aggressive and unapproachable (Vernarec 2001). This worsens their plight and individuals find themselves locked into a stress cycle.

Defence mechanisms

In response to stress an individual may attempt to cope by adopting mental defence mechanisms. These were originally identified by Freud (1934), who claimed that they were used to defend the self against conflict; however, they have been developed subsequently by many other psychologists. Defence mechanisms are unconscious processes used to cope with negative emotions. In the short term they are a healthy response and they help the individual to survive the immediate period following exposure to the stress. The major defence mechanisms are outlined in Table 8.2.

Defence mechanisms do not alter the cause of the stress, however; they only alter an individual's interpretation of it. They create an illusion and consequently involve a degree of self-deception. The prolonged use of mental defence mechanisms is therefore unhealthy.

SOCIAL CHANGES IN RESPONSE TO STRESS

In eustress, which is accompanied by a feeling of well-being, individuals feel confident and able to take on all tasks. As the level of stress increases, however, individuals begin to lose control and eustress is replaced by distress. Due to the fight or flight reaction that this invokes, individuals may appear aggressive and their social interactions may reflect this increased hostility. They may have frequent arguments with others and become intolerant. As the level of stress increases further they become overwhelmed and engrossed with the object causing their stress. They may reject all social contact, even with members of their family, and become isolated (Vernarec 2001).

Evidence based practice

Kittrel (1998), Norton et al (1998) and Carlson (1999) discovered associations between women's career development and family instability, particularly in younger age groups. These observations were reflected in Project 2000 students, where attempting to manage the demands of the course and their home lives led a very high number of students nurses to experience extreme difficulties in their relationships with their partners (Howard 2001).

Alternatively, because of the fight or flight reaction, individuals may become hostile and react aggressively as discussed in Chapter 11 on aggression. Eventually, in burnout, people become emotionally blunted and cynical. Their relationships with others will have already deteriorated and they may struggle to maintain the relationships they still have.

CAUSES OF STRESS

The causes of stress (stressors) are the result of an individual's interpretation of a social phenomenon. Holmes & Rahe (1967) found that stressors invoked stress according to their magnitude, and that their effects accumulated. They classified the significance of stressors in the Social Readjustment Rating Scale (Table 8.3). The greater amount of stress invoked by the stressor then the greater the weighting ascribed to it. Using the scale, the rating of each new stressor is added to those that have occurred within the previous year. It then becomes possible to assess an individual's level of stress by summating the ratings. Holmes & Rahe found that a final score of over 300 was associated with an increased occurrence of a stress related disease.

Table 8.3 The Social Readjustment Rating Scale (from Holmes & Rahe 1967 by kind permission)

1	Death of spouse	100
2	Divorce	73
3	Marital separation	65
4	Jail term	65
5	Death of close family member	63
6	Personal injury or illness	53
7	Marriage	50
8	Loss of job	47
9	Marital reconciliation	45
10	Retirement	45
11	Change in health of family member	44
12	Pregnancy	40
13	Sex difficulties	39
14	Gain of new family member	39
15	Business readjustment	39
16	Change in financial state	38
17	Death of close friend	37
18	Change to different line of work	36
19	Change in number of arguments with spouse	35
20	Mortgage over $10 000	31
21	Foreclosure of mortgage or loan	30
22	Change in responsibilities at work	29
23	Son or daughter leaving home	29
24	Trouble with in-laws	29
25	Outstanding personal achievement	28
26	Wife begins or stops work	26
27	Begin or end school	26
28	Change in living conditions	25
29	Revision of personal habits	24
30	Trouble with boss	23
31	Change in work hours or conditions	20
32	Change in residence	20
33	Change in school	20
34	Change in recreation	19
35	Change in church activities	19
36	Change in social activities	18
37	Mortgage or loan of less than $10 000	17
38	Change in sleeping habits	16
39	Change in the number of family get-togethers	15
40	Change in eating habits	15
41	Holiday	13
42	Christmas	12
43	Minor violations of the law	11

Evidence based practice

It has been observed that following the loss of a partner, particularly around retirement age, within 12 months the remaining spouse frequently becomes severely ill, or may die. Indeed, Lichtenstein et al (1998) found mortality rates of those most at risk was those bereaved between 60 and 70 years. Within the context of stressful life events, surviving partners within this age group are likely to have: recently experienced retirement and a reduction in income, adjusted to their own ill health, supported the deceased partner and the demands of their illness, experienced the death of the partner, met the financial and family demands following the death and undergone their own grieving, from both the loss of their partner and, according to Narayanasamy (1996), from feeling abandoned by their spiritual beliefs.

When experiencing similar life events, some individuals appear to be able to cope with stress better than others. Using Hebb's model of arousal (Hebb 1954) in conjunction with the social readjustment rating scale (Holmes & Rahe 1967) it is possible to see why one individual may be unaffected by an incident whereas to another individual the effect may be catastrophic. By reviewing events that occurred over the previous year, should one individual have an accumulation of stressors and another comparatively few then exposure to the same stressor will push the first individual into overload whereas the latter individual may have sufficient coping reserve.

Although the social readjustment rating scale was developed over 35 years ago, it remains a reliable instrument and enjoys extensive contemporary use (Hobson et al 1998). There are two major limitations of the scale, however. Firstly, it only addresses long-term stressors and fails to take into account short-term stressors such as being late for work or sitting in a traffic jam. Short-term stressors, or 'hassles', invoke a severe stress response but only for a short period (Lazarus et al 1985). Being out of the individual's control, however, they invoke distress and ultimately result in similar damaging effects to individuals' health as long-term distress. The second shortcoming of the social readjustment rating scale is forwarded by Cox (1978) who argues that it is difficult to generalize individuals' esoteric experiences of stress.

Holmes & Rahe (1967) assume that a stressor has more or less the same ability to cause the same amount of stress for everyone. This is the engineering model of stress and is demonstrated in Figure 8.4 where the spider is interpreted identically by subject A and subject B.

Cox (1978) argues this model is too simplistic, and that to gain a true understanding of the nature of stress the stressor must be appraised from the context of the perceived threat it poses to the individual. Thus, the severity of the stressor depends upon what degree of threat each individual thinks it poses. This is represented in Figure 8.5 where subjects A and B are exposed to the same stressor as before but, because of the meaning subject B attaches to the spider in that particular context, the interpretation of threat is greater for subject B than subject A.

Therefore, an assessment of an individual's stress should include a measure of an individual's hassles and an understanding of their interpretation of stressors (Cox 1978, Lazarus et al 1985, Narayanasamy & Owens 2001, Reich

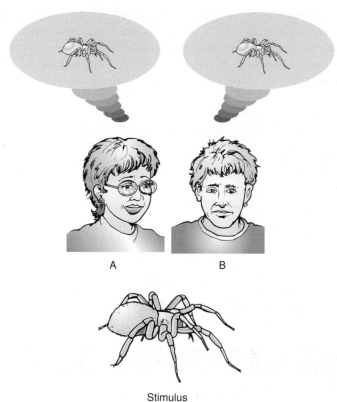

Stimulus

Figure 8.4   Interpreting the spider identically.

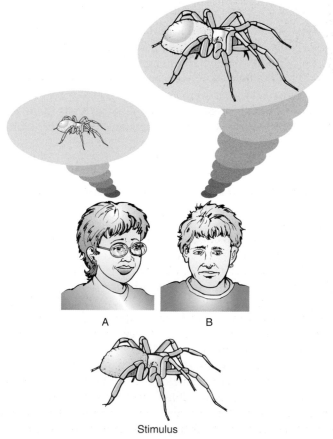

Stimulus

Figure 8.5   How each individual interprets the threat of the spider.

et al 1988). In an assessment the use of the social readjustment rating scale to measure long-term stresses is useful in so much as it identifies a baseline of background stresses. From this baseline, however, the effects of day-to-day stressors and the interpretation an individual attaches to the nature of stressful experiences must also be added.

THE STRESSFUL PERSONALITY

Although individuals' responses to stressors vary according to their interpretations, some individuals consistently respond to stressors in similar ways. Friedman & Rosenman (1974) classified these into two personality types: Type A and Type B. The Type A personality is characterized by extreme competitiveness and an inability to place stressors in perspective. They routinely work against the clock, find it difficult to say 'no', or to delegate, and consequently find themselves with multiple commitments. The end result is that they are unable to fit all tasks into the available time and they end up juggling tasks, switching from one to another, without completing any. This is compounded by a lack of direction. Rather than taking a systematic approach to problem solving, Type A individuals will attempt to solve problems without first identifying the goals. They are also fiercely competitive, leading them to appear aggressive, and they often react to minor irritations in the form of temper tantrums. By way of contrast, the second personality type, Type B, is the antithesis to Type A. They are almost unconcerned when confronted by stressors.

Type A and Type B are in reality two extreme points of a scale. Most people have traits of both personality types and fit on a point somewhere along it (Fig. 8.6). Significantly though, Friedman & Rosenman found that people with Type B characteristics were less susceptible to coronary heart disease (a common stress-related disease) than those with Type A, observations shared subsequently by Levi & Lunde-Jensen (1996).

BURNOUT

All healthcare workers experience long periods working with ill people, often with inadequate resources or support. This is a powerful stressor in the caring professions who become exhausted emotionally and, in turn, susceptible to develop burnout, particularly when the distress is prolonged, continuous and out of the individual's control (Janssen et al 1999, Maslach 1982). There are three major symptoms of burnout:

- emotional exhaustion – individuals are emotionally drained and feel unable to give more of themselves
- depersonalization – individuals become more isolated and hardened towards others
- trivialization of personal accomplishments – individuals are unable to deal with problems positively and trivialize any achievements they make.

Burnout is accompanied by profound psychological and social changes. Individuals become blunted emotionally, their cognitive ability decreases and, because they find it difficult to mix with others, they become isolated. This generally spills over into their personal lives where their relationships with their families and others deteriorate.

Individuals suffering from burnout often feel that it is a result of a weakness in their character, thus compounding their problem (Maslach 1982, Payne 2001). Some employers have encouraged this attitude, blaming the individual for being weak rather than addressing issues causing the distress (Confederation of Health Service Employees 1992). What must be remembered, however, is that burnout occurs as a result of external factors: 'No one burns out except in a climate that encourages burnout' (Welch et al 1982: 9).

To help individuals experiencing distress, many employers make counselling services available. The uptake of these services is likely to be small, however, and will only be used by those who are really desperate. Indeed, to utilize these services requires a degree of assertiveness. As individuals suffering from burnout are also likely to have a low self-esteem they are consequently unlikely to avail themselves of this support (Janssen et al 1999, Maslach 1982, Welch et al 1982). Additionally, although counselling interventions are effective for those who do use the service (Cooper et al 1996), they work at a tertiary level, i.e. after the event. To deal effectively with burnout requires the causes to be addressed.

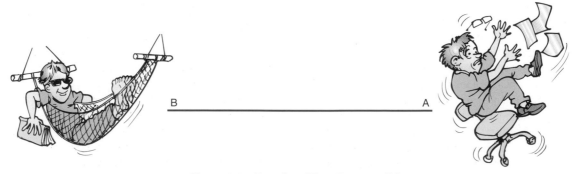

Figure 8.6 Type A and Type B personalities.

POST-TRAUMATIC STRESS DISORDER

Post-traumatic stress disorder (PTSD) is an extended response to an extremely threatening or catastrophic stressful event or situation (e.g. being a victim of a violent crime or witnessing a major disaster) that occurs within the 6 months of the triggering factor (World Health Organization 1992). Sometimes an individual may experience PTSD-like symptoms months or years following the triggering event, however. In this case it is called delayed PTSD.

The main features of PTSD are:

- flashbacks where individuals relive the experience during nightmares. Occasionally, when awake, they may also feel that the situation is about to recur
- emotional numbing with emotional blunting and detachment from others
- hypervigilance and an enhanced startle reaction
- avoidance of anything reminiscent of the triggering event
- confusion, anxiety and depression, and there may be attempts to commit suicide.

Additionally, a number of other symptoms can occur including insomnia, headaches, ulcers and circulatory problems. Sometimes individuals blame themselves for the incident and in addition they suffer fear and guilt. Often individuals feel abandoned by their faith, leading to spiritual distress (Narayanasamy 1996). Furthermore, to compensate individuals may abuse alcohol, or other drugs, which may lead on to dependence.

The most effective method of treatment for PTSD is early counselling intervention (Sims & Owens 1993). This focuses on individuals' unique problems, enabling them to make some sense out of their experience, adopt a problem solving strategy and to move through the initial period of crisis. In many areas of health care, following traumatic incidents, this is supplemented by debriefing exercises, clinical supervision and peer support (see Ch. 11).

RELAXATION, REST AND SLEEP

Relaxation

Relaxation is a complex concept to define, and is associated closely with social context. Sometimes relaxation is equated with tranquillity, rest and sleep. At other times, however, relaxation occurs through engaging in activities generating eustress, such as playing a sport or 'clubbing'. The inverted U hypothesis demonstrated that to function effectively an individual requires some stimulation. Too little stimulation is as distressing as too much (Sutherland & Cooper 1990). What is of fundamental importance, however, is that the activity is engaged in voluntarily. Being able to relax is therefore associated with retaining control of stressors. This is part of effective stress management, and is discussed later in this chapter.

Table 8.4 The five stages of sleep (adapted from Horne 1988 by kind permission of Oxford University Press)

Stage 1	Falling asleep. The individual becomes drowsy and barely conscious, although any slight sound would arouse him or her. Electroencephalograph (EEG) recordings show alpha waves that are associated with being awake
Stage 2	The individual is now asleep. Skeletal muscles are relaxed and movements are still; however, the individual can be roused easily. The EEG shows the appearance of slow waves called K-complexes, as well as bursts of rapid waves known as sleep spindles (Borbely 1987). Stage 2 accounts for more than half the time spent asleep
Stage 3	The individual is completely relaxed and is difficult to arouse. Familiar noises, such as a child crying, can awaken the individual, however. EEG waves become slower and larger and are known as delta waves (Borbely 1987)
Stage 4	Deep sleep. The individual rarely moves and is difficult to awaken. An increase in the percentage of delta waves is noted on EEG recording
Stage 5	Rapid eye movement (REM) or paradoxical sleep. This is characterized by a period of light sleep during which dreaming is thought to mainly occur. For Freudian analysts, dreaming is a symbolic process where the unconscious conflicts are brought to the conscious for resolution

Rest

While it is generally thought that resting is part of relaxation, it does not necessarily follow. Rest is a period of reduced physical activity during which the body repairs and restores itself. However, when people are forced into inactivity, such as when on bed rest as a result of illness, although in theory they are resting, they will probably not be relaxed. Indeed, apart from the concerns arising from their ill health, boredom from reduced stimulation will increase their level of distress (Sutherland & Cooper 1990).

Sleep

Sleep is associated with resting. It is a recurrent natural condition where consciousness is temporarily lost and bodily functions are partly suspended. It reverses, either by a natural return of consciousness or by external stimulation, for example by an alarm clock.

Horne (1988) identified five stages of sleep (Table 8.4). The five stages follow an organized cycle. Initially individuals move through Stages 1 to 4. A period of rapid eye movement (REM) sleep then occurs and the individual may change position in bed. The cycle then returns to Stage 2, progresses to Stage 5 and repeats until the individual awakens. Each cycle lasts around 90 minutes in an adult, but the length of time spent in each stage alters during the night. During the early part of the night the percentage spent in Stages 3 and 4 is larger in comparison with REM sleep, while in the later hours of sleep the proportion of REM sleep increases.

CIRCADIAN RHYTHM

The circadian rhythm is the daily pattern of life for humans. Experiments have demonstrated that when deprived of light, or other sources of time-keeping, humans adopt a sleep–wake routine that cycles approximately every 25 hours. This suggests that the circadian rhythm is set physiologically; however, in real life, it is modified in response to zeitgebers. These are external stimuli that synchronize the circadian rhythm of an individual with the environment, the most powerful of which are of an informative or social nature (Borbely 1987, Folkard 1991). Examples of zeitgebers are:

- the light/dark cycle
- knowledge of clock time
- the behaviour of others
- mealtimes.

Activity within circadian rhythm cycles also varies between two personality types:

- 'Morning types' who rise early and do much of their best work in the hours before noon, but become tired by early evening and do not then function as efficiently
- 'Evening types' who have difficulty rising in the morning, often have difficulty facing breakfast and do not really perform at their best until the afternoon – many are at their peak of alertness in the late evening and often settle late (Folkard 1991).

Reflection and portfolio exercise

Identify whether you are a 'morning type' or an 'evening type'. You can use this information when developing your time management programme, particularly when identifying the best time to study.

Patterns of sleep

Although sleeping once at night is the norm in most North European countries, one type of sleep pattern is not relevant for all cultures. For example, in some Mediterranean cultures a siesta is taken in the hottest part of the day and in China workers are expected to have a sleep in the middle of the day as part of the lunchtime break. Furthermore, the normal pattern of sleep changes with age (Table 8.5.).

Table 8.5   Pattern of sleep according to age

Age	2 months	3 years	25 years	75 years
Amount of sleep	18 hours	13 hours	8 hours	5 hours in 24 hours
Pattern of sleep	Asleep between daytime feeds	Night sleep and day nap	Night sleep	Night sleep and day nap(s)

Individuals' needs for sleep differ, though, and it is therefore impossible to generalize from the data given in Table 8.5. It is the individual who best knows whether or not they are receiving enough sleep.

CARE DELIVERY KNOWLEDGE

The previous section of this chapter demonstrated how the concepts of stress, relaxation and rest were closely entwined. These were all underpinned by psychological stress, however, and this is likely to affect nurses and their colleagues as well as clients and carers. Although individuals respond to stress in their own esoteric ways according to age, culture, gender and past experience, some responses are universal. By measuring these it is possible to assess the degree of stress an individual is experiencing, and to consider the ramifications on their ability to relax and rest. This section therefore begins by outlining tools to measure stress and progresses to examine common causes of stress affecting clients, carers and care professionals.

METHODS OF ASSESSMENT OF STRESS

Physiological measures

Because of the relationship between psychological stress and physiological disturbance, demonstrated by the General Adaptation Syndrome (Seyle 1984), it is possible to assess stress using physiological measures such as the electrical conductivity of the skin, heart rate and blood pressure. The disadvantage of physiological measures is that they do not explain why the individual feels stressed. Seyle (1984) found the immediate physiological effects of eustress and distress were identical. Consequently, similar recordings would be obtained for both positive and negative stressors. Therefore, although it is important to understand physiological indicators of stress, to understand the nature of the stress requires additional information.

Decision-making exercise

Immediately on admission most patients have their baseline observations recorded.

- Referring to the General Adaptation Syndrome, what are advantages and disadvantages of this?
- How might the disadvantages be addressed?

The Social Readjustment Rating Scale

The Social Readjustment Rating Scale (Holmes & Rahe 1967) was discussed in the Subject Knowledge section of this chapter. It is inappropriate to use only this instrument, as it may not record all the factors that are causing the current period of stress. Nor does it measure the amount of stress felt by the individual. However, this is an excellent instrument to gain insight into the background of an individual's situation, and to provide avenues for further exploration.

Stress scales and diaries

Similar to stress, another construct that is very difficult to measure is pain. Although pain usually derives from the physiological stimulus of pain receptors, individuals subjectively evaluate the amount and severity of the pain they experience. Because of its subjective nature, however, nurses have frequently misjudged the amount of pain patients experienced and, in consequence, have offered inadequate analgesia. This led to the development of pain scales where patients indicate the severity of pain they feel on a line ranging from 'No pain' at one end to 'Unbearable pain' at the other (see Ch. 10). Although these are not peremptory measures of pain, they indicate the effectiveness of pain management strategies, particularly if they include some form of scaling.

There are strong parallels between measuring pain and measuring stress. Stress is also a subjective phenomenon and shares similar difficulties of measurement. Therefore, to gain insight into stress from the individuals' perspectives, instruments should measure the nature, frequency and intensity of the experience. In research into the stress that student nurses experienced during their training, a modification of pain scales proved a very effective measure (Howard 2001). An instrument was designed around a 10-point scale. Prompts were included for guidance and ranged from 0, which indicated no stress at all, to 10 which indicated feeling totally overwhelmed; reflecting the Seyle's (1984) model of stress with lower scores indicating eustress and higher scores, distress. Over a period of time patterns of stress were generated for each student and by combining these data particularly stressful periods of the Project 2000 course were identified. When these data were supplemented by diary entries that were also supplied by the students, the reasons why the parts of the course were stressful also became apparent (Howard 2001). The ability of scales and diaries to indicate the time, nature and precipitating factors, however, make them useful instruments to assess the nature of stress that clients experience.

Identifying common stressors

Stress in clients

Clients may present when stress is:

- a primary reason for referral
- a cause of or a contributory factor to the client's condition
- occurring as a consequence of the client's illness.

Stress as a primary reason for referral

The purpose of the assessment is to gain understanding of the causes and the individual's experiences of stress.

Everybody's experience of stress is unique, depending on their interpretation of the stressors, the context of the stressors, and the number of stressors influencing the individual at any particular time. Similarly, individuals' responses to stress vary. Although the fight or flight syndrome classifies specific stress response behaviours, some individuals present as very anxious and apprehensive, some become very dependent on others to the point of automatic compliance, whereas others react with anger. Consequently, to be able to assist the client it is necessary to understand how that individual is experiencing stress and why he or she is reacting in that way. The purpose of assessment is to establish how the stress affects the individual's life and to identify recurrent patterns of events that act as triggers. From this baseline, interventions that are appropriate for that individual may be developed.

Stress as a cause of or a contributory factor to the client's condition

A high level of stress has adverse ramifications on physical health (Fawzy et al 1993, Totman 1990). Therefore, although the client's primary problem may be essentially physical the accompanying stress, if left unaddressed, will hinder recovery. This was demonstrated by Brosschot et al (1998) who found that when individuals were exposed to stressors they were unable to control, their immune systems became suppressed. Similarly, Pruessner et al (1999) reported that individuals who were in situations where they experienced high distress and low self-esteem had higher serum cortisol than would be expected which, in turn, would suppress their immune systems.

Clients may also be referred for a condition that is exacerbated by stress. This may take the form of a stress related mental or physical illness. The purpose of assessment in such an instance are to identify what the precipitating stressor was (e.g. becoming unemployed), when it happened, the context in which it happened, what other issues were occurring at the time, how quickly the illness developed and to establish how the client feels able to cope with the issues arising.

Stress occurring as a consequence of the client's illness

Clients may be concerned that they are going to die, that they are going to be in pain, that they may not wake up from an anaesthetic or that their prognosis is poor. To the nurse working on a busy ward these may appear to be unfounded fears. To the client they are very real. It is very easy for the nurse to become desensitized to clients' fears in a busy environment.

Waiting for results is a particularly stressful time. The insecurity inhibits positive thought processes, a situation exacerbated by the use of denial, particularly if the tests are to confirm a life-threatening disease. Uncertainty therefore moves the stressor out of the individual's control and they become distressed which, due to the fight or flight response, may be shown as denial or an aggressive attitude. Although it is possible to plan how to cope with the consequences of the test, it is only when the results of tests are known that the stressor can be isolated and positive steps taken to secure control.

Clients going into hospital may also worry about their continuing responsibilities. They may have dependent relatives and be uncertain about how they will be cared for. They may have a pet that requires care. They may worry about loss of income. They may be concerned that they will be unable to work again. The nurse, on identifying these problems, must spend time with the client and explore the issues from the client's perspective. It may sound obvious, but it is only when the client's problems have been identified that they can be addressed.

Clients may also experience spiritual distress, particularly when confronted with a poor prognosis. They may feel betrayed, asking 'Why me?' (Narayanasamy 1996), or may believe that they are being punished. This distress is compounded as many feel embarrassed for holding beliefs about God (Hay 1987). Indeed, even in clients who do not have religious beliefs, there is a need to make sense of life, and their situation, and it is this issue that provides a focus for nursing interventions.

Stress in clients' relatives

In a client's relatives, stress may result from concern about the client's illness, anger that the client is ill and guilt that they are unable to cope. This is a reaction of the grieving process (see Ch. 12). Some carers demonstrate this by avoiding the client and rarely, if ever, visiting. At face value this appears callous and uncaring. From within the context of individuals' reactions to stress, however, this can result from the fight or flight reaction or denial. Similarly, the fight or flight reaction explains why other relatives react aggressively. This is often projected onto the nurse where relatives may be hostile and constantly find fault with the care. In turn, this may result in the relative being labelled troublesome and treated with resentment by staff, thus perpetuating the situation. Alternatively, relatives may feel excluded from caring for their sick relative. This compounds their guilt and may increase the hostility to care staff. This emphasizes the importance of an understanding of the mechanisms of stress so as to recognize distress experienced by relatives and ameliorate their concerns. (For further information on managing hostility see Chapter 11 on aggression).

Stress in the workplace

Stress is a reaction of the individual to a stressful environment. Individuals may reason that if everybody else can cope then it is they who must be weak (Meadows et al 2000, Vernarec 2001). In turn, this leads the individual to develop a poor self-esteem. Consequently, it is important to understand how stress affects individuals in the workplace.

Working in health and social care is a stressful occupation. Staff are expected to cope in traumatic situations. They work unsocial hours and are expected to do more with limited resources. Remuneration is minimal and many do not have the security of a permanent contract of employment. In addition to daytime shift work, many staff are required to work periods of nights. Although research into circadian rhythms suggests that for short periods of time the body does not significantly alter its biological routines (Folkard 1991), this can be extremely disruptive to the individual's out-of-work commitments. In addition, care staff are regularly exposed to physiological stressors such as chemicals, solvents, poor lighting, poor heating, inadequate ventilation and excessive noise (Levi & Lunde-Jensen 1996).

Many inquiries into stress have focused on healthcare workers. Because of the wide range of staff working in health care, however, it is difficult to generalize findings obtained from one grade of staff to another. Harris (1989) developed the nurse stress index following a series of interviews with charge nurses and ward sisters. Although the instrument has received widespread use, it focused mainly on clinical and managerial issues, limiting its use with other grades of healthcare workers. There is an abundance of research into the stress experienced by qualified staff working in specialist areas, particularly the terminally ill. In student nurses, Rhead (1995) identified coursework, practice placements and confrontation with mortality particularly distressing, whereas Howard (2001) found financial difficulties, time management and relationship problems were significant causes of distress. Therefore, it becomes difficult to generalize all experiences of stress in health and social care to all grades of staff. However, the core issues of mortality, workload and role conflict are consistently cited, and these are strongly associated with burnout (Howard 2001, Janssen et al 1999, Maslach 1982, Meadows et al 2000, Payne 2001, Quine 1998).

Common indicators of excessive stress in the workplace are:

- bringing work home
- not being able to switch off from work
- feeling tense all of the time
- poor self-esteem
- difficulty in mixing with others
- deteriorating relationships
- an increase in arguments at work
- talking malevolently about colleagues
- feeling run down
- an increase in physical ailments.

Individuals are often unaware of these signs, which may then progress into a more serious problem. Using feedback from others, clinical supervision and developing greater self-awareness will help to identify these damaging events and take actions to limit them.

Assessing sleep

An assessment of sleep should examine sleep habits and routines. Hodgson (1991) suggests that the following aspects should be included:

- age
- normal pattern of sleep during health
- current pattern of sleep
- nutritional status
- emotional status
- daytime and night-time symptoms
- sleeping environment
- sleep-related rituals
- presence of dreams or nightmares
- present medication
- wake-time behaviour.

Assessments will be subjective as they will be based on individuals' perceptions; however, it is the clients who know if they feel refreshed after sleep or not. On occasions, a sleep chart may be completed to establish an individual's pattern of sleep, and reasons for waking. Finally, it is important to remember that the symptoms of the client's illness may contribute changes to sleep habits and it is possible for this to develop into a vicious circle.

PLANNING

Stress management

Stress, relaxation and rest are concepts that have a strong association; however, the centre of all is the ability to manage stress. Planning to enable relaxation and rest consequently focuses, in the first instance, on assisting the individual to manage stressors.

Stress management strategies fall into proactive and reactive methods. Reactive methods are used following a stressful event to help to manage the problem. Consequently, they work on the assumption that there is stress to be managed in the first place. In contrast, proactive strategies are taken to prevent or to minimize the number of stressful events experienced. Most methods of stress management can be used either proactively or reactively; however, to manage stress effectively, the aim should be to use all strategies proactively.

Physical interventions

Diet

Reactions to stress may lead to changes in eating habits such as in undereating or overeating. Commonly, when under prolonged stress (such as when completing assessments) individuals regress to a more secure developmental stage and engage in 'comfort eating' – consuming comfort foods which invariably contain high levels of sugar and fats. Additionally, many increase their consumption of alcohol. During the resistance stage of the General Adaptation

Syndrome, the body also retains sodium by excreting high levels of potassium. Left unchecked this could lead to exhaustion and, eventually, death. Although this is an extreme example, because of disturbances in diet and the adoption of unhealthy eating habits, a well-balanced diet is central to all stress management programmes.

> ### Reflection and portfolio evidence
>
> Keep a daily record of what you eat and drink, together with an indication of how stressed you felt.
> Use a scale of 0–10 where:
>
> 0   = No stress
> 1–4 = Positive stress
> 5–7 = Becoming distressed
> 8–9 = Very distressed
> 10   = Totally overwhelmed
>
> You might also like to note what of happened during the day to cause the way you felt.
>
> - Did your diet change as you became more stressed?
> - How did it make you feel on the day?
> - How does it make you feel now?
> - Could you adopt a healthier pattern of eating in the future?

Exercise

Exercise is often advocated as part of stress management. Engaging in a sporting activity means that attention is focused on playing the sport, thus diverting attention from the worrying recurrent thoughts that sustain the underlying stress. Sport also provides a safe, socially acceptable outlet for the aggressive drives that manifest during the fight or flight syndrome. When using sport as a method of stress management it needs to be remembered that people most susceptible to the negative effects of stress are the highly competitive Type A personality types (Friedman & Rosenman 1974). These individuals are likely to enter a sport and set ever-increasing goals that they strive to achieve. To counter this effect, some contemporary authors advocate engaging in non-competitive sports. As the nature of all sport is competition, however, the hollow 'politically correct' rhetoric of non-competitiveness becomes impossible to enact, and advocates of this strategy are likely to be ridiculed. What is important is that individuals retain control of the competitive element of the sport, playing for enjoyment rather than outright achievement.

Socialization

Time should be made for all commitments in life. When suffering from excessive work related stress in particular, individuals often find that they have little time for anything other than work and work related issues (Vernarec 2001), difficulties that are compounded should the individual work unsocial hours or shifts. In effective stress management, it is essential that individuals continue with existing social contacts, for example friends and family, in order to retain an appropriate perspective on new stressors in life.

PSYCHOSOCIAL INTERVENTIONS

Counselling

Earlier in this chapter it was seen that distress arises when individuals lose control of stressors. Counselling enables individuals to regain control of stressful situations by developing problem solving strategies for coping, thus limiting the amount of distress that stressors invoke (British Association of Counselling 1992). At times, though, this appears unrealistic. For example, a man may be diagnosed with human immunodeficiency virus (HIV). He is very likely to be extremely distressed regarding his condition and his prognosis. Although it is not possible to generalize for any individual, as everyone's circumstances are unique, it is likely that this man would use mental defence mechanisms, particularly denial, at this time (this is the first stage of the grieving process; see Chapter 12). Consequently, the initial focus of counselling would be to get him to accept the situation in which he finds himself, and the associated limitations. Once this is achieved a problem solving approach can be used to take control of events, as much as possible, which in turn will minimize the distress.

Spiritual care

In providing spiritual care, Narayanasamy & Owens (2001) found that nurses adopted personal and procedural approaches. Procedural approaches were to ensure that clients' religious beliefs were recorded, and involved arranging for the requirements of their faith to be observed. Personal approaches, however, were the most valuable and involved the nurse adopting a counselling type role. Although the nurse cannot provide solutions to clients' problems, by acting as a facilitator to help clients achieve realistic aims, clients are often able to achieve an inner peace. Narayanasamy (1999) identifies three skills for implementing spiritual care:

- Communication – Non-judgemental, active listening to facilitate clients to unburden their thoughts
- Trust building – Promoting security, showing genuine concern and keeping promises
- Giving hope – Supporting individuals who are struggling with questions of fear and faith by encouraging them to talk. Reflecting on memories of the good things that occurred in their lives, particularly when failure was defeated, can also help clients to face the future more positively.

Cognitive behavioural therapy

The purpose of cognitive behavioural therapy (CBT) is to replace negative, destructive thoughts with ones that are positive and constructive. CBT was developed as a treatment for negative thinking and low self-esteem in depression (Beck 1979). Similar to people with depression, however, individuals who feel overwhelmed through excessive stress also experience a low self-esteem, have negative thought processes and are often distracted by worrying thoughts. CBT can therefore be used successfully with these individuals (Fisher & Durham 1999) and it forms part of many stress management programmes.

Rehearsal

A CBT technique often used in assertiveness training is that of rehearsal. This technique is also very useful in the management of stress. Basically, it starts with defining the actual problem and considering the possible outcomes – desirable as well as undesirable. Individuals then consider strategies to achieve a desirable outcome from all alternatives. In this way, responses are practised, and confidence is developed, enabling the individual to take greater control of the situation when it happens in real life.

> **Reflection and portfolio exercise**
>
> Rehearsal can also be used when developing your portfolio. Think of a situation you are likely to encounter, but where you feel unconfident and anxious. An example might be attending a cardiac arrest. Write down your anxieties and talk to an experienced member of staff for guidance. It may be that you feel uncomfortable with handling the equipment, so try to negotiate some time to familiarize yourself with its location, when it is likely to be used, and practice handling the equipment (if possible). You might also be able to negotiate time with the school of nursing or resuscitation officer to practise using equipment on a mannikin in a clinical skills laboratory.
>
> Alternatively, many people use rehearsal when preparing for stressful events such as a job interview. In this situation, they try to predict the questions that they are likely to be asked, using the person specification and advice from colleagues, and they prepare and rehearse answers. If anxiety is really bad then it is useful to ask 'What's the worst thing that could happen?' to place the situation in perspective before analysing the feared situation further. Not only does this give individuals more confidence, it also prepares them with more insight into the demands of the post for which they are applying.

Group therapy

There are many variations of group therapy that may be used within a stress management programme. Local community mental health teams frequently facilitate these and they commonly include the following groups.

Anxiety management groups

These utilize a combination of education, social skills and self-help techniques. Their aim is to provide individuals with an understanding of the nature of stress and anxiety, and to help them to learn more effective skills of coping.

Assertiveness groups

Low self-esteem is generally accompanied by poor assertiveness skills. Many individuals are unable to refuse additional work, or fail to stand up for themselves, perpetuating their loss of control and leading to an increase in their level of stress. By developing assertiveness skills individuals are prepared to take more control of their life. In turn this allows better management of commitments, and subsequently of their stress.

Similarly, for people with Type A personalities, assertiveness groups can help them to learn less aggressive and more assertive modes of interaction. Their presence in groups containing people with low self-esteem should be carefully considered, however, as it is likely that Type A individuals would become very dominant in this situation, and their actions could become extremely destructive to the group process.

Social skills groups

Low self-esteem may contribute to individuals becoming socially isolated. In this instance social skills groups assist individuals to regain their ability of social interaction. They are particularly useful for people with Type A personality traits who are often impatient and aggressive (Friedman & Rosenman 1974). Consequently, these groups help individuals to learn more appropriate interpersonal skills.

Self-help groups

People with similar problems meet under the supervision of a trained facilitator. The intention of these groups is for members to support each other and to learn alternative ways of coping with their problems (Vernarec 2001).

Relaxation techniques

Relaxation techniques are used to control the symptoms of stress; predominantly increased muscle tension and recurrent worrying thoughts (Fisher & Durham 1999). Although this is a reactive measure, they are sometimes used to prevent a stressful period in an individual's life developing into a crisis. They are also helpful to assist individuals rest and prepare for sleep.

Meditation

The individual sits in a relaxed, balanced posture so that no muscular correction is needed to maintain position. Breathing rate is reduced to slow deep breaths, which counters the increased shallow respirations that occur under stress. When the correct body posture is achieved, individuals try to empty their minds of all thoughts or they may focus on a single object, such as a lighted candle. In effect, this stops the recurrent worrying thoughts that occur when people feel distressed. These actions assist the individual to experience a sense of calm and it is from this state that they may try to apply problem solving strategies to address their stressors.

Progressive muscle relaxation

In the fight or flight response, muscles contract in preparation for action. A prolonged increase in muscle tone leads to a feeling of tension, however, perpetuating the feeling of stress. Progressive muscle relaxation focuses the individual's attention on groups of muscles. The individual is asked to contract the muscle group, and then to relax the group, and then to compare the difference and to remember the feeling of relaxation. Each major muscle group is addressed in turn, leading to an overall reduction in muscle tone and, as relaxed muscles are incompatible with feelings of tension, the individual feels relaxed. Progressive muscle relaxation usually occurs when the individual is lying in a quiet room, with relaxing background music. However, for individuals experiencing difficulty sleeping, it may also be used when they retire to bed.

Relaxation in this way requires practice and clients are often given a tape to practise at home. Eventually, however, most will master the technique. It is usual for the initial relaxation sessions to be facilitated by a trained therapist though, as some individuals may react against the feelings of relaxation with panic as they perceive it as a loss of control.

Massage

This is an alternative method of muscle relaxation but is combined with touch. The use of touch during massage is a form of non-verbal communication suggesting that the person performing the massage cares about the individual receiving the massage. Sometimes this process is enhanced by the use of aromatic oils. Olfactory receptors are excited by these oils and in turn arouse the limbic centre (Cerrato 1998). In turn, the limbic centre stimulates the release of neurotransmitters, including endorphins, which produces a sense of well-being. Similar to relaxation therapy, the effect of massage often relaxes individuals sufficiently to enable them to discuss their main anxieties and from this foundation, problem solving strategies may be developed.

Biofeedback

This is a behavioural technique that uses operant conditioning to teach the individual how to manage the symptoms associated with stress. There are several variations to this method, all of which focus on the physiological symptoms of the fight or flight syndrome. At its simplest, patients are told to monitor their heart rate or to concentrate on their breathing. Utilizing methods of stress management similar to those of meditation, individuals are asked to try to reduce their pulse or respiration rate. Consequently, as these fall so does the feeling of stress.

A more sophisticated variation of this method uses a galvanometer to measure the electrical conductivity of the skin. As part of the fight or flight response, the rate of perspiration increases in proportion to the level of stress. In turn, this reduces the electrical resistance of the skin. The galvanometer measures this resistance and represents this audibly through a loudspeaker tone, a high tone indicating low resistance changing to a progressively lower tone as the resistance increases. Again, using methods of stress management similar to those used in meditation the individual attempts to reduce the pitch of the galvanometer and to maintain it at the low pitch. This gives feedback to the user who by this process learns to relax.

Drugs

Prescribed drugs

Contemporary prescribing practices do not advocate the routine use of drugs as part of stress management. In severe instances where pathologies develop, however, the use of medication is helpful. Two categories of drugs are commonly prescribed, anxiolytics such as diazepam or lorazepam, and antidepressants. Occasionally, medication may also be prescribed to aid sleep.

Anxiolytics   These drugs provide immediate relief from the unpleasant feelings associated with stress. This is a very short-term effect, although in periods of crisis they may be prescribed for a short period to reduce the level of anxiety and facilitate the return of problem solving thinking. Counselling may be used to aid this process as, should the underlying problems that caused the anxiety not be addressed, the unpleasant feelings will return as the effects of the drugs wear off. The danger that then occurs is for the individual to continue take the drug which in turn becomes a self-perpetuating cycle leading quickly to dependence.

Antidepressants   These drugs are sometimes prescribed when individuals experience prolonged periods of distress. Some types of antidepressants possess a sedative effect and these sometimes help to reduce recurrent worrying thoughts or, if given as a single night-time dose, to aid sleep. When individuals experience prolonged periods of distress, however, they also experience low self-esteem and the main reason antidepressants are prescribed is to help to improve this, so enabling positive thinking processes to return and aid individuals to address their problems.

Non-prescribed drugs   Increasing use is being made of non-prescribed preparations, particularly herbal remedies. These are claimed to possess similar properties as traditionally prescribed medication and are available without prescription. Generally, herbal preparations have received little empirical research and their exact mode of action is unknown. Furthermore, the quality of herbal preparations is variable as the active ingredients are often mixed with other constituents, making it difficult to draw conclusions for the benefits or of side effects (Linde 1996, Wong 1998). In particular, the safety of these preparations in pregnancy and during lactation is unknown and it follows that women should not take them during these times. Despite these cautions, however, herbal remedies are popular and in the management of stress the two most common remedies are valerian and hypericum.

Valerian   Valerian is used as an anxiolytic agent. While it is reported to possess sedative properties, it may also interact with other medication, particularly other sedatives, including alcohol. It is therefore, prudent to take similar precautions to other sedative medication when taking this preparation (Wong 1998).

***Hypericum perforatum* (St John's wort)**   Hypericum has a long history of use as an antidepressant and is the most investigated herbal remedy (Wong 1998). Linde (1996) notes that it is widely prescribed in Germany for the treatment of anxiety and depression. Within the UK, however, its use is mainly by self-medication. It is thought to work in a similar way to selective serotonin reuptake inhibitor type antidepressants, and is often referred to as the 'herbal Prozac'. Hypericum has fewer side effects than conventional antidepressants, with those reported being photodermatitis, gastrointestinal disturbance, dry mouth, restlessness or sedation (Wong 1998). Studies have compared hypericum to both placebo and antidepressant medication and found it successful in the treatment of mild depression (Linde 1996). Within stress management, the rationale for its use is similar to conventional antidepressants.

Other stress relieving substances

Many individuals use other substances to relieve stress. These include alcohol, nicotine and some illegal drugs. They are taken to provide immediate relief from the extreme unpleasant feelings associated with stress, or to help to induce sleep. This is a very short-term effect though and, as with all drugs, if the underlying problems that caused the distress are not addressed the unpleasant feelings will return as the effects of the drugs wear off. This may encourage the individual to take the drug again and a self-perpetuating cycle leading to dependence may quickly become established.

Aiding sleep

Particularly on admission to hospital, clients can have great difficulty in sleeping. The following approaches are useful to consider when planning strategies to aid sleep.

- Darkness. In hospital it is difficult to provide darkness as dim light is needed at night to promote safety. Many clients are used to sleeping in the dark, however, and may find that their pattern of sleep is disturbed by the light. In this situation, providing that safety is maintained, and that the client is able to tolerate them, blindfolds can be used to exclude unwanted light.
- Silence. Noise at night is a common problem for clients attempting to sleep, whether this is in hospital or at home. This can be addressed by staff turning down the volume of telephones and wearing quiet shoes. As a last resort, the use of earplugs may be helpful.
- Comfort. To be able to sleep, individuals need to be in a comfortable position. Although most people can achieve this independently, for those who a partially or totally immobile, assistance will need to be given.
- Not feeling tired. In illness, individuals who are used to being physically active may find that they are not tired and this can affect the time they take to settle to sleep.
- Food and drink. Many people settle to sleep following a light supper or snack or are in the habit of taking a night-time drink. Provision of a suitable drink or snack at an appropriate time can thus aid sleep.
- Temperature. People sleep less well if the ambient temperature is too warm or too cold. Although it is often difficult to adjust the temperature, this can be compensated for using more or fewer blankets and wearing appropriate nightclothes.
- Routines. The use of familiar bedtime routines can promote sleep. If a client is in hospital, retiring to bed at the usual time, having familiar objects from home (e.g. photographs or cuddly toys for children), and performing bedtime rituals may help to normalize the bedtime routine.
- Reading. Many people like to read before sleeping. While this may be unproblematic at home, in hospital this may

be achieved by using bed lights that do not disturb others and ensuring the client has access to books and magazines.

- Pillows. Some clients are used to sleeping with several pillows, while others are not. Additionally, some clients may have breathing difficulties if they have insufficient support. Consequently, the number of pillows needed should form part of the assessment and plan of care.
- Avoiding daytime naps if this is not a usual pattern of sleep. Often if there is little stimulation during the day it can be easy for clients to nap. In turn, though, this means that they will be less tired at bedtime and unable to sleep. This is particularly problematic for clients suffering from dementia who may reverse day and night time activities (see Ch. 16).

Medication to aid sleep This belongs to two main groups: hypnotics and anxiolytics. Hypnotics act on the central nervous system to induce sleep and include nitrazepam, temazepam and clomethiazole. Anxiolytics may also be given before major events such as surgery. The sedative properties of some antidepressants, such as dosulepin (dothiepin) can also be used to aid sleep. In this instance, medication will be prescribed as a single night-time dose.

Stress management for practitioners

Physical environmental stressors

These stressors should be addressed using the appropriate legislative framework such as the Health and Safety at Work Act 1974 and the Control of Substances Hazardous to Health regulations. They are discussed more fully in Chapter 2.

Clinical supervision

Clinical supervision provides a forum to discuss events that occur during clinical practice, to explore feelings towards them and to learn from the experience. The supervisor is usually an experienced professional whose role is to facilitate reflection on issues that occur in practice, consider alternative perspectives and to help the practitioner to develop confidence and self-esteem (Begat et al 1997). While this process helps to improve practice by maximizing control of stressors, it also assists in the management of stress (Quine 1998, Meadows et al 2000, White et al 1998). Begat et al (1997) reported that nurses felt emotionally refreshed following supervision. As emotional exhaustion is a major factor leading to the development of burnout (Janssen et al 1999, Payne 2001), it follows that clinical supervision should be available to all practitioners and incorporated within professional practice (UK Central Council 1996).

Individual supervision In individual supervision the supervisor's role is to listen, evaluate and teach. The practitioner and supervisor meet at least monthly at prearranged sessions lasting for around 1 hour. During these sessions there is time to reflect on issues that have occurred since the last supervision and time for planning a strategy for subsequent implementation. The value of supervision is that it provides an alternative perspective of events, it provides an outlet for the practitioner to discuss feelings held towards events, and it facilitates learning, via reflection, to enhance the practitioner's practice (UK Central Council 1996).

Group supervision In group supervision 6–10 professionals working in similar areas meet to reflect on their practice. The group is usually conducted by an experienced professional and the purposes, similar to individual supervision, are to provide a forum where practitioners can talk about their feelings, and to provide an environment to learn and improve practice. The advantage of group supervision is that a broad reflection is enabled and support can be offered from practitioners who have similar experiences (Begat et al 1997). This may be limited, however, due to the number of people sharing the time and because individuals may not feel safe to disclose as much in a group as they would during individual supervision. Group supervision should therefore be used to support rather than to replace individual supervision.

Reflection and portfolio evidence

Obtain a copy of *Position statement on clinical supervision for nursing, midwifery and health visiting* (UK Central Council 1996). Consider Key Statement 4: 'Every practitioner should have <u>access</u> to clinical supervision. Each supervisor should supervise a realistic number of practitioners.'

- What are your current clinical supervision arrangements?
- If you receive clinical supervision what have you gained from this?
- If you don't receive it then what do you think you could gain?
- What are your reservations?
- How can you use this to inform your negotiation of a supervision contract in the future as:
  (a) supervisee?
  (b) supervisor?

Time management

Under stress individuals may find that they have little time for anything other than work and work related issues. One of the problems that occur when individuals become overstressed is that their organizational ability declines. Individuals attempt to accommodate an ever increasing workload into an ever decreasing amount of available time, a situation which is compounded should the individual work unsocial hours or shifts. Because there is a finite amount of time, individuals then prioritize which tasks are to be given most energy and may end up leaving little time for family and social commitments. Life then loses structure and individuals become overwhelmed, a situation worsened by avoidance (Payne 2001). For example a student may have an assignment to complete; however, when it is time to begin work on it other tasks such as housework, ironing, etc. suddenly take priority.

Engaging in the work means engaging in the additional stress required to complete it. Thus, to avoid the immediate additional stress, the individual avoids the task. Unfortunately, this tactic worsens the situation as the task remains incomplete and must now be undertaken within an even more restricted time-frame. By providing structure through setting goals, targets and dates, time management helps to manage stressors. Underpinning time management strategies, however, must be the retention of existing social contacts, e.g. friends and family, in order to retain a proper perspective on life. Effective time management is therefore a fundamental part of stress management. By rigidly allocating time for all commitments in life, individuals can take control of stressors and prioritize what will and will not be achieved. This is returned to in the final part of this chapter, Personal and Reflective Knowledge.

PROFESSIONAL AND ETHICAL KNOWLEDGE

Traditionally within the UK, people requiring long-term health care were admitted into institutions. In contemporary society, however, many clients are cared for within the community, a consequence of changes to healthcare policy that have deliberately exploited the contributions of informal carers. Although the move towards community based care was the goal of governments from the 1950s, this policy accelerated during the Conservative administration of the 1980s and 1990s, and was continued by New Labour who were elected into office in 1997. To place stress within health and social care into context, from the perspectives of service users and providers of care, this section examines the sociopolitical context of caring within the UK.

THE INCREASED USE OF INFORMAL CARERS

Until the election of the Conservative administration of 1979, community care was thought a better option for many patients and carers. In reality though, progress towards community care was slow. After 1979, however, the view of community care changed to be seen as a cheaper option, and it was financial savings that accelerated the move to a community based service. The redefinition of care first appeared in the report *Growing Older* (Department of

Health and Social Security 1981):

> *The primary sources of support and care for elderly people are informal and voluntary. These spring from the personal ties of kinship, friendship and neighbourhood. They are irreplaceable. It is the role of public authorities to sustain, and, where necessary, develop – but never to displace – such support and care. Care in the community must increasingly mean care by the community.*
> *(Department of Health and Social Security 1981: 1.9)*

Thus formal care was replaced with informal (non-paid) care, and the roles of statutory services were changed to become facilitators rather than providers of care. The Griffiths Report on Community Care (Department of Health and Social Security 1988) hastened this position, advocating more care being delivered in the community using voluntary, not-for-profit and commercial sectors instead of statutory services. These proposals were subsequently embraced in the National Health Service and Community Care Act 1990 and are reflected by the reduction in the number of available hospital beds for the elderly from 46 000 in 1990–91 to 28 000 in the year 2000–01 (Department of Health 2003a) and, in adult mental illness and handicap from 52 000 available beds in 1995–96 to 39 000 in 2001–02 (Department of Health 2003b).

Following the election of the New Labour government in 1997 two documents were published that entrenched the reliance on unpaid carers. *Partnership in Action* (Department of Health 1998) was to improve collaborative care by requiring health authorities to plan services incorporating the views of local interested parties via Health Improvement Programmes. This was reinforced in *Caring about Carers* (Department of Health 1999a) which identified specific measures to assist unpaid carers to continue caring. What both papers failed to address, however, is whether informal carers actually wanted, or were able, to be carers. Indeed, in *Caring about Carers*, specific reference is made to enable support for young carers of school age.

Thus, as a result of successive policies, additional demands have been placed upon users and carers and these may well increase the amount of distress they experience. Clearly, there are profound ethical implications that must be considered by professionals offering support within the community.

CHANGES TO TERMS AND CONDITIONS OF EMPLOYMENT OF PAID CARERS

The National Health Service and Community Care Act 1990 introduced the concept of a market driven NHS. The service was split into purchasers, comprising GP fundholders and health authorities, and providers, in the form of NHS Trusts, private and not-for-profit organizations. Both trusts and fundholders were released from NHS conditions of employment and could set their own local employment terms for their staff. Providers drew their income from contracting their services to the purchasers, with these being negotiated annually. For many employees the removal of nationally

agreed terms and conditions of employment together with contract uncertainty resulted in unclear career pathways, a requirement for 'flexible working' patterns with removal of enhanced payments, and job insecurity. In addition, the workforce underwent a skill mix review, partly driven by difficulties in recruiting qualified medical and nursing staff, and many staff were required to develop new skills.

Additional demands were made with the introduction of the Health Act 1999. Although GP fundholders were replaced by Primary Care Trusts, contracting with providers remained, albeit for a 3-year rather than an annual contract. Implementation of the Health Act, together with meeting targets set in *Saving Lives: Our Healthier Nation* (Department of Health 1999b) and the National Service Frameworks, was formalized in the *NHS Plan* (Department of Health 2000a). Here, further targets, together with plans for partnership working between health and social services, were set. The result has been a period of great change and while many opportunities have been created, the workload and career structure of staff has been challenged. Again, this emphasizes the support that many will need to manage the additional stressors brought about by changes to their employment.

MANAGING EMPLOYMENT RELATED STRESS

It is easy for employers to claim that stress management is the responsibility of the individual as it is the individual who suffers the stress. It must be remembered, though, that stress arises from the individual's reaction to the environment. Although the individual has some responsibility in managing stress, managing stress also requires adaptation of the environment.

In addition to the adverse effects on front-line staff, the stressful workplace also affects the way in which line managers perform. Due to the competitive pressure within contemporary healthcare environments, managers may be hesitant to refuse extra work on already hard-pressed resources. In this situation staff subordinate to the manager find themselves pressurized and unable to control the situation. In the short term, productivity may appear to increase as staff draw on their reserve strengths to cope. Neglecting individual employees and promoting a stressful work environment leads to an increase in burnout, however (Janssen et al 1999, Payne 2001). Consequently, in the long term this strategy becomes counterproductive, as burned out staff result in decreased productivity. Indeed, it is easy for individual employees to become lost in the organization, feeling devalued and focusing on the negative aspects of work. This is compounded when managers concentrate on the underachievement of the organization rather than remembering to praise the good points (Meadows et al 2000), a situation highlighted in *An Organization with a Memory* (Department of Health 2000b) where oppressive environments were shown to inhibit the reporting of, and learning from, incidents.

The relationship between job satisfaction and employee behaviour was explored by Brunola (1996) who found a relationship between job satisfaction and burnout. As burnout decreases the productivity of staff, it is important, she argued, to develop strategies to address this. Similarly, Payne (2001) found a negative association between productivity and burnout, observing that individuals' problem solving abilities decreased under prolonged periods of extreme distress. Both argued for employers to implement stress awareness seminars, counselling and support groups for staff, an argument developed by Northcott (1996). Nothcott maintained that employers hold two contracts with employees. The first is the formal written contract detailing the terms and conditions of employment. The second is a hidden psychological contract within which employers should focus on their responsibilities to employees. He cited the 'macho management' culture that developed following the implementation of the National Health Service and Community Care Act 1990, as a result of which individuals' needs were often ignored, leading to poor morale, difficult recruitment and poor staff performance, observations that remain valid within contemporary healthcare environments (Meadows et al 2000, Quine 1998). Addressing employees' individual needs would accordingly provide mutual long-term benefit (Cooper et al 1996).

One of the reasons that the stressful workplace evolved, both in health and social care and in other areas of work, is that stress and stress induced diseases are not classified as industrial diseases. Traditionally industrial injuries have gained compensation only where the employer's negligence has resulted in an employee's physical injury. Earnshaw & Cooper (1994) noted that where injuries were not directly measurable, such as in repetitive strain injury, the success of employees to seek redress from employers was limited. Therefore individuals who find themselves unable to work through stress induced illness, even though it may have been caused by their employer, find it difficult to obtain compensation. Recently the way stress induced diseases are viewed in law has altered, though. An increasing number of claims against employers have been successful in securing compensation for stress induced disease (Earnshaw & Cooper 1994). Indeed, in the year 2000 there were 164 000 claims for stress related illnesses. Furthermore, stress is estimated to cost £7 billion annually in lost working days and NHS costs (Cooper 2001). Stressful workplaces lead to higher absences, attrition of staff and difficulty in recruiting replacements (Meadows et al 2000, Quine 1998), in turn exacerbating the situation for those who remain and making it difficult for managers to meet their targets. Therefore, should these trends continue, then there are potentially enormous costs for employers if they continue to ignore employee stress in the workplace.

PERSONAL AND REFLECTIVE KNOWLEDGE

Decision making exercise

Reflect on your life at work and at home.

- Overall, how stressed do you feel?

  (You might like to use a scale from 1 to 10. If you repeat this regularly you can monitor the pattern of stress in your life, which can be very useful if you can't identify all the causes.)

- What stressors do you encounter?

  (When do they occur? Do they create eustress or distress)?

- What coping mechanisms do you use?

  (Include positive and well as negative coping mechanisms here.)

- Could you reduce the amount of distress in your life?
- Can you find better coping strategies?
- What support facilities are available to you?

  (Peer support, clinical supervision, counselling services?)

- How does this knowledge enhance your personal and professional roles?

BECOME AWARE OF RESPONSES TO STRESS

To consolidate the knowledge gained from this chapter you should become more aware of your own response to stress and develop your individual stress management programme, using the guidelines that follow, to include in your portfolio of learning, as experiencing your own stress awareness and developing your own stress management programme will teach you many of the skills you will need to help others during your professional practice. Finally, if you have not already done so, work through the reflective exercises.

STRESS MANAGEMENT

Stress is exacerbated by losing control. In the Care Delivery Knowledge section it was shown how effective stress management programmes use problem solving approaches to enable individuals to take control of stressors. In personal stress management, this is underpinned by efficient time management. Essential equipment comprises:

- a diary
- a year planner
- a 'to do' list.

Make it a rule that you never make an appointment without your diary and when considering buying a diary it is important to select a format that will allow you to view at least one week at a time. Those that only allow you to view one or two days at a time are of limited use in personal time management as you are unable to see new appointments

Goal	To be completed by
Complete Physiology essay	10th October
Complete Sociology essay	21st October
Complete Psychology essay	7th November
Decorate kitchen	14th November
File holiday photos in album	20th November

Figure 8.7   Goal statements.

Physiology essay	To be completed by
Literature search	10th September
Write plan	15th September
First draft	25th September
Second draft	30th September
Read second draft	5th October
Final draft	10th October

Figure 8.8   Target dates for smaller goal components.

within the context of existing commitments. Personal organizers are very useful in this respect as they often contain yearly planners with monthly and yearly views that permit comprehensive views of other commitments. The disadvantage is that information has to be entered two or three times. Many electronic organizers are becoming affordable, however, and these will update all sections automatically. Although this seems an ideal solution, if you are buying one you should make sure that there is a facility to back up the data, ideally to a PC which can access the data though its own software. Otherwise, should the batteries (or even the organizer) fail, all of your information will be lost. *Caveat emptor!*

The first items that should be entered into your diary and year planner are holidays and time for yourself. These are the most important entries you will make and should not be altered – you will need to develop assertiveness skills here. All entries other than these will compete for the remaining space. Next enter dates and times that you know are committed into your diary, work days for example.

The second stage is to list all your objectives and construct a 'to do' list. It is also helpful to give each objective a priority rating. From this list identify end goals that will allow you to fulfil your objectives and the dates by which the goals must be achieved. Figure 8.7 shows a completed list of goal statements.

Take each goal statement and break it into smaller components. Set each component a target date for completion (Fig. 8.8).

Transfer these goals onto your yearly planner. In your diary set aside time to achieve these goals. A completed diary page may then look like Figure 8.9.

Things happen in life without warning and, due to its rigid structure, this approach to time management is often criticized for being idealistic. Although this approach is highly structured, it is not inflexible. The structure is necessary as events can quickly get out of hand; however, once you are aware of what your commitments are, you are able to make adjustments to your schedule to accommodate alterations in demands on your time.

CASE STUDIES RELATED TO STRESS

Four case studies now follow. Use the knowledge you have gained from this chapter to answer the questions at the end of each one.

September	September
Monday 11th 7.30–14.30 Early shift 19.30–21.00 Write plan for biology	Thursday 14th Visit Mum and Dad for the day
Tuesday 12th 7.30–14.30 Early shift 19.30–21.00 Write plan for biology	Friday 15th 9.00–12.30 Finish plan for biology Afternoon – gardening 21.00 Going out to pub
Wednesday 13th 7.30–14.30 Early shift 19.30–21.00 Write plan for biology	Saturday 16th 12.30–21.30 Late shift Sunday 17th 7.30–14.30 Early shift

Figure 8.9   Completed diary page.

Case study: Learning disability

Robin is 32 years of age and has a moderate learning disability which prevents him from managing daily activities of living independently. He lives with his elderly parents, attending a day centre twice a week and helping around the family home on other days. He is currently attending a well-man's clinic, run by the practice nurse who has been with the practice for over 20 years. The nurse notes that Robin has a BMI of 28 and a blood pressure of 160/90 mmHg. She curtly tells Robin that he is overweight and that he should go on a diet and exercise more to lower his blood pressure.

Before the clinic, you happened to be talking to Robin's father. He had disclosed to you that both he and Robin's mother had been unwell and it had been arranged for Robin to go into respite care for a month. This will be the first time that Robin has been separated from his parents and he is not keen to go. You feel that the distress may be contributing to Robin's hypertension and mention this to the practice nurse. She replies, however, that she has no time for 'psychobabble'.

- What physiological processes would lead the current social circumstances to affect Robin's physical condition?

- How would you manage Robin's condition differently?
- Why do you think the practice nurse rejects the influence of psychosocial factors on Robin's condition?

Case study: Child

Lucy is attending the health centre for examination of her baby, Britney, of 18 months. Lucy's partner was made redundant just before Britney's birth and this led the family to have severe financial problems. To worsen matters, Lucy's partner has been unable to secure further employment and has started to drink heavily. In consequence they have experienced several major arguments and their relationship deteriorated to such an extent that 3 months ago Lucy's partner walked out.

Lucy complains to the nurse that Britney does not seem to feed properly and that she keeps waking up during the night. This means that Lucy is not getting sufficient sleep and because of this she tends to become short tempered and ends up shouting at Britney. She feels unable to cope and finds looking after Britney, shopping, cooking and keeping the house tidy impossible to do on her own.

Weighing Britney at 12 months had shown that the target of treble birth weight had not been achieved. Regular weighing since then revealed a downward trend on the percentile scale. Britney is diagnosed as failing to thrive.

- Why do you think that Britney is failing to thrive?
- How would you assess Lucy's level of stress?
- What strategies would you utilize to help Lucy and Britney?

Case study: Adult

Following the advice from her occupational health nurse, Paula (aged 28) took up swimming once a week as a method of combating stress. She had always enjoyed swimming, and when she was younger had represented her school in swimming competitions.

Paula felt refreshed from swimming and found it a positive way of relieving her stress. One day she met an old schoolfriend at the pool who suggested that she join her swimming club.

Paula joined the club and soon was persuaded to enter competitions where she was successful in winning trophies. Paula needed to train intensively to maintain her competitiveness, however, and soon found herself training for five evenings each week with competitions most weekends. In contrast to her initial intention to use swimming as a method of stress management, Paula now found that swimming was an additional stress in her life.

- At which stage was Paula experiencing eustress from her swimming activities?
- At which stage was Paula experiencing distress?
- What advice should the nurse give clients who decide to use sport as a stress relieving activity?

Case study: Mental health

Kathleen is 43 years of age and married with two daughters aged 16 and 14 years. Over the previous fortnight she has gradually become withdrawn and insular. She neglects her personal appearance and is sleeping for prolonged, irregular periods.

During the assessment the nurse used the Social Readjustment Rating Scale to explore what issues had occurred in Kathleen's life over the previous year. It emerged that Kathleen's husband, who was employed as a fitter in the local car factory, had been told that the factory was to close and that he would be made redundant. The time that the factory closure was announced coincided with the onset of Kathleen's latest relapse.

Stress is often seen to precipitate a relapse of depression (World Health Organization 1992). The redundancy of her husband was seen as a major life event resulting in stress (Holmes & Rahe 1967). This, in turn, contributed to the recurrence of Kathleen's illness.

Using the Social Readjustment Rating Scale the nurse was able to quickly focus on the redundancy of her husband and, as Kathleen became able to enter into conversation, explore ways in which Kathleen and her family would cope.

- Is the redundancy of Kathleen's husband eustress or distress?
- Think of other reasons that may be contributing to Kathleen's level of stress (which may or may not be listed on the scale).
- What are the disadvantages of the Social Readjustment Rating Scale?

Summary

This chapter has examined the concepts of stress, relaxation and rest. It has included:

1. A demonstration that, although there is a relationship between them, they are independent concepts and in practice they need to be addressed as such.
2. Strategies for managing stress and promoting relaxation.
3. An exploration of the stressors encountered by professional and informal carers.

Annotated further reading and websites

Back K Back K 1999 Assertiveness at work: a practical guide to handling awkward situations, 3rd edn. McGraw Hill, New York. A self-training book that develops concepts of assertiveness and provides suggestions for nurturing assertiveness skills. Topics include negotiation skills, being able to say 'no', dealing with negative feelings and handling criticism. It is difficult to practise and develop these skills outside an assertiveness group; however, within this limitation, this is an extremely useful book.

Butterworth T, Faugier J, Burnard P (eds) 1998 Clinical supervision and mentorship in nursing, 2nd edn. Nelson Thornes, London. A fundamental text on using clinical supervision and mentorship. The book begins by examining the supervision relationship and how clinical supervision can assist in stress management. In the following chapters, the application of clinical supervision within all branches of nursing is addressed, these being clearly illustrated with examples from practice. This is an excellent resource for supervisors and supervisees.

Martin P 2002 Counting sheep: the science and pleasures of sleep and dreams. Harper Collins, London
An examination of the processes of sleep, and of the consequences of sleep deprivation. This is an easily read book that combines research with other literature to explore the nature of sleep and dreaming, and the possible consequences for an individual's health.

Quine L 1997 Solving children's sleep problems: a step by step guide for parents. Beckett Karlson, Huntingdon.
A book primarily aimed at parents. However, this material is also useful for professionals. Derived from research, the book helps parents to understand why their child is having sleeping difficulties and details strategies to help to resolve the problems.

Enter 'STRESS' or 'RELAXATION' into an internet search engine such as Google and you will receive pages and pages of links, many of which should be treated with extreme caution. Of those that are published by credible organizations, many are located in the USA. Although these contain interesting information, they tend to be USA specific and designed for access by US citizens. Consequently, should you want to obtain local services, you may need to restrict your search to sites within your own country.

http://www.howtomanagestress.co.uk/
A UK based stress management resource hosted by the Royal and Sun Alliance Insurance Group. This is divided into an area for adults and an area for children and adolescents. Each contains information and self-help resources, and there are valid links for further information.

http://www.lboro.ac.uk/departments/hu/groups/sleep/
The Loughborough Sleep Research Centre. Has information on sleep, and sleep research. Also links to other relevant websites.

http://www.mentalhealth.org.uk/
Home page of the Mental Health Foundation. This contains information and resources on a range of mental health issues and problems. It also has a good range of links.

http://www.samaritans.org
The website for Samaritans. It contains instructions for accessing services, resources and information. Samaritans is not a counselling service. What they do offer is to listen to people and hear their feelings in times of crisis, and they are available either on-line, by telephone 24 hours a day, or by a personal visit (within certain hours).

http://www.sleephomepages.org/
A comprehensive USA based site that has resources and links for sleep research and sleep disorders.

http://www.stress.org/
Home page of the American Institute of Stress. This organization was established in 1978 and contains a wealth of information on stress and stress-related diseases.

References

Beck A T 1979 Cognitive theory of depression. Guilford Press, New York

Begat I B E, Severinsson E I, Berggren I B 1997 Implementation of clinical supervision in a medical department: nurses' views of the effects. Journal of Clinical Nursing 6(5):389–394

Borbely A 1987 Secrets of sleep. Longman, Harlow

Bosma H, Marmor M, Hemingway H et al 1997 Low job control and the risk of coronary heart disease in Whitehall II (prospective cohort) study. British Medical Journal 314:558–565

British Association of Counselling 1992 Code of ethics and practice for counsellors. British Association of Counselling, Rugby

Brosschot J F, Godaert G L R, Benschop R J et al 1998 Experimental stress and immunologocal reactivity: a closer look at perceived uncontrollability. Psychosomatic Medicine 60(3):359–361

Carlson S L 1999 An exploration of complexity and generativity as explanations of midlife women's graduate school experiences and reasons for pursuit of a graduate degree. Journal of Women and Aging 11(1):39–51

Cerrato P L 1998 Aromatherapy: is it for real? RN 61(6):51–52

Confederation of Health Service Employees 1992 Tackling stress from health care work. Confederation of Health Service Employees, Banstead

Cooper C 2001 For pity's sake stop the work, I want to get off… Online. Available: http://www.depression.org.uk/main/pdf/ telegraph.pdf 28 Apr 2003

Cooper C L, Liukkonen P, Cartwright S 1996 Stress prevention in the workplace: assessing costs and benefits to organizations. European Foundation for the Improvement of Living and Working Conditions, Loughlinstown

Cox T 1978 Stress. Macmillan, London

Department of Health 1998 Partnership in action: new opportunities for joint working between health and social services. HMSO, London

Department of Health 1999a Caring about carers: a national strategy for carers. HMSO, London

Department of Health 1999b Saving lives: our healthier nation. HMSO, London

Department of Health 2000a The NHS plan: a plan for investment, a plan for reform. HMSO, London

Department of Health 2000b An organization with a memory: report of an expert group on learning from adverse events in the NHS. HMSO, London

Department of Health 2003a Health and personal social services statistics. Online. Available: http://www.doh.gov.uk/HPSSS/ TBL_B16.HTM 28 Apr 2003

Department of Health 2003b Health and personal social services statistics. Online. Available: http://www.doh.gov.uk/HPSSS/ TBL_B23.HTM 28 Apr 2003

Department of Health and Social Security 1981 Growing older. HMSO, London

Department of Health and Social Security 1988 Community care: agenda for action (Griffiths Report). HMSO, London

Earnshaw J, Cooper C L 1994 Employee stress litigation: the UK experience. Work and Stress 8(4):287–295

Fawzy F I, Fawzy N W, Hyun C S et al 1993 Malignant melanoma: effects of an early structured psychiatric intervention, coping, and affective state on recurrence and survival 6 years later. Archives of General Psychiatry 50(9):681–689

Fisher P L, Durham R C 1999 Recovery rates in generalized anxiety disorder following psychological therapy: an analysis of clinically significant change in the STAI-T across outcome studies since 1990. Psychological Medicine 29(6):1425–1434

Folkard S 1991 Circadian rhythms and hours of work. In: Warr P (ed) Psychology of work, 3rd edn. Penguin, Harmondsworth

Freud S 1934 The ego and the mechanisms of defence. Chatto & Windus, London

Friedman M, Rosenman R H 1974 Type A behaviour and your heart. Knopf, New York

Harris P E 1989 The nurse stress index. Work and Stress 3(4):335–346

Hay D 1987 Exploring inner space: scientists and religious experience. Mowbray, London

Health Act 1999 HMSO, London

Hebb D O 1954 Drives and the conceptual nervous system. In: Bindra D, Stewart J (eds) Motivation. Penguin, Harmondsworth

Hobson C J, Kamen J, Szostek J et al 1998 Stressful life events: a revision and update of the social readjustment rating scale. International Journal of Stress Management 5(1):1–23

Hodgson L A 1991 Why do we need sleep? Relating theory to nursing practice. Journal of Advanced Nursing 16:1503–1510

Holmes T H, Rahe R H 1967 The social readjustment rating scale. Journal of Psychosomatic Research 11:213–218

Horne J A 1988 Why we sleep: the functions of sleep in human and other mammals. Oxford University Press, Oxford

Howard D 2001 Changes in nursing students' out of college relationships arising from the Diploma of Higher Education in nursing. Active Learning in Higher Education 3(1):68–87

Janssen P M, Schaufeli W B, Houkes I 1999 Work-related and individual determinants of the three burnout dimensions. Work and Stress 13(1):74–86

Kitrell D 1998 A comparison of the evolution of men's and women's dreams in Daniel Levinson's theory of adult development. Journal of Adult Development 5(2):105–115

Kubler Ross E 1975 Death: the final stage of growth. Prentice Hall, London

Lazarus R S, Delongis A, Folkman S et al 1985 Stress and adaptational outcomes: the problem of confounded measures. American Psychologist 40:770–779

Legault S E, Freeman M R, Langer A et al 1995 Pathophysiology and time course of silent myocardial ischaemia during mental stress: clinical, anatomical, and physiological correlates. British Heart Journal 73(3):242–249

Levi L, Lunde-Jensen P 1996 A model for assessing the costs of stressors at national level: socioeconomic costs of work stress in two EU member states. European Foundation for the Improvement of Living and Working Conditions, Dublin

Lichtenstein P, Gatz M, Berg S 1998 A twin study of mortality after spousal bereavement. Psychological Medicine 28(3):635–643

Linde K M 1996 St John's wort for depression: an overview and meta-analysis of randomized clinical trials. British Medical Journal 313 (7052):253–258

Maslach C 1982 Burnout: the cost of caring. Prentice Hall, Englewood Cliffs

Matrunola P 1996 Is there a relationship between job satisfaction and absenteeism? Journal of Advanced Nursing 23:827–834

Meadows S, Levenson R, Baeza J 2000 The last straw: explaining the NHS nurse shortage. Kings Fund, London

Narayanasamy A 1996 Spiritual care of chronically ill patients. British Journal of Nursing 5(7):411–416

Narayanasamy A, Owens J 2001 A critical incident study of nurses' responses to the spiritual needs of their patients. Journal of Advanced Nursing 33(4):446–455

National Health Service and Community Care Act 1990 HMSO, London

Northcott N 1996 Contracts for good morale. Nursing Management 3(3):23

Norton L S, Thomas S, Morgan K et al 1998 Full-time studying and long-term relationships: make or break for mature students? British Journal of Guidance and Counselling 26(1):75–88

Payne N 2001 Occupational stressors and coping as determinants of burnout in female hospice nurses. Journal of Advanced Nursing 33(3):396–405

Pruessner J C, Hellhammer D H, Kirschbaum C 1999 Low self-esteem, induced failure and the adrenocortical stress response. Personality and Individual Differences 27(3):477–489

Quine L 1998 Effects of stress in an NHS trust: a study. Nursing Standard 13(3):36–41

Reich W P, Parrella D P, Filstead W J 1988 Unconfounding the hassle's scale: external sources versus internal responses to stress. Journal of Behavioral Medicine 11:239–250

Rhead M M 1995 Stress among student nurses: is it practical or academic? Journal of Clinical Nursing 4(6):369–376

Seyle H 1984 The stress of life. McGraw-Hill, New York

Sims A, Owens D 1993 Psychiatry, 6th edn. Baillière Tindall, London

Sutherland V J, Cooper C L 1990 Understanding stress: a psychological perspective for health professionals. Chapman & Hall, London

Totman R 1990 Mind stress and health. Souvenir Press, London

UK Central Council 1996 Position statement on clinical supervision for nursing, midwifery and health visiting. Online. Available: http://www.nmc-uk.org/cms/content/publications/Position%20statement%20on%20clinical%20supervision%20for%20nursing,%20etc.asp. 28 Apr 2003

Vernarec E 2001 How to cope with job stress. RN 64(3):44–46

Welch I D, Medeiros D C, Tate G A 1982 Beyond burnout: how to enjoy your job again when you've just about had enough. Prentice Hall, Englewood Cliffs

White E, Butterworth T, Bishop V et al 1998 Clinical supervision: insider reports of a private world. Journal of Advanced Nursing 28(1):185–192

Wong A H C 1998 Herbal remedies in psychiatric practice. Archives of General Psychiatry 55(11):1033–1044

World Health Organization 1992 The ICD-10 classification of mental and behavioural disorder. World Health Organization, Geneva

Chapter 9

Medicines

Carol Hall

KEY ISSUES

SUBJECT KNOWLEDGE

- A nursing definition of 'medicine'
- The action of medicine upon the body
- Potential non-therapeutic action by medicines
- Calculation of medicine dosages
- Routes of medicine administration

CARE DELIVERY KNOWLEDGE

- Practice knowledge for storage and administration of medicines in safety using application of research evidence
- Assessing clients in relation to medicine administration
- Planning to administer a medicine
- How medication administration can be evaluated

PROFESSIONAL AND ETHICAL KNOWLEDGE

- How errors in administration can be effectively managed
- The legal acts governing the storage and administration of medicines in the UK
- Prescribing medicines
- Moral and ethical dilemmas that can arise within the practice of medicines' administration

PERSONAL AND REFLECTIVE KNOWLEDGE

- Application of principles of medicines administration across all branches of nursing
- Awareness of personal position in both the giving and the using of medicines

INTRODUCTION

In most healthcare settings, medicines need to be administered to some of the client group for whom there is responsibility. This chapter explores the major issues in nurse decision making about administering medicines. It also introduces associated elements related to licensing, prescribing and dispensing medicinal treatment.

A broad concept of 'administration' includes many different component parts without which the nursing act of giving a medicine safely and effectively would be impossible. By this definition, there is a need to address issues related to the preparation required to give a medicine and also any follow-up management. This will include knowledge for understanding the way medicines are able to enter the body and the effects that may occur both therapeutically and non-therapeutically as a result of treatment. Although it is not possible to offer comprehensive advice related to individual medications in this respect, some common groups of medicines will be considered. For more detail, annotated further reading is provided. Administration may involve educating other carers to give medicines or educating clients to self-administer medicines. There is also a role in health promotion with regard to the safe handling and storage of medicines in both hospital and community settings. Finally, the nurse can facilitate understanding of the effects of the use of medicines socially, including public use of both 'over the counter' preparations and illegal substances. Legal and professional issues also need to be taken into consideration. The position of the nurse as both a professional and a member of the public is thus explored.

OVERVIEW

Subject knowledge

The physical aspects related to treatment with medicines are introduced, with a particular emphasis upon the mechanical and biological bases. Here, classification of medication by type is examined, followed by a consideration of the possible routes of administration, calculation of correct doses and how the body deals with medication. Further reading is offered and viewed as an essential development.

Wider psychosocial aspects of medicine use are included, with a consideration of the potential for abuse of medication and the societal impact of drugs today.

Care delivery knowledge

The role of the nurse in the provision of medicines for clients is explored. The discussion relates specifically to decision making in the assessment, planning, implementing and evaluation of total care. It is intended that this section should lead to a deeper understanding of a nursing practice role.

Professional and ethical knowledge

This part addresses issues related to legality and accountability, as well as examining ethical issues in the administration of medicines. Incidents such as errors in medication are explored and discussed in detail. Contemporary guidance relating to the eligibility of nurses to prescribe medicines is outlined, and resources are offered for further knowledge development in this area.

Personal and reflective knowledge

Throughout the chapter you are encouraged to think reflectively over issues related to the care of clients. It is anticipated that concepts raised throughout the chapter will be applied as a knowledge base for nursing practice.

As a starting point, application of these principles is facilitated through exemplar case studies with reflective questions. On pages 217–218 there are four case studies, each relating to one of the branches of nursing. You may find it helpful to read one of them before you start the chapter and use it as a focus for your reflections while reading. Of course, you should also explore examples from your own experience.

SUBJECT KNOWLEDGE

BIOLOGICAL

THE PHYSICAL BASIS OF MEDICINE ADMINISTRATION

Defining a medicine

When examining nursing issues related to the medicinal treatment of clients, it is found that there has been much debate about what constitutes a medicine, and also what constitutes an appropriate role for nurses in treating their clients. Indeed, such was the confusion over terminology and definition in this area of nursing practice, the Department of Health in their first Review of Prescribing, Supply and Administration of Medicines (1999) produced a glossary of

terminology to help facilitate a clear definition of what a medicine might be. Most authors now, however, recognize that a medicine is a substance that is used for therapeutic, diagnostic or preventative purposes (Hopkins 1999, Mallett & Doughty 2000). This definition thus provides a simple base for discussion.

Product licensing

Medications are issued a licence by law in the UK and similar arrangements are in place elsewhere in the world. The product licence stipulates which routes of administration are considered to be safe for its given strength and constitution and the client group who are considered within the licence. Details of any product licence agreement can be found within the guidance details included in the medicine packaging, and these should be adhered to in order to ensure clients' safety. If, as may happen, a medicine is prescribed that has no national product licence then this is considered to be prescribed 'off licence'. If a medicine is prescribed outside of the guidance included within the national licence, then this is considered to be 'off label'. Whilst the use of off licence and off label medication is generally not advised, it is accepted by the healthcare professions to be occasionally inevitable. There are implications in accepting this kind of prescribing, and these are addressed within professional issues later in this chapter. However, advice is given to nurses about such use within *Guidance for Administration of Medicines* (Nursing and Midwifery Council 2002a).

In addition to the product licence, all medications are issued with both a generic and a brand name. The brand name is the one by which the product is marketed, while the generic name is the name used in prescribing. Health carers should use the generic names, whilst being mindful of different brands.

Classification of medicines

Medicines can be classified two ways. Firstly, there is the legal classification of medicines, which categorizes medicines according to requirements governing their supply to the general public. This type of classification derives from the Medicines Act 1968, and will be addressed in more detail in the Professional Knowledge part of this chapter.

Secondly, and less formally, there have been attempts to classify medicines into groups that indicate the effect on a body system, the symptoms relieved, or the desired effect of the medication (e.g. Downie et al 1999, Hopkins 1999, Trounce 2000). In fact it probably does not matter, and is as much personal preference as anything else.

A comprehensive list of medicines and their side effects would be inappropriate in a chapter such as this and indeed reference to formularies such as the *British National Formulary* (BNF) (British Medical Association and the Royal Pharmaceutical Society of Great Britain 2003), the *Nurse*

Table 9.1 A framework for classifying medicines

Type of treatment or area	Name of medicine and brief notes for future reference
Cardiovascular	
Respiratory	
Gastrointestinal tract	
Renal	
Central nervous system	
Analgesic	
Hypnotic	
Psychotropic	
Anaesthetic	
Blood	
Infection	
Antibiotic (or bactericidal/ bacteriostatic/antiseptic)	
Antifungal	
Antiviral	
Immunization	
Vitamin, fluid or electrolyte imbalance	
Hormone or endocrine imbalance	
Cytotoxic treatment	

Prescriber's Formulary (British Medical Association 2002), or *Medicines for Children* (Royal College of Paediatrics and Child Health 2003) is recommended. However, it is acknowledged that a clear framework for categorizing drugs for further reference can be useful. The framework in Table 9.1 has been devised to assist nurses and students working and studying in practice. Although it must be emphasized that no nurse should give medications they are not familiar with, it is sometimes helpful to jot down notes about medications. By carrying this framework into the practice area, medicines may be noted down as you discover them in use, allowing access for revision and more in-depth study at a later date.

Decision making exercise

1. In your practice identify one medicine used within each of the classifications in the framework in Table 9.1 and find out all you can about it using the references for further reading identified at the end of the chapter. If possible, reflect on the exercise with colleagues.
2. Use your findings to discuss what factors may influence a nursing decision not to give an identified medicine to a client.
3. Although a useful way of identifying individual uses for medications, the above framework categories are not mutually exclusive.

Looking at your list, can you identify any medication that may fit into more than one of the above categories? What does this tell you about using this drug therapeutically?

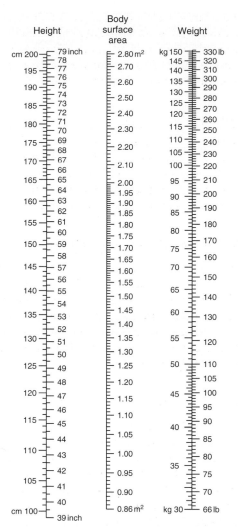

Figure 9.1 A nomogram of body surface area for adults. Directions: (1) find the patient's height; (2) find weight; (3) draw straight line connecting height and weight; (4) the point at which this line intersects the BSA column gives the patient's body surface area in square metres. (Reproduced with kind permission from Geigy Scientific Tables 1990, 8th edn, vol. 5, p. 105, © Novartis.)

CALCULATING MEDICINE DOSES

Calculation of a therapeutic yet safe dose of any medication is achieved by weighing the client and determining a safe dose per kilogram or by calculating the client's body surface area. In critical care areas a nomogram (see example: Fig. 9.1) can be used to determine surface area.

Medicines prescribed regularly in an adult setting may be appropriate for a wide range of clients and are often prescribed in a form that is held as stock by the pharmacist. For instance, an antibiotic such as ampicillin may be prescribed as a 250 milligram (mg) dose. The pharmacist sends stock capsules, which are 250 mg in strength so that the client requires one capsule. However, where children or the elderly are concerned, or where medication is particularly toxic, the dose can be calculated according to the weight of the client in milligrams per kilogram as recommended by the pharmaceutical

$$\frac{\text{What is required (prescribed dose)}}{\text{What is available (stock dose)}} \times \frac{\text{Available dilution}}{\text{(stock volume)}}$$

So if the dose prescribed is 500 mg of amoxicillin and the stock dose is 250 mg per one tablet (volume), the calculation is:

$$\frac{500}{250} \times 1 = 2 \text{, so two tablets are given}$$

Figure 9.2   Dose calculation formula.

$$\frac{\text{Fluid volume prescribed (ml)} \times \text{Drops per ml (on giving set)}}{\text{Duration of infusion (minutes)}} = \text{Drops per minute}$$

For example, if a man was prescribed 120 ml of medication over 1 hour delivered using an administration set giving 15 drops ml:

$$\frac{120 \times 15}{60} = 30 \text{ drops per minute}$$

If a child was prescribed 60 ml of medication over 1 hour through a set giving 20 drops per ml then:

$$\frac{60 \times 20}{60} = 20 \text{ drops per minute}$$

Figure 9.3   Calculating infusion rate.

company. This may not conveniently fall into a stock dose. Once a dose has been ascertained, it is up to the nurse to decide that the prescription is correct and ensure that it is given. This means a further calculation may be necessary. A formula for calculating medicines is shown in Figure 9.2.

Medicine doses are calculated using the metric system and are described in units of this system. When performing any calculation it is important that you ensure that the same unit is used for the stock and the prescribed dose. If the prescribed dose is in milligrams and the stock dose is only available in grams (g), then the stock dose needs to be converted into milligrams before a calculation can take place (see Annotated Further Reading for more information).

In summary it is essential to apply principles of mathematics in developing skills in administering medicines. Some elements that must be achieved effectively include:

- adding and subtracting
- multiplication and division
- conversion of Standardized International (SI) units (e.g. converting from micrograms to milligrams)
- conversion of SI units to fractions
- estimation, proportion and rounding
- using formulae to calculate drug doses and milligrams of medication per kilogram body weight.

It is true to say that many nurses find mathematics quite difficult. However, help is at hand. It is most important for a safe practitioner to be aware of their strengths and weaknesses and seek out help when necessary. Sources of help

might include personal tutors or mentors in placement, an online facility, such as that offered by learndirectuk (see section on websites at the end of the chapter) or one of the many text books written specifically for nurses (e.g. Gatford & Philips 2002). Universities and colleges also have study support facilities that can be accessed by students.

Calculating intravenous infusion rate

Once the correct dose of medicine is calculated, it may be necessary to make a last calculation to ensure the correct rate of delivery to the client, particularly if administration is via infusion, where a flow valve or an infusion pump may be used. If an infusion pump is available, the rate of delivery can be set and the nurse's role is primarily concerned with observing the client and monitoring the equipment. However, if there is no pump available, the rate of infusion may be set manually. To do this, the volume in millilitres (mL) contained in each droplet must be identified. Division of the rate required per hour by the volume of the droplets and then by 60 will enable determination of millilitres to be administered per minute and this can then be counted out (Fig. 9.3). Note that administration sets vary in droplet volume and it is extremely important to check details on the packaging of the administration set.

Decision making exercise

1. Mrs Johnson, an elderly lady, is found to be unwell while taking prescribed digoxin. The dose is reduced from 125 micrograms (μg) to 62.5 micrograms twice daily. On the ward the stock solution of digoxin is 50 micrograms/mL.

   Try to decide how much Mrs Johnson should receive at one dose.

2. Mrs Johnson is later prescribed intravenous antibiotics for a chest infection. She is to receive amikacin sulphate 150 mg infused in 100 mL of dextrose saline over 1 hour via a volumetric pump.

   At what rate should the infusion pump be set? (Check your answers with a nurse or nurse teacher to see if you are right.)

MEDICINES ADMINISTRATION

Routes of administration

Nurses have a useful contribution to make in their knowledge of what preparations of medication are available and appropriate for their clients, and they are uniquely aware of their clients' needs as a result of client assessment. When selecting a route for administration the nurses and doctors must work with the client to provide an optimum treatment programme that is safe and acceptable (Table 9.2).

Table 9.2 Routes for administration of medicine

Route	Notes
Oral	Including anything swallowed to the stomach or via nasogastric tubes
Sublingual/buccal	Allowed to dissolve under the tongue or in the cheek
Topical/local application	Including application into eyes, ears, or insertion into vagina, rectum
Transdermal	Through slow release patches adhered to the skin
Inhalation	Including via masks, nebulizers, breathing tubes
Intravenously/ intra-arterially	Administered into a vein or artery by a doctor or nurse with appropriate advanced qualifications
Subcutaneously/ subdermal	By injection under the cutaneous or dermal skin layers
Intramuscularly	By injection into muscle layers
Intrathecally	Administered by a doctor into the thecal cavity via a lumbar puncture procedure
Intraosseously	Administered by doctor into bone cavity (used for urgent access)
Other	It is possible for doctors to use other routes (e.g. into body cavities such as the pleural space or peritoneal cavity) in specific circumstances

Reflection and portfolio evidence

There are many different routes that can be selected for administration, as shown in Table 9.2. Think about a recent practice experience where a medication was given.

- What route was used?
- Was this the only possible way to give this medicine or could other routes have been selected?
- What are the issues if more than one route were possible?
- Record your findings in your portfolio.

Pharmacokinetics

The study of pharmacokinetics considers how a drug is processed as it passes through the body. The main phases of pharmacokinetic action are:

- absorption
- distribution
- metabolism
- excretion.

Absorption

Medication given is absorbed from the point of administration and into the cardiovascular system. Unless the medication is given by another route (thus bypassing this phase), nurses must be aware of the effects of the medicine in the effectiveness of absorption, and also the potential effect of the medicine at the site where it is being absorbed. With oral medication, consideration must include the effects of gastric secretion upon the efficacy of the drug and the potential effects of the medication upon the client's gastrointestinal tract.

Absorption of topical medications

With the administration of topical medications, there is usually an expectation that the desired effect will predominate at the local site. However, the potential for long-acting absorption of medication systemically is recognized in some situations. Transdermal patches are one example; these slowly release medications such as progesterone and oestrogens for hormone replacement therapy, or nicotine to aid in the cessation of smoking. Nurses caring for patients using topically applied products must consider what effect (if any) the absorption of such medication may have upon a client's systemic well-being, especially if the intended action is purely a local one.

Distribution

Once in the cardiovascular circulation, the medication is carried to its site of action. Again, there are areas of nursing knowledge that are important for consideration. It is useful to understand how the treatment is carried in the blood, since many medicines are bound tightly to plasma proteins while others are not. If a medicine has a high affinity for plasma proteins it may be necessary to give a large dose of the medication to achieve a therapeutic effect since only the proportion of the medicine that is not bound to the plasma proteins can be used effectively. Commonly used medicines with a high affinity for plasma proteins (more than 80% bound) include the antidepressant amitriptyline, and the anxiolytic diazepam. Other medicines with a high affinity for plasma proteins are propanolol, warfarin, furosemide (frusemide) and the antibiotics erythromycin and rifampicin. A comprehensive review of protein bound medications is offered by Kee & Hayes (1993).

When planning to administer medicines, a factor that may affect the client's concentration of plasma proteins should be considered. This is because an individual with a reduced albumin concentration may be at risk of toxicity if a dose of medication with a high affinity for plasma protein is given. In a classic study, increasing age was shown to reduce the amount of plasma protein by up to 20% (Loi & Vestel 1988) while malnutrition is also implicated in the reduction of circulating plasma proteins.

Other issues that should be considered in relation to the distribution of medication via the cardiovascular system include the rate and volume of perfusion to the desired area as any reduction in access to the required site may reduce the impact of the treatment offered. Additionally some areas of the body are protected from receiving many medications as a result of physiological barriers. The brain is one such area as the meninges around the central nervous system create a blood–brain barrier. Another area that selectively reduces the passage of substances is evident during pregnancy when the placenta offers a barrier between mother and baby. However, it should be noted that some substances may pass through these barriers. In nursing, the implications of the effectiveness of such barriers must be addressed when making informed decisions about nursing care. It is critical to assess the possibility of pregnancy in all premenopausal women who require medicinal treatment, with particular awareness of the potentially hazardous effects in causing fetal abnormalities of drugs such as phenytoin and tetracyclines, which can pass the placental barrier. Finally, the distribution of medication to infants via maternal breastmilk must also be acknowledged. In some cases medication given to the mother may be safe for her, but can have toxic effects on the baby. For more information about the effects of specific medications in breastfeeding please refer to the Annotated Further Reading at the end of the chapter.

Decision making exercise

Jack Harvey, aged 85 years, is in hospital following a recent diagnosis of congestive cardiac failure. He has been prescribed propanolol, but after a few days his heart rate drops to less than 60 beats/min (compared to a more usual 80 beats/min) and he complains of feeling unwell.

1. What may be wrong with Jack?
2. Within coronary care, there is a variety of medicines that act upon the heart in different ways. Propanolol is a beta blocker. Find out how beta blockers work and compare their action with that of the digitalis group of medicines.
3. What special considerations might you need to remember when administering medicines to clients who are elderly?

Metabolism

Metabolism (or breakdown) of any medication usually occurs in the liver (hepatic system). This may be therapeutic, in aiding the removal of active medication from the body by rendering it to inactive waste metabolites, or may hinder the effects of treatment, depending upon when such metabolism takes place. This issue is particularly pertinent when considering medicines that are administered orally, since much absorption via the gastrointestinal tract results in direct passage to the liver through the hepatic portal vein. In this situation the liver metabolizes a proportion of the medication (which varies between medications), before the medication reaches the cardiovascular circulation and is transported to the site of therapeutic benefit. This is known as 'first pass' metabolism, and although sometimes such a metabolism may be beneficial, as the metabolites themselves may have a therapeutic function, often it reduces the available therapeutic dose of medication by inactivating it. First pass metabolism is reduced in individuals with impaired hepatic function, and this is vital knowledge for nursing consideration in order to maintain the safety and well-being of the patient.

Finally, it is important to understand that it is possible to overload the liver with toxins resulting from the breakdown of medication as well as other substances such as alcohol, and this leads initially to an inability of the liver to cope effectively. If the liver continues to be overloaded with toxins over a prolonged period or is subjected to recurrent episodes of overload, damage may occur. This creates a permanently reduced hepatic function.

When considering administration to infants and young children, it is essential to recognize that in the young the ability to detoxify medicines is not mature, and therefore extreme caution should be taken when checking for an appropriate dose.

Excretion

After a variable period of time in the body the medication given to the client will be excreted. This is mostly via the kidneys, although other routes of excretion include the lungs, via bile into faeces, and in lactating mothers, breastmilk. There may also be some excretion through sweat glands onto the skin surface (Downie et al 1999). Perhaps the most important factor in medicine excretion, however, is the speed at which it is lost from the body. The balance between absorption and excretion determines the half-life of a medicine. This is the time it takes for the concentration of the medicine in the plasma to fall by 50% (Hopkins 1999). Clearly, a medicine with a long half-life can accumulate easily within the plasma. Those medicines that are particularly problematic are monitored carefully through checking blood plasma levels to ensure that plasma levels do not become dangerously high.

An important consideration for nurses, therefore, relates to factors about the client that may affect the response and half-life of a medicine. For example, clients who are at the extremes of the age continuum or have renal impairment require particular consideration. The infant does not develop full renal and urinary tract function until after the first year of life, while the renal function of the elderly (over 80 years of age) deteriorates to about half the capacity of a young adult (Trounce 2000).

Renal impairment can affect the excretion of medicines from the body, resulting in a build-up of metabolites, or in some instances medicines, in the circulation. A knowledge of such possibilities may alert you to making a decision to include specific points for observation related to medication in the client's plan of care. The Nursing and Midwifery Council (2002a) identify that knowledge of the client's history and plan of care combined with an awareness of the way in which specific medications may act is vital in providing safe nursing care in all areas of practice.

A full introduction to factors that may affect the response of medication can be found in Trounce (2000: Chs 1 and 22) and Downie et al (1999: Ch. 2).

Decision making exercise

Simon is severely learning disabled and has difficulty in maintaining urinary continence due to poor bladder tone causing retention of urine and dribbling incontinence. He is cared for by his mother who maintains that clean intermittent catheterization techniques aid Simon's urinary continence, but he occasionally develops urinary tract infections. Simon's mother, whilst managing his infection, comments to the practice nurse that Simon's urine smells of the current antibiotic treatment and wonders why.

1. How could you reassure Simon's mother that all is well?
2. Find out how antibiotics work and what broad classifications can be identified.
3. In a society that does not tolerate ill health, people are inclined to ask for antibiotics for minor infections. Reflect for a few minutes about the impact this may have in the long term.

Pharmacodynamics

Once a medicine has reached the site of therapeutic benefit it is able to exert a physiological effect before being excreted by the body. This is identified as pharmacodynamic action, and examination of this action of medicines in the body is comprehensively addressed within specific pharmacology texts such as Downie et al (1999). A more detailed consideration is presented by Waller et al (2001). It is important to realize, however, that even with today's rapidly advancing understanding of medical science, the frontiers of clinical pharmacology are still being extended (Trounce 2000).

POTENTIAL ADVERSE EFFECTS OF ADMINISTERING MEDICINES TO CLIENTS

Although the aim of using medicinal treatments for clients may be therapeutic, diagnostic or preventive, it is simplistic to believe that all medicines given are completely therapeutic in all cases. For both nursing and medicine the aim has always been recognized as 'To do the client no harm' (Nightingale 1859) or to 'First do no harm' (Hippocrates, cited by Manley et al 1994). This next section will explore potential threats to such ideals.

Gaining a therapeutic dose

In order for medicine to be effective, the dose for your client must be sufficient to be effective, but not too much, in which case the client may risk toxicity or poisoning. Factors in achieving a therapeutic dose are related to nursing and medical skill in prescribing and calculating the correct dose of medication and also the pharmacokinetic and pharmacodynamic capacity of the client. This may be related to their age, lifestyle or health condition, as highlighted above. However, even with a therapeutically assessed dose of medication, the response of individual clients can vary significantly, and thus a potentially useful medicine may be harmful. Nurse decision making contributes to risk reduction associated with the administration of medicines, and the identification of potential adverse effects is essential. Some potential adverse effects arising when giving a therapeutic medication are identified in Table 9.3.

As well as the adverse effects of giving any single medication to an individual, external influences may also cause damage. Clients may already be taking other medications that could interact with new treatment, causing adverse effects or altering the pharmacokinetic or pharmacodynamic action of either medication. A common outcome is a reduced or halted action (antagonism), which may be useful for use as an antidote, preventing the action of a medication once it has been given, or a potentiated action (synergism). Other reactions are also possible and for a comprehensive listing of currently known interactions see the *British National Formulary* (British Medical Association 2003).

Polypharmacy

An interaction between different drugs, as described above, may not be restricted to two substances, but may involve a multiplicity of medical treatments. This type of interaction is known as 'polypharmacy', and is documented in the healthcare literature, particularly in relation to the elderly (Hohl et al 2001).

Evidence based practice

Hohl et al (2001) examined the 300 patients aged over 65 years attending an Accident and Emergency department. They found that 90.8% were taking one or more medications prescribed over the counter. The average number of medications taken was 4.2 but the number varied between 0 and 17. Adverse drug related events were also reviewed as a reason for A and E department attendance. It was found that 10.6% of admissions had this reason cited for their attendance. The researchers concluded that adverse drug related incidents were an expensive and challenging public health problem, and a significant cause of admission to A and E departments.

Table 9.3   Potential adverse effects of medicines

Adverse effect/side effect	Nature of reaction
Idiosyncrasy	Often genetically determined
Hypersensitivity/allergy	May be life-threatening (anaphylaxis)
Skin reactions	Pruritus (itching) Urticaria (nettle rash) Erythematous eruptions (flushing and skin rashes) Skin peeling Eczematous lesions
Blood dyscrasias	Aplastic anaemia (due to bone marrow suppression) Thrombocytopenia (loss of platelets) Agranulocytosis (loss of white blood cells)
Gastrointestinal upset	Diarrhoea Dyspepsia Ulceration Nausea Vomiting Sore or dry mouth Anal pruritus Flatulence Abdominal pain
Central nervous system upset	Drowsiness Headache Dizziness Nausea Vomiting Tinnitus
Photosensitivity	Acute ocular sensitivity to light
Tolerance	The client responds increasingly less effectively to a regular dose of medication
Dependence	The client may become addicted to the medication

Although polypharmacy is more commonly identified in the older population because an increase in medicinal treatment is perhaps more linked to age related problems, it is not exclusive to this age group. There are therefore implications for all nursing personnel involved in taking client histories or in starting a new programme of medicinal treatment. Decisions regarding the likely response to treatment must be made in an informed and reflective way, and in order to do this the nurse's assessment must involve a thorough understanding of the information gained. In the case of the administration of multiple medicines to treat a client, this may mean close collaboration between medical, nursing and pharmacy teams as well as using databases such as the

British National Formulary, and the *Nurse Prescriber's Formulary* in order to become fully informed about the specific risks of polypharmacy to individual clients.

The role of the pharmacist

The responsibility of the pharmacist both in hospital and in the community is to ensure that any medications dispensed can be taken safely by the individual for whom they are prescribed. Within the hospital setting the pharmacist checks the client's prescription and can observe any possible effects of combining prescribed medications inappropriately. However, this is much more difficult within the community. Pharmacists must ask clients about other medications and point out any specific care that should be taken when using a prescribed medication. Many pharmacies have a computerized database of medicines dispensed for clients, thus allowing them to build up a clearer picture of a client's overall treatment. However, this type of system relies on the client using the same pharmacy outlet to obtain all their prescriptions. Ultimately, the client is responsible for informing those prescribing, dispensing or managing their medicinal treatment about any other medicines already being used.

Decision making exercise

Mrs Johnson was found to be nutritionally anaemic although she had been taking iron preparations prescribed by her general practitioner for some months. When informed about her anaemia, Mrs Johnson was adamant that she took her iron supplements and seemed quite angry that they did not appear to work. She complained that they gave her terrible indigestion leading her to take yet more medicine, and she showed her nurse a bottle of magnesium trisilicate, which she had bought from her local pharmacy without prescription. Since she had not thought it to be a 'proper' medicine she had not mentioned its use.

1. Identify the significance of the relationship between the two medicines taken by Mrs Johnson.
2. How could you use this information to offer health education to Mrs Johnson?
3. Reflect over the times when you have taken prescribed medications: have you ever taken any over the counter medication at the same time? Did you inform your doctor about what you were taking? Did your doctor or the dispensing pharmacist ask you if you were taking any other medicines?

Teratogenesis and iatrogenesis

When considering the possible effects of medicines on the body, it is not just the interaction between the client and medicine or between two medicines that can cause problems. Additionally there may be occasions when other factors such as the current health state of the client or issues associated with lifestyle may engender hidden dangers when combined with an otherwise acceptable treatment. The outcome of such problems may be described in two ways. First there is teratogenesis, which occurs in the treatment of women during or before pregnancy. The teratogenic outcome would be malformation or death of the unborn child. Perhaps the best-known example of this situation was the treatment of women with the anti-emetic thalidomide in the early 1960s for morning sickness. Although a highly effective anti-emetic, thalidomide was found to cause amelia (absence of limbs) during fetal development, leading to tragedy for many families whose children suffered as a result of this treatment.

A second problem is iatrogenesis, or the causing of sickness or injury as a result of treatment. Any side effect may be considered for inclusion, although usually more serious effects that may cause a need for treatment are highlighted. This situation may seem inconceivable to the nursing student who is advised about the benefits of treatment and assured that they should above all do no harm. However, this is a simplistic view of a complex issue and a balance of benefits versus harm may be a more reasonable stance to take. To ensure optimum safety and well-being for clients, you have a duty to understand the possible implications of treatment and to advise your clients so that they can make informed choices about proposed interventions.

Although nurses generally involve themselves in the use of prescription medicines for therapeutic, diagnostic or preventive benefit, many other substances may be used by clients. In this section, the use of substances that may not be prescribed by a medical practitioner are briefly explored, both in relation to the health of the individual and in relation to you as a nurse and as a member of society.

Decision making exercise

Ahmed, aged 6 years, was diagnosed as having leukaemia and his family wished him to receive current medicinal treatment as a potentially life-saving measure, although Ahmed said that he felt 'alright' before his treatment. After his treatment, however, Ahmed was sick and miserable, and his mouth became ulcerated and sore for a while. The doctors prescribed Ahmed further medicinal treatment to help alleviate his symptoms.

1. Was it right to offer Ahmed and his family treatment that would make him ill?
2. What are your personal beliefs about treatment for Ahmed?
3. How could your own personal beliefs affect the support you give Ahmed and his family through this difficult time in his treatment?

PSYCHOSOCIAL

CLIENT USE OF NON-PRESCRIBED SUBSTANCES

Whilst a medicine has been identified within this chapter as something that is for therapeutic, diagnostic or preventative purposes, there is an issue concerning who decides on such benefits. In hospital settings, medications are prescribed by nursing and medical staff whose qualifications permit them to make an informed decision and offer their clients appropriate advice about their treatment.

In modern society, however, many 'unprescribed' yet socially acceptable substances are used by the public. These may be used unwittingly as part of a social norm, or for a perceived therapeutic effect. Substances such as tobacco, coffee and alcohol, as well as over the counter preparations such as analgesics, cold cures, antihistamines or vitamins to name but a few are used commonly by the public. These substances may pose a risk to the health of particular individuals or may interact with prescribed medical treatments (Cnattingius et al 2000, Weathermon & Crabb 1999). Alternative therapies may also be adopted.

For nurses, pharmacists and doctors alike there is a challenge in ensuring that all clients receive health education about the medicines they receive and about the effects of interaction with other substances.

Reflection and portfolio exercise

Think back over the past week. How many times have you had:

- an alcoholic drink
- a cup of coffee or tea
- a cigarette or cigar
- a throat sweet or cough or cold cure
- an aspirin or paracetamol tablet
- a vitamin or iron tablet
- an oral contraceptive pill
- any non-prescription treatments?

Look at the above list. Reflect over which (if any) items:

1. Would be unsafe if inadvertently ingested by a child?
2. May, if taken in sustained amounts on a regular basis, eventually lead to physical damage to organs in the body?
3. May, if taken in sustained amounts on a regular basis lead to psychological dependence?

Use the formularies to find out whether you are right. Make a summary for your portfolio.

Poisoning

In nursing children, it is perhaps particularly important to be aware of the presence of medicinal substances in the home. There are also a myriad of other substances such as cleaning agents, especially those containing caustic soda (e.g. dishwasher powder), fertilizers and weedkillers (e.g. paraquat), which may be extremely dangerous to a child if accessed inappropriately. Many children are admitted to hospital every year following the inappropriate use of common substances leading to poisoning. Children's nurses and health visitors have a role in educating parents and families about safety in home storage of substances hazardous to health and may manage the care of children who have been poisoned.

Overdose

When considering the issue of overdose, it should be stressed that it may occur either intentionally or accidentally. Accidental overdose may result from the client misreading or misunderstanding the prescription label or failing to realize that more than one medication contains the same drug. Taking medicines containing the same drug concurrently would result in an overdose. This is perhaps most common with over the counter cold cures, many of which contain paracetamol. Accidental overdose may occur by proxy in the form of a medication error if a nurse fails to record that a medication has been given, thus allowing the dose to be unintentionally repeated.

Intentional overdose

An area common to all areas of nursing is the intentional abuse of medicines, whether prescribed or not, with intent to cause injury or death to oneself or another. Nurses in practice may find themselves working with victims of parasuicide or with relatives of those who have committed suicide through overdose. The physical nursing needs of para-suicide clients depend very much upon the type of medication taken and rely on multidisciplinary team working between the nurses, pharmacists and medical team involved in each individual's care. In most para-suicide cases there is an additional referral to a liaison psychiatrist for risk assessment and planning future management. It is likely that the nurse's role would involve monitoring and assessment of the client. A clear understanding of the substance taken and its likely effects of toxicity is essential. Those involved in such sad situations will require counselling and support. This is addressed further in Chapter 12 about death and dying.

> **Reflection and portfolio exercise**
>
> For nurses caring for those who have attempted to either seek help by taking an overdose or who have attempted to take their own lives, caring can be emotionally difficult. Consider how you might feel in this situation.
>
> 1. Would you feel cross that the person is taking up a bed by making themselves ill?
> 2. Would you feel confused or unable to understand?
> 3. Would you simply feel sorry for the person?
> 4. Could your feelings affect your care for that person?
> 5. Think about your own experience of caring for patients. Write a short reflective summary for your portfolio.

Use of illegal substances

A definition of an illegal substance is one that is classified within the schedules outlined in the Misuse of Drugs Act 1971, and is being manufactured, supplied or possessed by anyone not legally authorized to do so. The use of illegal substances cannot be ignored as it is an increasing problem in our society.

> **Evidence based practice**
>
> Drugs are an increasing national and international problem within society. Within the UK, contemporary evidence has identified the following:
>
> - Drug use is increasing, especially in young people
> - Drug prices are falling, making drugs more accessible
> - There is a strong relationship between criminality and drug misuse
> - Drug related deaths across the UK are rising.
>
> These findings are in Annual Report on the Drug Situation 2001 (Department of Health 2001).

Although it is not suggested that the use of illicit drugs should be encouraged or condoned by nurses, it is important to be aware of the nature and use of such substances by all clients in your care. Use must be assessed as part of the individual's lifestyle so that any prescribed medication can be given to best effect, since it is possible for non-prescription substances to interact with prescribed medications with serious consequences.

Assessment may reveal areas where individuals need help with managing the consumption of addictive substances, and nurses may have a role in helping find appropriate support and advice. However, issues associated with maintaining confidentiality when a client is pursuing an illegal activity are complex and extend beyond the remit of this chapter. Dimond (2002) explores these issues in more depth in her text *Legal Aspects of Nursing*.

ALTERNATIVE OR COMPLEMENTARY THERAPIES

The use of complementary or alternative medicines is within the rights of any client. However, the nurse must be aware of what is being used and must also be aware of any possible interactions between this and any proposed orthodox treatment. Nurses are able to use complementary therapies provided that they have successfully undertaken training to do so, take full professional accountability for their actions, have the informed consent of the client who is to receive such treatment, and have considered the appropriateness of the therapy to both the condition of the client and any coexisting treatments (Nursing and Midwifery Council 2002a).

HEALTH PROMOTION

Nurses have a unique position in society in their capacity to offer appropriate health education to a wide range of individuals and their families. A practice nurse's knowledge about the effects of smoking on the health of unborn children may be an essential contribution in helping a pregnant woman reduce the number of cigarettes she smokes (or better still stop smoking altogether), while the combined skills and knowledge employed by mental health nurses in drug and alcohol dependency units may offer a healthier future for their clients. Many more examples could be cited in relation to all nursing specialities.

Reflection and portfolio evidence

Reflect upon a recent day in practice.

- Can you identify any times when you or your mentor were involved in an activity associated with administering medicines but not actually giving a medicine to a client?
- What aspects included assessment and planning for giving medicines to clients?
- Record what you learned from these situations in your portfolio and discuss with your mentor.

Finally, there is the issue of the use of non-prescribed medicines by nurses themselves. After all, in spite of professional accountability, health carers are human and part of the wider society in which we all live. Social use of 'medicines' and difficulties surrounding abuse of substances are a very real issue, particularly in the stressful occupation of nursing. Recognition of personal problems are all important, for nurses and their professional colleagues. Indeed, as stated in the Nursing and Midwifery Council's Code of Professional Conduct, there is an obligation for any nurse 'to act quickly to protect patients from risk if you have good reason to believe that you or a colleague, from your own or another profession may not be fit to practice for reasons of conduct, health or competence' (Nursing and Midwifery Council 2002b: Section 8.2).

CARE DELIVERY KNOWLEDGE

Nurses are accountable for the safe administration of medicines in whatever setting they may be working. To do this

effectively they must be able to apply the knowledge discussed above according to the client's individual needs. Nursing skills are required that relate to assessment, planning of proposed nursing intervention, and the implementation and evaluation of any therapy prescribed. Additionally, the role of the nurse extends more broadly in ensuring the safety and well-being of clients when considered in relation to the guidance advocated within *Guidance for the Administration of Medicines* (Nursing and Midwifery Council 2002a). This document assumes a much wider role for the nurse both before and after a medicine is actually given. It is useful to explore the subject knowledge about medicines and administration above in relation to the organizational context and the intertwined roles of the nurse, multidisciplinary team and the clients themselves.

ORGANIZING ADMINISTRATION OF MEDICINES

The role of the nurse may vary practically according to the type of nursing situation. For instance, in areas with responsibility for groups of dependent clients, a different role in medicines administration will operate as compared to a situation where clients are independent and able to self-administer their treatment. Nurses may directly give prescribed medicines, or be involved with administration through education and supervision of the clients or their carers. In some settings the nurse's remit will extend to a role that will include the prescription of medicines from the *Nurse Prescriber's Formulary* or through a supplementary agreement or a client group direction. This type of involvement is discussed further within the professional and ethical section of this chapter.

THE ROLE OF THE NURSE IN THE ADMINISTRATION OF MEDICINES TO CLIENTS

In practice, nurses are accountable for any medication they administer, and to do this safely they must use knowledge gained through education and experience in a personalized way with each of their clients. It is helpful to consider the nursing role systematically. This includes assessing, planning, implementing and evaluating care. This can be applied in conjunction with a conceptual framework in accordance with an individual practitioner's philosophy of care. Areas that may be addressed before giving a medicine to a client are revealed by the questions below:

- What is the age of the client?
- What is the client's weight and baseline observations?
- What is the client's past medical history?
- What is the diagnosis of the client?
- Has the client consented to this treatment?
- Is the client currently taking any medications? If so, what are they?
- Has the client taken this medication before? If so was it tolerated and was it effective?

- How does the client prefer to take medication (i.e can they take tablets?)
- What is the preferred route for the medication prescribed?
- Is the client allergic to any medication?
- Does the client (and if appropriate, carer) understand why the medicine has been prescribed?
- Does the client (and carer) know about potential side effects that may occur?
- Who is going to administer the medicine? Do they know how to do this to gain optimum benefit?
- Is there any reason why the client should not receive the medicine prescribed?

Decision making exercise

Mr James, aged 62 years, lives in a council-owned flat, and is attended by the local community psychiatric nursing team for treatment of paranoid schizophrenia. A loner, he has no close family and few friends. He resorts to alcohol when he feels unable to cope with his situation.

Discuss with your colleagues what health promotion role the community psychiatric nurse might have in helping Mr James.

1. Find out why each of the questions listed above can be important.
2. Take one client in your next practice placement and use these questions to help you to find out as much as your can about your client's medicinal treatment.
3. Consider the ways in which the results of your assessment would help you in providing care for your client, and make some notes for your portfolio.

All of these considerations need to be taken into account when reviewing prescriptions and drug record sheets. Indeed, the nurse must ensure that such records contain all information relevant to the administration of a medication to the client, and that information is clearly documented without illegibility or ambiguity. This is recognized within government recommendations relating to safety in medicine administration practice, as a priority in maintaining a safe system (Department of Health 2000a). The nurse must also ensure that the drug record is checked thoroughly prior to the administration of a medicine in accordance with local policy. This can be complex, as abbreviations and Latin terminology are used by prescribers despite recommendations that this is not acceptable (British Medical Association and the Royal Pharmaceutical Society of Great Britain 2003). Whilst some texts offer a range of abbreviations, it is advised that any prescription containing information that is not fully understood by the nurse should not be acted upon until it has been rewritten or appropriately clarified to the satisfaction of all parties. Poorly written prescriptions contribute to medicine administration error, and nurses should not administer any medication about which they are not fully informed. After a medication is administered the event must be recorded according to local policy.

Planning nursing care

When planning care, all the information derived from the medicines assessment by the nurse and other members of the multidisciplinary team needs to be combined. This information must be used to identify common goals for the administration of the medicine prescribed and outline an individualized plan of care for the client. This can be followed by implementing care that can be evaluated regularly to determine the effect of the intervention, as illustrated by the following case:

While in hospital for treatment of congestive cardiac failure, Mrs Johnson's needs are individually assessed by her nurses and a specific plan is made to assess the effects of her treatment:

- *The problem: Mrs Johnson has congestive heart failure which requires treatment with digoxin 62.5 micrograms/day*
- *The outcome: Mrs Johnson will gain a steady pulse rate of 80–120 beats/min and appear well*
- *Nursing action: Observe Mrs Johnson for a lowered pulse rate of less than 60 beats/min, coupling of heart beats (felt at the wrist as double beats) or nausea and vomiting. In the event of any of these, contact the medical staff for advice.*

In relation to planning, there may be other issues taken into account that are related more to individual preferences; for instance, if a medicine needs to be taken with food, when is the usual mealtime for the client? Although in hospital meals may be delivered at set times, mealtimes can vary widely for individuals in their own homes; and for neonates who are fed on demand, it would be difficult to write up a medication to be taken with food at a set time! With planning and negotiation between the client, nurse and medical staff, a solution to such problems may be reached that meets the needs of all parties in providing optimum treatment.

Planning also needs to take place within the work organization, and this requires knowledge and skill on behalf of the nurse. If a medicine needs to be given at a specific time, the nurse needs to ensure that both the medicines and the client are available and prepared. The medication may require retrieving from a locked cupboard, reconstituting (if it is a dry powder to be made into solution) and offered in an acceptable way for the client, according to the route for which it is prescribed. Procedures need to be followed and the medicine must be given in accordance with the law, local policy and the nurses' *Code of Professional Conduct* (Nursing and Midwifery Council 2002b) (see the Professional Knowledge section of this chapter). In the case of the client, skin may have to be prepared for topical creams or it may simply be necessary to ensure that the client has a drink ready to swallow tablets.

Safety in medicine administration

It is also important for the practice of medicine administration to be safe for the administrator. Since all medication is given for the therapeutic or diagnostic effect it is going to have on the client, it is important to remember that carelessness or inappropriate handling of medicine can lead to the nurse and (possibly others) inadvertently receiving treatment. Illustrations of this include the administration of skin creams. If the nurse does not wear gloves to protect the skin, then the cream will be applied to her hand as well as the client. Where medicines are drawn up in a syringe by nurses before administration to a client, carelessness can lead to aerosol inhalation during this activity. Many cytotoxic medicines are reconstituted by the pharmacist in laminar air flow cubicles to draw any particles of the medication away.

Finally, in the case of liquids care should be taken to avoid splashing the medicine, which could be absorbed through the skin or inhaled.

With all medicine administration, careful handwashing before and after the procedure is essential in order to avoid cross-infection contamination from the nurse's hand to the client and potential ingestion of particles of medicine by the nurse. Where medications are particularly toxic the pharmacist may advise extra protective measures when handling, such as safety glasses or a protective gown, and these should be adhered to.

Within this text it is inappropriate to dwell upon the many specific practical skills and procedures required in administering medicines. However, there are texts with a skills development focus that do this well; particular examples include Mallett & Doughty (2000) or Nicol et al (2000).

All of the above considerations require planning on the part of the nurse as an outcome of an informed assessment of the situation.

Planning for client discharge

There is a considerable role for the nurse in planning a client's discharge from the care setting. There is a responsibility to ensure that prescribed medications to take home are available by liaising with the pharmacy department. Additionally the nurse must ensure that the client or carer will be able to manage the prescribed treatment effectively once they return home.

The nurse's role may simply involve advising a client about the frequency with which tablets should be taken or it could be more complex, involving education and assessment of the ability to perform a skill such as the instillation of eye drops. In either case, the nurse must evaluate the ability of those continuing care and be certain that care will continue after discharge. If this cannot be achieved alternative support may need to be planned, for instance a hospital based nurse discharging a client to the community may need to plan for intervention by the community nursing staff.

Evidence based practice

Parkin et al (1976) assessed the actual use of medicines prescribed to take home by 130 clients. They found that 66 clients failed to follow the instructions they were given in hospital, and of these 46 said that they were unable to understand the instructions. A more recent study by Latter et al (2000) identified that nurses were still not always performing their role in patient education related to medicine well. Communication is clearly a fundamental part of medicine administration practice and it is vital that both nursing practice and its effectiveness in client care are regularly evaluated.

Evidence based practice

A small study conducted by Sutherland et al (1995) tried out client self-medication for 1 month for some adult clients in a medical ward and a dermatology ward. They reported that 'a self-administration scheme would be possible and beneficial in acute medical wards', and a decision has been taken to extend the project hospital-wide to all appropriate areas. Further research evaluated self-administration in two children's wards. The researchers found that this method was well received by children and their families as well as nursing staff who reported improvements in facilitating care and improving comfort and access to medication (Wright et al 2002).

Implementing nursing care

In the act of giving a medicine all the assessment, planning and background knowledge comes together to permit safe and accountable action. Additionally, the nurse has to acknowledge and respect the rights of the client in receiving their medication (as discussed in the professional knowledge section of this chapter).

Although delivery systems in nursing may differ, the nurse's responsibility in administering medicines to clients is constant. One starting point is identified by Hall (2002) within 'eight rights' in drug administration (Fig. 9.4). The Nursing and Midwifery Council (2002a) offers further advice relating to the professional accountability of the nurse administering a medicine, and it is wise to refer to this guidance also.

Although these references offer a useful start, the nurse may need to be flexible about how such guidance is achieved. For instance, it cannot be assumed that the nurse will always give a client his or her medicine. Self-medication by clients is recognized as one way of empowering clients and improving safety (Audit Commission 2001, Wright et al 2002). In children's nursing, nurses work in partnership

The nurse must ensure that:

THE RIGHT MEDICATION

is given to

THE RIGHT CLIENT

at

THE RIGHT TIME

on

THE RIGHT DATE

in

THE RIGHT DOSE

via

THE RIGHT ROUTE

in

THE RIGHT PREPARATION

and

THE RIGHT DOCUMENTATION

is completed

Figure 9.4   The eight rights of medicines administration.

Reflection and portfolio evidence

In your practice placement, try to observe one situation where a nurse ensures that a client receives their medicines. Note in detail what you see, including the nurse's actions and the client's actions.

1. How did the administration of this medicine integrate with the total care of the client and with the nurse's total role?
2. What knowledge did the nurse need to have to ensure that the medicine was received safely?
3. What new knowledge did you gain from the situation? Record your learning in your portfolio.

Evidence based practice

A study of children's nurses' roles on administering medicine found that nurses identified 201 activities that were considered to be part of a nurse's role ensuring a medicine was to be administered safely (Hall 2002). Key themes that emerged in relation to these roles included client and family education and information, management and knowledge acquisition, and admission and discharge planning as well as more commonly acknowledged skills and practices associated with the rights of administering.

with parents and the children, and in the community, nurses may be responsible for overseeing their clients who are self-administering medicines in their own homes.

Practical considerations in giving medicines

Additionally, some practical issues fall outside the above rights and professional guidance, and must be addressed when implementing the administration of a medicine. Failure to acknowledge these would not perhaps be considered as a medication error, but would make the difference between unacceptable and optimum practice. Such issues are considered elsewhere in this book, but may include for instance the management of infection control (see Ch. 4), an issue that is particularly pertinent in relation to the administration of intravenous medication. If a client becomes septicaemic due to contamination during the administration of a medication, their safety could be as much compromised as if they were given the wrong dose.

A final aspect to consider is the nurse's knowledge of resuscitation techniques and equipment in the event of an anaphylactic reaction to a medication (see Ch. 3). When any medicine is given, it is the responsibility of the nurse to know what possible side effects may occur and to observe for these once the medication has been administered. This aspect will be addressed further in the next section, on evaluation of care.

EVALUATION OF NURSING CARE IN RELATION TO MEDICINES

In relation to clients, all treatment with medication requires evaluation regarding its effect (beneficial or otherwise) for the client. The nurse must use both general and clinical skills of observation as well as communication skills, and must be able to record and communicate findings to other members of the multidisciplinary team appropriately. A fundamental part of the nurse's decision making role with regard to medicine administration is related to identifying whether a medication is effective or sufficient for the client's needs. Within this, a major aspect is the evaluation and assessment of pain control (see Ch. 10). Evaluation requires the use of many clinical monitoring skills (e.g. temperature control, respiratory rate, patient's colour, mood and behaviour) in determining outcomes. The therapeutic effects of any medication given must be reviewed and any untoward reactions that may have occurred as a result of treatment must be managed.

All registered nurses are beholden to administer medicines for therapeutic, diagnostic or preventive benefit, but there are many ways in which client's optimum health and safety can be compromised in spite of the intentions behind the planned treatment with medicines. The qualified nurse therefore plays an important part in promoting the health and safety of clients with regard to the evaluation of the administration of their treatment as well as in the more recognized areas of health and safety already outlined and included in Chapter 2.

PROFESSIONAL AND ETHICAL KNOWLEDGE

In this section the nurse's role in the prescribing and administering of medicine is considered in relation to British law currently governing practice, the nurses' *Code of Professional Conduct* (Nursing and Midwifery Council 2002b), and the impact of local policy. Clients' rights will be considered regarding their consent to treatment and the right to refuse medicinal treatment will be explored. Finally, the nurse's role in the management of medication error is addressed.

LEGAL CONSIDERATIONS IN PRESCRIBING AND ADMINISTERING MEDICINES

In Britain, the manufacture, prescription, safe handling, storage and custody of medicines are all subject to legislative control arising from two main acts of parliament and a set of guiding regulations as follows:

- Medicines Act 1968
- Misuse of Drugs Act 1971
- Misuse of Drugs Regulations 1985.

Each of the Acts determines different legal controls which must be observed by the nurse in daily practice.

Legal classification of medicines

Under the Medicines Act 1968 drugs are classified into three main groups:

1. Pharmacy-only products: those only to be sold through a registered pharmacy under the supervision of a pharmacist.
2. General sales list: medicines that may be sold from a retail outlet without a pharmacist or registration as a pharmacy provided certain conditions relating to the security of the premises are adhered to.
3. Prescription-only medicines: medicines that are only available on a practitioner's prescription. This group is divided to identify those drugs that are simply to be prescribed by a practitioner and those that are further governed by additional requirements under the Misuse of Drugs Act 1971.

A clear knowledge of the classification of medications is essential for the nurse who has responsibility for ensuring the safe and legal administration of medicines to clients.

Within the Misuse of Drugs Act 1971 and the Misuse of Drugs Regulations 1985, controlled drugs are identified and categorized according to requirements governing their import, export, supply, possession, prescribing and record keeping (Dimond 2002). For hospital based nurses, knowledge regarding these Acts is essential in understanding the

way controlled drugs are stored and handled in the practice setting. Strict regulations govern where a controlled drug should be kept, how it may be ordered and transported from pharmacy, where it must be kept, who holds the keys to access controlled medicines, and how the prescription checking and use of such drugs must be documented. In non-institutional settings, however, the nurse is not permitted to keep any stock-controlled drugs. Controlled drugs may only be obtained for those who are named on a prescription.

Decision making exercise

You are working as a nurse in charge at a respite home for clients with severe learning disability. One morning, Simon, a short-stay client in the home, develops signs and symptoms of a urinary tract infection. You call Simon's general practitioner, but he is unable to see him until the afternoon. You know that another client has been prescribed antibiotics for a similar diagnosis. A colleague suggests that if you borrowed some of this client's antibiotics for Simon then he could begin treatment right away.

1. How should you react to this suggestion?
2. What knowledge and legal rationale would influence your response?

Reflection and portfolio evidence

In your practice, find a controlled drug prescription. Try to identify the following:

1. How does a controlled medicine prescription differ from prescriptions that are not for controlled medicines?
2. What is special about the cupboard where controlled medicines are stored? Who has the keys?
3. What governs the administration and storage of controlled medicines?
4. What does the nurse need to know in order to give a controlled drug safely?
5. What is included in the controlled record of administration?

Record your findings in your portfolio.

NURSE PRESCRIBING

Following the publication of the Department of Health Report of the Advisory Group on Nurse Prescribing (1989), the Medicinal Products: Prescriptions by Nurses etc. Act 1992 has enabled provision in law for district nurses and health visitors to prescribe a number of commonly used medications from a nurses' formulary without recourse to a medical practitioner.

This began initially within a number of demonstration sites, but in 1998, a national roll-out of nurse prescribing was announced, which was completed in 2001. The role of the nurse as a prescriber has been supported by the *NHS Plan* (Department of Health 2000b) which proposed that by 2004, nurses should be able to prescribe medicines either independently from the *Nurse Prescriber's Formulary* or as supplementary prescribers.

Alternatively, nurses may also be able to supply medicines to a specified client group under Patient Group Directions. Within the last 2 years the UK government has announced plans for how nurse prescribing might be extended in line with the *NHS Plan* (Department of Health 2002b). This has led to the inclusion of a wider eligibility for nurse prescribers. Prescribers may now include a range of practitioners and not just those with district nursing or health visiting qualifications.

For new nurses, prescribing may remain a future plan for their role, as to prescribe independently or supplementarily requires post-registration experience and training. However, it is increasingly likely that they will be working with team members who are trained to prescribe, and they may encounter the need to supply medicines using patient group directions. It is therefore essential to know what the different types of prescribing involve.

Types of nurse prescriber under the Department of Health (2001a) arrangements

Independent prescribers

In this role, nurses who are appropriately trained through a recognized and accredited course can prescribe medications independently from the *Nurse Prescriber's Extended Formulary* (Department of Health 2003b). The areas in which independent prescription may take place according to current government recommendation are:

- minor illness
- minor injury
- health promotion
- palliative care.

A number of prescribers prepared prior to these arrangements, may independently prescribe to the more limited *Nurse Prescriber's Formulary*.

Supplementary prescribers

This category of prescribing has been introduced in 2003 for nurses working with more complex conditions. Supplementary prescribers once again must complete an accredited post-registration training course. They can prescribe for a client once the client has been assessed by a doctor and a treatment plan has been established. They can alter dosages, frequency, and active ingredients of medication within the limits of the agreed treatment plan.

Patient Group Directions

These directions enable nurses to supply prescription only medicines to clients under generalized directions of a doctor. Examples may include provision of vaccines, or specific medicines out of hours. Patient Group Directions are also used in hospital. An example might be the supply of topical anaesthetic creams prior to theatre admission or blood sampling.

Further information about nurse prescribing see section on websites at the end of this chapter.

Medicine administration and the *Code of Professional Conduct* for the nurse, midwife and health visitor

As well as working within the law and within professional training, the nurse is also accountable to the Nursing and Midwifery Council, which is the nurses' governing body for professional practice. The *Code of Professional Conduct* and its supplementary guidance paper *Guidance for the Administration of Medicines* (Nursing and Midwifery Council 2002a,b) assist the nurse in fulfilling the expectations the Council has of them as a professional body. Additional advice can also be gained from the *Guidance for Professional Practice* (UK Central Council 1996, adopted by the Nursing and Midwifery Council 2002b), especially in relation to the extended role in medicines administration. Although the law will instigate criminal proceedings in the event of a breach, the Council's guidance adheres to the general principles of law and to regulations regarding the management of drugs.

The Nursing and Midwifery Council has the power to remove practitioners who fail to meet professional standards from the professional register, thus removing an individual's right to practice in the UK. The Nursing and Midwifery Council's regulations are more comprehensive and detailed in relation to nursing clients than those required by law, but they also assist the nurse in interpreting the law.

Local policies for medicines storage and administration

Local policies are established within individual health trusts and care settings and set the expectations of the employer with respect to their employed practitioners. Nurses must be aware of the contents of their local policy, because it is unlikely that an individual nurse who becomes involved in any legal action with a client would receive support or insurance if the employer's policy had been contravened during the incident. This would be irrespective of whether the practice is acceptable to the Nursing and Midwifery Council or legal standards. This is particularly important in relation to the administration of medicines because there are variations between individual employers in what is deemed to be acceptable practice. This is particularly well illustrated in relation to the checking of medicines by individual practitioners. The law holds an individual accountable for medicine administered irrespective of qualification, but the Nursing and Midwifery Council states that only a qualified practitioner can give medicines, and advocates that:

in the majority of circumstances a first level registered nurse, a midwife or a second level nurse, each of whom has demonstrated the necessary knowledge and competence, should be able to administer medicines without involving a second person.

Local policies, however, vary with regard to how many (one or two) nurses are required to check a medicine, and where a second checker is required, there is variation as to who that person is to be. For nurses who change employment or who participate in agency employment, an awareness of local variations in policy is essential.

Clients' rights

As with any form of treatment all clients have a right to be fully informed about the medicines they receive and most have a right to refuse treatment if it is against their wishes. There are, however, some exceptions to this rule, and for nursing this has moral and ethical implications, which require consideration.

Treatment of children

In the treatment of children, it is beholden to the nurse to ensure that the child client and their family receive information about their treatment that is appropriate to their understanding. If it is considered that the child client is old enough and mature enough to understand the implications of his or her treatment then his or her decision should be allowed by the health carer. This is supported in law by the precedent set by the Gillick case in which a general practitioner won his case to prescribe a child under the age of 16 years contraceptive medication without recourse to her parents for permission. For a child who is under 16 years of age, however, any decision for treatment is usually made with the joint consent of the parents. This is commonly incorporated into hospital policy as a guideline for health carers. Finally, the Children Act 1989 has also influenced treatment

Decision making exercise

Six-year-old Ahmed is undergoing treatment for leukaemia. While you are in practice he is to have oral medication, which he hates intensely. On this particular occasion he refuses to take his medicine, which is a vital part of his treatment.

- Does Ahmed have any right to refuse his treatment?
- Discuss this with your peers and record the responses you conclude.

for children in stating that any course of treatment must be in the best interests of the child concerned. In a few cases this may have implications if a parent refuses to consent to treatment for a child where the child is too young to consent for themselves, and where the treatment is unanimously considered by medical professionals to be in the best interests of the child. As a last resort, the child may be made a ward of court in order to allow treatment to be given without parental consent. Similar assessments must be made for those with learning disabilities. The administration of medicines for children and those with learning disabilities can cause ethical dilemmas in practice.

A second major consideration in children's nursing relates to the high number of medicines that are administered either off label or off licence. There are obvious ethical dilemmas here because it is the licensing restriction that mitigates in ensuring the research tested safety of the medicine. Since in the past, access for research with children has been complex, many medicine licences have only been requested for use with adult clients. Over time, these medicines have become used within child health, although no licence has been agreed. This is a position children's nurses must be aware of, indeed in the *National Service Framework for Children's Hospital Services* (Department of Health 2003a), a section is devoted to this problem. In a professional role, health carers should not have to choose to give medicines where the effects of their use is unknown. However, children's nurses may have the dilemma of choosing whether to administer a prescription off licence or off label, or refusing a child a treatment that may be therapeutic. If guidance from the Nursing and Midwifery Council (2002a) is taken into account then the consideration may be to act in the best interest of the child, and to be fully aware of the evidence that would support administration of such medication.

Treatment of the mentally ill

Most mentally ill clients do have a right to consent to or refuse treatment. In some situations, however, treatment is obliged by law and is involuntary. This is usually because the client's illness indicates a risk to themselves or to the community unless treatment is maintained. Again issues may be raised regarding the rights of the client and the role of the nurse in protecting such rights, especially if the treatment given benefits the community rather than the client himself, for instance the use of medication to subdue noisy or aggressive clients.

Other considerations related to the management of all clients, but especially pertinent to those taking medicines for chronic illness, include the validity of an initial consent if a client changes his or her mind or wishes to stop treatment. Issues that require consideration include what rights a dangerously aggressive client has to stop treatment if the medication is successful. Many medications that affect mood also have side effects, which may be uncomfortable or inconvenient to the client, but if treatment is stopped, will their aggression make them a danger to society? Do such clients have a right to refuse?

Whilst there is both legal and ethical controversy surrounding the individual's rights versus the rights of the community for safety, the Nursing and Midwifery Council (2003) does identify for nurses that giving medication to patients without their knowledge and consent may occasionally be necessary. The Council's position statement acknowledges that whilst disguising medicine in the absence of informed consent must always be regarded as deception, a clear distinction should always be made between those who have the capacity to refuse medication and those who lack such a capacity. Within this distinction, they further identify that there are those who have not got the capacity to know they are receiving medicinal treatment and those who would have if they were not being deceived by covert administration. They advise that in any situation the nurse will need to be sure that 'what they are doing is in the best interests of the client and be accountable for this decision' (UK Central Council position statement on the covert administration of medicines, 2001, Section 4. 6, adopted by the Nursing and Midwifery Council 2002a).

Additionally, the effect of stopping medicines without planning must be considered, and clients should be advised if considering refusal. Medicines such as fluphenazine decanoate (Modecate) have a long-acting effect, which cannot be reversed quickly. There are also implications for withdrawing treatment where a medicine creates a dependence because it is addictive or it reduces the body's ability to produce a similar substance naturally (e.g. glucocorticosteroids). Rapid withdrawal of such substances could be dangerous or cause discomfort.

The client's position

Finally, when caring for individuals requiring treatment with medications there is also the possibility that they may not wish to disclose their use of other medicines. This may occur in all branches of nursing and for many different reasons. In childrens' nursing for instance, a teenage girl may not wish her family to know that she is taking oral contraceptives, or another situation may arise if a client is using a substance considered to be illegal. Many issues arise from these scenarios which merit reflection and discussion.

MANAGEMENT OF MEDICATION ERRORS

Medication errors occur in the event of a client not receiving their medicine (error of omission) or receiving it when there is reason to withhold it, or in a manner that is not appropriate (error of commission). When errors do occur, they may have a devastating effect; at the least they demonstrate the fallibility of systems and individuals, and at worst they can cause discomfort, pain or be potentially fatal for the clients

involved. Given the seriousness of such errors, it is perhaps surprising to learn how commonly they occur (Department of Health 2000a).

In the event of an error occurring, the nurse concerned must ensure the safety of the client and staff. This would usually involve immediately contacting members of medical and pharmacy teams and explaining what has happened in the incident so that an appropriate course of action can be taken.

After the practical management of any error, the nurse must complete documentation to record the incident. The nature of further action then depends upon the type of error made and on whether the error is in contravention of the *Code of Professional Conduct* (Nursing and Midwifery Council, 2002b) or the law, or local policy.

> ### Evidence based practice
>
> Ridge et al (1995) used covert observation to look at single-nurse administration in one NHS trust hospital. They observed a 3.5% total error rate and comment that this is too high. There must also be concern that wrong doses accounted for 15% of maladministration in their study. This error rate for medicines is identified within the Department of Health (2000) document *An Organization with a Memory*, but this also recognized a need to understand error as part of a system of practice rather than blaming individuals. This has led to changes in political thinking about incident reporting and management of incidents such as medication error (Department of Health 2001b).

> ### Evidence based practice
>
> Arndt (1994) explored nurses' experiences with medication errors using a qualitative approach. She analysed discourse from two group discussions, 12 unstructured interviews and six self-written reports where nurses described their experiences with medication errors.
>
> She concluded that medication errors caused nurses to feel ashamed and humiliated, and they forced situations of conflict, which demanded that nurses make moral decisions. She also suggested that nurses' ability to cope depends heavily upon the support of colleagues at the time of the incident. Think about this evidence.
>
> Ask yourself whether all medication errors are wrong or should the potential severity of outcome be taken into consideration when planning disciplinary action?

PERSONAL AND REFLECTIVE KNOWLEDGE

AWARENESS OF PERSONAL POSITION IN EVERY ASPECT OF MEDICINES

In conclusion, this chapter has introduced you to many facets of knowledge required to make effective nursing decisions when planning the storage and administration of medicines to clients. The chapter demonstrates the need for a wide range of nursing skills, from understanding the complexities of medicines' law and physiological action to the more practical elements such as perceptual and communication skills required when working with both clients and other members of the nursing and multidisciplinary team. The safe and effective administration of medicine requires nurses to be knowledgeable, and importantly, vigilant in their practice, and as with other areas of practice highlighted in this book, also requires you to be aware of the latest developments in research related to of all the areas addressed. This chapter has introduced research based evidence in medicine administration supporting rationale for the care to be offered. It is not intended to be a complete record of all applicable research or necessarily the most up to date and relevant to your own specific practice area, but it serves as an illustration of the work that is available and can be used to enhance care in practice.

CASE STUDIES RELATING TO THE USE OF MEDICINES

In summary, case studies are provided to enable the application of concepts presented in this chapter. In each one, issues will be raised that are meaningful to that individual situation, but may also be transferable to other settings with different clients.

Case study: Adult

Julia Hargreaves is 26 years old and lives alone in a flat in the centre of a large city. She moved 5 years ago from her parents' house in the country to find work after graduating from university. Julia is admitted to hospital after a car knocks her off her bike as she is cycling home one evening. On admission Julia is adamant that she wishes to have no treatment with medicines as she is in early pregnancy and does not wish to hurt her baby. Julia is found to have a compound fracture of her left tibia and is in considerable pain. Without antibiotics she risks seriously complicating her injury by developing osteomyelitis.

- What factors would you need to take into account when planning care for Julia?
- Discuss what you consider the nurse's role might be in the above situation?
- If Julia persisted in her request for no medical treatment, what dilemmas may face carers who are looking after her and her unborn child?

Case study: Mental health

Mohammed Shah is 20 years old and newly diagnosed as having mental illness, which requires long-term treatment with antipsychotic drugs to prevent deluded, aggressive and occasionally violent behaviour. He has been treated now for 6 months and feels that he is cured and no longer requires his fortnightly injections. Although Mohammed continues to attend the clinic for these, he is becoming increasingly dissatisfied with the nurses, and is starting to suggest that he may not come any more.

- As the practice nurse, how might you respond to Mohammed?
- What would be the dilemmas to be solved in making your response?
- Mohammed was being treated with the antipsychotic fluphenazine decanoate (Modecate). What are the therapeutic benefits and side effects of antipsychotic medications such as this?

Case study: Child

Chloe Jackson is 6 years old and lives at home with her mother and father and 2-year-old brother Caspar. She has had severe eczema since she was a baby and this frequently becomes inflamed with open lesions. At a visit to the surgery Mrs Jackson is advised by her general practitioner to accept a prescription for glucocorticosteroid treatment for Chloe. Mrs Jackson is very anxious about the prospect of this treatment since she has heard that glucocorticosteroids have bad side effects.

- What information should be offered to Mrs Jackson about the benefits and effects of glucocorticosteroid treatment?
- What advice should be given if Chloe is to receive glucocorticosteroid treatment for her eczema?
- The glucocorticosteroid treatment is to be administered at home in the form of a topical cream. What education should be included regarding administration and storage?
- Mrs Jackson comments that she has heard that alternative medicine is an effective way of managing eczema. She asks the practice nurse for an opinion. What advice could the practice nurse offer?

Case study: Learning disabilities

Sam Doppler is a 30-year-old man with mild learning disability. He manages to live alone and works as a kitchen assistant in a small café. One day he cuts his hand on an unwashed knife at work. After a few days the cut becomes inflamed and sore and Sam is unable to use his hand and so he attends his general practitioner. Sam is prescribed a course of oral antibiotics and advised not to return to work until his hand has healed.

- What advice should Sam receive about taking his antibiotics?
- Given his learning disability, what strategies may be employed to ensure that Sam understands the prescription he is given?

- Sam asks the practice nurse to explain why the doctor has given him tablets when it is his hand that is sore. Discuss the pharmacokinetic action of oral antibiotic treatment from taking the medication to its therapeutic action at the required site.

Summary

This chapter has drawn together theoretical concepts relating to the use of medicines. It has applied this knowledge in relation to the practice of caring for individuals. The chapter has included:

1. An outline of medicinal action on the body, and also consideration of non-therapeutic action by medicines.
2. Consideration relating to the administration of medicines including the calculation of medicine dosages, routes by which medicines may be administered and knowledge for storage and administration of medicines in safety using application of research evidence.
3. Nursing care of clients who require medicines, including the assessment of clients in relation to medicine administration, planning to administer a medicine and how medication administration can be evaluated.
4. Professional and ethical knowledge relating to the legal acts governing the storage and administration of medicines in the UK. Moral and ethical dilemmas that can arise within the practice of medicines prescribing and administration.
5. Effective management of errors in administration.

Knowledge illuminated within this chapter has been combined with evidence from other referenced sources and applied within a range of situations. Suggestions have been made for portfolio development in relation to medicines management.

Annotated further reading and websites

British Medical Association and the Pharmaceutical Society of Great Britain 2003 British National Formulary no. 45. British Medical Association, London
A useful formulary for identifying types and effects of medication.

Dimond B 2002 Legal aspects of nursing. Prentice Hall, New York
In a specific chapter on law as it applies to medicine administration, the nurse's duty of care to the client is considered.

Downie G, Mackenzie J, Williams A 1999 Pharmacology and drug management for nurses, 2nd edn. Churchill Livingstone, Edinburgh
This book offers a comprehensive explanation of current theories regarding pharmacodynamics in a complete chapter on this subject.

Kee J L, Hayes E R 1993 Pharmacology: a nursing process approach. Saunders, Philadelphia
Chapter 4 of this book offers a clear and comprehensive review of the metric system, calculating medicines and determining body weight and surface area. Although an older text, the information relating to calculation of medicines is relevant and easy to use.

Royal College of Paediatrics and Child Health 2003 Medicines for children. Royal College of Paediatrics and Child Health, London
A national formulary for identifying types and effects of medication for children. This includes the Royal College of Paediatrics and Child Health's position statement on use of unlicenced medicines for children. A second edition is due at the time of writing.

http://www.bnf.org.uk/
The website of the British National Formulary produced by the British Medical Association. The most up-to-date evidence relating to medicines licenced within the UK can be accessed here.

http://www.nmc-uk.org/
The website of the Nursing and Midwifery Council, this offers professional guidance to nurses on their role in administering medicines.

http://www.doh.gov.uk/
This is the Department of Health website. It holds a wealth of information, and reports on all aspects of health. It contains current plans for extending and developing nurse prescribing.

http://www.npc.co.uk/
The website of the Nurse Prescribing Centre. Although designed for nurses who are prescribers, it holds useful information for all interested in prescribing and administering medicines.

http://www.learndirect.co.uk/
This is the website of a national adult education initiative. It holds useful resources for numeracy assessment and development.

References

Arndt M 1994 Nurses medication errors. Journal of Advanced Nursing 19:519–526

Audit Commission 2002 Medicines management. HMSO, London

British Medical Association 2002 Nurse Prescriber's Formulary 2002/2003. British Medical Association, London

British Medical Association and the Royal Pharmaceutical Society of Great Britain 2003 British National Formulary no. 45. British Medical Association, London. Online. Available: http://www.bnf. org.uk/

Children Act 1989 HMSO, London

Cnattingius S, Signorello L B, Anneren G et al 2000 Caffeine intake and the risk of first-trimester spontaneous abortion. New England Journal of Medicine 343(25):1839–1845

Department of Health 1989 Report of the Advisory Group on nurse prescribing. HMSO, London

Department of Health 1999 Review of prescribing, supply and administration of medicines. HMSO, London. Online. Available: http://www.doh.gov.uk/

Department of Health 2000a An organization with a memory. HMSO, London. Online. Available: http://www.doh.gov.uk/

Department of Health 2000b The NHS Plan. HMSO, London

Department of Health 2001a Annual report on the drug situation 2001. HMSO, London. Online. Available: http://www.doh.gov.uk/

Department of Health 2001b Building a safer NHS. HMSO, London. Online. Available: http://www.doh.gov.uk 12 Aug 2003

Department of Health 2003a The National Service Framework for children: acute and hospital services. HMSO, London. Online. Available: http://www.doh.gov.uk/

Department of Health 2003b Items prescribable by nurses through the Nurse Prescriber's Extended Formulary. Online. Available: http://www.doh.gov.uk/nurseprescribing/pomlist.htm 15 Aug 2003

Dimond B 2002 Legal aspects of nursing, 3rd edn. Prentice Hall, New York

Downie G, MacKenzie J, Williams A 1999 Pharmacology and drug management for nurses, 2nd edn. Churchill Livingstone, Edinburgh

Gatford J D, Philips N 2002 Nursing calculations, 6th edn. Elsevier, London

Hall C 2002 An evaluation of nurse preparation and practice in administering medicine to children. PhD thesis. University of Nottingham School of Education, Nottingham

Hohl C M, Dankoff J, Colacone A et al 2001 Polypharmacy, adverse drug related events, and potential adverse interactions in elderly patients presenting to an emergency department. Annals of Emergency Medicine 38(6):666–671

Hopkins S J 1999 Drugs and pharmacology for nurses, 13th edn. Churchill Livingstone, Edinburgh

Kee J L, Hayes E R 1993 Pharmacology: a nursing process approach. Saunders, Philadelphia

Latter S, Rycroft-Malone J, Yerrell P et al 2000 Evaluating education preparation for a health education in practice: the case of medication education. Journal of Advanced Nursing 32(5):1282–1290

Loi, C-M, Vestel R E 1988 Drug metabolism in the elderly. Pharmacology Therapy 36:131–149

Manley G, Sheiham A, Eadsforth W 1994 Sugar coated care? Nursing Times 90:7

Mallett J, Doughty L (eds) 2000 The Royal Marsden Hospital manual of clinical procedures. Blackwell, Oxford

Medicinal Products: Prescriptions by Nurses etc. Act 1992 HMSO, London

Medicines Act 1968 HMSO, London

Misuse of Drugs Act 1971 HMSO, London

Misuse of Drugs Regulations S.I. 1985/2066 1985 HMSO, London

Nicol M, Bavin C, Bedford Turner S et al 2000 Essential nursing skills. Mosby, London

Nightingale F 1859 Notes on nursing: what it is and what it is not (1980 reprint of 1st edn). Churchill Livingstone, Edinburgh

Nursing and Midwifery Council 1996 Guidance for professional practice. Nursing and Midwifery Council, London

Nursing and Midwifery Council 2001 UK Central Council position statement on the covert administration of medicines. Nursing and Midwifery Council, London

Nursing and Midwifery Council 2002a Guidance for the administration of medicines. Nursing and Midwifery Council, London

Nursing and Midwifery Council 2002b Code of professional conduct. Nursing and Midwifery Council, London

Nursing and Midwifery Council 2003 Position statement on the covert administration of medicines. Online. Available: http://www.nmc-uk/org 12 Aug 2003

Parkin D M, Henney C R, Quirk J et al 1976 Deviation from prescribed treatment after discharge from hospital. British Medical Journal 2:686–688

Ridge K W, Jenkins D B, Noyce P R et al 1995 Medication errors during hospital drug rounds. Quality in Health Care 4:240–243

Royal College of Paediatrics and Child Health 2003 Medicines for children. Royal College of Paediatrics and Child Health, London

Sutherland K, Morgan J, Semple S 1995 Self administration of drugs: an introduction. Nursing Times 91:23

Trounce J 2000 Clinical pharmacology for nurses, 16th edn. Churchill Livingstone, Edinburgh

Waller D G, Renwick A G, Hillier K 2001 Medical pharmacology and therapeutics. Saunders, Edinburgh

Weathermon R, Crabb D W 1999 Alcohol and medication interactions. Alcohol Research and Health 23(1):40–51

Wright A, Falconer J, Newman C 2002 Self-administration and re-use of medicines. Paediatric Nursing 14(6):14–17

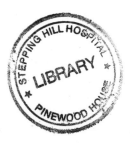

Chapter 10

Pain

Karen Jackson

KEY ISSUES

SUBJECT KNOWLEDGE
- The physiology of pain
- The evolution of pain theories
- Physiological signs of pain
- Psychosocial elements of pain
- Behavioural responses to acute pain and adaptation
- Cultural and spiritual influences on pain

CARE DELIVERY KNOWLEDGE
- Assessment of pain
- Assessment of pain in children
- Planning effective management
- Complementary therapies

PROFESSIONAL AND ETHICAL KNOWLEDGE
- Role of the nurse in relation to pain
- The multidisciplinary team in pain management
- The role of the specialist nurse
- Ethico-legal issues in pain management

PERSONAL AND REFLECTIVE KNOWLEDGE
- Understanding the theories of pain
- Awareness of your own beliefs and values about pain

INTRODUCTION

Treating pain is a basic humanitarian concern (Park et al 2000) and it is unacceptable for patients to suffer pain unnecessarily (Carroll & Bowsher 1993). Pain is a key responsibility for the nurse as a member of a multidisciplinary team and therefore up-to-date knowledge of pain is essential throughout your nursing career. Pain is a problem in its own right, but may be associated with other areas of care. Pain is also a symptom common to many illnesses and therefore nursing knowledge in this field is vital. It has been found that nurses often lack knowledge and awareness of the resources available for the effective management of pain. Such nurses are therefore unable to perform their role effectively. Pain can have harmful effects on many aspects of the body's normal functioning and repair processes (Munafò & Trim 2000). Chronic pain has many serious adverse effects and has been linked with suppressing immune function (McCaffery & Pasero 1999). This chapter will explore how pain might be experienced. Although most people can readily identify with the concept of physical pain, other areas such as the emotional, mental and psychological elements of pain are often overlooked.

This chapter is designed to further your knowledge and to encourage you to continue to explore this subject. The activities incorporated here are intended to act as a starting point for your development. It will help you explore the issues involved in the pain experience from a broad perspective. The approaches will encourage you to use other resources, including your personal and practical experience in various settings, library resources and interactions with your peers. Additional reading is suggested to enable you to develop your knowledge and skills further.

OVERVIEW

This chapter is divided into four parts, each with a specific focus in relation to pain.

Subject knowledge

This section considers the physiology of pain, pain transmission, physiological signs of pain, theories of pain, and psychosocial elements of pain.

Care delivery knowledge

This section considers the assessment of pain. Related symptoms relevant to pain assessment, the use of pain assessment tools, and the use of carers to aid assessment are also considered. Effective pain management, pharmacological interventions and modes of delivery, and non-pharmacological interventions are explored.

Professional and ethical knowledge

This section explores the nurse's role in effective pain care in a plural society. The nurse's specialist role and multidisciplinary team role in pain management are also examined. Ethical considerations around the delivery and management of pain are reviewed in the light of documents such as the Human Rights Act 1998, 2000 and the Children Act 1989.

Personal and reflective knowledge

In this section you are able to bring together the issues covered by the previous three sections as well as your existing knowledge and experiences to explore the care of four individuals related to the specialist branches of nursing. You therefore have the opportunity to apply existing knowledge in the area of effective decision making and to increase your knowledge by a wider investigation of the issues involved in the nursing care of these individuals. It is also relevant to consider your personal gain in relation to your knowledge base and evidence of learning.

On pages 240–241 there are four case studies, each one relating to one of the branches of nursing. You may find it helpful to read one of them before you start the chapter and use it as a focus for your reflections while reading.

SUBJECT KNOWLEDGE

BIOLOGICAL

This section explores the physiology of pain. Theories of pain transmission are discussed and you are encouraged to apply these to your own experiences.

THE PHYSIOLOGY OF PAIN

It is necessary to consider several factors in relation to how pain is evoked and perceived. The relationships between the major components need to be understood and recognized.

Table 10.1 The evolution and major contributions of pain theories (adapted from Stevens & Johnston 1993 with kind permission of Lippincott, Williams & Wilkins)

Theory	Theorist	Major contribution
Specificity	Descartes (1664/1972)	Pain is a distinct sensation mediated by nerves designed for nociceptive processing with physiological specialization
Intensity	Erasmus Darwin (1794)	Pain is the result of intense stimulation of nerve fibres in any sensory organ
Pattern theories		Several conceptualizations of pain stimulus intensity and central summation are key concepts
(a) Central	Livingstone (1943)	Central mechanisms for summating peripheral summation pain impulses and pathological stimulation of sensory nerves initiates activity in reverberating circuits between central and peripheral processes
(b) Sensory	Bishop (1946, 1959) Nordenbos (1959)	Rapidly conducting fibre system excite, and inhibit, synaptic transmission in the slowly conducting system for pain. From this evolved the theories of myelinated and unmyelinated fibre systems, functions of nerve fibres, and the multisynaptic afferent system
Affect	Marshall (1894)	Emotional quality of pain distorts all sensory events
	Melzack & Wall (1965, 1973, 1982, 1988)	Global theory accounting for the sensory, affective and cognitive dimensions of pain – pain processing not rigid, but flexible

In 1970, Merskey offered a definition of pain as 'an unpleasant experience which we primarily associate with tissue damage or describe in terms of such damage or both'. This definition allows for the concept of pain to be evoked even if there is no direct indication of tissue damage, and seems to agree with the everyday definition of pain. The exact mechanism for the transmission of pain is unknown, but several theories have been put forward.

Pain transmission theories include:

- that pain is an emotion rather than a sensation
- that pain is a specific entity
- that pain is produced by stimulation of non-specific receptors given a nerve impulse pattern (McCready et al 1991).

Several theories of pain have evolved and guide the conceptualization of pain (Table 10.1).

THE EVOLUTION OF PAIN THEORIES

Although pain theories enable some understanding of pain an examination of how pain messages may be transmitted is necessary to develop understanding and further conceptualization.

Pain transmission

Pain fibres or nociceptors (noxious sensation receptors) are specialized neurones located throughout the body, particularly in the skin (Fig. 10.1). These specialized nerve endings recognize tissue damage. Pain results when the impulses from these nerves reach consciousness. The nerve endings are stimulated by a chemical substance that is released or formed as a result of cell disruption. When the peripheral nerve fibres carrying impulses generated by the painful stimuli enter the spinal cord, they enter the dorsal horn of the spinal grey matter, passing through the dorsal root of the spinal nerve. When a nerve fibre ends it is involved in a synapse where the nerve message is chemically transmitted to the next nerve cell and its fibre. Many different chemicals

are involved in transmission at different synapses and no one transmitter substance is confined to a single functional system. The primary actions and functions of some of these neurotransmitters are listed in Table 10.2.

A sound introduction to pain perception/transmission can be found in Wood (2002), a *Nursing Times* special feature on pain.

Reflection and portfolio exercise

- Reflect and try to describe in your own words how you as an individual are able to perceive pain.
- Given this description consider factors that would affect your perception of pain. It may be helpful here to compare the differing perceptions of pain when 'banging your thumb' or having a headache or having a toothache.
- Use this exercise to write a short summary for your portfolio, demonstrating your understanding of your own pain experience.

Gate theory

One of the most widely accepted theories of pain is the gate theory, which suggests that pain is determined by interactions between three spinal cord systems (Melzack & Wall 1996). It proposes that pain impulses arrive at a gate, thought to be the substantia gelatinosa. When open the impulses easily pass through, if partially open only some pain impulses can pass through, and if closed none can pass through. It further suggests that the gate position depends on the degree of small or large fibre firing. Accordingly, when large fibre firing predominates, the gate closes, and when small fibre firing predominates the pain message is transmitted (Fig. 10.2). For more detailed information see Melzack (1996) or Wood (2002).

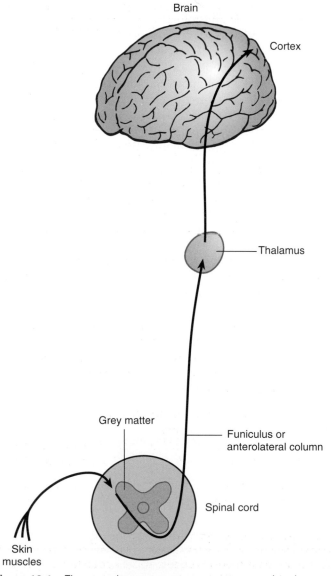

Figure 10.1   The central nervous system, structures and pathways.

Table 10.2   Functional relationships of neurotransmitters

Neurotransmitter	Action
Substance P	Is thought to be the neurotransmitter substance released that results in increasing pain perception
Enkephalins	Produce analgesia, euphoria and nausea
5-Hydroxytryptamine	Enhances pain transmission at local level, but inhibits pain when acting on central nervous system structures such as the dorsal horn
Beta endorphins	Probably responsible for dulling pain perception from injuries

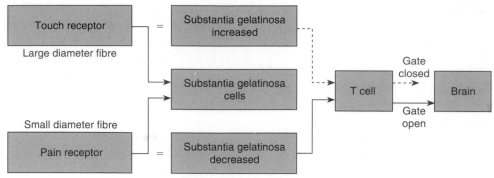

Figure 10.2   Gate theory. (Adapted from Melzack & Wall 1965.)

PHYSIOLOGICAL SIGNS OF PAIN

In sudden acute pain certain physiological signs of pain may exist (Table 10.3); these are linked to the fight or flight mechanism of the adrenaline (epinephrine) and noradrenaline (norepinephrine) functions as an initial response to the experience of pain. However, over time the body seeks equilibrium physiologically as these responses cannot be maintained without causing physical harm. The major problem with physiological indicators of pain is that they may be due to other factors such as stress. Also these physiological responses are short-lived and return to near normal as the body's systems acclimatize (Hawley 1984). Therefore although they may be indicators of acute and sudden pain, they are of little use as indicators of chronic pain.

Table 10.3   Physiological manifestations of acute pain and adaptations

Physiological response to acute pain	Adaptation over time (chronic pain)
Increased blood pressure	Normal blood pressure
Increased pulse rate	Normal pulse rate
Increased respiration rate	Normal respiration rate
Dilated pupils	Normal pupil size
Perspiration	Dry skin

Physiological manifestation of acute pain and adaptation

There are differences between acute and chronic pain and this has an impact on the individual experiencing pain, since not only the physiological responses, but also the psychological and social consequences differ. Acute pain is associated with a well-defined cause. There is an expectation that it is time bound and will disappear when healing has occurred. Chronic pain continues long after an injury has healed. It is a situation for the person experiencing it rather than an event (Munafò & Trim 2000). Chronic pain can be further subdivided as either malignant or non-malignant. Chronic non-malignant pain is persistent and has no end point. It has far-reaching effects and may cause problems with partners, family, friends and employers. Treatment philosophies centre around helping patients to take responsibility for their pain and helping them to cope with it using a variety of strategies, such as in the care of a person with arthritis. In contrast chronic malignant pain may have an end point; treatment approaches include sufficient analgesic to relieve pain and techniques such as relaxation. Such differences in definition reflect the multidimensional nature of the pain.

PSYCHOSOCIAL

PSYCHOSOCIAL ELEMENTS OF PAIN

In this section definitions and ideologies are explored along with misconceptions of the experience of pain for the individual.

Pain is a difficult concept to understand. The assumption that there is a simple and direct relationship between a noxious stimulus and subsequent pain has been disputed by the realization that many environmental and internal factors modify pain perception (Main & Spanswick 2000, Melzak & Wall 1996). There are numerous causes of pain. The threshold (level at which pain is felt) varies between individuals, and can vary within the same person at different times (Gillies 1993). This is further complicated by factors such as emotion, culture and previous experience, the end result being a unique experience for that individual. Therefore, pain should be regarded as a subjective phenomenon (Devine 1990). It is important then that the nurse working with a person experiencing pain is able to accept that pain is both physical and psychological. Thus pain is both biologically and phenomenologically embodied. Moreover culture intercedes in the pain experience and therefore transcends the mind–body divide.

Some of the recognized behavioural responses to both acute and chronic pain are listed in Table 10.4. These may be used as cues by nurses in their quest to determine the pain experience of the patient.

Reflection and portfolio exercise

- In your own words try to define the term pain.
- Looking at this definition, explore how you view pain and from this try to consider on what your views are based. For example, you may have had a particularly painful experience that influences your views of pain or you may never have experienced pain.
- Consider whether these views affect your beliefs about other people in pain. If they do, in what way?
- Reflect on how your personal beliefs could affect your decision making when a patient or client requests pain relief.

Table 10.4 Behavioural responses to acute pain and adaptations

Behavioural response	Adaptation over time
Observable signs of discomfort	Decrease in observable signs, though pain intensity unchanged
Focuses on pain	Turns attention to things other than pain
Reports pain	No report of pain unless questioned
Cries and moans	Quiet; sleeps or rests
Rubs painful part	Physical inactivity or immobility
Frowns and grimaces	Blank or normal facial expression
Increased muscle tension	

BEHAVIOURAL RESPONSES TO ACUTE PAIN AND ADAPTATION

Pain has been defined as whatever the person experiencing it says it is, existing whenever the person says it does (McCaffery 1972). This definition allows for the complexity of pain, but in some ways limits its understanding. The literature indicates that the definition of pain depends upon the one person defining it. Wall (1977) produced the definition 'Pain is'. Such a wide definition allows freedom for the practitioner to consider the individual phenomenon but may also be problematic due to individual attitudes and beliefs about pain. The International Association for the Study of Pain (IASP) has attempted to recognize the problem in multiple definitions of pain-related terms. It has sought to establish a universal definition of pain as 'an unpleasant sensory and emotional experience associated with actual or potential tissue damage, or described in terms of such damage' (International Association for the Study of Pain 1979, Merskey & Bogduk 1994). These definitions may not, however, be appropriate or useful for young children who are often unable to describe or say what or where the pain is, people with communication difficulties, or sedated patients. Anand & Craig (1996) attempted to increase awareness of pain definitions and their appropriateness in relation to infants, young children, verbally and mentally disabled people and those who are comatosed. Pain causes powerful emotions in its sufferers; fear, anxiety, anger and depression are frequently cited. These emotions have a great impact on the individual's understanding and control of the pain.

Pain in any individual has to be judged by indirect evidence, and the appearance, non-verbal behaviour, physiological status and circumstance of the pain need to be interpreted (Fordham & Dunn 1994). Many misconceptions can be problematic in the interpretation of pain. The amount of tissue damage is not an exact prediction of the intensity of pain. It is easy to suppose that individuals receiving the same surgery, appendicectomy for example, will experience the same pain. The evidence, however, is that the pain experience is individual and varies from both person to person and situation to situation. McCready et al (1991) suggest that an individual's reaction to pain is determined by past experiences, state of health and level of growth and development. More recently Skevington (1995) identified that the environment and the social context in which patients find themselves influence their reaction to pain.

When examining behavioural responses it is essential that vulnerable individuals, for whom behaviour may be a major characteristic, are considered. Vulnerable individuals would include young children and infants and people with impaired vocal ability. Historically children's pain was ignored (Carter 1998). However, recently there has been a rise in concern in relation to the provision of care services for children and their families. It is necessary to explore some of the myths and assumptions that have prevailed regarding infants and young children's pain. Price (1990) stated that these unproved assumptions exist as a consequence of the limited knowledge about children's experience of pain. But some years later in many areas these assumptions continue (Woodgate & Kristjanson 1996). However, with the advent of pain teams, clinical nurse specialists and guidelines for clinical practice such as those produced by the Royal College of Nursing (1999a), there is hope that children's pain will be managed more appropriately.

There is evidence that erroneous beliefs have been used to justify regrettable clinical practices (Craig 1992). Furthermore healthcare professionals have acted as if they believed claims about the insensitivity of infants to pain (Craig 1992).

Common beliefs/assumptions are:

- infants are incapable of feeling pain
- infants are incapable of expressing pain
- children do not feel as much pain as adults
- children tolerate pain better than adults
- the neural system of infants is different from that of adults, so they do not experience or perceive pain as acutely or as meaningfully as adults
- children do not have past experiences of pain so do not experience or perceive it in the same negative way as adults

(Broome & Slack 1990, Lloyd-Thomas 1990, McCaffery & Pasero 1999, McConnan 1992, McCready et al 1991, Stevens & Johnston 1992).

Evidence based practice

Hamers et al (1998) carried out a literature search and found that some studies suggest that nurses undermedicate children and that their postoperative pain is not sufficiently relieved. They also suggested that the *pro re nata* (PRN) 'as required' prescription could be a strategy for enabling nursing staff to make decisions as to the child's need for analgesia. On the basis of this review the authors suggest a standard prescription of pain medication rather than PRN is necessary and that further research is warranted in this area.

Another study by Colwell et al (1996) examined the use of paediatric pain scales postoperatively by nurses; they compared the nurse's estimates of pain intensity and the child's self-report. Few nurses had used a paediatric pain scale prior to their involvement in the study. Those who were taught how to use them matched the children's self-report far more closely that those who, in the control group, were not. They concluded that the nurse can, with the use of appropriate pain tools, discriminate between pain and anxiety and make more proven decisions about pain management.

Reflection and portfolio exercise

- Think about a painful experience you have had and try to write a description about it.
- Include thoughts about how it made you feel and how people close to you responded to your pain.
- Try to remember if the pain altered your lifestyle. Were there some activities, for example, that you felt unable to take part in?

Children may not have past experience of pain, but they learn quickly. Ethological theory supports this: an expression of emotion that is helpful to the survival of the organism is likely to emerge (Charlesworth 1982). Therefore an expression of distress in relation to tissue damage is of extreme importance to the infant's survival. Pain would logically become one of the first emotions to emerge. It has been found that tolerance to pain increases with age, so the child is more likely to have an intense pain experience. In relation to the neural system of infants, it is now believed that the process of myelination occurs *in utero* and by birth myelination of the sensory roots has begun. Therefore the ability to experience and perceive pain has been established.

Many factors influence the way pain is perceived by the individual. Past experience of pain, the personality of the individual experiencing the pain, anxiety related to the pain experience and cultural influences all affect the pain sensation. Most of us grow up thinking in certain ways that cause us to erroneously doubt others who indicate they have pain (McCaffery & Beebe 1994). We need to be aware of this and by this awareness prevent ourselves from acting on these misconceptions.

Any past experience of pain or pain relief can affect the intensity of the pain (Carr & Mann 2000, Main & Spanswick 2000, Wells 1984). Pain can be influenced by the meaning it has to the individual. For example, the headache that you previously have dismissed as nothing may with a limited knowledge of medical theory be interpreted as being due to a brain tumour. This associated meaning will influence the way you perceive the pain. Anxiety, fear and depression can all increase pain sensation. Pain is reported to be more intense when an individual is anxious and reduced when anxiety levels are reduced (Akinsanya 1985, Vingoe 1994).

Reflection and portfolio exercise

During a child placement experience you are observing a physical education session. Peter Smith is known to dislike physical exercise. He appears to slip down a climbing rope, landing heavily on his right foot. He immediately begins to cry and crumples to the floor clutching his ankle. The teacher in charge asks him what is wrong. 'I've hurt my foot,' he says, 'It really hurts, I don't think I can walk on it'.

- What are your first thoughts about Peter's pain?

Note the questions that are going through your mind about the situation. What other facts do you need to know here? You may quite naturally assume that Peter is trying to get out of the exercise or you might feel genuine concern for his welfare, but it is likely that some of that concern will be coloured by your perception of Peter not enjoying the class.

- You may be shocked to see a boy cry. Depending on your own personal beliefs and value systems, you may find it acceptable or unacceptable for a boy to cry.
- You may find yourself wondering what Peter's background is. Has he had previous experience with pain? What are his cultural norms and his perception of the situation?
- You will probably come to some decision about Peter and his pain. Make some brief notes of the points that influence your decision.

Evidence based practice

Wakefield (1995) examined how nurses talk about patients' pain and pain management. She conducted a series of in-depth unstructured group interviews with nurses during which they were encouraged to discuss postoperative pain management and its effectiveness. This revealed that nurses tended to categorize patients according to their symptoms or overt pain behaviours. Essentially this led to patients not being believed when they signalled that pain was becoming a distressing symptom.

Psychiatric/mental pain

This complex issue has undergone considerable deliberation by many writers in recent years. The terms 'hysterical pain' and 'operant pain' have been used to describe the experience of patients who appear to be experiencing pain for psychological rather physical reasons. It is important to consider that the patient's expression of pain is as real to them as to those who have pain due to an accepted cause such as surgery or fractured bones. Wall & Melzack (1999) write that they 'have reservations of the use of this term in relation to its application to the theory of pain and psychological illness … Since those grouped under it include people whose pain is related to anxiety, depression and many psychiatric conditions' (Wall & Melzack 1999: 931). They further state that it is important to distinguish these phenomena in order to apply appropriate treatment, whether antidepressants, psychotherapy or rehabilitative measures. This area

deserves a far greater consideration than can be presented within this chapter; see section on Further Reading.

CULTURAL AND SPIRITUAL INFLUENCES ON PAIN

The cultures within the profession of nursing or the institution of a hospital affect the way that pain is assessed, the way that decisions are made about the possible treatments, and the way that pain is managed.

Ethnicity in pain management is of particular significance in a multicultural country, such as the UK. Each individual has intrinsic associations with culture: it socializes us to know what is expected of us and of others. Culture shapes beliefs and constrains behaviours. In such an environment the nurse must constantly be aware of professional issues in providing culturally appropriate care, and also of constraints on other practitioners due to their cultural beliefs and values. Research has found that initiatives by the National Health Service to meet the healthcare needs of the ethnic minority groups in Britain are inadequate and their specific needs are not fully recognized (Papadopoulos 1999, Thomas & Dines 1994, Vydelingum 2000). The process of the nurse–patient interaction occurs within the context of the demands and culture of the workplace (Walker et al 1995). It has been argued that investigation of the basis of ethnic differences in pain experience is important in order to develop efficient pain control regimes for all sections of the population (Thomas & Rose 1991).

There are theological overtones in the pain experience as pain plays a central part in religious thought. The Christian concept is of pain as a paradox: Christ healed others in pain, but allowed himself to be crucified and endured agonizing pain. Pain is viewed as a challenge to be overcome. Buddha has been cited as a warrior, a saint and a victim. Examples of pain control can be found in many cultures, for example, the Indian fakir who controls pain while lying on a bed of nails and the African tribes that practice lip or cheek piercing as ritualistic ceremonies do not appear to experience pain. Where stoicism is a cultural value, the behavioural expression of distress is generally less acceptable. Older people may view pain as a preliminary to death. Each culture has its own set of beliefs and attitudes with respect to the way people react to pain. These are passed on through the generations and acquired by socialization (Parsons 1992).

Care must be taken not to stereotype people, remembering that there is variability within cultures as well as between cultures. These misleading effects of cultural stereotypes, and the belief by nurses and doctors that they are the experts regarding the patient's pain, lead to problems in assessing the patient's pain. Also the ethnicity of both the individual in pain, and those attempting to assess the pain, clouds the perceptions of health professionals (Walker et al 1995). Many of the early works investigating the sociocultural dimensions of pain have been criticized for reinforcing ethnic stereotypes, for example Zola's study into the reactions of Italian-Americans and Irish-Americans to illness

(Zola 1966) or the Zborowski study into the cultural components of experiencing pain among Italian-Americans and Jewish-Americans (Zborowski 1952). Professionals should consider the fact that the more difference there is between the patient and themselves the more difficult it is for them to assess and treat the patient.

Helman (2001) suggests that:

- not all cultural or social groups respond to pain in the same way
- cultural background can influence how people perceive and respond to pain, both in themselves and others
- cultural factors can influence how and whether people reveal their pain to health professionals and others.

Gender is also an issue in the pain experience. Both male and female subjects believe that females have an innate ability to cope with pain and this is generally linked to reproduction (Bendelow 1993). In the available literature the views are that gender is of no significance or that females have lower pain thresholds than males. Work by Faucett et al (1994) found that the men reported less severe pain than the women. Gender differences in the pain experience are usually recorded in terms of sensitivity to experimentally induced pain (Bendelow & Williams 1995).

CARE DELIVERY KNOWLEDGE

Brown et al (1999) found that nurses have inadequate knowledge and unacceptable attitudes regarding pain management. In order to make the most of decision making skills in practice, the nurse must access appropriate knowledge to support and rationalize these actions. This section applies knowledge about the areas of pain assessment and relief of pain to the practice of nursing. You are encouraged to examine and apply this knowledge to exercises that will help you develop decision making skills.

Nurses are the gatekeepers of medication usage and as such have a responsibility to increase their knowledge in pharmacological as well as non-pharmacological techniques for pain management. The prescribing of analgesia by physicians on an 'as required' basis leaves the responsibility for the decision to give analgesia firmly with the nurse (Carr & Mann 2000, Craig 1992). Nurses can therefore be instrumental in pain management in all settings. Many writers have stressed the need for nurses to assess an individual's beliefs and attitudes about pain and pain management accurately (Bonica 1990, McCaffery & Pasero 1999, Sofaer 1998). Because of its subjective nature, the individual in pain is the only one who can assess the pain accurately.

The routine and traditional practices of many care institutions can pose difficulties in the assessment of pain. The use of 'drug rounds' may cause patients to comply, accepting analgesia at this time and feeling unable to ask for it at a more appropriate time for them. Skilful assessment techniques will limit this problem, identifying both the individual nature of the pain and its recurrence at more frequent intervals than the 'drug round' timing. An awareness of pain should therefore be a routine matter in caring for patients.

Reflection and portfolio exercise

Rituals in nursing practice can become entrenched, and in many healthcare institutions drugs are still administered via a 'drug round'.

- During your practice placements compare the experiences of patients on the unit or ward that links pain relief to drug rounds and those where self-administration of drugs is the norm.
- To what extent do drug round practices need to be modified to suit individual needs for pain relief?
- How might ritualistic practices affect your decision making in relation to pain management?

ASSESSMENT OF PAIN

Pain expression

Assessment is a process by which a conclusion is reached about the nature of a problem. Planning effective pain management is a crucial part of the nurse's role. In order to achieve this it is necessary to assess the level of the individual's discomfort in an attempt to identify a potential course of action. Thus the cycle of the nursing process becomes part of the equation. The nurse needs to be able to draw conclusions about the individual's pain to assess the level and intensity of the pain based on information from the patient. Once this has been achieved it is then possible to plan a course of action to alleviate the pain, implement this and evaluate the action. Although this is possible without the patient's cooperation, it is better to involve the individual in the assessment of their pain. Otherwise nurses are simply applying their own beliefs and values to the situation and making assumptions about patients' pain levels. The nurse must therefore be proactive and skilled in recognizing potentially painful situations, particularly in those instances where the patient may not be able to communicate verbally. To achieve this we need to ascertain whether pain assessment is an appropriate action, believe that the person has pain, and be committed to assessing the pain. This should lead to a clarification of the extent of pain and its treatment. In some circumstances, this assessment will need to be not only accurate, but also swift, for example when dealing with a patient suffering the pain of a myocardial infarction (heart attack), where the need for immediate and effective pain relief is a priority.

Although the nurse's role in this area is paramount, the only individual who is truly able to assess the pain is the person who is suffering it. So wherever possible the patient should be assessing the pain and not the nursing staff. In circumstances where the patient is unconscious, has a communication difficulty or is a child, the nurse must use their observational skills and make an informed decision based on the evidence presented by the patient, bearing in mind that the family and other carers can be asked for further clarification.

The accurate assessment of an individual's pain is an inherently difficult process. The nurse must be able to establish a trusting relationship with the patient and his or her family or carers. The nurse must also be aware of their own beliefs and prejudices about pain. Timing of pain assessment is very important and dependent upon many factors, not least of which is the desire of the patient to participate in the assessment, the severity of the pain and the potential pain treatment. Such assessment involves the skills of observation so that the non-verbal pain behaviours can be seen and recognized (Table 10.5). It must be remembered that these behaviours are influenced by the individual's social and cultural norms. Your interpretation will also be influenced by these factors. Therefore it is not possible to make assumptions based on the absence of a recognized non-verbal pain behaviour since each pain experience for the individual is unique.

The nurse may conclude that someone is in pain if:

- an individual states that this is the case
- an individual's behaviour is indicative of pain
- an individual has undergone some experience that we would consider to be painful.

Decision making exercise

Mrs Singh is an elderly widow living in a maisonette. Her family live close by and have very regular contact with her. She is receiving treatment for glaucoma and the community nurse has been asked by her general practitioner to assess her needs as her family are unable to instil her eye drops at lunchtime. She speaks very little English and has limited mobility. When the nurse arrives Mrs Singh is accompanied by her niece who says she has just arrived and is worried about her aunt who does not appear to be herself today. On meeting Mrs Singh she is sitting hunched in a chair and is moaning and rocking back and forth slightly.

- Consider the appropriate nursing actions in this instance.
- Using the list of aspects related to pain assessment in Table 10.5 decide what factors you would take into account in Mrs Singh's case.
- Using a friend, role-playing Mrs Singh's niece, complete an assessment of her pain.
- What more do you need to know that might help you in effective decision making about Mrs Singh's care?

Table 10.5 Aspects of pain assessment

Pain	Nature, intensity and site Likely cause Precipitating factors and circumstances (e.g. time of day, movement, eating)
Examples of non-verbal pain behaviours	Facial expression Change in mood Crying, screaming, wailing, weeping Lack of appetite Nausea, vomiting Pale or flushed skin colour Reluctance to move Increased activity Unusual behaviour Unusual posture Holding, pressing on the part that hurts
Related symptoms	Nausea, anxiety, breathlessness
Resources	Patient's coping strategies Nursing knowledge and skills in using and teaching non-pharmacological methods of pain relief Medical and pharmacological knowledge and skills in both pharmacological and non-pharmacological methods of pain relief Availability of resources such as time, equipment, privacy and so on
Meaning and significance to patient	Purpose and consequences

Related symptoms

An initial assessment should include some information about the history of the pain as follows:

1. Information about the initial onset of the pain. This includes a comparison of the medical history with the patient's own version and allows similarities and discrepancies to be addressed. This may be linked to surgery, illness, trauma or an unknown cause. The patient may believe that something totally unrelated to the identified clinical cause of the pain is responsible.
2. Position of the pain. A body outline may be used for this purpose and then used as a baseline to chart any improvement or deterioration in the pain.
3. A description of the pain. The patient should be encouraged to use his or her own words for this exercise. Children have a limited vocabulary and may well use words that an adult would not normally use, such as 'owie', 'squidgy' or a 'headache in my tummy'.
4. Elements affecting the pain. These can include position, eating, activity, and time of day.
5. Previous treatment. The success or otherwise of past treatments helps the nurse plan effectively in this pain experience.
6. Any other medical history.

Psychological aspects

The possibility of stress, changes in lifestyle, depression or behavioural disorders in the individual and their relevance to the pain experience need to be considered, and specialist referral may be necessary (see also Ch. 8 covering stress and relaxation).

Social aspects

Information about the family, housing, employment and other interests are relevant in a pain assessment as often these positively or negatively influence a pain problem.

Observation

The most natural reactions are seen when observation is informal and carried out when the patient is unaware of being observed. Formal observation usually involves the use of some form of documentation or pain chart.

Decision making exercise

Mrs Singh, whom you met in the earlier exercise, has now been assessed. There is nothing physically wrong with her. It transpires that she has received bad news from her family in India and a very dear nephew has been killed in a road traffic accident.

- Reflect on whether this information would make a difference to your initial thoughts about your nursing actions.
- Would the use of any of the pain assessment tools discussed below have been helpful in this case?
- From information already covered in the section on Subject Knowledge, what might be the most important part of a pain managment strategy for Mrs Singh?
- How might you use this experience in caring for patients in practice?
- Jot down your ideas for inclusion in your portfolio.

Use of pain assessment tools

There are many formal pain assessment tools to aid in assessing the patient's pain, from a simple visual analogue scale to the more complex. When using the visual analogue scale the patient is asked to rate the pain along a line between no pain and the worst pain imaginable (Fig. 10.3). An intensity rating can also be used, in which case the patient picks the description that most closely relates to the pain they are experiencing (Fig. 10.4). Other pain tools use a variety of other ways in an attempt to clarify the patient's pain.

For clients in the community the use of a personal pain diary has been recommended. The patient records the pain, describes it and includes comments about how it has changed, if at all, how it affects their daily lifestyle and any effective pain relief. Writing down this information allows the opportunity to organize potential triggers and patterns of pain that emerge (Chaitow 2002). The patient needs to get into a routine of recording in this diary, since it is likely that more accurate information is achieved with the recent experience of pain. The patient therefore records the information as it occurs, if possible, within their normal lifestyle. Questions might include:

- Is the pain constant or intermittent?
- After what activities does it hurt?
- What sort of pain is it?
- Is there swelling, redness or heat in the area of pain?
- Is the pain affected by emotion?
- If you are female, is the pain made better or worse by aspects of your menstrual cycle?

The method of pain measurement should be bias-free and there must be a particular focus on practicality and versatility (Main & Spanswick 2000, McGrath 1989, Twycross et al 1998). However, although these are desirable aims they may be difficult to achieve. An array of pain assessment

---

Reflection and portfolio exercise

Pain assessment tools in the practice situation vary in use according to the client group and the evidence about their reliability and validity. In relation to specific client groups or specific healthcare situations that you have experienced during your practice placements:

- Find out what pain assessment tools are available for use and review how they are used.
- Have any of these tools been tested as valid and reliable? You may have to look at the research literature to find this out.
- Using these practice experiences and the case studies at the end of this chapter decide which pain assessment tool is appropriate for each patient. Try to justify your choice.

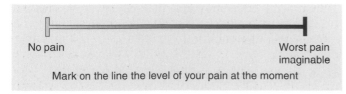

Figure 10.3   A visual analogue scale.

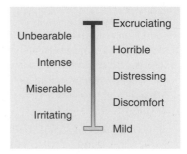

Figure 10.4   An intensity rating scale.

tools has been developed for adults, but most rely on communication and cognitive abilities not mastered by young children (Stevens et al 1987, Twycross et al 1998). Their use is also restricted for people with some learning disabilities or those who are unable to communicate verbally. These people continue to be especially vulnerable to poor pain management (Carter et al 2002). Specific tools to assess the pain of young children and infants are available, e.g. the Liverpool Infant Distress Score (LIDS) (Horgan et al 1996) and Face, Legs, Activity, Cry, Consolability (FLACC) score (Merkel et al 1997). However nurses need to understand how such tools can be used.

ASSESSMENT OF PAIN IN CHILDREN

The current awareness of children's pain has resulted both from a deeper professional commitment, and from a consciousness of pain overall; it is also reflective of changing social concerns (Carter 1998). Many tools are now available to assess children's pain. Practitioners need to understand how these instruments can be used appropriately with the individual child in their care. There is strong evidence that pain assessment in children must be multidimensional. Not only is pain expression individual for children, it is also affected by their chronological age and cognitive development (Woodgate & Kristjanson 1995). Children as young as 3 years old are able to provide adequate information of their pain experience (Abu-Saad 2001). Behavioural observation methods circumvent the possible difficulties of comprehension that are inherent in any paediatric self-reporting scale (Goodenough et al 1997, Lloyd-Thomas 1990). Pain measurement is based on three components: behavioural indicators, physiological parameters, and the child's report of his pain (Hamers et al 1998, Royal College of Nursing 1999a).

Although the assessment of a child's pain is an important issue, the effective relief of that pain must be achieved. Nurses should be enabled to anticipate pain in the child and manage this based on obvious alterations in anatomical or physiological integrity (Broome & Slack 1990). For example, it would seem inevitable that pain will occur following a surgical procedure, therefore pain relief should be provided in anticipation of this pain.

Parents and others as aids in assessing children's pain

Pain behaviours in children can be misinterpreted as separation anxiety, fear or distress due to immobilization. A number of studies have identified that nurses use behavioural cues to aid pain identification (Fuller & Conner 1996), that infants displayed behavioural responses to painful stimuli (Rushforth 1994), and that many children cannot or will not report pain to those providing health care (Woodgate & Kristjanson 1995). Since nurses have reported that they rely on non-verbal cues in paediatric pain assessment, although this is appropriate, assumptions made by nurses about behaviour should be validated with the child if possible, or the parents or carers.

Children identify their parents and carers as the most important source of comfort when in pain (Royal College of Nursing 1999b). However, nurses do not appear to use the parents and carers as a source of information in pain management. It must be a consideration that the parents and carers themselves are in a stressful situation and may need to be enabled to perform this role. Usually parents are reliable sources of information about their child's behaviour during hospitalization (Wilson & Doyle 1996). They can give an indication of the child's experience of pain and ways of coping with it, thus providing baseline information on which the nursing staff can build. Parents should be adequately prepared to meet the challenges of their child's pain (Finley et al 1996, McCready et al 1991). This is a further role of the children's nurse who needs to ensure that the parents are as informed as possible so that they can help their child manage the pain (Royal College of Nursing 1999a).

Evidence based practice

Gillies et al (1995) found that young children's pain after surgery is often poorly recognized and consequently poorly treated. This study also found that staff required more focused training in the accurate assessment and management of children's pain. The study looked at 40 children under 5 years of age who had received surgery. Parents and staff also participated and the study further concluded that mothers had an important role in assessing and managing their child's pain.

PLANNING EFFECTIVE PAIN MANAGEMENT

It has been suggested that the management of pain should be diverse enough to take account of the various dimensions of the pain experience. It must then be an important issue for nurses in their professional role, a part of clinical decision making and professional reflection in action. Nurses are responsible for the administration of drugs to patients. They are also responsible for educating patients and their families or carers, as appropriate, in the management of their prescribed medications (see Ch. 9 on medicines). The nurse can be instrumental in ensuring a more personalized approach to the individual's pain management, but to achieve this the nurse needs a sound knowledge of the various methods of managing pain. Such actions are usually considered in terms of pharmacological and non-pharmacological interventions.

Decision making exercise

Mr Phil O'Reilly has been admitted suffering from chest pain. This is thought to be due to a severe angina attack. He is grey, sweating profusely and is complaining of chest and left arm pain. He is obviously frightened and has asked you to contact a priest as he is convinced that he is about to die. His partner has been contacted and is on the way to the hospital from work. Accurate and quick assessment is required in this case of acute pain.

- What areas of pain assessment would take priority in this case?
- Consider the additional information you would require from Mr O'Reilly's partner to enable you to liaise effectively between the patient and the doctor managing Mr O'Reilly's pain.
- Once adequate pain relief has been achieved what health promotion strategy would be necessary from the nurse to help Mr O'Reilly prevent or reduce the frequency of recurrence of the chest pain in the future?

Pharmacological interventions

The correct use of medication is essential for effective pain management, but has been shown to be an area where nurses often fail to excel. Most commonly problems occur due to inaccurate assessment of pain as the presenting problem and a lack of insight into which drugs to use in the treatment of different types of pain (Latham 1991). Nurses are now able to prescribe certain drugs, but this is limited and often drugs required for treatment of severe pain will need a medical prescription. Nurses need knowledge of the methods of administration of analgesia and how these drugs are applicable to the patient's pain experience. For example the preferred route of opioid administration for cancer patients is oral (Vortherms et al 1992) or in relation to children, many report the pain of injections as the worst pain therefore the use of such routes should be minimized. Some medicines have been found to be more effective for certain types of pain. The nurse interacts with both the patient and the doctor responsible for prescribing analgesia and is therefore in an ideal position to influence appropriate prescribing. This will result in an individualized and consequently more effective regimen to aid the patient's pain management. A sound knowledge base and experience will enhance the recognition of the implications of the information yielded by the assessment (Fordham & Dunn 1994). Also the patient should understand the medicines they are taking and the reasons they are taking them, particularly in cases of chronic pain management where the patient may have available to them a variety of analgesic agents.

Types of analgesia

There are three categories of analgesics: opioid drugs, non-opioid drugs and co-analgesic drugs, and their usage is generally based upon their method of action.

1. Opioid drugs (e.g. morphine, pethidine, codeine) mainly work in the brain and spinal cord to inhibit the transmission of pain. They are generally used to relieve severe pain and associated effects include a sense of well-being in the individual. They are therefore linked with a tendency to produce mental and physical dependence. They are subject to the Misuse of Drugs Act 1971 and have to be prescribed by a medical or dental practitioner.
2. Non-opioid drugs (e.g. aspirin, paracetamol, ibuprofen, indometacin) mainly work in the peripheral tissues by interfering with chemicals that stimulate pain endings. Useful in the relief of musculoskeletal pain and mild to moderate pain.
3. Co-analgesic drugs have a variety of actions, for example muscle relaxant or sedative (diazepam), antidepressant (amitriptyline), or suppressor of inflammatory reactions (corticosteroids).

A range of issues are relevant in considering appropriate analgesic therapy. Drugs can be used alone or in combination to produce pain relief. The intensity of pain should influence the type of analgesic prescribed. The effective dose varies for each individual and therefore the effect of the drug given should be carefully monitored. There is a ceiling with non-opioid drugs so that beyond a certain dose there will be no increased analgesic effect, but with opioid drugs the limitations of dosage appear to be the associated side effects. Repeated administration of narcotic (opioid) drugs have been shown to cause tolerance and dependence. This is no deterrent, however, in the control of pain in terminal disease. Recommended practice is to adjust both the dose and the frequency of administration so that the patient never suffers pain.

Ideally, an optimum level of pain control is achieved by using analgesic agents. However, this may take time, and because of the uniqueness of the individual pain experience, pain relief should be constantly evaluated and updated. The duration of action of the analgesic is an important issue since the ideal is to maintain an acceptable level of pain relief for the patient. The nurse therefore needs an awareness of both the effectiveness of the drug and its duration. In this way the nurse will be able to limit the delay between the time when the patient needs pain relief and the time when the administered drug becomes effective. Analgesic ladders are frequently used in practice situations to achieve this aim (Fig. 10.5).

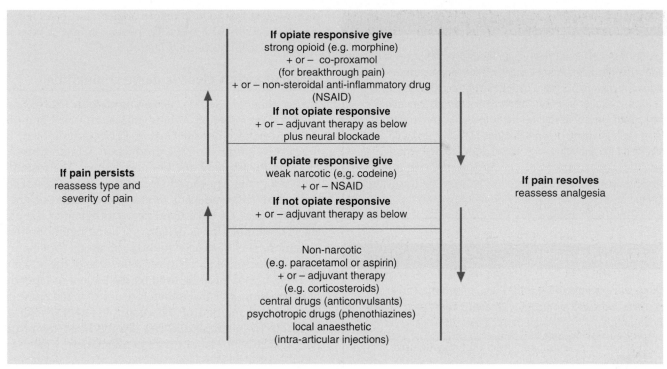

If opiate responsive give
strong opioid (e.g. morphine)
+ or − co-proxamol
(for breakthrough pain)
+ or − non-steroidal anti-inflammatory drug
(NSAID)
If not opiate responsive
+ or − adjuvant therapy as below
plus neural blockade

If opiate responsive give
weak narcotic (e.g. codeine)
+ or − NSAID
If not opiate responsive
+ or − adjuvant therapy as below

Non-narcotic
(e.g. paracetamol or aspirin)
+ or − adjuvant therapy
(e.g. corticosteroids)
central drugs (anticonvulsants)
psychotropic drugs (phenothiazines)
local anaesthetic
(intra-articular injections)

If pain persists
reassess type and
severity of pain

If pain resolves
reassess analgesia

Figure 10.5   An analgesic ladder.

Reflection and portfolio exercise

Consider the drugs that may be given to an individual in mild, moderate or severe pain.

- Investigate the use of each of the following analgesic drugs – paracetamol, ibuprofen, dihydrocodeine tartrate, morphine – from your textbooks and reflect on how you have seen them used in practice. Establish how each drug works and its common side effects and make notes of these.

Reflect over the following:

- Consider how side effects affect your decision making in the choice of drugs to administer to a particular client group (e.g. children, adults or the elderly).
- Now consider how side effects will affect your decision making in the choice of drugs to administer in a particular pain context (e.g. postoperative pain, cancer pain, chronic pain).
- Will the client's locality make a difference to your decision making (e.g. whether at home or in hospital)?
- Write a summary of your learning and how it will help your practice for your portfolio.

Modes of delivery

Many routes are available for the administration of medicines (see also Ch. 9) and it is now necessary to explore some of these routes in relation to the administration of analgesics. Opioid and non-opioid analgesics can be given by various routes including orally, intramuscularly, intravenously, rectally and subcutaneously.

Infusion pumps are often used for the administration of analgesics and can be:

- intravenous (commonly used for acute postoperative pain)
- subcutaneous (commonly used for palliative care)
- epidural, that is, a nerve block (commonly used for labour pain).

Pumps can also be operated by the patient to provide patient controlled analgesia (PCA). The analgesic is prescribed as for the infusion pump and the nurse sets up the system as required. The patient is then able to take control of their pain in a positive way. There is usually a button control and when the patient depresses the button he or she receives a bolus dose of the analgesic to limit the pain. Each PCA pump has a 'lock out' time between doses so that the patient cannot overdose. There are also security features such as a key to lock the pump to limit the risk of interference once the prescribed rate has been set.

Whatever the mode of delivery a careful explanation is required for the patient and their family or carers as appropriate so that they can take an active part in the pain control.

Non-pharmacological interventions

There are many strategies that do not involve drugs that can be used to help relieve pain. These non-pharmacological interventions can be used successfully with most client groups and include distraction, cutaneous stimulation and relaxation techniques (May 1992). For the infant, distraction can include holding and cuddling or using a dummy or comforter. Older children may be encouraged to count or talk about other more pleasant experiences to help distract them. Play therapy can also be useful in taking the child's mind away from the pain. Cutaneous stimulation includes gentle massage or rubbing of the skin, which may be used for all age groups. Relaxation techniques can be used effectively with older children who have the cognitive skills to understand instructions as well as with adults. It has been shown to be a beneficial method in pain management (Main & Spanswick 2000). Deep breathing and counting can be used to take the focus off the pain and can result in a lessening of the pain experience. Meditation is one of the most effective means of counteracting the stress associated with pain and anxiety by producing a relaxation response (Chaitow 2002). Visual stimuli have also been shown to be successful in increasing pain thresholds and pain tolerance. In 2002 Tse et al found that the use of visual stimuli could be a successful adjunct to pain relief. In their experiment they used a soundless video display of natural scenery, such as a mountainous area, river flow and a waterfall, which significantly increased both pain thresholds and pain tolerance in their subjects. In their conclusions they suggest that to help relieve anxiety and pain, the provision of windows with views for patients might be very useful within the hospital complex (Tse et al 2002).

Transcutaneous electric nerve stimulation

Transcutaneous electric nerve stimulation (TENS) can be used for the relief of chronic and acute pain. The precise mechanism of pain relief using TENS is unknown, but it may act by stimulating the production of endorphins or by blocking the primary afferent nerve fibres. The system consists of a battery-powered electrical pulse generator that is connected via some leads to electrodes placed on the skin over the area of a peripheral nerve innervating the painful site. The stimulation is usually felt as a tingling or buzzing sensation. TENS has been found to be useful for labour pain and postoperative and chronic pain. One of the advantages of TENS is that it can be used by the patient independently of the nursing staff and is therefore useful in the home environment as a method of pain control. TENS machines are available to purchase and can also be hired for a specific period such as for labour pain in pregnancy.

Massage

Massage is a therapeutic manipulation of the soft tissue of the body. It is believed that it limits the pain experience by stimulation that 'closes the gate' on the pain or alternatively stimulation of the skin may result in the release of endorphins (Chaitow 2002). It can also be viewed as a form of relaxation or distraction, drawing attention from the pain and altering the perception of pain.

The massage is usually carried out over and around the site of the pain. However, massage should not take place in areas that are actively inflamed, or where there are open wounds or damaged skin. Care should be taken with this therapy, since it is a form of communication and may be open to various interpretations. Culturally the intimacy involved in this technique must be handled sensitively, and an acceptable approach must be sought. Sometimes a foot massage may be more acceptable than a body massage.

Complementary therapies

Over recent years interest in alternative therapies has grown. Complementary therapies are holistic natural therapies that may be used in conjunction with conventional medical or nursing treatments to enhance the physical and psychological well-being of the patient. The use of such therapy demands the practitioner to be autonomous in their practices. The practitioner in this instance need not necessarily be a nurse. The nurse in this situation will be answerable for the choices made in the treatment delivered and will be accountable under the *Code of Professional Conduct* (Nursing and Midwifery Council 2002) for such actions. The therapies require a hands-on approach by the practitioner and the therapies need time as well as privacy in which the practitioner and patient can communicate. These approaches need careful handling, since some nurses may believe that they can learn all there is to learn about a complementary therapy in a half day's study. They may then go on to put the patient at risk because of a lack of competence. Complementary therapies could offer the patient benefits by focusing on the process of promoting health and healing (Armstrong & Waldron 1991). However, there is also a need for the patient to appreciate the potential benefits of such treatments, as belief in treatment is vital for success (Chaitow 2002). Armstrong & Waldron (1991) suggested criteria for the practice of complementary therapies. These include:

- consent from the patient, relative or carer before treatment
- consultation with a relevant medical practitioner
- authorization agreed between the nurse and nurse manager
- documentation with a record of the treatment in the patient care plan.

The UK Central Council (1996) included a section about complementary and alternative therapies in their *Guidelines for Professional Practice*. This document has been adopted by the Nursing and Midwifery Council. They recommend that nurses ensure that the introduction of these therapies is always in the best interests and safety of the patient or client. Further, they suggest a team approach where it should be part of professional teamwork to discuss the use of complementary therapies with medical and other members of the healthcare team. Furthermore practitioners are reminded that we can be called to account for any activities carried out outside conventional practice.

Aromatherapy

Aromatherapy is the use of essential oils in the treatment of medical conditions or as relaxing agents, and has been in use over many centuries. The exact way aromatherapy works is unknown, but it has been found to be effective for enhancing well-being, relieving stress and rejuvenating and regenerating the body. Treatment usually involves massage and can take several hours. Aromatherapy has been particularly used in the treatment of:

- stress-related conditions (e.g. anxiety, depression, insomnia)
- digestive disorders (e.g. colic and constipation)
- skin conditions (e.g. acne and eczema)
- minor infections (e.g. cystitis).

Acupuncture

Acupuncture was developed by the ancient Chinese. Fine needles are used that pierce the skin at points on the body where particular effects can be obtained. These needles may then be rotated or stimulated. Certain types of acupuncture are thought to promote release of endogenous opiate (endorphins and enkephalins) (Wall & Melzack 1999). Other theories are that nerve fibres carry and transmit the acupuncture effect or that the meridians are electrically distinct and that changes within them are responsible for triggering the neural and hormonal responses (Chaitow 1993, Jessel-Kenyon et al 1992).

Acupressure

Acupressure has evolved from the same Oriental roots as acupuncture. Acupressure uses finger pressure on the acupuncture points to manipulate the energy imbalances. Acupressure is a versatile treatment that can be given wherever and whenever it is convenient. Acupressure should not be used around an open wound or where there is inflammation or swelling.

Reflexology

Reflexology is based on the belief that the body's natural healing mechanisms can be enhanced by the application of pressure to certain areas of the feet and hands. The areas are connected to different parts of the body by a flow of energy.

Treatment usually involves the patient sitting with their legs raised, while the feet are examined. Pressure is then applied to all areas on both feet. The therapist uses the feel of certain areas to establish which areas need attention. It is usual for a treatment to last between 30 and 60 minutes. Transient effects may be noticed as the body heals itself, where unresolved health problems may flare up temporarily. There have been attempts to relate the mode of action of reflexology to neurology, where the nerve supplies appear to be related in several areas of the body. Therefore stimulation of the body's surface can affect the functioning of internal organs. However, there is limited evidence of this to link the identified areas of the feet and all other parts of the body.

Homeopathy

Homeopathy is a treatment based on the belief that a substance that produces the symptoms of a health problem may also cure it (i.e. treating like with like). According to homeopaths, symptoms are a manifestation of the body's efforts to fight the process of disease. There is therefore no point in suppressing the symptoms. The aim is to establish the cause of the symptoms and to treat the whole person, allowing the body's natural defences to restore health. It is claimed that homeopathy can be used for any reversible illness and that it has other benefits including a preventive role and a strengthening role. By helping the body's natural defences homeopathy may complement the action of other medicines.

Homeopathy has been found to be particularly effective when used with:

- allergic conditions such as hay fever
- stress-related conditions such as eczema or migraine.

An example of homeopathic treatment of eczema is the use of petroleum, despite the knowledge that petrol and oil can cause cracks and itchiness in a person with sensitive skin exposed to them.

> **Evidence based practice**
>
> In 1995, Rogers, a mental health nurse, found that homeopathy proved useful for alcohol-dependent patients during detoxification when distress and mental 'pain' can be very acute. In a small scale pilot study he worked with the assumption that successful homeopathic treatment would reduce the frequency and length of relapses and help the patients maintain abstinence or control consumption. Of the seven clients who received treatment all reported benefits. In the case studies included, the benefits to the individual of the homeopathic treatments are clearly outlined. One of the major benefits was an improvement of sleep patterns; a disturbed sleep pattern is often the most intractable problem after detoxification.

Hypnotherapy

Hypnosis appears to be a relatively recent phenomenon, dating back to the late 18th century. Rhythmic dancing and drumming that induce a similar state have a long history in Africa and North America and something closely resembling hypnosis can be traced back to ancient Egypt, Greece and the Druids in the UK. Hypnotherapy is the use of hypnotic techniques in the treatment of certain conditions. The trance-like state allows the individual to become more compliant, relaxed and open to suggestion. Suggestions are implanted that can be triggered after the individual has come out of the trance, but it is probably impossible to make anyone do something against their will. The individual is usually induced into a hypnotic state by the therapist. People can be taught to induce the state themselves to help with relaxation, and tapes can be used to aid this process.

There is no adequate explanation of how hypnotherapy works. It is thought that on hypnosis the individual enters a mental state between wakefulness and unconsciousness, and electroencephalograms (EEGs) taken on hypnotized subjects support this. Hypnotherapy can be particularly useful in the treatment of physical conditions where there may be a large psychological element such as eczema, psoriasis, migraine and colitis. Insomnia and phobias, obsessions, some addictions and compulsions, for example smoking, eating disorders and compulsive gambling, can benefit from hypnotherapy. Care is needed, however, for those with severe psychological health problems such as depression or psychosis as hypnosis can lead to further disturbance.

> **Evidence based practice**
>
> A study found that hypnotherapy should be considered as a complementary treatment in dermatology (Stewart & Thomas 1995). The participants, 18 adults and 20 children with extensive atopic dermatitis that had proved resistant to conventional therapy, were given hypnotherapy and their conditions were monitored for up to 18 months. All except one showed an immediate improvement after the first treatment and this was maintained at the following two clinic appointments.
>
> A further study investigated the anti-emetic effect of hypnosis for children receiving chemotherapy (Coanch et al 1995). Children in the experimental group who were taught a self-hypnosis technique reported a significant decrease in the frequency, severity, amount and duration of nausea.

> **Reflection and portfolio exercise**
>
> - Consider how your professional role as a nurse may enable you to work together with the patient in the use of complementary treatments as part of conventional treatment.
> - Make notes of the various aspects of your role and how these may benefit patients in their choice of therapy.

PROFESSIONAL AND ETHICAL KNOWLEDGE

This section explores the areas of decision making in relation to your future professional role in practice, specifically in relation to teamwork and the specialist role of the nurse. Legal and ethical areas are highlighted, but these are not exclusive and you should explore the multifaceted professional role further.

ROLE OF THE NURSE IN RELATION TO PAIN

The Nursing and Midwifery Council's (2002) *Code of Professional Conduct* requires the nurse to 'protect and support the health of individual patients and clients' and also to 'assess the knowledge, skills and abilities required for lawful, safe and effective practice without direct supervision'. The nurse therefore has a responsibility to his or her patients and clients to increase their knowledge of pain and to use this knowledge in the implementation of pain care. A conceptual framework is necessary if the complexity of pain is to be understood.

Pain is a complex phenomenon involving physical, psychological, emotional and spiritual components. It is therefore vital that the nurse views each individual's situation holistically. The nurse's sphere of responsibility may be within a hospital or other establishment or more widely in the community. The role includes teaching the patient, administering medications and using non-pharmacological pain relief methods (McCaffery & Beebe 1994). Nurses should also take into account their own views about pain as these influence the way we interact with others. It is difficult to look at our own fears, myths and prejudices honestly, but without this we risk misinterpreting the experience of others (Fordham & Dunn 1994). It is therefore necessary to attempt to have a positive attitude to the person in pain and to accept overall what he or she is able to tell you about their pain.

In summary each individual nurse has many roles in the care of patients in pain. Figure 10.6 illustrates this multifaceted role and conceptualizes the discussion that has taken place.

Evidence based practice

A study by Baillie (1993) found that nurses give less priority to the relief of pain than other nursing duties. Later De Rond et al (2000) found that the implementation of a pain monitoring programme (PMP) consisting of two components – (1) education of nurses about pain, (2) assessment and management and implementing a daily pain assessment using a numerical scale – improved nurse assessment of patients' pain. It also improved the documentation of pain in the nursing records.

THE MULTIDISCIPLINARY TEAM IN PAIN MANAGEMENT

The nurse works as part of a team. Usually this team is working towards a common goal for the promotion of the ultimate good of the patient or client. In pain control many team members may be involved. Commonly these include:

- the patient or client and their family, carers, or significant others
- nurses – perhaps a specialist nurse with specific responsibility for pain management
- doctors – anaesthetists with their specialized skills in relation to local and regional block analgesia
- physiotherapists.

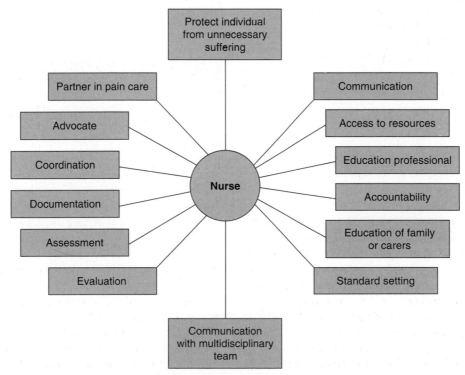

Figure 10.6 The role of the nurse in pain management.

Frequently other individuals are involved in the pain care, particularly in cases of chronic or uncontrolled pain, for example:

- an occupational therapist
- a pharmacist
- a radiotherapist
- a psychologist.

A complementary therapist, who may or may not be a nurse, may also be involved in the individual's pain care. Since the environment of care is commonly a hospital or the patient's home, the nurse is in the ideal position to act as the coordinator of the team approach to pain control. Thus the importance of effective communication is further highlighted.

The patient and their family or carers have a greater responsibility and control of the pain plan when the patient is cared for in the community. The patient and their family or carers must therefore be adequately prepared to carry out this responsibility. While in hospital patients adopt a routine that is part of the hospital environment, but in their own home they need the support to facilitate their abilities to deal effectively with their pain. The teaching role of the nurse is a major factor in ensuring the patient is able to manage at home.

All nurses have a role in health promotion in relation to the use and abuse of analgesic drugs by the public. Mild analgesics can be obtained without a medical prescription and can be overused for minor ailments. Prolonged and continued use can be detrimental to the long-term health of the individual. The public are often not aware of the 'hidden drug' element when advertising promotes a product under a user friendly name such as 'Night Nurse'. The actual content of analgesia within the drug may not be noticed. People have inadvertently overdosed themselves because of this problem.

Easy to obtain analgesics are often the most readily at hand when someone wishes to take an overdose, as in attempted suicide or deliberate self-harm (Carrigan 1994, Davenport 1993). The most dangerous drug in overdosage and also ironically one of the safest in its usual prescribed dose is paracetamol (Panadol). Because of its delayed effects on the liver a relatively small ingestion of this drug can have fatal consequences.

THE ROLE OF THE SPECIALIST NURSE

The growth of the clinical nurse specialist role and specialist practitioners is a relatively recent phenomenon in the UK. Essentially this came about as a result of the UK Central Council's papers considering the future and scope of professional practice (Department of Health 1999, UK Central Council 1992, 1994). The suggestion of these papers is to promote autonomous practice sensitive to changing healthcare needs. The development of the clinical nurse specialist stimulates the individual to become more involved in one area of nursing, applying their skills to identify problems and seek answers (McSharry 1995). A study undertaken in England in 1996 showed that pain was one of the most common areas of specialist nursing practice (McGee et al 1996). This pain specialist nursing role within a hospital or community unit has often been instigated within a multidisciplinary team. The pain specialist nurse gives advice to both healthcare professionals and the public on the effective management of pain. Thus health education and research are primary functions of such a team. The specialist nurse is a key member of the team and advises nurses, carers and the public, often through a system of links with individual representatives of a ward or unit or patient representative group. Through 'link nurse' schemes difficult individual cases can be referred directly to the specialist nurse for advice. Such schemes also allow for updating of all health professionals on recent research based evidence of practice (Elliott 1995), such as pain management.

ETHICO-LEGAL ISSUES IN PAIN MANAGEMENT

Moral thinking is primarily a matter of reflecting on past experiences and predicting future consequences (Kenworthy et al 2002). The main moral dilemmas in pain management are often focused around the care of the dying and in the day-to-day decision making about adequate levels of analgesia.

Thompson et al (2000) suggest three models that the nurse may adopt in terms of professional role:

- code based ethics – related to a code of conduct under which most nurses operate
- contractual ethics – usually apply where the patient or client approaches the carer before the start of treatment
- covenantal ethics – apply to long-term situations such as palliative care.

Providing prompt and adequate management of pain relief for adults is now a widely accepted philosophy, but there are still misconceptions when it comes to managing a child's pain. Misconceptions about the effects of analgesia on children can seriously affect the care of children in pain. Controversies exist over the safety of pharmacological interventions (Stevens & Johnston 1992). Specific reasons given for the undermedication of infants include the fear of addiction and respiratory depression and lack of knowledge concerning the physiological effects of opiates in the pain relief of infants (Craig 1992, Stevens & Johnston 1992). The nurse must have a clear understanding of the ways in which children and those with learning disabilities can experience and exhibit pain. Despite in some instances their limited ability to communicate we must recognize them as an authority about the nature and existence of their pain. A major role of the nurse must be to alleviate the individual's pain.

Problems also occur when there is confusion in understanding and acceptance of the patient's declaration of pain. Pain is an experience of the individual, body and mind

(Fordham & Dunn 1994). It is recognized that pain may have an emotional or psychological origin, termed psychogenic pain, but many individuals caring for patients have difficulty with this distinction. This in turn can be a source of confusion and inappropriate care delivery when this pain 'in the mind' is considered made up or imaginary pain. Patients may be labelled as timewasters or attention seeking. Psychogenic pain may be defined as a localized sensation of pain caused solely by mental events, with no physical findings to initiate or sustain the pain (McCaffery & Beebe 1994). Conventional attitudes to pain make it difficult to believe that mental states can result in physically perceived symptoms and this in turn influences the care provided. Essentially the nurse needs to identify their own preconceptions of pain and to accept the patient's declaration of pain, whatever the perceived cause, and seek to provide appropriate interventions.

This complex task requires developmental, societal and professional knowledge and skills. A further factor that influences the nurses' medication practice is their ability to assess the level and intensity of pain and then to intervene to manage that pain. Ideally the individual should receive pain relief before they develop severe pain. The nurse has this responsibility in her professional role. With the arrival of quality mechanisms of clinical areas that provide charters to improve the well-being and increase the rights of individuals in hospital, freedom from pain should become a priority. Pain care should be a nursing priority for all client groups. But generally any vulnerable client, the person with learning disabilities, a mental health problem or a child, is at risk of poor pain care due to their limited ability to communicate successfully with healthcare professionals coordinating their pain care management.

The rights of all patients, adult or child, are for high-quality care in all aspects of pain management. Nurses are accountable for their own individual level of knowledge, skills and attitudes. They will also, because of their position in the healthcare team, have a significant role in patient advocacy in relation to pain management (Mallik 1994, Royal College of Nursing 1995). In the broader professional arena the development of National Service Frameworks, Clinical Governance, standard setting and benchmarking are all moves toward equality in care provision and delivery.

Decision making exercise

Charles is a 60-year-old retired miner who has been diagnosed with lung cancer and had surgery, but now has symptoms of spread of the cancer to the spine. He has been discharged home to the care of the primary health care team. The district nurse has noted that Charles's pain, despite regular doses of morphine, is not being controlled adequately. The general practitioner has been reluctant to increase the drug dosage any further and stated that he 'considered the dosage adequate for the stage of the disease'.

- Decide on how the district nurse should approach this situation if she is to remain accountable for providing Charles with adequate pain relief.
- Review the moral dilemma for the nurse if the general practitioner refuses to increase the dosage and review Charles's case in order to provide pain relief at this stage of his illness.

PERSONAL AND REFLECTIVE KNOWLEDGE

AWARENESS OF YOUR OWN BELIEFS AND VALUES ABOUT PAIN

To make effective decisions in relation to the patient in pain the nurse requires knowledge and skills in the area of pain management. An understanding of the theories of pain and pain transmission is necessary to help conceptualize the experience for the patient. Nurses have an important part to play in pain management by individualizing the assessment of pain and acting as advocates for their patients. They should be proactive and anticipatory in the care and assessment of their patients' pain. Involving the individual, if possible, and his or her family or carers, in the assessment, management and evaluation of pain, and using a partnership approach will provide holistic and theory based nursing care. To provide optimum care for your patient you must be aware of influences such as your own beliefs and values about pain, cultural norms, behaviours and stereotyping. This awareness should enable you to be less biased and lead to effective treatment of the patient's pain. Nurses have a responsibility to constantly improve and update their knowledge and skills in all areas of pain management.

The experience you gain in practice placements is of vital importance to your learning about pain management. Keeping a reflective diary will help you isolate those experiences that are relevant to the knowledge base provided by this chapter and the further reading necessary to solve specific problems you have encountered. The recording and analysis of this will also provide processes for your use in your portfolio development. The exercises throughout this chapter can prompt you to take a reflective and questioning approach to your practice experience.

CASE STUDIES IN PAIN MANAGEMENT

The following case studies will help you consolidate the knowledge gained from the chapter and further your reading and practice experience.

Case study: Adult

Miss Prudence Allison has been admitted for rehabilitative treatment after a fall at home. She has sustained a fractured right femur and a dislocation of her right shoulder. She has osteoporosis of the spine that has recently deteriorated. She has a great deal of pain and distress from this condition and she has frequently stated that she feels it's time her life came to an end. She has been prescribed analgesia of dihydrocodeine (DF118) on a pro re nata (PRN) basis. She has now been hospitalized for 4 weeks and has developed a chest infection.

The nurse is not in a position to address Miss Allison's request to end her life, but should seek to interpret the reason why this request may have been made. Miss Allison is in continual pain and lately her injuries and now her chest infection have combined to cause her added distress and discomfort.

Social, educational, racial, gender, religious and family circumstances can impact upon the behaviour and attitudes of the patient. The nurse should be aware of and able to judge the effect of these factors in assessing the patient and formulating the best approach to treatment.

- There are many areas within Miss Allison's care for an ethical debate. In the light of the information you have about Miss Allison, consider the request that she has made.
- What might be the reason for this request?
- How is your role as a nurse affected by the ethical and legal issues that surround this request?
- What might be considered the difference between effective pain relief for Miss Allison and her request to end her suffering?
- Miss Allison is suffering with her long-term condition. Consider the actions the nurse may be able to take to help Miss Allison cope more effectively with it.
- What advice and resources may be available to Miss Allison to limit her pain?

Case study: Mental health

Malique King is a 45-year-old man, of no fixed address with an itinerant lifestyle. He suffers from schizophrenia and is also an alcoholic. He has been brought into the Accident and Emergency department on several occasions in the last few weeks. He has usually been found collapsed in a drunken state in the street or park. Previously, despite attempts to refer Malique for appropriate mental health and medical consultation, he has disappeared from the department after a couple of hours. He has come into the department this evening of his own accord, smelling strongly of alcohol. He is dirty and unkempt and is complaining of 'bellyache'. His baseline observations of pulse and respiration are slightly elevated. The doctors have been informed, but they appear to believe that Malique is looking for a bed for the night. Malique has never complained of pain before when he has been brought into the department; in fact he has always appeared very unhappy at being in the department and has not been very communicative.

- Consider the reasons why the doctors may not believe Malique's complaints of pain.
- Consider the appropriate action that the nurse should take to assess Malique and to ensure his needs are met.
- What are the grounds for these actions?
- What are the responsibilities of the nurse?
- Write a short account of your actions in relation to the theory that supports the accountability role of the nurse in this instance. This will help you to rationalize the decisions you have made in relation to Malique's needs.

Case study: Learning disabilities

Louise Freeman is 29 years old. She has cerebral palsy that arose as the result of trauma during her birth. She is quadriplegic with developmental delay and has very little communication, though is usually able to vocalize whether she is happy or sad. She has some difficulty swallowing and eating has always been difficult. She has been cared for at home by her elderly parents. Recently Louise has developed pressure sores on her buttocks and elbows and her parents are finding it increasingly difficult to maintain her normal eating pattern. She has been admitted to hospital to give some support to her parents and to assess the difficulty with feeding. She has recently lost weight and on admission she weighs 4 stone 10 lbs (30 kg). Mrs Freeman tells you that she thinks Louise is not comfortable.

- You need to be able to assess the level of Louise's pain so that you can make decisions to carry out appropriate nursing care. Find out what tools are available to you and if they are suitable to assess Louise's pain.
- Consider the factors involved here so that the pain can be accurately assessed.
- What members of the multidisciplinary team may be involved in Louise's pain care and why would they be included?
- Louise is now able to return home. She has been prescribed pentazocine (Fortral) suppositories to help control her pain. Consider the information her parents will need about her analgesia to keep her pain under control.
- Louise's mother is reluctant to give her the analgesic as she does not want her to be sleepy in the daytime. How would you explain to her the way that the drug works and its effects?

Case study: Child

Jordan Simpson is 14 years old. He has sickle cell anaemia and has been admitted to the ward in crisis. Jordan is the eldest of three children and his mother, Joan, who is a single parent, relies on him to help with the care of his brother and sister. Joan works in a local public house and in the evenings Jordan babysits. Joan has had trouble paying the bills and Jordan has been very worried about this. It is felt that this stress has brought on the current crisis.

On admission Jordan is in severe pain. He is quiet and uncommunicative. His facial expression is a grimace. His mother has accompanied him, but she needs to return home very shortly to collect her other children from school. PCA has been commenced with a morphine infusion.

- Consider the care decisions that have to be made to achieve optimum pain relief for Jordan.
- Find out about sickle cell anaemia and the precipitating factors.
- Are there any special observations to be made when Jordan is receiving morphine?
- Make a decision about how you may be able to help Jordan and his family prevent further crises.
- Consider the various roles of the nurse here to provide Jordan with appropriate care and support.

Summary

This chapter has drawn together theoretical concepts of pain and applied this knowledge in relation to the practice of caring for individuals. It has included:

1. Theories of pain and how pain is transmitted within the individual. Physiological and psychological signs and symptoms of the pain experience have also been examined.
2. Factors influencing decision making by nurses in relation to pain assessment and management have been considered.
3. The use of pain assessment tools in practice and different ways of reducing pain in an individual have been explored, including the use of pharmacological and non-pharmacological intervention and the inclusion of complementary therapies.
4. The professional role of the nurse in pain management has been discussed, both as an individual and as a member of a multidisciplinary team.

5. Knowledge illuminated within this chapter has been combined with evidence from other referenced sources and applied within a range of situations. Suggestions have been made for portfolio development in relation to pain management.

Annotated further reading and websites

Carter B (ed) 1998 Perspectives on pain: mapping the territory. Arnold, London
For an excellent account of the cultural aspects of pain, see the chapter 'Cultural dimensions of pain', by Bryn Davis.

Wall P D, Melzack R 1999 Textbook of pain, 4th edn. Churchill Livingstone, Edinburgh
An excellent general textbook. See especially the discussion on psychiatric/mental pain, pp 931–949.

http://www.painsociety.org/
This is the site of the British Chapter of the International Association for the Study of Pain. It includes recommendations of the society for nursing practice in pain management.

http://nmap.ac.uk/
This website contains resources related to many aspects of pain including management and assessment but also relating to current evidence for practice in this area.

http://www.uclan.ac.uk/
This website includes national benchmarking standards for the assessment of pain.

http://www.doh.gov.org/
The Department of Health's website contains details of the paper *Essence of Care* relating to benchmarking standards, which include pain assesssment and management.

http://www.ich.ucl.ac.uk/
This website includes details of the Children's Pain Assessment Project, and also standards for pain audit and best practice in pain assessment in children.

References

Abu-Saad H H 2001 Evidence based palliative care across the lifespan. Blackwell Science, Oxford

Anand K J S, Craig K D 1996 New perspectives on the definition of pain. Pain 67(1):3–6

Akinsanya C Y 1985 The use of knowledge in the management of pain. Nurse Education Today 5:41–46

Armstrong F, Waldron R 1991 A complementary strategy. Nursing Times 87(11):34–35

Baillie L 1993 A review of pain assessment tools. Nursing Standard 7(23):25–29

Bendelow G 1993 Pain perceptions, gender and emotion. Sociology of Health and Illness 15(3):273–294

Bendelow G, Williams S 1995 Pain and the mind–body dualism: a sociological approach. Body and Society 1(2):83–103

Bishop G 1946 Neural mechanisms of cutaneous sense. Physiology Review 26:77–102

Bishop G 1959 The relationship between nerve fibre size and sensory modality: phylogenetic implications of the afferent innervation of the cortex. Journal of Nervous and Mental Disorders 128:89–114

Bonica J L 1990 The management of pain, 2nd edn. Lea & Febiger, Philadelphia

Broome M E, Slack J F 1990 Influences on nurses management of pain in children. American Journal of Maternal Child Nursing 15(3):158–162

Brown S Y, Bowman J M, Eason F R 1999 Assessment of nurses' attitudes and knowledge regarding pain management. Journal of Continuing Education in Nursing 30(3):132–139

Carr E C J, Mann E M 2000 Pain: creative approaches to effective management. Macmillan, Basingstoke

Carrigan J T 1994 The psychosocial needs of patients who have attempted suicide by overdose. Journal of Advanced Nursing 20(4):635–642

Carroll D, Bowsher D 1993 Pain management and nursing care. Butterworth-Heinemann, Oxford

Carter B (ed) 1998 Perspectives on pain: mapping the territory. Arnold, London

Carter B, McArthur E, Cunliffe M 2002 Dealing with uncertainty: parental assessment of pain in their children with profound special needs. Journal of Advanced Nursing 38(5):449–457

Chaitow L 1993 Holistic pain relief: how to ease muscles, joints and other painful conditions. Thorsons, London

Chaitow L 2002 Conquer pain: the natural way. Duncan Baird, London

Charlesworth W R 1982 An ethological approach to research on facial expressions. In: Izard C E (ed) Measuring emotions in infants and children. Cambridge University Press, Cambridge, pp 317–334

Children Act 1989 HMSO, London

Coanch P, Hockenbery M, Herman S 1995 Self-hypnosis as antiemetic therapy in children receiving chemotherapy. Oncology Nursing Forum 12(4):41–46

Colwell C, Clark L, Perkins R 1996 Postoperative use of pediatric pain scales: children's self-report versus nurse assessment of pain intensity and affect. Journal of Pediatric Nursing 11(6):375–382

Craig K D 1992 Pleasure and pain: a scientist/professional looks at organized psychology. Canadian Psychology 33(1):45–60

Darwin E 1794 Cited in Dallenbach K 1939 Pain: history and present status. Journal of Psychiatry 52:331–347

Davenport D 1993 Structured support at a time of crisis: treatment of paracetamol overdose. Professional Nurse 8(9):558–562

Department of Health 1999 Making a difference: strengthening the nursing, midwifery and health visiting contribution to health and healthcare. Department of Health, London

De Rond M E J, De Wit R, Van Dam F S A M et al 2000 A pain monitoring programme for nurses: effects on communication, assessment and documentation of patients' pain. Journal of Pain and Symptom Management 20(6):424–439

Descartes R (1664/1972) Treatise on Man (M Foster trans.). Harvard University Press, Cambridge

Devine, T 1990 Pain management in paediatric oncology. Paediatric Nursing 2(7):11–13

Elliott P A 1995 The development of advanced nursing practice. British Journal of Nursing 4(11):633–636

Faucett J, Gordon N, Levin J 1994 Differences in postoperative pain severity among four ethnic groups. Journal of Pain and Symptom Management 9(6):383–389

Finley G A, McGrath P J, Forward S P et al 1996 Parents' management of children's pain following minor surgery. Pain 64:83–87

Fordham M, Dunn V 1994 Alongside the person in pain: holistic care and nursing practice. Baillière Tindall, London

Fuller B F, Conner D A 1996 Distribution cues across assesses levels of infant pain. Clinical Nursing Research 5(2):167–184

Gillies M L 1993 Postoperative pain in children: a review of the literature. Journal of Clinical Nursing 2:5–10

Gillies M L, Parry-Jones W L, Smith L N 1995 The pain we overlook: postoperative pain in children under five years. Child Health 3(1):31–33

Goodenough B, Addicoat L, Champion G D et al 1997 Pain in 4–6-year-old children receiving intramuscular injections: a comparison of the Faces Pain Scale with other self-report and behavioural measures. Clinical Journal of Pain 13(1):60–73

Hamers J P, Abu-Saad H H, Van Den Hout M A et al 1998 The influence of children's vocal expressions, age, medical diagnosis and information obtained from parents on nurses' pain assessment and decisions regarding interventions. Pain 65:53–61

Hawley D 1984 Postoperative pain in children: misconceptions, descriptions and interventions. Pediatric Nursing 10:20–23

Helman C 2001 Culture, health and illness, 4th edn. Arnold, London

Horgan M, Choonara I, Al-Waidh Sambrookes J et al 1996 Measuring pain in neonates: an objective score. Paediatric Nursing 8(10):24–27

Human Rights Act 1998 HMSO, London

International Association for the Study of Pain 1979 Pain terms: a list with definitions and notes on usage. Pain 6:249–252

Jessel-Kenyon J, Cheng N I, Blott B et al 1992 Studies with acupuncture using a SQUID bio-magnetometer: a preliminary report. Complementary Medical Research 6(3):142–151

Kenworthy N, Snowley G, Gilling C (eds) 2002 Common foundation studies in nursing, 3rd edn. Churchill Livingstone, Edinburgh

Knapp-Spooner C, Karlik B A, Pontieri-Lewis V et al 1995 Efficacy of patient-controlled analgesia in women cholecystectomy patients. International Journal of Nursing Studies 32(5):434

Latham J 1991 Pain control, 2nd edn. Mosby, London

Livingstone W 1943 The mechanism of pain. Macmillan, New York

Lloyd-Thomas A R 1990 Pain management in paediatric patients. British Journal of Anaesthesia 64:85–104

McCaffery M 1972 Nursing management of the patient in pain. Lippincott, Philadelphia

McCaffery M, Beebe A 1994 Pain: clinical manual for nursing practice, UK edn. Mosby, London

McCaffery M, Pasero C 1999 Pain: clinical manual, 2nd edn. Mosby, St Louis

McConnan L 1992 Measuring a child's pain. Canadian Nurse 88(6):20–22

McCready M, MacDavitt K, O'Sullivan K 1991 Children and pain: easing the hurt. Orthopaedic Nursing 10(6):33–42

McGee P, Castledine G, Brown R 1996 Survey of specialist and advanced nursing practice in England. British Journal of Nursing 5(11):682–686

McGrath P A 1989 Evaluating a child's pain. Journal of Pain and Symptom Management 4(4):198–214

McSharry M 1995 The evolving role of the clinical nurse specialist. British Journal of Nursing 4(11):641–646

Main C J, Spanswick C C 2000 Pain management: an interdisciplinary approach. Churchill Livingstone, Edinburgh

Mallik M 1994 An impossible ideal? The role of the child advocate. Child Health 2(3):105–109

Marshall H 1894 Pain, pleasure and aesthetics. Macmillan, London

May L 1992 Reducing pain and anxiety in children. Nursing Standard 6(44):25–28

Melzack R 1996 Gate control theory on the evolution of pain concepts. Pain Forum 5(1):128–138

Melzack R, Wall P 1965 Pain mechanisms: a new theory. Science 150:971–979

Melzack R, Wall P 1973 Psychophysiology of pain. International Anaesthesiology Clinics 8:3–34

Melzack R, Wall P 1982 The challenge of pain, vol. 1. Penguin, Harmondsworth

Melzack R, Wall P 1988 The challenge of pain, vol. 2. Penguin, Harmondsworth

Melzack R, Wall P 1996 The challenge of pain. Penguin, Harmondsworth

Merskey H 1970 On the development of pain. Headache 10:116–123

Merskey H, Bogduk N (eds) 1994 Classification of chronic pain, 2nd edn. ASP Press, Seattle

Merkel S, Voepel-Lewis T, Shayevitz J R et al 1997 The FLACC: a behavioural scale for scoring postoperative pain in young children. Pediatric Nursing 23(3):293–297

Misuse of Drugs Act 1971 HMSO, London

Munafò M, Trim J 2000 Chronic pain: a handbook for nurses. Butterworth-Heinemann, Oxford

Nordenbos W 1959 Pain. Elsevier, Amsterdam

Nursing and Midwifery Council 2002 Code of Professional Conduct. Nursing and Midwifery Council, London

Papadopoulos I 1999 Health and illness beliefs of Greek Cypriots living in London. Journal of Advanced Nursing 29(5):1097–1104

Park G, Fulton B, Senthuran S 2000 The management of acute pain, 2nd edn. Oxford University Press, Oxford

Parsons E P 1992 Cultural aspects of pain. Surgical Nurse 5(2):14–16

Price S 1990 Pain: its experience, assessment and management in children. Nursing Times 86(9):42–45

Rogers J 1995 Remedy of detox. Nursing Times 91(38):44–46

Royal College of Nursing 1995 Advocacy and the nurse: Paper 22 – Issues in nursing. Royal College of Nursing, London

Royal College of Nursing 1999a Clinical practice guidelines: the recognition and assessment of acute pain in children: recommendations. Royal College of Nursing, London

Royal College of Nursing 1999b Ouch! Sort it out: children's experiences of pain: report. Royal College of Nursing, London

Rushforth L 1994 Behavioural response to pain in healthy neonates. Archives of Disease in Childhood 70:174–176

Sofaer B 1998 Pain: principles, practice and patients, 3rd edn. Stanley Thornes, Cheltenham

Skevington S M 1995 Psychology of pain. John Wiley, Chichester

Stevens B, Johnston C C 1992 Assessment and management of pain in infants. Canadian Nurse 88:31–34

Stevens B, Johnston C C 1993 Pain in the infant: theoretical and conceptual issues. Maternal Child Nursing Journal 21(1):3–14

Stevens B, Hunsberger M, Browne G 1987 Pain in children: theoretical, research and practice dilemmas. Journal of Pediatric Nursing 2(3): 154–166

Stewart A C, Thomas S E 1995 Hypnotherapy as a treatment for atopic dermatitis in adults and children. British Journal of Dermatology 132(5):778–783

Thomas V J, Dines A 1994 The health care needs of ethnic minority groups: are nurses playing their part? Journal of Advanced Nursing 20:802–808

Thomas V J, Rose F D 1991 Ethnic differences in the experience of pain. Social Science and Medicine 32(9):1063–1066

Thompson I E, Melia K M, Boyd K M 2000 Nursing ethics, 4th edn. Churchill Livingstone, Edinburgh

Tse M M Y, Jacobus K F, Chung J W Y et al 2002 The effect of visual stimuli on pain threshold and tolerance. Journal of Clinical Nursing 11:462–469

Twycross A, Moriarty A, Betts T 1998 Pediatric pain management: a multidisciplinary approach. Radcliffe Medical Press, Oxford

UK Central Council 1992 The scope of professional practice. UK Central Council, London

UK Central Council 1994 The future of professional practice: the Council's standards for education and practice following registration. UK Central Council, London

UK Central Council 1996 Guidelines for professional practice. UK Central Council, London

Vingoe F J 1994 Anxiety and pain: terrible twins or supportive siblings? In: Gibson H B (ed) Psychology, pain and anaesthesia. Stanley Thornes, Cheltenham, pp 282–307

Vortherms R, Ryan P, Ward S 1992 Knowledge of attitude toward, and barriers to pharmacological management of cancer pain in a statewide random sample of nurses. Research in Nursing and Health 15:459–466

Vydelingum V 2000 South Asian patients' lived experience of acute care in an English hospital: a phenomenological study. Journal of Advanced Nursing 32(1):100–107

Wakefield A B 1995 Pain: an account of nurses' talk. Journal of Advanced Nursing 21(5):905–910

Walker A C, Tan L, George S 1995 Impact of culture on pain management: an Australian nursing perspective. Holistic Nurse Practitioner 9(2):48–57

Wall P D 1977 Why do we not understand pain? In: Duncan R, Weston-Smith M (eds) The encyclopaedia of ignorance. Pergamon Press, Oxford, pp 361–368

Wall P D, Melzack R 1999 Textbook of pain, 4th edn. Churchill Livingstone, Edinburgh

Wells N 1984 Responses to acute pain and the nursing implications. Journal of Advanced Nursing 9:51–58

Wilson G A M, Doyle E 1996 Validation of three paediatric pain scores for use by parents. Anaesthesia 51:1005–1007

Wood S 2002 Nursing Times Special focus: Pain. Part 1. Nursing Times 98(38):41–45

Woodgate R, Kristjanson L J 1995 Young children's behavioural responses to acute pain: strategies for getting better. Journal of Advanced Nursing 22:243–249

Woodgate R, Kristjanson L J 1996 A young child's pain: how parents and nurses 'Take Care'. International Journal of Nursing Studies 33(3):271–284

Zborowski M 1952 Cultural components in response to pain. Journal of Social Issues 8:16–30

Zola I 1966 Culture and symptoms: an analysis of patients' presenting complaints. American Sociological Review 31:615–630

Chapter 11

Aggression

Paul Linsley

KEY ISSUES

SUBJECT KNOWLEDGE
- How aggression arises
- Precursors to aggression
- Factors that inhibit aggression
- Clients who may be liable to aggressive expression

CARE DELIVERY KNOWLEDGE
- Methods to minimize the risk of aggression and violent incidents
- Ways to manage an aggressive client or incident
- Management following an aggressive incident
- How nursing care can minimize the incidence of aggression
- Methods to limit the incidence of aggression and violence in the working situation

PROFESSIONAL AND ETHICAL KNOWLEDGE
- Legal issues concerning nurses, clients and the workplace
- Zero tolerance for aggression

PERSONAL AND REFLECTIVE KNOWLEDGE
- Become aware of your own aggressive responses
- Become aware of your own precipitants to aggression
- Apply the principles of aggression management to professional nursing practice in all branches of nursing

INTRODUCTION

This chapter addresses the topic of aggression and how nurses respond to this danger. It does this by explaining aggression from its theoretical and practical aspects. An important feature of the chapter is the application to nursing care of the concepts discussed.

OVERVIEW

Subject knowledge

This part of the chapter explores what is understood by the term aggression and the situations in which it occurs. Aggression is considered in terms of its biological and psychological explanations.

Care delivery knowledge

This section explores the management of aggression. Models of aggression management are considered and applied to clinical practice. Aggression management and methods to reduce the aggressive actions are key elements of this section.

Professional and ethical knowledge

Here there is a discussion of the professional issues that stem from aggression. This section includes management of aggression as well as legal, preventative and safety issues.

Personal and reflective knowledge

Within this section is an extended exercise for you to complete, to increase awareness of your own responses to aggression and to provide you with evidence for your learning portfolio. In addition, this section contains four case studies (pp. 258–259) that explore issues of aggression management in each of the four branches of nursing. You may find it helpful to read one of them before you start the chapter and use it as a focus for your reflections while reading.

SUBJECT KNOWLEDGE

DEFINITIONS OF AGGRESSION AND VIOLENCE

Aggression can be seen as any form of behaviour used with the intention to harm or injure another person (Health Services Advisory Committee 1997). This definition includes violence and destructive acts carried out with the intent to cause physical harm, directed either outwardly towards others or inwardly at the individual (self-mutilation). Thus, aggressive acts range on a continuum from verbal or emotional acts to serious physical harm (Shepherd 1994).

Aggression in health care

Bibby (1995) defines health related aggressive actions as those occurring when a health worker feels threatened or abused or is assaulted by a member of the public during the course of their duties. Aggression within the healthcare setting has been extensively reported as a major area of concern. Acts of aggression within health care increasingly reflect similar findings within society at large, and the growing perception that violent crime is more common (Whittington 1997), although how much of this results from better reporting mechanisms within the National Health Service and a heightened awareness amongst staff that such behaviour need not be tolerated is unclear (Department of Health 2000).

Nurses have many stresses to face during the course of their work. They work unsociable and long hours in often difficult and trying conditions. They care for people who are in distress, maybe chronically ill or perhaps with a host of other problems. Likewise, it could be that the client's relatives or friends express their frustration or distress through aggression towards staff. Whilst these factors do not excuse acts of aggression it is easy to understand why nurses and those that they care for occasionally come into conflict. Rarely does aggression take place in a vacuum; the people who assault nurses are often the very people that they are caring for. Despite this nurses are often expected to face their assailants and even to continue to provide and care for them following an attack. This situation is likely to test the nurse's ability to cope with the psychological consequences of threats and assaults even further, and in a way the cycle becomes self-perpetuating.

Aggressive actions can also originate from colleagues (Geen 2001). Many tensions can occur within work teams, and in healthy organizational cultures those tensions can be a valuable force for initiating change (Royal College of Nursing 2001). But if unhealthy tensions are not resolved swiftly, bullying behaviour can start to occur. Bullying turns to harassment when it is targeted repeatedly toward the same person and the victim is to some extent defenceless in the face of the perpetrator (Leymann 1990). Bullying is a very real problem within the health service (Royal College of Nursing 2001) causing many nurses to take sickness absence or early retirement and to leave the service altogether.

This situation is clearly undesirable and every practical measure should be undertaken in order to stamp out bullying and harassment in the workplace, including disciplinary measures, and if need be, dismissal.

Many theories of aggression have been developed, suggesting that there are many different causes of aggression. Each has its support and its criticism but although there is no unanimously accepted explanation, each theory helps to develop insight into the build up and display of aggression.

BIOLOGICAL THEORIES OF AGGRESSION

Biological theories focus upon somatic phenomena underpinning aggression. Three major theories are examined in this section: the role of neurotransmitters, the endocrine system and genetic influences.

Neurotransmitters

Two neurotransmitters, noradrenaline (norepinephrine) and serotonin, have been the prime focus of studies into aggression (Fig. 11.1). Low serum concentrations of serotonin and high serum noradrenaline concentrations have been found in aggressive individuals (Hollin 1992). Unfortunately, though, a simple cause and effect relationship between these neurotransmitters and aggression has not in fact been found. So, while they do not cause aggression on their own, they may contribute to the severity of the aggressive episode (Hollin 1992, Owens & Ashcroft 1985).

The endocrine system

Most research into hormones and the aggressive response has concerned the sex hormones. These are thought to act at two levels:

- first, by predisposing the individual to become biologically developed in terms of muscular and other body systems to enable aggression to be used in the pursuit of sexual or other drives

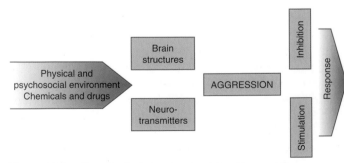

Figure 11.1 Neurological structure and function and the occurrence of aggression. This shows how environmental factors provide input to the brain structures and how the neurotransmitter state of the individual can give rise to aggression or inhibition of aggression.

second, by the direct incitement to act aggressively under the influence of sexual hormones.

Owens & Ashcroft (1985) noted how the male sex hormone, androgen, influenced aggressive responses. They discussed how castrated rats became less aggressive – probably due to their removed androgen supply – and how monkeys with high serum androgen concentrations were associated with higher levels of aggressive responses. The problem is that it is difficult to replicate these findings in human subjects. Although it can be shown that males are more involved in violent and sexual crimes and that male delinquency is associated with the onset of puberty (Hollin 1992), attributing such behaviour to high androgen levels has not been proven in human subjects.

One other area of hormonal influence on aggressive behaviour is the role of hormones in the menstrual cycle (Prentky 1985). This was promoted by women attributing violent or aggressive actions to the premenstrual stage of their menstrual cycle. Again problems establishing a definite causal linkage is the major issue and as yet this has not been established.

Genetic factors

Owens & Ashcroft (1985) identified three major genetic influences on aggressive behaviour:

- certain abnormal chromosome patterns influence aggressive behaviour
- personality has been considered to be genetically determined
- specific sex chromosomal abnormalities are associated with aggression, with some patterns increasing and others decreasing aggressive behaviour

Eysenck & Gudjonsson (1989) argued for a genetic influence in offending, as monozygotic (identical) twins were found to be more likely to offend than dizygotic (fraternal) twins. Although this may be explained by similarities of upbringing rather than genetic factors, Bouchard et al (1990) found that twins raised apart demonstrated similar behaviour.

Jeffery (1979) also attributed aggressive behaviour to genetic make-up. He considered that an extra Y chromosome in male prisoners was associated with aggressive behaviour. Additionally, he considered there was also a greater proportion of such individuals in secure mental hospitals. The findings of this research have been questioned, however, as other studies have found that such individuals commit crime against property rather than against people (Casey et al 1973, Price 1978). Consequently, a similar problem emerges to that of other biological explanations of aggression. It is difficult to separate factors like genetic make-up from the complex variables that make up human individuals.

Consequently, while biological theories provide an interesting context into the nature and severity of aggression, to adhere strictly to a biological causation of aggression is

unsafe. Aggressive behaviour always occurs within a social context and it is this factor that must also be examined.

ETHOLOGICAL THEORIES OF AGGRESSION

Biological theories of aggression have also been advanced by ethologists, researchers who study the behaviour of animals in their natural environments. In doing so several have advanced views about aggression in humans based on their observations of animal behaviour. This is done with the assumption that observations derived from the study of organisms below humans in the evolutionary scale will provide insights into human behaviour as well.

When ethologists consider any class of behaviour, they are, according to Hinde (1982), concerned with four issues:

1. What immediately causes it.
2. How such behaviour has developed over the animal's life cycle.
3. What were the consequences of such behaviour.
4. How behaviour has evolved within the species.

This view of aggression as an innate instinct in both humans and animals was popularized in three widely read books of the 1960s: *On Aggression* by Konrad Lorenz (1966), *The Territorial Imperative* by Robert Ardrey (1969), and *The Naked Ape* by Desmond Morris (1967). The aggressive instinct postulated by these authors builds up spontaneously – with or without outside provocation – until it is likely to be discharged with minimal or no provocation from outside stimuli. In addition, Lorenz (1966) suggested that man's social evolution meant that aggressive tendencies and feelings of aggression build up inside us and are not released through everyday activities as they were in our evolutionary past in activities such as hunting. He argued that we expend very little energy just staying alive and get a build-up of aggression by thinking about life's problems and stressors.

PSYCHOSOCIAL THEORIES OF AGGRESSION

Three major psychosocial theories of aggression are considered:

- psychoanalytic theory
- frustration–aggression hypothesis
- social learning theory.

Figure 11.2 shows an outline of the psychosocial view of aggression.

The psychoanalytic theory

Freud's model of the person comprised a bipolar model (Frankl 1990):

- at one pole is an Eros drive – the instinct for life
- at the other pole is a Thanatos drive – the death or destructive instinct.

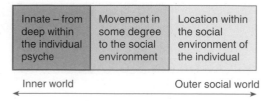

Figure 11.2   Location of aggressive impulses.

The assumption behind this theory is that two primitive forces, the life and death instincts, oppose each other in our subconscious, and this incongruence is the origin of aggression. Freud asserted that this is a process void of thought patterns, and is driven solely and entirely by our instincts, the aim being satisfaction. This model would seem to have a crucial flaw, however; having defined the general aims of the life and death instincts, Freud failed to determine their source.

Frustration–aggression hypothesis

The frustration–aggression hypothesis was first set out in the 1930s by Dollard et al (1939). This theory proposes that aggression, rather than occuring spontaneously for no reason, is a response to the frustration of some goal-directed behaviour by an outside source. Goals may include such basics needs as food, water, sleep, sex, love and recognition. Contributions to frustration–aggression research further established that an environmental stimulus must produce not just frustration but anger in order for aggression to follow (e.g. Berkowitz 1990, Geen 2001), and that the anger can be the result of stimuli other than frustrating situations, such as verbal abuse (Cohen et al 1998). That is not say that anger will always lead to aggression, however, as anger can be displayed in a number of ways and conversely act as a motivator and medium for positive change (Berkowitz 2001).

Social learning theory

In contrast to instinct theories, social learning theory focuses on aggression as a learned behaviour. This approach stresses the roles that social influences, such as models and reinforcement, play in the acquisition of aggressive behaviour (e.g. Anderson & Dill 2000; Bandura et al 1963; Bandura 1969, 1973, 1977; Carlson et al 1990).

Social learning has three principal components:

1. Behaviour: an observer sees a model perform a particular behaviour.
2. Learning or acquisition phase: the observer attends to important features of the behaviour, remembering what was seen and done.
3. Performance: imitates the behaviour at a later time.

Accordingly children learn social skills through a fundamental developmental process called modelling. This involves being attentive to the following: remembering, imitating and being rewarded by people, television, books and magazines (Bushman 1998). A correlation has been found between the viewing of violence and increased interpersonal aggression, both in childhood and later, in adolescence (Atkinson et al 1987, Gross 1992). Viewing violence can elicit aggressive behaviour by desensitizing a person's view of violence, whereby the greater the frequency of aggression and violence witnessed, the less disturbing they become (Anderson & Dill 2000, Bushman 1998). Reducing restraints on aggressive behaviour through modelling can reduce the inhibitions against behaving aggressively by coming to believe that this is a typical or permissible way of solving problems or attaining goals, and in turn, distort a person's views about conflict resolution (Bushman 1995, 1998; Geen 2001).

CARE DELIVERY KNOWLDGE

THE NATURE OF AGGRESSION

Aggression can take many different forms and guises. Physical aggression inflicts harm through deed or act, whereas verbal aggression creates harm through words. Aggression can also be expressed directly or indirectly (Kaukiainen et al 2001). Direct means of aggression take place in face-to-face situations, whereas indirect aggression is delivered via the negative reactions of others (Buss 1995). Often, indirect aggression is a kind of social manipulation, like spreading malicious rumours about the target person or trying to persuade others not to associate with him or her.

Bullying and harassment are two types of aggression commonly found in the workplace (Royal College of Nursing 2001) that encompass the type of behaviour described above. Not only are such behaviours upsetting for those directly involved, but also for those who witness and have to deal with it. Most organizations now have policies and procedures for dealing with bullying and harassment that outline what is and what is not acceptable behaviour. Penalties for transgression can result in dismissal. However, proving that someone has been a bully is difficult, particular if it has been done in a covert way. Baron & Neuman (1996) and Geddes & Baron (1997) found that in work settings, verbal and passive forms of aggression were rated as more frequent than physical and active forms.

Reflection and portfolio exercise

As we have seen, aggression means different things to different people. Make a list of behaviours that *you* associate with aggression using the following headings:
words and phrases
behaviour
moods and emotions
body language.

- Which of these behaviours do you attribute to yourself?
- Which of these behaviours do you attribute to others?
- Are there similarities between the two lists?

In 1995 the Policy Studies Institute found that up to two-thirds of ethnic minority nurses reported racial abuse or other forms of harassment from clients or their families, and more than one-third said that they had been racially harassed by work colleagues (Royal College of Nursing 2001).

In a survey of 6000 Royal College of Nursing members conducted in the year 2000, one in six nurses reported that they had been bullied or harassed by colleagues. Almost half of these nurses said a manager or supervisor was responsible. More than one in three nurses reported they had been bullied or harassed by clients and their relatives, and only one-third reported the incident to a senior manager (Royal College of Nursing 2001).

● Look up your employer's policy on *Bullying and Harassment* and see what it has to say in relation to the above findings.

Table 11.1 Prediction of aggression: the individual (adapted from Pollock et al 1989, Hinde 1993 and Farrington 1994)

Prediction category	Examples
Personality factors	Low threshold of frustration or impulsivity Increased liability to become aroused An antisocial personality such as someone who is habitually aggressive or undercontrolled Substance abusers
Previous history of aggression or violence	An institutional record where violence has been a factor may mean an increased risk of violence A genetic constitution that tends towards a lack of control
Biological factors	Disinhibitory factors such as caused by brain damage, and some organic mental illnesses
Mental disorder	Psychotic individuals who experience a build-up of tension before a violent outburst Some depressed individuals may attempt to kill others for altruistic reasons, to relieve their supposed suffering Frustration, fear or pain may lead to aggressive responses

Table 11.2 Prediction of aggression: the social environment (adapted from Pollock et al 1989, Hinde 1993 and Farrington 1994)

Prediction category	Examples
Peer influences and group pressures	Peer and group pressures to act aggressively may be exerted on individuals Certain geographical areas may process more aggressive cues than others School influences can occur with some schools processing relatively more offenders in their pupils compared with other schools Generally, the culture that individuals may have been exposed to that do not denigrate aggression may be predispose certain individuals to an aggressive response pattern
Economic, social and environmental influences	Economic and social deprivation tend to be associated with offending and sometime aggressive responses There may be an association between situational influences and aggressive behaviour, such as the availability of weapons Additional social factors include extrafamilial roles, peer group and media influences Uncomfortable or stressful social or physical conditions can predispose to aggression
The presence of a victim	As a subject upon whom aggression is expressed is necessary, so victims are essential in the expression of aggression; the assertion is made here that aggression is not likely to occur without the presence of someone on whom to carry out the aggressive act

It would be wrong to rely solely on polices and procedures to protect the individual from aggression. One possible way of combating aggression such as bullying is to develop skills of assertiveness (Burnard 1991). It is suggested that those people who are singled out for bullying and harassment are those that lack the ability to stand up for themselves and their rights. Briggs (1986) suggests that assertiveness is about the individual standing up for their rights in such a way as not to violate the rights of others. Being assertive can help the individual to develop a belief and confidence in herself or himself. The more that individuals stand up for their rights and act in a manner that is respectful of themselves and others, the higher their self-esteem. Assertion can help a person to grow in confidence so that they can tackle such situations when they chose to.

Minimizing the risk of aggression

Research into aggression focuses on discovering the biological, environmental, psychological and social factors that influence aggressive behaviour. These factors can be categorized as features of the situation or as features of the person in the situation. Pollock et al (1989), Hinde (1993) and Farrington (1994) identified factors implicated in aggressive behaviour (Tables 11.1 and 11.2). Table 11.1 focuses on the individual whereas Table 11.2 focuses on the individual's interaction with the environment. Either of these factors may lead an individual to aggress. An awareness of such predisposing factors is therefore necessary in the assessment and management of aggression risk.

Perhaps the biggest cause of aggression is interpersonal provocation (Berkowitz 1993, Geen 2001). Provocations include insults, slights, other forms of verbal aggression, physical aggression, and interference with an individual's attempts to attain an important goal.

IDENTIFYING CUES THAT WARN OF IMMINENT AGGRESSION

At times, for whatever reason, interventions between service users and care staff go wrong. When this occurs, there are three possible types of outcome. The conflict may be resolved peacefully and may even result in positive learning and action; the conflict may be left unresolved and perhaps cause greater trouble at a later stage; or the conflict may escalate and result in some form of aggressive behaviour. Escalating aggression places clients and staff at risk, thus it is essential that timely, sound interventions are initiated (Richardson 1994).

Behaviour is the first glimpse into aggression in others. Individuals usually give warning that an act of aggression is about to happen. Morrison (1992) listed a series of behaviours associated with aggression (Fig. 11.3).

Staff may ignore such signals owing to a lack of confidence in their own skills to deal with the situation and fear that they could make matters worse rather than better. Avoidance of potential aggression is likely to increase the danger, however. Consequently, an awareness of the escalation of aggression is essential. Once the danger signals are recognized, limiting action can be taken, and the earlier the probability of a satisfactory outcome is increased.

Motor agitation
Pacing
Inability to sit still
Clenching or pounding of fists
Jaw tightening
Increased respirations

Verbalizations
Verbal threats
Intrusive demands for attention
Loud, pressured speech
Evidence of delusional or paranoid thought content

Affect
Anger
Hostility
Extreme anxiety
Irritability
Inappropriate or excessive euphoria

Level of consciousness
Confusion
Sudden change in mental status
Disorientation
Memory impairment
Inability to be redirected

Figure 11.3 Behaviours associated with aggression. (From Morrison 1992.)

WAYS TO MANAGE AN AGGRESSIVE INCIDENT

What follows here is intended as a general guide. Specific interventions and procedures will be provided by individual employers and these should be used for final guidance.

The immediate response to an aggressive incident

Personal safety is priority. Professional codes of conduct do not require individuals to jeopardize their own safety; it is better to leave and find alternative ways of providing care. If there is no choice but to intervene, however, as would happen if you were unable to remove yourself and needed to defend yourself, colleagues should be alerted, via a panic button, call system, emergency telephone or panic alarm. Similarly, bystanders should be asked to leave the area and move to a place of safety.

Containing an aggressive incident: the assault cycle

If the point has been reached where the potential for aggressive acts has been reached then an assault cycle is entered. Rowett & Breakwell (1992) and Leadbetter & Paterson (1995) describe how this is structured (Fig. 11.4). Using this five-stage model helps to identify how the aggression has occurred and the type of intervention that would be most appropriate.

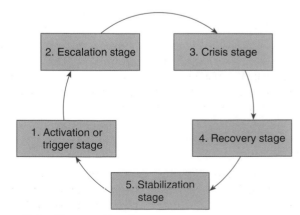

Figure 11.4 The assault cycle.

Activation or trigger stage

In this stage some event or interpersonal situation arouses the person. It could be as the result of one thing or an accumulation of things.

> ### Decision making exercise
>
> Judith woke up late for her morning shift. She went to the kitchen for coffee and breakfast and found that she had run out of milk. Hungry, she left the house, intending to buy a snack from the local shop, only to find when she arrived that she had forgotten her purse. As she could not do without her purse she had to return to her house to collect it. She was now very late and became entangled in morning traffic. Arriving late for work someone said the 'wrong thing' to her and she responded by 'biting their head off!'
>
> Referring to the fight or flight response and the effect of hassles (see Ch. 8 on relaxation and stress) offer a possible explanation for Judith's reaction.

Escalation stage

Stress and frustration increase. Calming measures need to be used. Feelings, emotions, attitudes and posture all influence the way that people view and listen to each other. Explaining something to someone who is feeling upset, angry or indignant is difficult until the person's feelings have been relieved. Consequently, the person's feelings need to be recognized and acknowledged. A return to the previous stage is possible, and this should be the aim of interventions. However, in areas of low support, such as working in the community, the practitioner should aim to extract themselves from this situation and to return to base.

Crisis stage

Physical, emotional and psychological impulses are expressed. If escalation to the crisis stage occurs communication is more difficult. Communication remains a priority. However, if the situation becomes unsafe then personal safety and that of others in the immediate vicinity is of paramount importance. Consequently, the area around the aggressive individual should be evacuated and help should be sought from appropriately qualified staff in sufficient numbers to safely contain the situation.

Recovery stage

Agitation decreases, anxiety lessens, and communication becomes possible. At this stage the acute crisis has ended. However, caution still needs to be maintained as the individual may feel upset at how they have been treated and can still revert to the crisis stage. It is necessary that staff maintain control of the situation and contain the risk of further aggression. Depending on the area, this may require the use of sedation or seclusion, in which case local policies for observation will need to be implemented. Other staff that were called to help may also need to maintain their presence. Alternatively, the individual may be detained by the police.

Stabilization

The client is able to regain control of outward behaviour. Often a post-crisis depression occurs and the individual becomes guarded and uncertain. At this stage he or she is most likely to be receptive to clinical interventions and may feel remorse, guilt or shame for their behaviour. It is important to maintain communication with the client and to investigate with them the reasons why the crisis occurred. The client needs to know that he or she is still accepted and the emphasis needs to be on how the client can be helped to avoid future repetition of the aggression. The role of nursing staff is not to judge or punish such clients, but to assist them to live more effective and less problematic lives.

FOLLOWING AN AGGRESSIVE INCIDENT

The nursing management following an aggressive incident falls into two main areas: the first immediately following the incident and the second concerning the time thereafter.

Immediately following the incident

During this time it is important that things are allowed to return to normal. Practical assistance should be given in terms of getting the victim home or to hospital, alerting significant others, retrieving possessions and the like. The immediate concerns of staff should be addressed as far as is possible, even if the incident seems to have been minor. Persistent low-level violence can produce psychological effects as damaging as more serious individual incidents. Likewise staff should be encouraged to fill out formal report forms, including those incidents that appear minor, as 'near misses' can be the precursors to more serious incidents.

Burton (1998) states that prompt and accurate recording of an aggressive incident is essential and should include every relevant detail, even from before the incident occurred. He provides a set of questions that are useful when writing up a report on an aggressive incident (Fig. 11.5).

Whilst it is important to record an aggressive incident near the time it happened for purposes of accuracy, more important is the support of those involved in the incident itself. No member of staff should be should be left to go home alone as though nothing had happened. Violence should not be seen as 'part of the job'; it cannot always be prevented or avoided, but it can be handled properly, with due regard for the safety and well-being of clients and staff alike. A violent confrontation or attack is an extremely

- Who was involved?
- Where did it take place?
- What was/were the trigger factor(s)?
- What was the context?
- What was said, and by whom?
- What behaviours were displayed?
- What was the response of those intervening?
- How was the situation handled?
- What were the outcomes?
- What means finally ended the situation?
- What took place following the incident?
- What steps should be taken to prevent such an incident occuring again?

Figure 11.5   Useful questions for writing a report. (From Burton 1998.)

upsetting experience, as well as being very frightening. It is only right that a great deal of thought goes into supporting people who have been subject of an aggressive incident.

Up to a few days following the incident: debriefing

Healthcare staff who have encountered a violent or aggressive incident can experience various feelings. Usually, there is a psychological numbing immediately following an attack in which the person begins to try and make sense of what it is they have just been through. This is followed by feelings of exhaustion, tension, anger and frustration which, over time, may come to develop feelings of guilt about the incident. Often people ask 'Could I have done things differently?' or 'Was I to blame for the incident?' There may be a loss of confidence associated with feelings of fear, wariness and apprehension and an overestimation of future violence. In the long term the staff member might experience flashbacks and intrusive memories of the event and may reach a state of burnout. There might be a loss of vocation and the person may go off sick or leave the profession altogether.

These feelings and thoughts are normal responses to abnormal circumstances and are generally short-lived. However, there is always the possibility that such feelings and thoughts could develop into something more disabling as in post-traumatic stress disorder. The disorder consists of three main types of symptoms, high arousal (e.g. irritability, startle response), avoidance (e.g. avoiding situations or people associated with an aggressive event) and re-experiencing (e.g. upsetting and repeated thoughts of the event) (Wykes & Mezey 1994).

It is important that having been involved in a violent or aggressive incident, individuals are allowed to recover and receive practical help and support. Even after minor incidents, feelings may be difficult to control and may affect the ability to return to deal with further problems. Therefore, all incidents must be followed with debriefing.

A debrief should be conducted with all staff involved in the incident to establish the facts and to allow time for staff to talk about the incident. This should be conducted as near

as is practical to the time at which the incident took place, certainly no longer than a few days following the event (Robb 1995). Debriefing allows individuals to deal with the aggressive incident and examine how procedures might be improved to prevent a reoccurrence (Royal College of Psychiatrists 1998). The aim of a debrief is not to apportion blame, but to offer support (Cembrowicz & Ritter 1994). If appropriate a debrief should be conducted with the client involved in order to reduce the negative impact for future contacts. All staff should be provided the opportunity to vent their emotions and thoughts on the matter and to be reassured that support will be available to them in the future if they so need it.

How a debriefing is conducted and the form it takes will be very much down to the individuals involved and the resources available to them. Conducting a debriefing requires skills and knowledge and should be led by someone competent in such matters. Disclosure of the kind described within an aggressive incident can be a painful experience for the individual involved, bringing things to consciousness that need dealing with. The memory of a challenging situation often includes an affective component, so the people involved in the debrief should be aware of and comfortable with the affective responses of others (Rich & Parker 1995). Some incidents may be so challenging that they create a great deal of uncontrolled emotion, and cathartic support may be necessary before an attempt to think positively or constructively becomes possible (Heron 1986). Another important point is to know when to refer on. If someone has been either physically or psychologically damaged then psychological support from skilled professionals may need to be arranged.

Reflective practice

An adjunct to the debriefing session is the use of reflective practice. Reflective practice allows the nurse to consciously consider their experiences through the integration of theory with practice and in turn with praxis, through experience (Atkins & Murphy 1993, Rich & Parker 1995). Reflection involves defining a problem, asking questions, examining evidence, analysing assumptions and biases, confronting emotional unease, considering other interpretations and tolerating ambiguity. It requires constructing new knowledge by perceiving a dilemma, exploring the differing perspectives, integrating existing and new knowledge and considering new alternatives (Paterson 1995). Reflection can be undertaken on an individual basis or through clinical supervision.

Reviewing the incident

The purpose of a review is to take positive learning from the incident to reduce the likelihood of similar situations happening again and to see how such incidents could be managed more effectively, if at all. Littlechild (1996) suggests that strategies for managing aggression should exist at three levels: with practitioners, with managers and at an agency level. This structure should form the basis of a review:

1. At practitioner level opportunities are present for individuals to learn from their experience and they need to adopt different or modified personal strategies.
2. At manager level learning points can be identified and questions concerning issues such as the availability and skill of help provided and the speed of response should be asked.
3. At agency level issues of policy amendment or change may need to be addressed and the effectiveness and availability of post-incident support can be identified.

Decision making exercise

Your colleague appears down during her clinical placement in the operating theatre. You ask what the problem is and she discloses that a particular consultant appears to be picking on her and ridiculing her for her inexperience at every opportunity. Recently he rapped her across the knuckles with a swab-holder because she held a retractor the wrong way during an operation. She has complained to the theatre manager but was told: 'He is like it with all new nurses until he gets to know them.'

- How does your trust/workplace/unit go about reporting incidences of violence and aggression?
- What constitutes an aggressive act on the part of a
  — client?
  — relative?
  — member of staff?
- What would you advise your colleague to do next?

The nursing interventions so far have provided understanding of some of the possible ways to deal with an aggressor. The following sections consider the wider issues involved in the professional management of aggression. The following topics will be explored in the light of nursing care:

- skills used in managing an aggressive incident
- risk management.

SKILLS USED IN MANAGING AN AGGRESSIVE INCIDENT

Communication skills

An aggressive person may be upset, frightened or confused, not understanding their situation or what is happening to them. The immediate response to someone escalating towards violence is to try to restore calm and stabilize their emotional state. However, before this can be done an assessment of the situation needs to be made. Following this assessment, the subsequent interventions are determined by a number of seemingly competing factors.

Evidence based practice

In 2000 the Department of Health conducted a national survey into the reported incidences of violence and aggression in NHS Trusts and Authorities in England. A total number of 84 273 violent or abusive incidents were reported. This was an increase of some 24 000 over the previous year 1998/99 (the only other occasion on which this sort of information had been collected on a national basis).

The survey found that the number of violent incidents varied by trust type; for example, the average for mental health/learning disabilities trusts was two and a half times the average for all trusts. It found that there was a significant underreporting of violence directed at staff working in the NHS and that this was historical. The survey also found that there were differences in the way that data on violent incidents were collected. For example, the definition of a violent incident in one trust might include verbal abuse, and in another trust it might be excluded. Such information is vital if the true level of risk faced by NHS staff is to be identified.

Generally three things are considered (Delaney et al 2001, Janelli 1995):

1. The individual's characteristics (level of orientation, age, presenting features, diagnosis and level of risk to self and others).
2. The resources available to the nurse at the time of the incident (staffing levels and other tasks needing completion).
3. The requirements of the organization for which the nurse works (particularly policies and procedures regarding the management and control of aggression and violence).

Talking to an aggressive person: verbal responses

An important step in an interaction is to calm the individual's anger in an attempt to bring about a more rational discussion of the situation (Burton 1998, Nursing and

---

Reflection and portfolio exercise

The use of good communication skills when dealing with someone who is aggressive is highlighted throughout the chapter. Carry out a SWOT (strengths, weaknesses, opportunities, threats) analysis of your own communication skills to see where your strengths and weaknesses in communicating with clients lie, and identify the opportunities and threats which may aid or obstruct effective communication with an aggressive client. It is important that you are honest with yourself and again it might be interesting to ask a trusted colleague to complete a separate SWOT analysis of your communication skills, and to compare their perceptions with your own.

Midwifery Council 2002). There are a number of strategies that can help here:

- acknowledge the existence of the problem
- use active listening skills
- show genuine concern and understanding
- give reassurance and support as appropriate.

Problem solving When the situation is calmer, encourage the individual to identify and explain the nature of the problem, and to try and identify a solution (Garnham 2001). Do not agree or disagree and be careful not to get drawn into an argument, or to promise anything that can not be delivered, as this could escalate the situation.

Supportiveness Be supportive and avoid defensiveness. Accept that the person is angry, and avoid retaliatory remarks. Ask questions that focus on the aggressor (Leadbetter & Paterson 1995). For example: 'Tell me more about how you feel.' Be prepared to accept criticism. You may even seek it by asking: 'What is it about my behaviour that is annoying you?' Allow the person time to express how they feel, and do not be in a hurry to resolve the encounter (Garnham 2001).

Reflection and portfolio exercise

The meaning behind words is conveyed by the way in which they are spoken. We have a degree of control over what we say, but much less control over the way that we speak. If we are to appear calm in the face of an aggressor then we need to give some thought as to how we present ourselves verbally to another. Considering the following:
- Clarity – clear or indecipherable?
- Volume – too quiet or too loud?
- Tone – appropriate, soft, sarcastic?
- Modulation – adjustment of tone and pitch
- Stress – pressure and/or emphasis
- Silences – pauses and hesitations
- Respirations and sighing.

Information giving When giving information:

- repeat and stress important points
- give important messages first
- try to be consistent, avoid confusing or conflicting messages.

Certain phrases may be provocative and make an aggressive individual even angrier. Examples include: 'Now don't be silly', 'Pull yourself together', 'This is no way for an adult to behave', or even 'You're not the only person with a problem!'

Depersonalize the situation Depersonalize the issues in circumstances where you have no personal influence over

decisions, refusing requests, etc. Let the person know it is not your personal decision, but is due to the policy of the organization. Provide information about complaint procedures and alternative sources of help, if appropriate (Burton 1998, Farrell 1992).

Talking to an aggressive person: non-verbal communication

Every time verbal communication takes place it is complemented with a complex repertoire of movements and gestures. They are usually congruous to the verbal message but sometimes they may be conflicting (incongruous). Non-verbal communication helps to maintain the flow of communication and acts as a subtle indicator to show when a person has finished speaking. Appropriate use of non-verbal communication, then, can demonstrate interest and understanding of the individual's problems. Of particular use when working with aggressive individuals, correct interpretation of non-verbal communication provides considerable insight into the other person.

Not only is it important to be sensitive to the assailant's non-verbal communication, but sensitivity to and awareness of our own body signals is also vital. Using body language appropriately in a helping relationship can help to facilitate a client's trust and confidence in the nurse. The use of tone of voice, eye contact, touch, facial expression and posture can convey the qualities of genuineness and warmth. Using non-verbal communication effectively can help to relax the client and increase the likelihood of them exploring their problems in a more constructive manner. The following section will examine some of the common defusion strategies that can be employed using non-verbal communication when faced with an aggressor.

Mood matching This is where the arousal level is matched between all people in the interaction. For example, in a conversation with someone who feels depressed, people attempt to be slightly 'downbeat'. Similarly, the mood is reasonably cheerful when talking to someone who is happy or excited about something.

In contrast, when talking to somebody who is agitated people attempt to be calm, so not to inflame the situation. The danger of this is that it can be misinterpreted as indifference. One option is to match the other person with a similar level of energy. However, in this instance, energy would not be a displayed as aggression. Rather it would be shown by concern, involvement and interest.

Mirroring This is the physical equivalent of mood matching. Mirroring is exactly as it says: it is where one person physically reflects the way the other person is sitting or standing. Normally this occurs entirely spontaneously; if one person sits back then so does the other one, if one person comes forward then the other does likewise, and so forth. Observational research shows that people who are mirroring each other tend to get on better than those who don't ('getting on' being measured by the length of conversation they have) in spite of the fact that this is normally going on unconsciously.

It is possible to utilize this phenomenon and use it to enhance the interactions with the aggressor. This needs to be done with some caution, however, as if exaggerated, it may be seen to be mimicking or mocking.

Eye contact   This is also an important and sometimes misunderstood area (Argyle 1988). In an escalating aggressive situation there are various types of exchange:

- Stage 1 is before any aggressive interaction has taken place and the eye contact is of an ordinary pattern.
- Stage 2 is where either or both parties sense that the conversation is gradually becoming more heated and one or both attempt to minimize eye contact.
- Stage 3 is where the situation is unambiguously aggressive and almost out of hand. This is where eye contact is of a long duration, high intensity, challenging and aversive.

The task therefore, is to try to maintain the pattern of ordinary eye contact, appropriate to stage 1, apparently not noticing any changes in eye contact demonstrated by the other person. If eye contact is too threatening, however, averting the gaze to the shoulders is effective as it signifies non-confrontational interest, but it also allows the aggressor to be kept in full view.

Touch   Touch in the common course of treatment can be a sign of positive communication; aggression is also primarily expressed through bodily contact and therefore it is recommended to avoid touching clients who are aroused or angry. Likewise, invading a person's personal space can be perceived as a threat. Encroachment of this by anyone who is uninvited creates feelings of uneasiness and crowding. This is important to remember when addressing an aggressive person as there is the danger of invading the aggressor's personal space and escalating the situation. Therefore a distance should be maintained between the nurse and the potential aggressor, mindful of the need to keep a safe means of exit.

Communicating assertively

Farrell & Gray (1992) make the observation that being assertive is an effective way of dealing with aggression. Assertive people are confident in and relaxed when dealing with others. They have a clear idea of their personal rights and do not allow others to infringe on them. They are able to say 'no' clearly and directly to other people, to ask for what they want, and to negotiate an equitable compromise in a difficult situation. They can respond to criticism realistically, accept complaints and handle put-downs.

The application of assertiveness in situations that threaten aggression assumes that people are attacked or victimized, or are in danger of becoming aggressive themselves, partly because they do not express their wishes, or do so in a socially ineffective manner (McDonnell et al 1994). While assertiveness training may help people who are not confident to manage difficult situations more effectively, there are those that this approach does not suit and who are not comfortable with being assertive. Being assertive, like any other skill, needs to be practised and developed, and there is always the danger that if used inappropriately then it could exacerbate a situation rather than resolve it. A further drawback of this approach is that people may slip from being assertive to being aggressive (McDonnell et al 1994).

If nurses are to use assertiveness techniques then they need to be given proper training in their use. There are undoubtedly a number of benefits to be had from being assertive; however, in order to use such skills effectively, the nurse needs to appreciate and clearly understand the difference between being assertive and being aggressive.

> **Reflection and portfolio exercise**
>
> Experiment with assertive responses in situations that you find difficult. You could do this by the means of role play, enacting such situations with a colleague, trying out different responses and techniques. Likewise you could video the role play and make an analysis of your assertive skills with a view to bringing about change.

LIMITING THE INCIDENCE OF AGGRESSION

Prevention is always better than cure, and every effort should be made to reduce the incidence of aggression and violence. However, it would be impossible to eliminate aggression altogether and approaches used in reducing particular forms of aggression and violence may be counterproductive in dealing with different persons in different situations (Royal College of Nursing 1998).

RISK MANAGEMENT

With the current focus on risk management there is an increased impetus for managers and clinicians to identify risk assessment practice and develop preventative strategies in the control and management of violence and aggression (Royal College of Psychiatrists 1999). Professional competence is demonstrated by making an assessment of risk factors and instigating appropriate interventions (Erskine 1991) utilizing a theory based framework (Allen 1997). Current trends indicate that a continuous risk management approach to aggression, to accommodate changes in risk, is likely to be the most efficacious (Paterson et al 1999).

Two important points must be borne in mind when designing a risk assessment. First, it should be integrated with other risk assessments within health and safety, and can generally draw on their logic and methods. Second, the risk assessment should be fit for the purpose for which it was designed. As yet there are no well worked out and validated systems of risk assessment for work-related violence that are easily available; however, risk from violence and aggression can be regarded as a function of four factors (Royal College of Nursing 1998):

- the frequency of potential conflict situations
- the duration of the conflict situation
- the likelihood of the individuals involved acting in a violent or aggressive manner
- the magnitude of the harm caused.

One person alone can not do an adequate risk assessment and information should be gathered from a number of sources and shared. It should also be borne in mind that risk is dynamic and is largely dependent on circumstance, which can alter over a brief period of time. Because of this risk assessment needs to be predominantly short-term and subject to frequent review. Actions to reduce the identified risk can then be taken based on the findings of the risk assessment. These may include relatively small measures such as removing from a room ornaments that may be used as weapons, to more major measures such as providing closed circuit television units (CCTV) and the monitoring of clinical areas.

Reflection and portfolio exercise

Obtain a copy of the policy for dealing with violence and aggression for your workplace. List what it says about:
- prevention of aggression
- de-escalation
- handling a violent incident
- management following an aggressive incident.

Planning for non-aggressive units

Gould (1994) described several practical ways in which violence was reduced on a psychiatric continuing care ward. Among his recommendations were:

- allowing clients their privacy
- providing comfortable surroundings
- treating clients as partners in care
- listening and actively responding to client concerns and requests
- consistency of approach to clients by the nursing staff
- providing clear leadership.

Undoubtedly, if these recommendations are not implemented clients will be more likely to resort to aggressive acts in order to make themselves heard. Contrast the above list with the precipitants to aggression identified by Burrow (1994):

- overcrowding
- inappropriate temperature
- restricted movement
- lack of available information
- inhospitable décor
- lack of facilities to occupy clients
- perception that clients are less of a priority than members of staff.

The Royal College of Psychiatrists (1999) made a number of recommendations with reference to the structure and layout of rooms used to interview clients and their relatives. These are worth considering for all clinical areas and are as follows:

1. Healthcare workers should have safe working conditions and should not be expected to interview clients in isolated rooms. Interview rooms should be situated close to main staff areas.
2. All interview rooms should have a readily accessible panic button or an emergency call system, with policies for staff to respond rapidly to the alarm when it is activated.
3. The exit to all interview rooms should be unimpeded. Doors must not require a key to exit. Ideally doors should open outwards.
4. The furniture should be suitable and the room should be free from clutter.
5. It is advisable to have an internal inspection window, to permit viewing when the room is occupied.

Excessive time spent waiting to be seen can sometimes lead clients to become aggressive. The policy should therefore be to prevent waiting times as far as possible. If clients must wait then it is important to try to engineer a situation whereby the time passes as easily as possible. Be honest about how long the person will have to wait. If you do not know how long it will be, then tell them so. Similarly, should additional delays suddenly occur, such as will happen in an emergency, explain the situation to those who are waiting and tell them how long a delay is expected.

During an interview, try to prevent unwarranted interruptions. Repeated interruptions of an interview either by telephone or by others coming into the room in which the nurse is seeing the client can easily unsettle some people. However, in preventing interruptions, be sure that nurses do not cut themselves off from those who might want to check on their safety.

PROFESSIONAL AND ETHICAL KNOWLEDGE

LEGAL ISSUES

Aggression is unacceptable and constitutes a fundamental violation of human and legal rights that can lead to criminal and civil law prosecution. Trusts, as employers, have duties, with respect to the management of work-related violent incidents, framed by both national and European health and safety legislation and in the UK by their common law duty of care (Royal College of Nursing 1998).

Health and safety

The obligations of employers

Under health and safety legislation an employer must take reasonable care to protect employees from risk of foreseeable injury, disease or death at work. The effect of this is that if an employer knows of a risk to the safety of their staff, or ought to know the existence of such a hazard, he or she will be liable if a member of staff is injured or killed, or suffers illness as a result of the risk, and if the employer has failed to take reasonable steps to avoid or protect against the risk. The requirements on employers, under the health and safety legislation, have been summarized by the Health Services Advisory Committee (1997) and the Royal College of Nursing (1998). They are as follows:

The Health and Safety and Welfare at Work Act 1974
Employers must:

- protect the health and safety of their employees
- protect the health and safety of others who might be affected by the way they go about their work.

The Management of Health and Safety at Work Regulations 1992 Employers must:

- assess all risks to the health and safety of their employees
- identify the precautions needed
- make arrangements for the effective management of precautions
- appoint competent people to advise them on health and safety
- provide information and training to employees.

Reporting of Injuries, Diseases and Dangerous Occurrences Regulations 1995 (RIDDOR 95) Employers must:

- report all cases in which employees have suffered death or major injury or have been off work for 3 days or more following an assault that has resulted in physical injury.

The Employment Rights Act 1996 Employers are also protected by the Employment Rights Act 1996, which says that they must not be disadvantaged or dismissed on particular health and safety grounds. These grounds include raising health and safety concerns with the employer and taking protective action such as leaving the workplace in the event of serious and imminent danger. For example, a community nurse is protected from any action by their employer if they leave a client's home because of abuse or violence from the client or relative.

The obligations of employees

While it is the responsibility of the employing organization to provide safe systems of work, individuals also have a responsibility to follow safe working practices. In their everyday work, employees need to remain watchful for their own safety and that of their colleagues.

However, the problem with the law is that it does not always explain clearly how far staff may go in dealing with violent and aggressive acts. Any direct and intentional application of force to another person without lawful justification is battery, which is criminal. In the healthcare setting battery might include the use of restraint or sedation (Gostin 1983) or forcibly searching a client. Often these methods can be justified, but nurses must be aware of the possible limitations to actions like these. The nurse is only within the law when there is lawful justification for their action. Under the doctrine of self-defence, any person can take all reasonable steps to ensure that he or she does not come to any harm and that harm does not befall another; in the eyes of the law self-defence can be carried out on behalf of someone else. Self-defence can also be used to discourage or prevent unlawful force and to avoid or escape from unlawful detention, although it is important to demonstrate to the aggressor that there is no desire to fight and a willingness to disengage.

The law gives the term 'reasonableness' the rider that force used is actually necessary. This suggests that if a client can usually be dealt with by non-physical means, the use of physical restraint would constitute an assault. In addition, the force must be proportionate to the harm to be avoided and the degree and duration of force or restraint used must be proportionate to the harm that is being avoided.

Zero Tolerance

The Department of Health launched the NHS Zero Tolerance campaign in October 1999 (Department of Health 1999) to inform the public that aggression, violence and threatening behaviour will not be tolerated by staff working in the health service. The guidance aims to balance staff protection with the duty to provide services and states that care will be denied to clients who abuse staff. The government says care is not to be denied to clients with severe mental health problems or other conditions that clinicians think leave the client incapable of taking responsibility for their actions. Understandably, a number of criteria must be met before treatment can be withdrawn.

The guidance is driven not just by health and safety requirements and the duty of care owed by employers but also by the Human Rights Act 1998. This act seeks above all others to protect the dignity and feelings of employees from 'inhuman' or 'degrading' treatment on the part of the employee (Article 3). In addition to this the campaign has been backed by new prosecution procedures for both staff and service users. This has resulted in closer working between NHS Trusts and other local agencies such as the police and the Crown Prosecution Service, accumulating in an increase of successful prosecutions against individuals for assaulting staff (Schwehr 2001).

Special considerations: community care

Although the issues raised so far in the chapter relate in some ways to the situation of community care, one important difference exists: that nurses working in the community often work on their own in clients' homes. To this end extra thought and consideration needs to be given over to the issue of safety. To avoid being isolated in a client's home it is recommended that the community nurse ensures that someone else within the community team knows of their visit, both in terms of where they are going and when they should return. To this end it is also important to let colleagues know of any change in itinerary and what is expected of them in the event of the community nurse not returning at the designated time.

Where possible the community nurse should arrange for contact with clients of particular concern to be made in a surgery or other health service premises where support staff will be available. Where a home visit cannot be avoided, however, the appointment should be scheduled for a time of day that affords extra security, such as the morning when parents are around taking their children to school, and when drug activity and drunkenness should be at a minimum. If necessary, the community nurse should be prepared to take a colleague with them and, if appropriate, ask the police for escort. In addition to this, the community nurse should be prepared to readdress the goals of their visit if the situation is not how they expected it to be and leave if they feel threatened or unsure.

Consideration should be given over to the type of shoes and clothes that are worn by the community nurse. Shoes and clothes should not hinder movement or the nurse's ability to run.

Likewise, thought should be given to where the nurse has parked his or her car as it is likely that this will be the only means of escape if things go wrong. To this end the nurse should ensure that their vehicle has sufficient petrol and is well maintained.

PERSONAL AND REFLECTIVE KNOWLEDGE

REFLECTION AND PORTFOLIO EVIDENCE: BECOME AWARE OF YOUR OWN REACTIONS TO AGGRESSION

Increasingly we are being encouraged to reflect on practice as a nurse. This exercise is intended to increase your analytical skills with regard to aggressive incidents. Using Johns' reflective model below draw on your own experience or from peers or from other professional nurses to look at an aggressive incident that took place in practice.

Christopher Johns' model for structured reflection

This model (Johns 1993) offers a series of questions for the nurse to help reflection on experience:

1. Can you describe your experience? What happened?
2. What caused the events to happen as they did?
3. What significant background factors were there? What was the context of the event?
4. Can you reflect on your experience? Try considering the following:
   (a) What were you trying to achieve?
   (b) Why did you intervene as you did?
   (c) What were the consequences for you, the client, relatives and colleagues?
   (d) How did you feel about the experience when it was happening?
   (e) How did the client feel about it and how do you know this?
   (f) What factors or knowledge influenced your decisions and actions?
5. Did you have any options and what would have been their consequences?
6. What have you learned from the experience? For example:
   (a) How do you feel about the experience *now*?
   (b) Could you have dealt better with the situation?

Once you have completed this exercise you can include it in your portfolio.

CASE STUDIES INVOLVING AGGRESSIVE BEHAVIOUR

There now follow four case studies, one from each branch of nursing. Using the evidence presented in this chapter, try to answer the questions at the end of each scenario.

Case study: Adult

Staff Nurse Clare Marsden works on a medical admission ward. Following the new admission of an elderly lady the lady's husband requests to see Clare in private. The lady's husband explains that he has been looking after his wife since she had a stroke several months ago and that he had been 'forced into bringing her into hospital by their GP!' He becomes more and more angry as he relates to Clare his concerns for his wife's well-being. He is worried that his wife 'won't get the attention in hospital that she did at home', 'that she won't have company', 'that she'll be left to rot in bed', and that 'she would never get home again!' Whilst expressing his concerns for his wife he invades Clare's personal space making her feel ill at ease. He starts to raise his voice and becomes animated in both his speech and behaviour, punctuating his sentences with a pointing finger.

- What factors may underlie Mr Marsden's behaviour?
- What strategies could Clare possibly adopt to meet the situation?
- Should the incident be reported? If so, to whom and in what format?

Case study: Child

Max is aged 9 years. Following the recent death of his father in a car accident Max has become increasing hostile in his manner. He has physically fought with friends to the point that they will no longer play with him, and he now argues with his mother on a frequent basis.

On one occasion he spat at her and on another lashed out with his fists and feet. Max's mother confides in you during a visit to the well woman's clinic that she feels unable to control Max's behaviour and that he is 'escalating out of control!' She feels that 'she has not only lost her husband but her son as well'.

- How might Max's mother seek to address his anger and aggressive manner?
- What support could you offer Max's mother?
- What agencies within your local area could you refer Max and his mother to for more specialist help if needed?

Case study: Learning disabilities

Barbara is a woman in her early forties who had been resident in a long-stay hospital for people with learning disabilities. Although Barbara had a history of aggression, the incidences and severity of these outbursts were not as marked as they had been in the past. In fact everything seemed to be going well for Barbara until she was moved to a small community home run largely by mental health nurses following a merger of local healthcare services. Shortly after her transfer, Barbara's behaviour has deteriorated, resulting in her lashing out and striking a member of staff.

- With reference to knowledge gained in this chapter, offer possible explanations as to why Barbara's behaviour might have deteriorated.
- How could this situation have been better managed to prevent distress and aggression?
- What strategies might the staff of the new unit employ to bring the situation under control and address Barbara's needs?

Case study: Mental health

Mr Smith is a young man of 25 years. He has a medical diagnosis of paranoid personality disorder. He was 'persuaded' to come into hospital by the local community psychiatric nurse after he had voiced thoughts of harming his neighbours, who he believed to be 'out to get him'.

Following admission Mr Smith decides that he is not staying, as he now believes the nurses to be in league with his neighbours. On attempting to make his exit from the ward he threatens to 'punch the lights out' of a male staff nurse who tries to converse with him and encourage him to stay 'until he has seen the doctor'.

- What should the immediate actions of the staff nurse be?
- What factors should be taken into consideration when addressing Mr Smith's safety and well-being?
- What factors should be taken into consideration when addressing the needs of the other clients on the ward and staff members?

Summary

This chapter has emphasized the need to be aware of potential outbursts of aggression in nursing practice. A wide range of issues relating to the management of aggression was explored, including:

1. Through various approaches, several challenging areas of nursing practice were highlighted in relation to the control and management of aggression, for example, communication skills, assessment skills and practices, documentation requirements, policies and procedures and support available.
2. Key concepts include maintaining a therapeutic milieu, preventing escalation, identifying aggressive patterns of behaviour, and using appropriate interventions.
3. Properly trained staff can improve the quality of life within the healthcare environment by decreasing frustration and fear for staff and clients alike.
4. Further recommendations include the need to adopt a risk management approach to working with potentially aggressive individuals, as well as the development of guidelines in aggressive management.
5. It is from this base that professional decision making can develop.

Annotated further reading and websites

Bibby P 1995 Personal safety for health care workers. Arena, Aldershot
The book on personal safety for healthcare workers by Pauline Bibby from the Suzy Lamplugh Trust offers a more personally orientated approach and gives advice for personal safety. Very useful chapters include assertiveness and practical steps to safety, as well as guidelines for travelling. This book also contains a chapter devoted to trainers in the management of violence.

Breakwell G 1995 General and specific clues and dangerousness checklist. In: Kidd B, Stark C (eds) Management of violence and aggression in health care. Gaskell, London
For a concise account of the current theories concerning aggression this chapter is an excellent resource of recent developments. The chapter also contains an account of the assault cycle.

Kidd B, Stark C 1995 Management of violence and aggression in health care. Gaskell, London
This book offers useful chapters on the practical management of aggression.

Royal College of Nursing 1998 Dealing with violence against nursing staff. Royal College of Nursing, London
This publication is concerned with the nature and management of violent incidents that NHS staff may encounter in the course of their work. Full of practical hints and advice.

Storr A 1992 Human aggression. Penguin, Harmondsworth
For a wider view of aggression in terms of social, individual and interpersonal factors, this book makes interesting and useful reading.

http://www.nhs.uk/zerotolerance /downloads/index-htm
Department of Health 1999 NHS Zero Tolerance: We Don't Have To Take This. HMSO, London
A useful resource that reminds the healthcare worker that they need not put up with violence and aggression in the workplace.

http://www.fnrh.freeserve.co.uk/index1.html
The Forensic Nursing Resource Homepage maintained by Phil Woods, Senior Lecturer in Forensic Mental Health Nursing, Florence Nightingale School of Nursing and Midwifery, King's College London. An excellent resource that includes research papers, articles, assessment tools and links to other relevant websites.

http://www.suzylamplugh.org/home/index.shtml
The Suzy Lamplugh Trust homepage. This contains links to resource packs, many of which need to be purchased. You can jump from this site to the trust's training department who can organize personal safety conferences. There is also a shop section selling personal safety equipment on-line.

http://www.homeoffice.gov.uk/crimprev/personalsafety.htm
Home Office guidance on personal safety. Advice for maintaining personal safety in a range of situations, and what to do if you have been attacked.

http://www.successunlimited.co.uk/bully/index.htm
A resource targeted at supporting those who suffer from workplace bullying. A useful resource; however, if you do feel that you are being bullied then your professional organization or union representative should be your first contact.

References

Anderson C A, Dill K E 2000 Video games and aggressive thoughts, feelings and behaviour in the laboratory and in life. Journal of Personality and Social Psychology 78:772–790

Allen J 1997 Assessing and managing risk and violence in the mentally disordered. Journal of Psychiatric and Mental Health Nursing 4:369–378

Ardrey R 1969 The territorial imperative. Fontana, London

Argyle M 1988 Bodily communication. Methuen, London

Atkins S, Murphy K 1993 Reflection: a review of the literature. Journal of Advanced Nursing 18:1188–1192

Atkinson R L, Atkinson R C, Smith E E et al 1987 Imitation of film-mediated aggressive models. Journal of Abnormal and Social Psychology 66:3–11

Bandura A 1969 Principles of behaviour modification. Holt, New York

Bandura A 1973 Aggression: a social learning analysis. Prentice-Hall, Englewood Cliffs

Bandura A 1977 Social learning theory. Prentice-Hall, Englewood Cliffs

Bandura A, Ross D, Ross S A 1963 Imitation of film-mediated aggressive models. Journal of Abnormal and Social Psychology 42:63–66

Baron R A, Neuman J 1996 Workplace violence and workplace aggression: evidence on their relative frequency and potential causes. Aggressive Behaviour 22:161–173

Berkowitz L 1990 On the formation and regulation of anger and aggression: a cognitive–neoassociationist analysis. American Psychologist 45:494–503

Berkowitz L 1993 Pain and aggression: some findings and implications. Psychological Bulletin 106:59–73

Berkowitz L 2001 Affect, aggression and antisocial behaviour. In: Davidson R J, Scherer K, Goldsmith H H (eds) Handbook of affective sciences. Oxford University Press, Oxford

Bibby P 1995 Personal safety for health care workers. Arena, Aldershot

Bouchard T J, Lykken D T, McGue M et al 1990 Sources of human psychological differences: the Minnesota study of twins reared apart. Science 350:223–228

Breakwell G 1995 General and specific clues and dangerousness checklist. In: Kidd B, Stark C (eds) Management of violence and aggression in health care. Gaskell, London

Briggs K 1986 Assertiveness: speak your mind. Nursing Times 82(26):24–26

Burnard P 1991 Assertiveness and clinical practice. Nursing Standard 5(33):37–39

Burrow S 1994 Nurse-aid management of psychiatric emergencies: 3. British Journal of Nursing 3(3):121–125

Burton R 1998 Violence and aggression in the workplace. Mental Health Care 2(3):105–108

Buss A 1995 Personality: temperament, social behaviour and the self. Allyn & Bacon, Boston

Bushman B J 1995 Moderating role of trait aggressiveness in the effects of violent media on aggression. Journal of Personal and Social Psychology 69:950–960

Bushman B J 1998 Priming effects of violent media on the accessibility of aggressive constructs in the memory. Personality and Social Psychology Bulletin 24:537–545

Carlson M, Marcus-Newhall A, Miller N 1990 Effects of situational aggression cues: a quantitative review. Journal of Personal and Social Psychology 58:622–633

Casey M D, Blank C E, McLean T M et al 1973 Male patients with chromosome abnormality in the state hospitals. Journal of Mental Deficiency Research 16:215–256

Cembrowicz S, Ritter S 1994 Attacks on doctors and nurses. In: Shepherd J (ed) Violence in health care: a practical guide to coping with violence and caring for victims. Oxford University Press, Oxford

Cohen D J, Eckhardt C I, Schagat K D 1998 Attention allocation and habituation to anger-related stimuli during a visual search task. Aggressive Behaviour 24:399–409

Delaney J, Cleary M, Jordan R et al 2001 An exploratory investigation into the nursing management of aggression in acute psychiatric settings. Journal of Psychiatric and Mental Health Nursing 8:77–84

Department of Health 1999 We don't have to take this: NHS guidance on zero tolerance. Department of Health, London

Department of Health 2000 2000/2001 Survey of reported violent or abusive incidents, accidents involving staff and sickness absence in NHS Authorities, in England. Department of Health, London

Dollard J, Doob L W, Miller N E et al 1939 Frustration and aggression. Yale University Press, New Haven

Employment Rights Act 1996 HMSO, London

Eysenck H J, Gudjonsson G H 1989 The causes and cures of criminality. Plenum, New York

Farrell G 1992 Therapeutic response to verbal abuse. Nursing Standard 6(47):29–31

Farrell G A, Gray C 1992 Aggression: a nurse's guide to therapeutic management. Scutari Press, London

Farrington D P 1994 The causes and prevention of offending, with special reference to violence. In: Shepherd J (ed) Violence in health care: a practical guide to coping with violence and caring for victims. Oxford University Press, Oxford, pp 149–177

Frankl G 1990 The unknown self. Open Gate Press, London

Garnham P 2001 Understanding and dealing with anger, aggression and violence. Nursing Standard 16(6):37–42

Geddes D, Baron R A 1997 Workplace aggression as a consequence of negative performance feedback. Management Communication Quarterly 10:433–455

Geen R G 2001 Human aggression, 2nd edn. Taylor & Francis, London

Gostin L 1983 A practical guide to mental health law. MIND, London

Gould J 1994 The impact of change on violent patients. Nursing Standard 8(19):38–40

Gross R 1992 Psychology: the science of mind and behaviour. Hodder & Stoughton, London

Health and Safety and Welfare at Work Act 1974 HMSO, London

Health Services Advisory Committee 1997 Violence and aggression to staff in health services: guidance on assessment and management. HSE Books, Sudbury

Heron J 1986 Six category intervention analysis. University of Surrey, Guildford

Hinde R A 1982 Ethology. In: Brennan W (ed) 1998 Aggression and violence: examining the theories. Nursing Standard 12(27):36–38

Hinde R A 1993 Aggression at different levels of social complexity. In: Taylor P J (ed) Violence in society. Royal College of Physicians, London

Hollin C R 1992 Criminal behaviour. Falmer Press, Brighton

Human Rights Act 1998 HMSO, London

Janelli L M 1995 Physical restraint use in acute care settings. Journal of Nursing Care Quality 9(3):86–92

Jeffery C R 1979 Biology and crime. Sage, London

Johns C 1993 Professional supervision. Journal of Nursing Management 1(1):9–18

Kaukiainen A, Salmivalli C, Bjorkqvist K et al 2001 Overt and covert aggression in work settings in relation to the subjective well-being of employees. Aggressive Behaviour 27:360–371

Leadbetter D, Paterson B 1995 De-escalating aggressive behaviour. In: Kidd B, Stark C (eds) Management of violence and aggression in health care. Gaskill, London

Leymann H 1990 Mobbing and psychological terror at workplaces. Violence Victims 5:119–126

Littlechild B 1996 The risk of violence and aggression to social work and social work staff. In: Kemshall H, Pritchard H (eds) Good practice in risk assessment and risk management. Jessica Kingsley, London

Lorenz K 1966 On aggression. Methuen, London

Management of Health and Safety at Work Regulations 1992 HMSO, London

McDonnell A, McEvoy J, Dearden R L 1994 Coping with violent situations in the caring environment. In: Wykes T (ed) Violence and health care professionals. Chapman & Hall, London, pp 189–207

Morris D 1967 The naked ape. McGraw-Hill, New York

Morrison E 1992 A hierarchy of aggressive and violent behaviours among psychiatric inpatients. Hospital and Community Psychiatry 43:505

Nursing and Midwifery Council 2002 Code of professional conduct. Nursing and Midwifery Council, London

Owens R G, Ashcroft J B (eds) 1985 Violence: a guide for the caring professions. Croom Helm, London

Paterson B L, McCornish A, Bradley P 1999 Violence at work. Nursing Standard 13(21):43–46

Pollock N, McBain I, Webster C D 1989 Clinical decision making and the assessment of dangerousness. In: Howells K, Hollin C R (eds) Clinical approaches to violence. John Wiley, Chichester

Prentky R 1985 The neurochemistry and neuroendocrinology of sexual aggression. In: Farrington D P, Gunn J (eds) Aggression and dangerousness. John Wiley, Chichester

Price W H 1978 Sex chromosome abnormalities in special hospital patients. In: Owens R G, Ashcroft J B (eds) Violence: a guide for the caring professions. Croom Helm, London

Reporting of Injuries, Diseases and Dangerous Occurrences Regulations 1995 HMSO, London

Rich A, Parker D 1995 Reflection and critical incident analysis: ethical and moral implications of their use within nursing and midwifery education. Journal of Advanced Nursing 22:1050–1057

Richardson C 1994 Management of aggressive incidents by psychiatric nurses. Australian and New Zealand College of Mental Health Nursing Inc, Annual Conference Proceedings Brisbane, pp 214–221

Robb E 1995 Post-incident care and support for assaulted staff. In: Kidd B, Stark C (eds) Violence in health care: a practical guide to coping with violence and caring for victims. Oxford University Press, Oxford

Rowett C, Breakwell G M 1992 Managing violence at work. National Foundation for Educational Research, Slough

Royal College of Nursing 1998 Safer working in the community: a guide for NHS managers and staff on reducing the risks of violence and aggression. Royal College of Nursing, London

Royal College of Nursing 2001 Challenging harassment and bullying: guidance for RCN representatives, stewards and officers. Royal College of Nursing, London

Royal College of Psychiatrists 1998 Management of imminent violence: clinical practice guidelines: quick reference guide. Royal College of Psychiatrists, London

Royal College of Psychiatrists 1999 Safety for trainees in psychiatry: Council report CR78. Royal College of Psychiatrists, London

Schwehr B 2001 Zero tolerance: drawing the line in health and social care. Online. Available: http://www.CareandHealth.Com 24 June 2002

Shepherd J (ed) 1994 Violence in health care: a practical guide to coping with violence and caring for victims. Oxford University Press, Oxford

Siann G 1985 Accounting for aggression: perspectives on aggression and violence. In: Brennan W (ed) 1998 Aggression and violence: examining the theories. Nursing Standard 12(27):36–38

Whittington R 1997 Violence to nurses: prevalence and risk factors. Nursing Standard 12(5):49–56

Wykes T (ed) 1994 Violence and healthcare professionals. Chapman & Hall, London

Wykes T, Mezey G 1994 Counselling for victims of violence. In: Wykes T (ed) 1994 Violence and healthcare professionals. Chapman & Hall, London, pp 207–225

Chapter 12

Death and dying

Linda Wilson

KEY ISSUES

SUBJECT KNOWLEDGE
- Different forms of death from death of the cell through to cortical and brain stem death
- Concept of ontological death and the 'near death experience'
- Differing cultural perspectives on death
- The grieving process and coping with loss

CARE DELIVERY KNOWLEDGE
- The dying process
- Breaking bad news
- Physical signs of an approaching death
- Managing the care of the dying client

PROFESSIONAL AND ETHICAL KNOWLEDGE
- Trends in the location of death in today's society
- Issues in the professional coping with death
- New challenges: living wills, the rights of dying clients to request help to die, euthanasia
- The role of the coroner in certain deaths
- Organ donation

PERSONAL AND REFLECTIVE KNOWLEDGE
- Personal fears and misgivings about own death and that of others
- Consolidate knowledge through case study exercises

INTRODUCTION

Death is a unique experience for each person and, unlike certain other nursing and medical interventions where we can improve on our initial care, we have no second chance in this situation. It is vital that the death event is never seen as a routine experience. The care of dying people is an issue within the care of clients in a broad spectrum of settings.

There is no right way to die or to grieve and it is vitally important in health care that we offer unconditional support to individuals and families having the experience. It is useful to clarify what the terminology means and what is meant by palliative and terminal care:

- Palliative care or palliation is a broad band of care of indeterminate length that should start from the moment a client is diagnosed as having a disease for which there is no cure, and the focus of the care of the client moves from curing to caring (i.e. symptom relief as opposed to curative treatment).
- Terminal care is the management of the end of life (i.e. the last hours or days before death).

It has been argued that health professionals have difficulty managing clients who require palliative care, partly because of the conflict in cure versus care. As medicine is very much concerned with cure, a dying patient is often seen as a failure and this may lead to treatment being offered that is no longer of benefit to the individual (Cassell 1974). Virginia Henderson (1966) in her definition of nursing identified caring for the dying as a key part of the nurse's function, carrying equal weight with the curative element of care. The British Medical Association guidance *Withholding and Withdrawing Life Prolonging Treatment* (British Medical Association 2001) was developed to address this and is discussed further with other ethical issues. The registered nurse is often in a position to help junior medical staff cope with the loss of the client and, handled sensitively, the nurse can have a marked influence on the subsequent care of others.

OVERVIEW

Subject knowledge

In the biological part, the definitions of death, what it is and how it may impinge on practice are explored. The physical manifestations of death, the life cycle of the cell and types of death are addressed. In the psychosocial section, societal and cultural attitudes to death are explored, the determinants and processes of grieving are examined, and finally the stages in the dying process are outlined.

Care delivery knowledge

The role of the nurse in managing the care of the dying is discussed. The care and support needed by relatives is also considered.

Professional and ethical knowledge

In this part the role of the coroner, managing the death, the necessary formalities and the legal and ethical problems associated with the dying individual are examined.

Personal and reflective knowledge

Here you are asked to explore your own personal responses to death and dying and to record these in your portfolio of learning. You have an opportunity to consider four case studies on page 277 using your personal experience and the chapter content. You may also find it helpful to read one of them before you start the chapter and use it as a focus for your reflections while reading.

SUBJECT KNOWLEDGE

BIOLOGICAL

What is death? On a microscopic level, cells in the body die and are renewed constantly from birth. At a macro level, however, regulated changes in groups of cells occur as part of the normal ageing process. This section therefore begins by examining the life cycle of the cell from its inception to its death. In turn, this provides the foundation from which the life cycle of the human organism can be understood.

CELL LIFE AND DEATH

Normal cells undergo orderly regular periods of mitosis (cell reproduction) and normal cell growth occurs in two phases:

1. From birth to maturity where the total number of cells is constantly increasing as the person develops to full size.
2. From maturity to death when the number of cells produced equals the number of cells that die and overall body size remains relatively constant.

Consequently, in adults, whether cell growth is fast or slow, the overall number of cells does not increase (Sinclair 1989).

Cells are created by the process of either:

- mitosis, where the parent cell reproduces itself to produce two daughter cells identical to the parent cell, or
- meiosis, which occurs only in spermatozoa or egg cells where each daughter cell has the haploid number of chromosomes.

The lifespan of a cell varies according to its type. A neurone does not reproduce in a lifetime whereas an epithelial cell in the gut wall may reproduce every day. Additionally, tissues composed of relatively undifferentiated cells, for example bones and the liver, are able to regenerate themselves easily. At the other extreme, a cell can become so specialized that it cannot reproduce itself, for example the erythrocyte (Montague & Knight 1996). There is normally strict control over the rate of growth of cells in any body tissue by the integrated actions of hormones and growth factors. Loss of such control leads to tumour growth, and in cancer the life cycle of the cell is somewhat different. The spreading of a malignant disease is due to the increased lifespan of cells rather than the proliferation of cancer cells. Priestman (1989) points out that only 50–60% of cancer cells die during the span of the disease.

When a cell is injured or is dying, the lysosomes (from the Greek words 'lysis', dissolution, and 'soma', body) release enzymes which break down the cell. Lysosomes are vital for phagocytosis to occur and large numbers of them are present in leucocytes.

LIFE, AGEING AND DEATH OF THE HUMAN ORGANISM

Regulated changes occur as individuals advance in chronological age, and this phenomenon is referred to as the normal ageing process. Normal life expectancy, which refers to the average length of survival of a species, is determined by environmental factors, whereas lifespan denotes the maximum age reached and appears to depend upon genes (Montague & Knight 1996). Although life expectancy can improve when the environment improves, lifespan for an individual may remain unchanged. Several theories have been proposed to explain how cellular ageing occurs (Brookbank 1990, Cunningham & Brookbank 1988), but none is conclusive (see Annotated Further Reading on p. 277). Generalized changes with ageing involve all organ systems resulting in a loss of reserve function, which will eventually lead to total system failure and death. The rate at which this occurs naturally varies with each individual. However, if there is acute damage to organs at any age, as in multiple trauma, which leads to shock and loss of circulation to vital tissues, then multiple organ failure becomes a feature in the dying process of that individual (Viney 1996).

Cessation of respiration
Absent heart and pulse sounds
Lack of spontaneous activity
Absence of reflexes and response to stimuli
Dilated fixed pupils
Persistent distortion of the pupil and eyeball on pressure
Segmentation of blood in the retinal arteries when viewed
  by ophthalmoscope
Rigor mortis

Figure 12.1   Criteria for cardiorespiratory death.

Fixed pupils
Absent corneal reflex
Absent vestibulo-ocular reflexes: no eye movements during or
  after slow injection of ice cold water into each ear
No motor cranial nerve responses
No gag reflex or response to bronchial stimulation by catheter
No respiratory effort off the respirator with the PCO_2 @ 6.7 kPa

Figure 12.2   Criteria for brain stem death. (From Hinds & Watson 1996.)

Cardiorespiratory death

Most people regard death as cardiorespiratory death; that is when the heart and lungs no longer function, and the majority of people who die are judged against the cardio respiratory criteria outlined in Figure 12.1. However, with the advent of resuscitation and ventilation, cardiorespiratory conditions for death are no longer adequate. Consequently, other diagnostic criteria have had to be identified to allow death to be determined in individuals being ventilated artificially.

Brain stem death

The criteria to establish brain stem death (Fig. 12.2) were devised to provide clear parameters for clinical staff when making decisions about discontinuing life support (Pallis 1983, Pallis & Harley 1996).

Brain stem death was initially identified at the Conference of Medical Colleges and Faculties of the United Kingdom in 1976 (Jennett 1982). Hinds & Watson (1996) discuss this concept and suggest that it relates to the destruction of the brain stem, which makes independent functioning impossible. The criteria by which brain stem death can be diagnosed have been the subject of debate and review since brain stem death was recognized and identified as a specific form of death (Day 1995, Fisher 1991, Norton 1992, Pallis 1983). Doctors must ensure that the individual being tested for brain stem death is not under the influence of any paralysing drugs such as vecuronium bromide and atracurium besylate, which may be used to sedate clients while they are ventilated. These drugs act by competing with acetylcholine at the receptor site at the neuromuscular junction. The action

of these muscle relaxants can be reversed with anticholinesterases such as neostigmine (British Medical Association and Pharmaceutical Society 2002). Likewise clients who have overdosed on barbiturates (although now rare) require a careful assessment to ensure that the sedative effects of the drug do not mask the client's reaction to the brain stem death criteria. The same caution applies if barbiturates have been used to treat intractable cerebral oedema (Louis et al 1993) and sufficient time should be given after the cessation of treatment before undertaking the brain stem tests. Similar problems arise with clients suffering from myxoedema and hypothermia as their reactions will be very sluggish and may even be imperceptible.

Reflection and portfolio exercise

A number of other endocrine and metabolic disorders also need to be excluded and these are clearly identified within the guidelines available at your hospital, which will be based on the national guidelines.

● Find out what these are and add them to your portfolio of learning.

The brain stem death tests are carried out by two medical practitioners, one of whom is the anaesthetist or physician in charge of the case while the other must not be involved with either the care of the client or the transplant team (if an organ transplant is being considered). Brain stem tests are repeated 4–48 hours later. If both are negative, ventilator support maintaining respiratory function is discontinued.

Cortical brain death

The concept of cortical brain death was first proposed in the USA with the Nancy Cruzan case and subsequently in the UK with the Tony Bland case (Jennett & Dyer 1991), in which the clients were in a persistent vegetative state (PVS) and had suffered irreversible cortical brain damage, which had destroyed the higher senses. This situation does not mean,

Reflection and portfolio exercise

Find out if your practice placement areas have any local guidelines for diagnosing brain stem death.

● Compare these local guidelines with what has been outlined in this chapter.
● Reflect on what the feelings of relatives might be if their relative is diagnosed as dead and yet the body remains ventilated.
● Discuss with your peers how you feel and how healthcare professionals cope with these situations.

however, that the client's death is imminent. With feeding and skilled nursing management such an individual can exist for many years. It is difficult to class this as living as this suggests a life of which one is aware. The fact remains that unlike in the event of brain stem death, the life of these clients can be sustained. The ethical dilemmas related to the concept of cortical brain death are discussed more fully later.

Ontological death

A highly controversial notion is that of ontological death. Philosophers in the USA have suggested that once the personhood of an individual has been irretrievably destroyed, that person is to all intents and purposes dead and can be used as an organ donor. Personhood concerns the essence of the individual not the biological being – it is consciousness, recognition of self as an entity, reasoning, moral coding and the many other attributes we associate with being 'ourselves'. Loss of personhood is seen as loss of the self. This theory would have significant repercussions for the severely handicapped, people suffering from dementia, and other vulnerable individuals if the inherent dignity of the individual, however damaged, was seen as less than human.

PSYCHOSOCIAL

THE NEAR DEATH EXPERIENCE

Throughout history, individuals have described experiences of having glimpsed the hereafter; one of the more interesting descriptions can be found in the Book of Revelations in the Bible (Revelations: 21), which theologians believe must have included this phenomenon. Cole (1993) cites an American opinion poll that suggests that near death experiences (NDEs) are not rare occurrences. Some 38–50% of those who come close to death recount experiences consistent with an NDE.

Physiologists have claimed that such experiences can be replicated in the laboratory by the use of mind altering drugs and brain stimulation. Blackmore (1988) gives a detailed breakdown of the process, but fails to explain why only some clients experience an NDE. The salient features of any NDE are similar regardless of culture, age, sex, educational background, financial status or psychiatric history (Osis & Haraldsson 1986). Simpson (2001) discusses the concept and applies it to nursing practice. According to Ring (1980) the features of NDE are:

- an initial phase linked to feelings of extraordinary peace, calm, warmth and comfort
- separation from the physical body with a bird's-eye view of the body – the so-called 'out of body experience'
- movement through a cylindrical dark space, which ends with a bright light
- meeting a being of light, which is often the appropriate deity for the individual

- emerging into a beautiful place such as a garden or a 'heaven-like' place where those who are already dead are encountered.

The vast majority of NDEs are described as joyous and not alarming. However, for a few the experience is very distressing, these same features creating a hell-like environment rather than the reassuring one described above. Given that at least 20% of clients undergoing a cardiac arrest procedure experience an NDE, nurses need to recognize their role in allowing clients to discuss what they have experienced.

It is likely that clients worry that they will not be believed, or worse still that they are hallucinating, and feel a considerable sense of relief when they realize that they are not alone in what they have seen and felt. It is useful within the documentation following a cardiac arrest with the subsequent survival of the client to include the potential problem of the client having had an NDE.

Reflection and portfolio exercise

- Have you or any of your relatives or friends experienced what has been described above as an NDE?
- Were you or they able to describe their experiences to others?
- What was the reaction of others to your or their experience?
- Reflect on what your reactions and feelings are about this phenomenon.
- How might your reactions influence your response and decision making if confronted with a client who recounts an NDE to you?

A change in behaviour may lead health professionals to suspect that a client has had an NDE, by the client becoming either agitated or, conversely, withdrawn and quiet. The client should be encouraged, but never pressed, to talk about what happened and whether they saw or experienced anything while they were very ill. It is essential that anything confided by the client is not dismissed, though it may appear extremely bizarre. These episodes may be interpreted as confusion on occasions. Children also have these experiences.

For information on grieving in children see Hill (1994).

ATTITUDES TOWARDS DEATH

Attitudes towards death and dying have changed dramatically in the UK and the developed world, particularly in the years since World War II. With the improvement in infant mortality rate and increasing life expectancy, however, death is no longer a commonplace experience among the public. Consequently, many people have not had contact with a death. Care of the deceased is now left largely to the professional, namely funeral directors. The lack of familiarity with death makes people fearful and anxious about their own death and that of their family members.

Attitudes towards the type of death that is preferable have also changed. In Victorian times, a slow, lingering death would have been preferred to a sudden death because of the need to settle affairs and gather everyone together. Conversely, research suggests that people nowadays would prefer to die in their sleep or suddenly (Peberdy 1992). Attitudes are very much culturally determined and depend upon the beliefs that people have about for example the afterlife, retribution and reincarnation.

Recognizing the spiritual needs of clients as opposed to their religious beliefs is vital; we all have a spiritual dimension linked to our beliefs about life, death, hope, etc., and not having religious views should not be equated with a lack of spiritual need. Demonstrating an understanding and respecting the views of clients and their relatives facilitates the grieving process instead of making them angry or defensive.

There are marked religious norms in relation to the grieving process. For example, whereas in Western culture a dying individual is visited by only close family and friends, within some Asian groups and Romany families, large numbers of visitors may arrive to pay their respects and may wish to stay night and day. Alternatively, a dying Buddhist may wish to forego pain relief and to lie on the floor to be near to Mother Earth and to meditate. Such behaviour can be interpreted as confusion and caring staff may put the client back to bed several times because they do not understand the significance of what is happening. If a religion is cyclical (e.g. Hinduism and Buddhism), and individuals believe in a continuous series of lives, the death will only be a means of transfer to a new life. This belief may explain in part the more readily accepting manner in which death is approached by both the family and the client.

Religious beliefs and references to the practice and customs of different ethnic groups are numerous and diverse and should therefore be explored in depth (Green 1989;

Narayanasamy, 1993, 1995; Praill 1995). It is always useful to record a contact name and number for the religious representative, as well as recording religious affiliation, so that if the client suffers an unexpected collapse the appropriate people can be contacted to provide support for both the client and family. A knowledge of where people can find support is valuable for both the dying person and the dying person's friends and relatives. The aim of care must be to meet the holistic needs of the client – physical, psychological, social and spiritual – if we are to make a significant contribution towards the client's 'good death'. Sadly many of our standards of care for the dying client fall far short of what we would personally find acceptable or desirable for ourselves or our relatives (Copp 1994).

An appropriate death

Most people have an idea of what they consider to be the ideal way to die and may have discussed this 'ideal' with relatives and friends in terms of 'wishes'. Likewise they have goals they would like to achieve before they die. These become more acute and important when a person is given an estimate of how long he or she will live when diagnosed with an incurable disease. Weisman (1988) speaks of an 'appropriate' death which includes:

- reducing, but not necessarily eliminating, conflict
- making dying compatible with the dying person's own view of him or herself and his or her achievements
- preserving or restoring relationships as much as possible
- fulfilling some of the dying person's expressed aims.

Expectations of when death is appropriate also affect the way in which people react to it. For an adult the death of a parent is seen as a great sadness, but it is within the natural scheme of things – that is the elders leaving room for the new generation. However, the death of a child is a death of the future, the life that would have been rather than the life that has been. Sudden death, although it may be preferred by the individual, is particularly stressful because it challenges all our established coping strategies (Wright 1996). There are numerous factors influencing how people manage the unmanageable, and the overwhelming nature of sudden death needs to be brought down to manageable proportions, for example where a young mother has died, who will look after the children and who can collect them from school? The bereaved individual needs to work in small steps initially to cope. These coping strategies in relation to death are usually referred to in terms of the 'grieving process'.

Evidence based practice

In the paper 'A review of current theories of death and dying' *Journal of Advanced Nursing* (1998) 28(2) 382–390 Copp reviews theories of grief and gives a detailed overview of Kubler Ross (1969), Buckman (1993) and Copp's own 'readiness to die' theory (1998) which involves considering the bodily readiness and the person readiness.

- Reflect critically on these theories to see how they apply to your work in clinical practice.

GRIEF

Grief and its expression are very individual phenomena and each person who is suffering must be helped in the ways most suited to his or her needs. Many studies have been carried out in order to investigate common patterns that contribute to grief as a concept and a reality (Parkes 1975, 1987; Parkes & Parkes 1984) and in turn have identified the determinants of grief. These are listed in Figure 12.3 and form the basis of discussion within this section.

The mode of death

How a person dies can be extremely important, especially if death was unexpected. Questions such as 'Did he or she suffer?' 'Was he or she involved in an accident?' 'Was it his or her fault?' puzzle and concern grieving relatives as they look for meaning. Most people wish to die in familiar surroundings and if death occurs in a strange environment it gives an added dimension to the grief. Suicide produces particular problems because those who are left look for reasons and apportion blame in order to try to make sense of what has happened (Stone 1995). A suicide in adolescence is particularly hard to bear as it is difficult to accept that a young person with all of life's potential before them should choose to end it. Suicide can also be seen as a massive rejection of the parents who conceived and nurtured that life

---

Mode of death
Nature of the attachment
Who the person was
Historical antecedents
Personality variables
Social variables

Figure 12.3   Determinants of grief.

(Hindmarch 1993). Likewise there is a stigma in being the spouse of a suicide. Where murder is involved, there is the added intrusiveness of press and media interest.

The nature of the attachment

The natural peaks and troughs of any relationship will affect the way in which the death is perceived. The feelings will not be the same if the relationship was strong and supportive as those if the couple were ambivalent towards each other. Where a family member has HIV or, at a later stage someone is dying of AIDS, there can be great difficulty in discussing the illness because of the stigma attached to it. The fact that the person's personal behaviour may have contributed to their contracting the disease should not colour health care anymore than smoking, drinking or overeating contribute to disease. Blaming in this context is unhelpful; however, family members may need to vent these feelings as a safety valve.

Who the person was

The position of the deceased within the family will significantly affect the grief that is felt at their demise. The strong matriarch, the downtrodden wife, the domineering husband are but a few examples of the relative influence and position of the dead person within the family circle. The dependence upon the deceased may give some pointers as to the progress of grief. For example, the death of a spouse may give the surviving partner freedom once again and may be seen as a good thing.

Historical antecedents

How the bereaved individual has coped with crisis previously will have an effect on this bereavement. If he or she did not work the grief through in the past, the current problems may well be compounded and this will complicate the grieving process.

Personality variables

Problems occur more readily if the bereaved person had a particularly dependent and clinging relationship with the deceased.

Social variables

Religious beliefs and responses of communities to grief may help or hinder the grieving process. Wright (1991) cites the case of a Jewish woman who had great difficulty coping with the death of her baby son because of the tradition of burial within 24 hours and her subsequent feelings of not being able to say goodbye.

THE GRIEVING PROCESS

Engel (1964) takes the view that losing a loved one is as psychologically traumatic as being seriously injured oneself. He argues that normal grief reactions are a threat to one's mental health. Thus, in the same way that physical healing is necessary to help the body restore its equilibrium, a time is required to allow grieving to occur.

Stages in the grieving process apply equally to anticipatory (before the event) grief and the feelings experienced when a loved one actually dies. The reactions of relatives to a poor prognosis and the death of their loved one can be many and varied, ranging from frozen to histrionics. Judging the relative who does not appear unduly moved as coping well is often erroneous.

Worden (1991) identified the tasks of mourning as being able to:

- accept the reality of loss
- experience the pain of loss
- adjust to the environment where the deceased is missing
- move on with life.

According to Worden (1991) the first step is to accept the reality of the loss. Where a death has been anticipated and the family has observed the gradual decline in health of the significant person who is dying, the loss is an observable phenomenon. In the case of sudden death, particularly where there is no body, as in a major maritime disaster, accepting the loss can be extremely difficult. Parents bereaved through cot death often return to the hospital to see the baby several times to reassure themselves that it is their baby who has died. Parents may find it difficult to hand the baby over to the staff to be moved to the mortuary and hospital staff have said that they find it difficult to put the baby's body in the refrigerator without wrapping it in a blanket. Laakso & Paunonen-Ilmonen (2001) discuss the issue of maternal grief in their study which identified that the ability of staff to meet the needs of the grieving mothers was often inadequate because many feelings and experiences were not identified and were thus unmet.

Decision making exercise

Mrs Feeney had been married for 37 years to Charles when he collapsed with a massive stroke and died. Mrs Feeney's daughter was very worried by the overwhelming nature of the grief and asked the general practitioner to call. He prescribed a course of antidepressants and Mrs Feeney remained on the tablets for several years, not feeling very much pleasure or pain. When Mrs Feeney became aware of the problems of tranquilliser addiction, she decided to try to stop and sought help from her general practitioner. He referred her to a community psychiatric nurse, who is now helping her with in-depth counselling and support as Mrs Feeney is now battling dependence and coping with her unresolved grief. She has had two short admissions to the psychiatric department.

- How could Mrs Feeney have been helped to cope with her grief immediately after her husband's death?
- Debate the issue of prescribing drug therapy in order to help people cope with loss in any form.
- Explore the specific counselling approaches that the community psychiatric nurse could take in helping Mrs Feeney.

Worden (1991) states that individuals need to experience the pain of the loss, but watching individuals who are suffering and not being able to stop the hurt is very difficult. However, severe psychological problems can result if someone is not allowed to grieve. Unresolved grief can lead to psychological disturbance and mental ill health. The pain is therefore needed to allow healing. Many employers allow 3 days' compassionate leave on bereavement and this can suggest that the acute grief can be dealt with within this time-frame. However, Parkes & Parkes (1984) suggest that 2 years is a more realistic period of mourning.

The third task in mourning involves adjusting to an environment in which the deceased is missing. The survivor has to learn skills that were previously the responsibility of the deceased. By doing this, though, the bereaved person may well restore the damage to their feelings of self-worth. Worden (1991) recognizes that the survivor does not always realize all of the roles performed by the deceased until around 3 months from the time of the death.

Finally the survivor needs to relocate the deceased within their past and continue with their life (Worden 1991). The deceased will always be remembered and significant, but the time has now come to love and live again. Worden (1991) cites a case from Alexy (1982: 503) where a mother is talking about her dead son as a good example of moving on:

Only recently have I begun to take notice of things in life that are still open to me. You know things that can bring me pleasure. I know that I will continue to grieve for Robbie for the rest of my life, and that I will keep his loving memory alive. But life goes on, and like it or not I am part of it. Lately there have been times when I notice how well I seem to be doing on some project at home, or even taking part in some activity with friends.

Grief in children, especially when grieving for a brother or sister, can get mixed up with feelings of guilt that something they have done has caused the illness and death. Relationships with parents can also be affected as children may blame the parents for their sibling's illness and death (Sourkes 1987). There is a concurrent need to allow the grieving child space and time to question and talk about their feelings as well as for parents to share their grief with the child or children that remain (Cowlishaw 1993). Models used with adults do not fit very well. Tonkin (1996) suggests that rather than grief diminishing over time, life expands. One of her clients, discussing the death of her daughter, describes thinking that the grief would become 'neatly encapsulated in a small and manageable way' and she was distressed when this did not happen, but what she discovered was that although on significant dates, her grief was still as prominent, at other times, her life had grown to allow her to re-engage with life and this had been really helpful.

Reflection and portfolio exercise

An organization that provides practical help and support to bereaved children and their families is Winston's Wish. They also provide a range of materials to health professionals dealing in this very difficult area.

http://www.winstonswish.org.uk

- Visit this site and see what resources you can add to your portfolio to draw on when working with bereaved children.

CARE DELIVERY KNOWLEDGE

THE DYING PROCESS

So far this chapter has focused on societal and cultural attitudes to death and on coping with grief. The focus has been on the bereaved, outside what the actual experience of dying might mean for the individual. In this section, the focus is on the dying process itself. One of the best recognized approaches to the dying process was devised by Kubler Ross (1975) (Fig. 12.4). She postulated a series of steps or stages through which dying people frequently pass. These stages do not apply to everyone and are frequently not followed in a clear orderly sequence. They serve as a guide as to where people are in terms of their understanding and acceptance of the situation in which they find themselves.

The denial stage is a reaction to being given bad news. Therefore, this section begins by considering the skills needed for breaking bad news before outlining in more detail the physical needs of the client who is dying.

Denial	'They can't mean me'
Anger	'Why should this be happening to me'
Bargaining	'What can I do to take this weight away from me'
Depression	'Everything is useless, I wish I were dead'
Acceptance	'Let me enjoy what time I have left'

Figure 12.4 Stages in the dying process. (From Kubler Ross 1975.)

BREAKING BAD NEWS

Decision making exercise

Mrs Monk was a 67-year-old widow who had multiple myeloma diagnosed for more than 1 year. She attended the ward for frequent blood transfusions, but appeared totally unwilling to explore what was wrong with her. Having asked several very leading questions to the students on the ward, the registrar decided to discuss her diagnosis with her. He explained frankly and clearly to her the type of illness she had, the likely prognosis and the treatment. She appeared to be very grateful to him and expressed this as he left. However, within 15 minutes, she was heard expressing serious doubts about his knowledge and competence. Mrs Monk knew, but had not been thrilled at having what she had already guessed confirmed.

- Using Kubler Ross's model, can you identify which stage (if any) of the dying process Mrs Monk is expressing?
- Explore Kubler Ross's model in more detail and discuss how well it fits with your practice experiences to date.
- Can this model be applied to your personal experiences of loss of any kind?

The breaking of bad news requires special skills, which can be learnt rather than being a natural feature of that person's interactions with clients. Buckman (1992) identifies the key stages as follows:

- get the physical environment right
- find out what the client already knows
- find out what the client wants to know
- share the information
- respond to the client's feelings
- plan any coping strategies and follow these up.

A review by Leliopoulo et al (2001) looks at the effects of truth telling on palliative care clients and is useful in terms of providing the theoretical underpinning for evidence based practice. The fact is that bad news is bad news no matter how sensitively or carefully it is broken, but the long-term outcome of breaking bad news in a sensitive and appropriate way will be apparent in the way in which the client copes with the information. The practice of telling relatives before the client or instead of the client is one that often causes alarm among nursing students (Kiger 1994, Saunders & Valente 1994). There is a notion that deceiving people protects them and that the truth will harm them. Ian Ainsworth Smith, a hospital chaplain and author, was interviewed on this theme and made the rejoinder that finally it is the truth that heals (Ainsworth Smith & Speck 1982). Nurses need to be wary of colluding with relatives to deceive clients. When relatives say that the client would not cope with the news, more often it is the relative saying 'I cannot cope with the news' (Buckman 1992).

RECOGNIZING THAT DEATH IS APPROACHING

Many experienced nurses may say that being able to recognize that death will occur soon is intuitive, a 'gut feeling'. However, it is a number of events that jointly suggest to the experienced nurse that this is the case. Lindley Davis (1991) discusses the physiological changes that occur, using a systems based approach.

Cardiovascular system

The heart rate initially increases, but as hypoxia increases then the heart rate and the blood pressure decrease. As peripheral perfusion fails, the client becomes clammy due to failure of the insensible loss to evaporate from the skin. Because of a decrease in metabolic functioning, the heat lost from the body decreases, but the temperature of vital organs is maintained. The client is cyanosed, cold and clammy when touched, and the skin appears mottled.

Respiratory system

With failing cardiac output and greatly reduced lymphatic drainage, the lungs become congested, resulting in hypoxia. Breathing decreases and the rhythm can become irregular. As the levels of circulating carbon dioxide increase, so the brain becomes less sensitive and the periods of apnoea increase. This pattern of breathing is often referred to by experienced nurses as Cheyne–Stokes respiration, even if at times this may not be strictly physiologically true.

Musculoskeletal system

Severe muscle weakness can occur due to the failing circulation and the frequently reduced intake of nutrients by the dying person. The muscles of the tongue and tissues of the soft palate may fall back into the throat, resulting in a loud snoring sound commonly called the 'death rattle'.

The sphincters controlling the bladder and bowels relax leading to a loss of bowel and bladder function and subsequent soiling in the last hours before death. Walker (1973) discussed her observation that in the moments before death, clients became restless and appeared to struggle even when they had previously been moribund, and that this was followed by a period of calm.

Special senses

As the level of hypoxia increases, all the special senses are affected and their sensitivity is decreased, in particular the ability of the eyes to focus and distinguish in poor light. As the sensations of taste, smell, hearing and vision fail, the client may experience changes in mental state. It has been believed that the sense of hearing is the last to fade and that nurses and relatives should continue to communicate verbally with the client right up to the moment of death.

Renal system

With the fall in cardiac output, there is a corresponding drop in kidney perfusion. This prevents the kidney from functioning efficiently and therefore the amount of urine produced decreases.

Pain

Although pain is often associated in the mind of the public with dying, it is generally the case that pain, if present at all, is well controlled. We usually think of pain as a physical sensation, but if the client is in mental anguish, their family's perceptions about the level of pain and distress the client may have are enhanced; because they are in the terminal stages of an illness and will soon die. One of the greatest wishes surrounding death is not to die alone or in pain. Many of the features of pain can be recognized through the verbal and non-verbal responses of the client. Pain may manifest itself as a physical symptom, but may have psychological, spiritual or other roots when it may be unrelieved by analgesia – the concept of 'total pain' as outlined by Saunders (1990) (see also Ch. 10 for a fuller discussion on pain and its management).

CARING FOR THE INDIVIDUAL WHO IS DYING

In order to manage the care of the client, nurses need to develop their listening skills and be familiar with symptom relief methods. The management of care has been greatly influenced by the hospice movement (Parkes & Parkes 1984) and by nursing development units such as that run by Dr Jessica Corner at the Royal Marsden Hospital. To promote good quality care, the approach taken by professionals should be empowering so that the client's wishes matter until they die. To fulfil wishes there should be non-judgemental advocacy so that all requests are met and the team should work closely together to ensure that all understand and comply with the client and the family's wishes.

Caring for the dying child's symptom control follows the same pattern as that for adults with the need for a particular sensitivity to the child's wishes regardless of age or mental ability (Brady 1994).

Breathing

The symptoms of breathlessness are distressing and unnecessary in many dying clients. Giving antibiotics to treat chest infections can ease the condition, but will not have any significant effect on the outcome for the client. Regnard & Tempest (1992) suggest administering 100% oxygen if the client is hypoxic and has no previous respiratory disease. This will help to manage the client's fear, which is very distressing and acute if he or she continues to fight for breath. Hyoscine hydrobromide can be introduced via the syringe driver to reduce the 'death rattle' as it will reduce secretions that the client has not the energy to expectorate. Sedation should never be seen as an easy option, but is used if more appropriate and if the client is less aware of the problem. Ideally, drugs are used with the client's permission. Positioning is often significant while the client remains conscious, but the client should be encouraged to adopt the position he or she finds most helpful. Sitting in a well-padded chair may be more comfortable than being bed-bound.

Nutrition

The notion of feeding dying people is controversial. As a general rule of thumb, if the client wants to eat, food should be provided in a manageable form, including enteral feeding if the client wishes. Anorexia is a fairly common problem, and nausea and vomiting are experienced by 40% of dying people with cancer (Regnard & Tempest 1992). In the final stages of dying, many individuals do not want to eat or drink, but controversy has arisen where discontinuing feeding has led to the death of the individual, for example in the Tony Bland case (Airedale National Health Service Trust *v*. Bland 1993). This whole area is discussed by writers in both the ethics and the medical field (Jennett 1996).

More common in everyday nursing practice is the discontinuation of hydration. However, in such cases, the continuance of mouth care is vital to the client's sense of well-being. According to Gallagher-Allred (1993) dehydration is a natural anaesthesia for terminally ill clients because it appears to decrease the client's perception of suffering by reducing the level of consciousness. However, the nurse must be sensitive to when a client may be thirsty and wish to drink, especially if too weak to hold a glass and take the drink for him or herself (Hall 1994).

Movement

The use of corticosteroids to control the pressure symptoms of an encapsulated tumour coupled with poor nutritional status and limited mobility may lead to the development of pressure sores. Keeping the client dry and clean can assist the person's sense of well-being. Where the client has advanced bronchitic or cardiac problems then the poor gaseous exchange rather than corticosteroids are a major contributory factor to pressure sore development. Within hospice units, clients are nursed on pressure-relieving beds to obviate the need for turning. Routines and rituals in turning should give way to client comfort and the client's wishes are paramount.

Constipation

This is a major consideration with all terminally ill people because of their reduced mobility and reduced intake of food and fluids. It is even more of a problem for terminally ill individuals who are receiving opiates for pain management. The appropriate aperient must always be given with these drugs as the feeling of fullness and discomfort is a further cause of anorexia in the dying individual.

Weakness and lethargy

The combination of weakness and lethargy is possibly one of the most frustrating combinations of symptoms. The individual wants to do more, but is exhausted by minimal effort. Research is ongoing into this area and the issue of muscular weakness predominates (Regnard & Tempest 1992). Physiotherapy and hydrotherapy can help to keep the client mobile, but weakness remains one of the most difficult symptoms to treat individuals who are terminally ill.

PROFESSIONAL AND ETHICAL KNOWLEDGE

This part of the chapter primarily focuses on the ethical and legal issues related to the care of the dying individual. However, it is important to discuss the issue of where a client should die first. This part will also briefly explore the personal reactions and beliefs of nurses and how these reactions can affect their professional role in caring for the dying. The 'emotional labour' of nursing in the field of hospice care needs to be recognized.

THE LOCATION OF DEATH

Whereas death at home is the preferred option of most clients (Wilkinson et al 1999), the family may not be able to cope with the level of care involved. Hospice care is available to a limited number of people but often only for short respite periods to allow the family to have a rest. A significant number of clients still die in a hospital bed. While dying in hospital may not be the ideal, nurses need to integrate aspects of what makes hospice care desirable into the ward. Unlike the situation with other ailments, the client only dies once and a poorly managed death is like a pebble in a pond – it has effects far beyond the client and his or her

Table 12.1   The advantages and disadvantages of death at home, in the hospital, or in the hospice

Location	Advantages	Disadvantages
Home	Familiar and family involved Atmosphere routine Freedom to have visitors More control for person Less feeling of helplessness for relatives	Relatives can become resentful or exhausted Disruption to family life Lack of facilities Care fragmented Isolation Difficulty in getting help quickly
Hospital	24–hour access to care Rapid response to changes Multidisciplinary approach Eases burden on relative(s) Equipment readily available	Inflexible routine Alien environment Relatives can feel excluded Care can be very technical Lack of continuity
Hospice	Home from home Highly skilled and motivated staff Expertise in all aspects of care High staff/volunteer ratio to client	Lack of availability Bias towards middle class Christianity Limited available treatment services on site Possibility of overnursing the client

family. Table 12.1 lists some of the possible advantages and disadvantages of dying in each location. You may be able to add equally valid advantages and disadvantages to the list.

For each individual client the resources available may limit the fulfilment of their wishes. Much has been done in recent years to bridge the gap between home, hospital and hospice care by developing many specialist nursing services. There are numerous voluntary groups who provide support, in addition to numerous health professionals within the community and hospital. The community nursing staff have a vital role to play not only in providing care, but also in their ability to support the family and coordinate the involvement of other care workers. They keep the primary healthcare team informed about the client's progress and assess need. Extra care packages can be available to provide enhanced resources for a finite period of time to assist the client to go home to die. The development of the Macmillan Nursing Service has provided specialist support and guidance to assist those who are involved with the care of the client. They do not deliver hands-on care themselves, but are a resource for those involved with the client. This includes family members, general practitioners, and community staff. Some Macmillan nurses are very specialist, for example specializing in breast care, lymphoedema, haematology or paediatrics, while others work on a locality basis or are hospital based. Services are also provided by the Marie Curie nurses, and they can also provide a sitter service to allow the primary carer to have a break. In some areas there is access to 'hospice at home', but this is at present still sporadic. Day hospices are often available for those who wish to attend on a daily basis. All offer social support for the client and the family, and some provide ongoing assessment of the client and can provide emergency admission to sort out troublesome symptoms. Berenthal (1994) also discusses the role of the voluntary sector in helping to meet the needs of dying people and their families.

PROFESSIONAL COPING

Nurses need to maintain their own psychological well-being as well as that of the client. Becoming dysfunctional in grief at the death of a client is of little benefit to anyone. Thankfully, the idea that the nurse who is upset at the death of a client is acting in an unprofessional manner has largely disappeared from professional practice. In order to care for an individual, practitioners naturally invest emotional energy. What needs to be considered is the degree of involvement that can reasonably be given to meet the needs of the client without depleting our reserves for other clients.

Evidence based practice

Through questionnaires and interviews, Spencer (1994) carried out research aimed at identifying how nurses manage their grief in an intensive care unit. The results showed that 41.2% felt guilty when a client died. Further insight was given by Demmer (2000) who demonstrated a statistically significant relationship between personal death-related experience and death anxiety and attitudes toward dying patients.

Informal discussion and peer support are very useful in coping strategies (Adey 1987, Little 1992) while Demmer (2000) argued for the development of appropriate training and support programmes in death and dying issues that are tailored to meet the needs of different levels of nursing staff.

Nurses have problems in admitting that they have difficulties in coping with their feelings and find consulting outside agencies difficult. Spencer's study revealed that many nurses had received little training in how to deal with grief and this was similar to findings in Hockley's work (Hockley 1989). When asked what form of support would be most helpful, 15.7% replied that a counsellor might be of use, but Adey's study (Adey 1987) suggests that a counsellor is of only limited benefit. Most respondents favoured an informal discussion and one-to-one chats. Clinical supervision has frequently been put forward as a method to enable professionals to cope in these situations. However, while clinical supervision has this potential, the close and confiding nature of supervisory relationship can also arouse feelings of discomfort which, in turn, must be addressed by an experienced supervisor (Jones 1999).

Any death where the client is in hospital for less than 24 hours
Any death where the client has not been treated by a doctor during the last illness or has not been seen by a doctor within the 14 days before death
Any death due to violent or unnatural circumstances
Any death occurring while undergoing a surgical procedure or before recovering from the effects of the anaesthetic
Death following a surgical procedure if the procedure could have a bearing on the cause of death
Death caused by an industrial disease
Death of a person in receipt of a war pension
Death where the cause is uncertain
Any sudden or unexplained death

Figure 12.5 Deaths that have to be reported to the coroner.

Fisher (1991) states that grief can be turned into growth and suggests the use of structured bereavement counselling as a way in which it can be handled positively. She suggests that many nurses come to palliative care settings because death has been managed badly where they have worked previously. She also sees early identification of those who need help as vital in promoting mental well-being. Similarly Kubler Ross (1975), Parkes (1972) and Morris (1986) are cited by Fisher (1991) as having identified the growth potential in grief. Saunders & Valente (1994) suggest that nurses who care for a terminally ill client need to develop an 'emotional muscle'. This can be achieved by understanding theory, recognizing their own mortality and using whatever support is available. The most common source of distress to student nurses is how the clients die. Wilkes (1993) addresses the issues relating to how students perceive death, the so-called good or bad death:

These nurses see a 'good' death as one where the client is comfortable, alert and pain free and where the person is accepting of the situation and is surrounded by loved ones in a personally determined environment. On the other hand nurses' descriptions of a 'bad' death include images of pain, loneliness, distress, unacceptance and unpreparedness.

To this end, clinical supervision is an extremely useful tool for enabling inexperienced staff to reflect on their experiences and share difficult situations, thus developing their skills while recognizing future educational requirements.

LEGAL AND ETHICAL ISSUES

Because of technological advances and increased expectations of clients, an understanding of the legal issues surrounding death is vital to sound practice. Within this section, the role of the coroner is explored as are some very pertinent ethical issues, namely living wills, the 'right to die' and euthanasia.

The role of the coroner

The coroner is appointed by the local authority, but totally independent of them, to investigate sudden and unexplained deaths. Coroners are drawn from the ranks of solicitors or medical doctors of 5 or more years experience.

Coroners are supported by coroner's officers, which are civilian posts, but the majority of whom are former police officers. Their role is to investigate the circumstances surrounding the death and report back to the coroner.

The coroner convenes an inquest, calls evidence, questions witnesses and brings in a verdict. The coroner can be supported by a jury or act alone. Coroners are appointed for life, there is no statutory retirement age and the decision of a coroner is final. Figure 12.5 lists the circumstances under which a doctor must legally report a death to the coroner.

The coroner may ask for a postmortem and the request cannot be refused despite religious objections, but the issue is dealt with sensitively. The coroner's officer attends each postmortem. If the death of an organ donor has to be referred to the coroner, then the coroner must be asked to give consent to the removal of the organ, since the removal could affect some important evidence. In this instance, consent is usually given quickly.

If the death may be due to murder, manslaughter or infanticide, the coroner must send the papers to the Director of Public Prosecutions. The coroner sits with a jury for certain cases such as deaths in custody, industrial accidents or those caused by police officers in the course of their duties.

Coroners are empowered to rule on the cause of death as being as follows:

- natural causes
- open verdict
- accident
- misadventure
- suicide
- unlawful killing.

Coroners' inquests are open to the public and if you wish to attend one it is best to contact the coroner's officer at your local police station.

Withholding treatment

With the increasing expectations of medicine and health care, the ethical implications for doctors and nurses of withdrawing, or not offering, treatment are great. The debate about whether or not to resuscitate clients is very current. Clients may fear they will not be offered all treatments available to treat their disorder on the grounds of cost, and new treatments tend to be much more costly than standard treatment. To address this, and to try and reduce the inequalities, the National Institute for Clinical Excellence (NICE) was established to identify and evaluate best treatment in a range of conditions. Many are relevant here and their deliberations can be found on their website (National Institute for Clinical Excellence 2003). It is worthwhile keeping abreast of their ongoing work as some of their proposals, e.g. their advice on the use of beta interferon in multiple sclerosis, has caused controversy, and clients may ask about their work.

The case of Miss B in 2002 who asked for ventilation to be discontinued on the grounds that she was competent to do so raised many questions. That a client's belief differs from that of the medical/nursing staff as to what is in 'the client's best interest' can cause much distress. Miss B had made a living will in 1999 when she had suffered a spinal haemorrhage. Having had a further bleed in February 2001, she was left virtually totally paralysed. Dame Elizabeth Butler Sloss, in her recommendations, reminded the medical profession that they should remember that the seriously disabled person who is mentally competent has the same right to make decisions and have personal autonomy as any other person with mental capacity. These principles are contained in the guidelines *Withholding and Withdrawing Life Prolonging Treatment* (British Medical Association 2001) which incorporate the Human Rights Act 1998.

The living will

Living wills or advance directives were first developed in the USA and derive from the work of Kutner (1969). In 1976, the State of California passed the Natural Death Act 1977, which recognized the principle of living wills. The purpose of a living will is to allow autonomous individuals to make decisions while in good health about the care or withholding of care that they would wish to receive in the event of suffering from a prescribed list of illnesses within clearly defined boundaries. The will can include the appointment of a healthcare proxy, that is someone who is well acquainted with the client's wishes and can apply them in situations where the advance directives are felt to be ambiguous.

Respecting a client's autonomy consequently causes several ethical dilemmas for healthcare professionals. If we remain competent to the end of our lives, then we can clearly state what we would wish or not wish to happen to us. Jean Harlow, the famous film actress, died of a treatable infection because she was a Christian Scientist who refused orthodox medical treatment. If we are to allow people to make their own choices, then we need to remember that they will not always choose as we would.

Progressive mental illness can make this very difficult, though. People with certain types of mental disorder who are subject to delusions can make 'a valid and legally binding (at common law) advance statement as long as they are clear about the consequences of the particular decision they wish to make' (British Medical Association and Royal College of Nursing 1995).

Although living wills are legally binding in common law in the UK they are sometimes overruled by family members and clinicians. As the client is no longer able to act for themselves, it is important to be aware of the legal status of such documents and to work with the proxy decision maker to ensure that the wishes of the client are respected. This is particularly true in decision making about resuscitation.

EUTHANASIA

Within the remit of a living will, the individual concerned cannot ask for assistance in dying as this is euthanasia which is illegal in most countries. In Australia, euthanasia legislation was enacted in 1995 (Voluntary Euthanasia Society – Northern Territories) although this has since been suspended to prevent several other states taking similar action. In Holland, euthanasia legislation was passed in 2002, and doctors are not prosecuted if they follow the clearly defined criteria and report the death to the coroner as euthanasia.

In palliative care there is a paradox that the treatment used may actually hasten a client's death. However, what distinguishes this from euthanasia is that the primary intention is to treat the client, not to bring about their death. This is the doctrine of double effect, and is most commonly seen in the administration of narcotic analgesia. The desired effect is to alleviate the pain; the unwanted effect is that it may cause respiratory depression.

Euthanasia has sometimes been practised illegally in Britain, as demonstrated by the case of Dr Cox in the treatment of Lilian Boyes (case of R v. Cox 1992). This elderly lady was crippled with both rheumatoid arthritis and osteoarthritis and begged her consultant, whom she had known for many years, to end her suffering. Having already tried very large doses of morphine, which sadly increased aspects of her pain, he resorted to intravenous potassium chloride, which has no therapeutic value, and she swiftly died. This case is certainly not an isolated one – the physician attending King George VI later admitted performing euthanasia on him. Research by Ward & Tate (1994), surveying the attitudes of NHS doctors, found that 32% confirmed that they had complied with a request from a patient to hasten their death. McLean & Britton (1996), in a survey of 1000 doctors, found that 28% had been asked to assist but only 3% had agreed to help. The legal system, while abhorring euthanasia, has obvious sympathy with medical practitioners who are involved with 'mercy killing'. A survey cited by the Voluntary Euthanasia Society in 1995 into doctors' attitudes towards euthanasia set the figure higher, with 30% of practitioners admitting to it. Nurses who are in the clinical area face a dilemma and may be perceived as trouble makers if they 'whistle blow'.

Euthanasia as a term was linked with the Nazi atrocities during World War II. Opponents of the concept cite this as the reason that no liberalization of the legislation should occur. The critical feature to be considered is the intention with which the act is carried out. In the literature, euthanasia (from the Greek 'eu', good, 'thanatos', death) is categorized at its simplest, in four different ways:

- involuntary active
- involuntary passive
- voluntary active
- voluntary passive.

The case of Lilian Boyes, who was given voluntary active euthanasia by Dr Cox has been discussed. An example of involuntary active euthanasia would be where a doctor increases the narcotics given to a postoperative client without the client's consent and with the express purpose of killing the client from respiratory depression. This is obviously totally unacceptable and is not supported by any campaigning body whatsoever. The case of Tony Bland (Jennett & Dyer 1991) was involuntary passive euthanasia, involuntary in that he did not request it, and passive in that it involved withholding treatment rather than administering a noxious substance. Voluntary passive euthanasia would be the situation where a client decides to refuse further treatment, for example refuses resuscitation in the case of a further cardiac arrest (or the case of Miss B discussed above).

The most contentious issue for medical practitioners and nurses is voluntary euthanasia (Johnstone 1994) (see Annotated further reading, p. 278). The main argument centres on the right of the dying individual to choose and maintain control over his or her dying. By managing death, the individual may have choices about the location, manner and timing of the event. What is so noble about a painful lingering death? The pro-life campaign centres on the sanctity of life issues and the 'slippery slope' argument. The 'slippery slope' refers to the risks associated with any liberalization of the law. Pro-life campaigners fear that allowing euthanasia to be legalized would open the floodgates and that it would rapidly take on a life of its own like that resulting from the passing of the Abortion Act 1967. The public would be at risk of devaluing the lives of disabled people and risk genocide.

There are also moves to legalize physician assisted suicide. Suicide has been legal since 1961 but aiding and abetting a suicide is still a criminal offence. Legalization would allow a physician to prescribe a lethal dose of drugs which the client would then take without the doctor's assistance. The arguments for and against are very similar to those for and against euthanasia.

ORGAN DONATION

Organ donation and receipt remains the only hope for survival to many individuals in end stage organ failure. The problem of asking very distressed individuals if they will consent to their relative's organs being used is largely due to an absence of a clear expression of the individual's wishes. The living will and the new computerized register of donors can with adequate public information be much more user friendly than the previous card system and should provide the basis for discussion with the family (Dimond 1993).

PERSONAL AND REFLECTIVE KNOWLEDGE

It is inevitable that in both your personal and professional life you will need to cope with death and dying. As stated at the beginning of this chapter, dying is a unique experience for each person. In your professional capacity as a nurse in whichever field you specialize you can make a difference to the experiences of dying clients and their families by providing informed and sensitive care. Through your knowledge of the contents of this chapter, your exploration of issues arising from the exercises, and your personal and reflective experiences in practice, you will be able to provide a high quality of care for the dying in whatever setting is appropriate for that person.

SUGGESTIONS FOR PORTFOLIO EVIDENCE: PERSONAL FEARS AND MISGIVINGS

Having read the contents of this chapter, it is important for you to consider what death means to you personally. It is often difficult to cope with negative attitudes towards dying.

Personally, for me, it has sometimes been difficult to deal with my negative feelings about dying individuals. I had always assumed that caring for the dying would be rewarding and fulfilling, and in the majority of cases it is. Dying, however, does not make people saint-like, and we should not feel guilty that we are not drawn to every dying person, but what is vital is that we deliver a high standard of 'appropriate care' to our client. Nurses need to care for themselves and take their own good advice about coping with stress. Coping with the stress of caring is discussed in more depth in Chapter 8.

Think back to Worden's tasks of mourning (Worden 1991) discussed previously (p. 269). In your own life can you identify using these or do you tend to put problems that carry a high cost in terms of emotion out of sight? Some writers refer to this latter method of coping as 'shelving problems'. Sadly we can only do this for a time depending on our coping ability; eventually a significant loss will trigger memories of other losses and this can lead to severe depression and withdrawal, even breakdown.

Your answers in the above reflective exercise will be unique, but it may help to discuss and share them with a colleague or in clinical supervision. This is after all how we grow as human beings and develop the skills of nursing clients who are dying and who are receiving palliative care.

CASE STUDIES RELATED TO DEATH AND DYING

The following case studies are included so that you can consolidate the knowledge gained from reading this chapter and from the learning that has taken place through your experience in the practice of nursing.

Case study: Learning disabilities

A 60-year-old man with Down syndrome suffered a massive stroke and was dying in a supported living bungalow. He and his fellow residents had previously lived in a large institution for most of their lives. Some residents displayed challenging behaviour during the period up to and immediately following his death.

- Can you identify the particular challenges of nursing the client and his fellow residents both during and after the death?
- How can nurses help those with learning difficulties understand the concept of death?

Case study: Adult

Sarah Warner was a 41-year-old lady with two young children aged 10 and 6 years. Her husband, Peter, was a haemophiliac and contracted human immunodeficiency virus (HIV) from untreated factor VIII in 1990. Peter died in 1992 and Sarah died in 1994, after a short hospital stay, from *Pneumocystis carinii* pneumonia. The nurses caring for Sarah felt it was so unfair as neither Sarah nor her husband had done anything wrong and now the children were orphans.

- How can nurses ensure that they do not blame people for their illnesses?
- How might nurses' attitudes to the possible cause of death affect how they provide appropriate individualized care?
- What special support do children need to help them to grieve at their parent's death?

Case study: Mental health

Mrs Groves was a 70-year-old lady who had been a long-stay client in a large psychiatric institution. She had schizophrenia as a young woman and this had become compounded in her later years by dementia. As she had become increasingly frail and unsteady on her feet she fell, fracturing her right femur, and required a period of bed rest to recover. She subsequently developed a chest infection, which did not respond to antibiotics or chest physiotherapy. As it became apparent that she was dying, the nursing staff endeavoured to have a constant presence with her and she had a very peaceful and dignified death.

- What difficulties do you think you will have when dealing with clients who appear to have no insight into their condition?
- What is our role as nurses in such cases? (You might like to look at the *Code of Professional Conduct* (Nursing and Midwifery Council 2002).)

Case study: Child

Sarah Lee was a 6-year-old girl with bacterial meningitis. Sadly, despite a rapid diagnosis and rapid hospitalization, she died 48 hours later after initially showing some signs of improvement. Shortly afterwards her 4-year-old brother developed the same symptoms, but he recovered with minimal damage and was soon allowed home.

- Using the tasks of mourning and the antecedents of death, can you give any view on the reason why Sarah's little brother may have suffered in the period following his sister's death?
- How far should doctors go to save the life of a child?
- Would you be happy to allow your child to have experimental therapy that offers a chance of recovery?
- When should we stop resuscitating? (The answers here may well be financial as well as moral.)

Summary

This chapter has explored definitions of death, ranging from the physiological cardiorespiratory death, through cortical and brain stem death to the concept of ontological death. It has included:

1. The processes of dying and grieving were considered and the different cultural perspectives contrasted.
2. The implications for nurses, including strategies and rationales for care to support clients, and their families, in a dignified death.
3. Ethical issues were debated and these were contrasted with the legal arguments.
4. Finally, readers were asked to consider their own attitudes towards death, and to consolidate their knowledge within their own portfolio of learning.
5. A wide range of further reading and internet resources accompany this chapter. The internet sites were valid at the time of writing; however, since the time of publication there may be changes to the content, or availability, as these are beyond the publisher's control.

Annotated further reading and websites

British Medical Association 2001 Withholding and withdrawing life prolonging treatment, 2nd edn. British Medical Journal, London
An essential text for all health professionals which gives clear guidance for making decisions in this very difficult area.

Hill L (ed) 1994 Caring for dying children and their families. Chapman & Hall, London
This is a comprehensive multi-authored book on care of dying children and their families. Many chapters give research based

evidence and Chapter 9 by Michael Brady gives a comprehensive outline of symptom control in the dying child.

Jennett B 1996 Managing clients in a persistent vegetative state since Airedale NHS Trust vs. Bland. In: McLean S (ed) Death, dying and the law. Dartmouth Press, Aldershot
A good exposition of the Tony Bland case can be found in this chapter by Brian Jennett. An interesting overview of this debate can also be found in Hall (1994), which the reader might care to peruse.

Johnstone M J 1994 Bioethics: a nursing perspective, 2nd edn. Saunders, Sydney
Johnstone argues the case both for and against euthanasia in a systematic way, which will provide useful material for follow up reading.

Voluntary euthanasia: the facts. Voluntary Euthanasia Society of England and Wales, London
This video is available from the Voluntary Euthanasia Society of England and Wales, 13 Prince of Wales Terrace, London W8 5PG. The main arguments on both sides are well explored. The society is also willing to provide living wills and information about their campaigns and can be contacted by writing to the above address.

Wilson L 1999. Living wills. Nursing Times Monographs, London
In this paper I explore some of the issues surrounding living wills and suggest additional reading.

Wright B 1996 Sudden death, 2nd edn. Churchill Livingstone, Edinburgh
Wright has written several books on sudden death from his perspective as clinical nurse specialist in crisis care based at Leeds Royal Infirmary and writes from extensive experience. I would particularly recommend this book for perusal and because it contains a clear commonsense approach based on work by Caplan (1964) and Worden (1991) (see also Ch. 3 in this book, on resuscitation).

ALERT http://www.donoharm.org.uk
HOPE (Healthcare Opposed To Euthanasia), 58 Hanover Gardens, London SE11 5TN. Society for the Protection of the Unborn Child, 5–6 St Matthew Street, London SW1P 2JT, Tel: 020 7222 5845. Also on http://www.spuc.org.uk. Organisations to contact for pro-life views.

http://www.doh.gov.uk/consent
Department of Health 2000 Reference guide to consent for examination and treatment. Gives some very useful information in relation to clients/clients rights, which will enhance your reading in relation to this chapter.

http://www.funeralcare.co-op.co.uk/index.asp
The website of the Co-operative Funeral Service. This is a valuable resource containing information of what do to when someone dies, who to contact and how to arrange a funeral.

http://www.homeoffice.gov.uk/ccpd/coroner.htm
A government website detailing the work of the coroner's office.

http://www.childdeathhelpline.org.uk/index.html
The national child death helpline website. This is a support service, run by volunteer parents, with helplines open 365 days a year.

http://www.crusebereavementcare.org.uk/
Offers support and counselling to bereaved people. Website has contact numbers and online resources and information.

References

Abortion Act 1967 HMSO, London

Adey C 1987 Stress: who cares? Nursing Times 83(4):52–53

Ainsworth Smith I, Speck P 1982 Letting go, 2nd edn. Society for the Propagation of Christian Knowledge, London

Airedale National Health Service Trust v. Bland 1993 2 WLR 316,343

Alexy W D 1991 Dimensions of psychological counseling that facilitate the grieving process of bereaved parents. In: Worden J W Grief counselling and grief therapy, 2nd edn. Routledge, London, pp 498–507

Berenthal J A 1994 A welcome break for the carers. Professional Nurse 9(4):267–270

Blackmore S 1988 Visions from the dying brain. New Scientist 118:1161

Brady M 1994 Symptom control in dying children. In: Hill L (ed) Caring for dying children and their families. Chapman & Hall, London

British Medical Association 2001 Withholding and withdrawing life prolonging medical treatment guidance for decision making, 2nd edn. British Medical Journal, London

British Medical Association and Pharmaceutical Society 2002 British National Formulary, 44th edn. British Medical Association, London

British Medical Association and Royal College of Nursing 1995 The older person: consent and care. British Medical Association, London

Brookbank J W 1990 The biology of aging. Harper & Row, New York

Buckman R 1992 How to break bad news. Macmillan, London

Caplan G 1964 Principles of preventive psychiatry. Cited in: Wright B 1996 Sudden death intervention skills for the caring professions, 2nd edn. Churchill Livingstone, London

Cassell E 1974 Death inside out: dying in a technological age. In: Steinfels P, Veatch R M (eds) Death inside out. Harper & Row, New York

Cole E J 1993 The near death experience. Intensive and Critical Care Nursing 9:157–161

Copp G 1994 Palliative care nursing education: a review of research findings. Journal of Advanced Nursing 19:552–557

Copp G 1998 A review of current theories of death and dying. Journal of Advanced Nursing 28(2):382–390

Cowlishaw S 1993 When my little sister died. Merlin, Derby

Cunningham W R, Brookbank J W 1988 Gerontology: the biology, psychology and sociology of aging. Harper & Row, New York

Day L 1995 Ethics and law: practical limits to the uniform determination of death act. Journal of Neuroscience Nursing 27(5):319–322

Demmer C 2000 The relationship between death-related experiences, death anxiety, and patient care attitudes among AIDS nursing staff. Journal for Nurses in Staff Development 16(3):118–123

Department of Health 1998 Our healthier nation. HMSO, London

Department of Health 2000 Reference guide to consent to examination or treatment. HMSO, London

Dimond B 1993 Transplants and donor cards. Accident and Emergency Nursing 1:49–52

Engel G 1964 Grief and grieving. American Journal of Nursing 64:9

Fisher M 1991 Can grief be turned into growth? Professional Nurse 7:178–182

Gallagher-Allred C 1993 Nutrition and hydration in hospice care: needs, strategies, ethics. Hospice Journal: Physical, Psychosocial and Pastoral Care of the Dying 9:2–3

Green J 1989 Death with dignity: meeting the needs of clients in a multi-ethnic society. Nursing Times 85

Hall J K 1994 Caring for corpses or killing clients. Nursing Management 25(10):81–82

Henderson V 1966 The nature of nursing. Collier Macmillan, London

Hill L (ed) 1994 Caring for dying children and their families. Chapman & Hall, London

Hindmarch C 1993 On the death of a child. Radcliffe Medical Press, Oxford

Hinds C J, Watson D 1996 Intensive care: a concise textbook, 2nd edn. Saunders, London

Hockley J 1989 Caring for the dying in acute hospitals. Nursing Times 85(39):47–50

Human Rights Act 1998 HMSO, London

Jennett B 1982 Brain death. Intensive Care Medicine 8(1):1–3

Jennett B 1996 Managing clients in a persistent vegetative state since Airedale NHS Trust v Bland. In: McLean S (ed) Death, dying and the law. Dartmouth Press, Aldershot

Jennett B, Dyer C 1991 Persistent vegetative state and the right to die. British Medical Journal 302(6787):1256–1258

Johnstone M J 1994 Bioethics: a nursing perspective, 2nd edn. Saunders, Sydney

Jones A 1999 'A heavy and blessed experience': a psychoanalytic study of community Macmillan nurses and their roles in serious illness and palliative care. Journal of Advanced Nursing 30(6):1297–1303

Kiger A 1994 Student nurse involvement with death. Journal of Advanced Nursing 20(4):679–686

Kubler Ross E 1975 Death: the final stage of growth. Prentice Hall, London

Kutner L 1969 Due process of euthanasia. Cited in Lush D 1993 Advance directives and living wills. Journal of the Royal College of Physicians 27(3):274–277

Laakso H, Paunonen-Ilmonen M 2001 Mothers' grief following the death of a child. Journal of Advanced Nursing 36(1):69–77

Leliopoulo C, Wilkinson S M, Fellowes D 2001 Does truthtelling improve psychological distress of palliative care clients? A systematic review Evidence Based Medicine Reviews 2002: 1–20

Lindley Davis B 1991 Process of dying. Cancer Nursing 14:6

Little D 1992 Informal trauma support urged. Cited in: Spencer L 1994 How do nurses deal with their own grief? Journal of Advanced Nursing 19(6):1141–1150

Louis P T, Goddard-Finegold J, Fishman M A et al 1993 Barbiturates and hyperventilation during intracranial hypertension. Critical Care Medicine 21(8):1200–1206

McLean S (ed) 1996 Death, dying and the law. Dartmouth Press, Aldershot

McLean S A M, Britton A 1996 Sometimes a small victory. Institute of Law and Ethics, University of Glasgow, Glasgow

Montague S, Knight D 1996 Cell structure and function, growth and development. In: Hinchliff S, Montague S, Watson R (eds) Physiology for nursing practice, 2nd edn. Baillière Tindall, London

Morris P 1986 Loss and change. Cited in: Fisher M 1991 Can grief be turned into growth? Professional Nurse 7(3):178–182

Narayanasamy A 1993 Nurses' awareness and educational preparation in meeting their clients' spiritual needs. Nurse Education Today 13:3

Narayanasamy A 1995 Spiritual care of chronically ill clients. Journal of Clinical Nursing 4(6):397–398

National Institute for Clinical Excellence 2003 Recommendations. Online. Available: http://www.nice.org.uk 15 Aug 2003

Norton D J 1992 Clinical applications of brain stem death protocols. Journal of Neuroscience Nursing 24(6):354–358

Nursing and Midwifery Council 2002 Code of professional conduct. Nursing and Midwifery Council, London

Osis K, Haraldsson E 1986 At the hour of death, 2nd edn. Marmaroneck, New York

Pallis C 1983 ABC of brain stem death (articles from the BMJ, 1982–1983). British Medical Journal, London

Pallis C, Harley D H 1996 ABC of brain stem death, 2nd edn. British Medical Journal, London

Parkes C M 1972 Determinants of outcome following bereavement. Cited in: Fisher M 1991 Can grief be turned into growth? Professional Nurse 7(3):178–182

Parkes C M 1975 Bereavement: studies of grief in adult life. Penguin, Harmondsworth

Parkes C M 1987 Models of bereavement care. Death Studies 11(4):257–261

Parkes C M, Parkes J 1984 Hospice vs hospital care: reevaluation after 10 years as seen by the surviving spouse. Postgraduate Medical Journal 60:120–124

Peberdy A 1992 Death and dying workbook: life and death. Open University Press, Milton Keynes

Praill D 1995 Approaches to spiritual care. Nursing Times 91(34):55–57

Priestman T 1989 Cancer chemotherapy: an introduction. Pharmatalia Carlo Erba, London

R v. Cox 1992 12 BMLR 38 Winchester CC.

Regnard C, Tempest S 1992 A guide to symptom relief in advanced cancer care, 3rd edn. Haigh & Hockland, London

Ring K 1980 Life at death: a scientific investigation of the near death experience. Coward, McGann & Geoghegan, New York

Saunders C (ed) 1990 Hospice and palliative care: an interdisciplinary approach. Edward Arnold, London

Saunders J, Valente S 1994 Nurses' grief. Cancer Nursing 17:318–325

Simpson S 2001 Near death experience: a concept analysis as applied to nursing. Journal of Advanced Nursing 36(4):520–526

Sinclair D 1989 Human growth after birth, 5th edn. Oxford University Press, Oxford

Sourkes B 1987 Siblings of the child with a life-threatening illness. Journal of Children in Contemporary Society 19:159–184

Spencer L 1994 How do nurses deal with their own grief? Journal of Advanced Nursing 19(6):1141–1150

Stone H W 1995 Suicide and grief. In: Smith B, Mitchell M, Constantino R et al Exploring widows' feelings after the suicide of their spouse. Journal of Psychosocial Nursing 33:10–15

Tonkin L 1996 Growing around grief: another way of looking at grief and recovery. Bereavement Care 15(1)

Viney C 1996 Nursing the critically ill. Baillière Tindall, London

Walker M 1973 The last hour before death. American Journal of Nursing 73:1592–1593

Ward B J, Tate P A 1994 Attitudes among NHS doctors to requests for euthanasia. British Medical Journal 308(6940):1332–1334

Weisman A D 1988 Appropriate death and the hospice program. Hospice Journal 4:65–77

Wilkes L M 1993 Nurses' descriptions of death scenes. Journal of Cancer Care 93(2):11–16

Wilkinson E K, Salisbury C, Bosanquet N et al 1999 Patient and carer preference for, and satisfaction with, specialist models of palliative care: a systematic literature review. Palliative Medicine 13(3):197–216

Worden W J 1991 Grief counselling and grief therapy, 2nd edn. Routledge, London

Wright B 1996 Sudden death intervention skills for the caring professions, 2nd edn. Churchill Livingstone, London

Chapter 13

Hygiene

Maggie Mallik

KEY ISSUES

SUBJECT KNOWLEDGE

- Structure and functions of the skin, the mouth, the eyes, hair and nails as they relate to hygiene care
- History of hygiene care practices in society
- The impact of individual, cultural and spiritual beliefs on individual hygiene practices

CARE DELIVERY KNOWLEDGE

- Assessment of an individual's hygiene needs in relation to care of the body, mouth, hair and eyes
- Assessment tools and oral care
- Differing modes of delivery of hygiene care for all body parts

PROFESSIONAL AND ETHICAL KNOWLEDGE

- Hygiene care and the image of the nurse
- Privacy and dignity related to hygiene care
- Ritualization of hygiene care and skill mix
- Policy and hygiene care

PERSONAL AND REFLECTIVE KNOWLEDGE

- Personal feelings about giving hygiene care
- Consolidation of learning from the chapter through case study work

INTRODUCTION

Maintaining hygiene according to one's personal and cultural norms is a basic human need. Helping individuals maintain their own hygiene is recognized as a fundamental role for the nurse. In partnership with the client and carer, the nurse is the primary decision maker in this area of healthcare practice. Responsibility for promoting and maintaining excellence in the quality of hygiene care delivered is a key function of nursing (Department of Health 2001). However, the role of the nurse in the delivery of care will alter depending upon the particular context in which hygiene care is delivered and the specific needs of the individual.

Children and teenagers need varying levels of support and teaching to help them meet their hygiene needs. Health education for the child and the family is important for this client group in whatever context. Children and adults with deficits in learning ability need extra encouragement, time and teaching in order to meet their needs. The person with a mental illness who has become demotivated about maintaining personal appearances and hygiene needs the nurse to act as advisor and counsellor. The nurse has to be highly sensitive to the client's personal wishes while still encouraging normal hygiene behaviour. Adults whose health status is compromised by acute or chronic illness need specific support within a continuum from total self-care to being totally dependent upon the nurse for hygiene care. The dignity and privacy of all clients, especially the elderly, needs to be facilitated and protected by the nurse whatever the context of hygiene care delivery (Department of Health 2001).

The context of care has important implications for decision making about hygiene because of the environmental conditions in which the education, support and care are delivered. The nurse often has to adapt to the resources available. There may be a need to become active politically to obtain better resources or facilitate these resources through communicating and working closely with other professionals in health and social care.

The content of this chapter outlines both the scientific and practice based knowledge needed by the nurse to promote and deliver hygiene care. The aim of this chapter is to explore fully this domain of nursing and to outline clearly the knowledge base needed for decision making for all aspects of hygiene care.

OVERVIEW

General and specialist knowledge are needed in decision making on the delivery of hygiene care. Specialist knowledge is related to hygiene care for specific body parts. For this reason the Subject Knowledge and Care Delivery Knowledge subdivisions of the chapter are further divided into the relevant specialist sections involved in the administration of hygiene care. These sections include:

- body hygiene care
- oral hygiene care
- eye hygiene care
- hair and nails hygiene care
- perineal hygiene care.

Subject knowledge

Knowledge from the physical sciences is explored in relation to the skin, mouth, eyes, hair, nails and perineum. In each section the focus is on the applied knowledge needed to make decisions about hygiene care. The psychosocial knowledge base integrates these specific body parts in order to outline issues in hygiene care related to development and individuality. The historical and social dimensions of hygiene care and cultural and spiritual norms are explored.

Care delivery knowledge

This part follows a similar format as the Subject Knowledge section, but concentrates on the knowledge needed in the assessment and delivery of hygiene care to and with patients and clients.

Professional and ethical knowledge

The professional, ethical, political and social dimensions of hygiene care are addressed. Privacy and dignity issues are explored. Hygiene care as a ritual within nursing is discussed with a particular focus on the role of the nurse as the key decision maker in this area of healthcare practice.

Personal and reflective knowledge

There is a particular focus on the reflective experiences of students in the delivery of care that is intimate and private. Case studies are used to help consolidate knowledge gained from practice and the chapter content.

On pages 300–301 there are four case studies, each one relating to one of the branch programmes. You may find it helpful to read one of them before you start the chapter and use it as a focus for your reflections while reading.

SUBJECT KNOWLEDGE

BIOLOGICAL

STRUCTURE AND FUNCTION OF THE SKIN, HAIR, NAILS, PERINEUM, MOUTH AND EYES AS THEY RELATE TO HYGIENE CARE

The skin

The structure and functions of the skin are more fully outlined in Chapter 14 on skin integrity. Reference will be made here to some of the specific structures that are pertinent to skin and body hygiene. A key function of the skin is protection. Its unique structures protect the body from:

- undue entry or loss of water
- pressure and friction
- microorganisms
- chemicals (weak acids and alkalis)
- most gases
- physical trauma (alpha rays, beta rays to a limited extent, and ultraviolet radiation) (Hinchliff et al 1996).

The two layers of the skin, the epidermis and dermis, function as a single layer. However, the outer layer, the epidermis, has five layers of cell types, each of which has its own unique function. The innermost cell layer of the epidermis (the stratum basale) is important in skin regeneration as the cells are constantly dividing and reproducing, the life cycle of skin cells being approximately 35 days (see Ch. 14 on skin integrity). These new cells move through the epidermal layers to the surface of the skin. For the purposes of hygiene care, the stratum corneum, the outermost horny cell layer, is therefore of primary interest. The cells or squames of the stratum corneum are all dead and are constantly being shed from the surface of the body. According to Hinchliff et al (1996) up to 1 million of these cells are shed every 40 minutes through the process of desquamation or exfoliation.

Keratin helps the epidermis form a tough protective barrier. The process of keratinization, which begins in the basal layer, means that the horny cells of the stratum corneum are filled with this protein. Keratin is most evident in areas of the skin exposed to stress, for example the palms of the hands and soles of the feet. Both psoriasis (a skin condition characterized by rapid and excessive production of keratin cells) and dandruff (hyperplasia of the scalp) result in the exfoliation of flakes of keratin (Hinchliff et al 1996).

Certain bacteria are normally present on the skin's outer surface, for example *Staphylococcus epidermidis* and *Corynebacterium*. They are classified as normal flora (commensals) and are protective in function because they inhibit the multiplication of disease-causing organisms. These normal commensals, which inhabit the deeper layers of the stratum corneum, are not usually shed with exfoliation. Commensals use healthy skin scales as a source of food and also rely on the skin having a slightly acid pH in order to maintain their protective function in preventing disease (Hinchliff et al 1996).

The dermis layer of the skin contains collagen and elastic fibres, nerve fibres, blood vessels, sweat glands, sebaceous glands and hair follicles. The last three are particularly significant in relation to hygiene care.

Decision making exercise

Given that commensals are a normal feature of human skin investigate the following:

- How might the use of soaps affect the activity of normal skin flora?
- How will babies born with no resident skin commensals gain these normal bacteria?
- What will be the effect of lack of hygiene care on these skin commensals?
- What effect might alcoholic skin preparations used both in cosmetic preparations and surgical lotions have on the normal skin flora?

Sweat glands

Eccrine and apocrine glands are two types of sweat glands; they are distributed throughout the skin, and assist in temperature control. They produce sweat when the skin temperature rises above 35°C. Approximately 500 mL of sweat is produced each day in temperate climates. Secretion of sweat also occurs in response to stress and anxiety as well as to certain spicy foods. Both the production of sweat and its evaporation from the skin assist in heat loss from the body, and the rate of evaporation is particularly important in the patient with pyrexia (raised body temperature) (see Ch. 6 on homeostasis).

Sweat left on the skin, especially if from the apocrine glands of the axilla and genital areas, is responsible for body odour through the process of bacterial decomposition (Hinchliff et al 1996). There are genetic differences in the structure of apocrine glands, which are more developed in populations of African origin than of Asian origin (Bolander 1994). The apocrine glands are dormant during childhood, but begin to actively secrete sweat during puberty and continue to do so throughout adult life. The widespread use of deodorants in developed countries is based on the principle that these solutions will kill the bacteria and mask any odour produced. Antiperspirant sprays block the openings of the ducts to the sweat glands with metal salts such as aluminium (Hinchliff et al 1996).

Sebaceous glands

Sebaceous glands secrete sebum into the hair follicles. This sebum is an oily odourless fluid containing cholesterol, triglycerides, waxes and paraffins that lubricates the skin and keeps it supple and pliant. Sebum also has a role in waterproofing the skin. Sebaceous glands are found in highest numbers over the scalp and face, the middle of the back, the genitalia, and in the auditory canal.

Babies and young children have relatively fewer and less active sebaceous glands and are therefore more prone to skin redness and excoriation in damp conditions, while the loss of sebaceous glands in old age also makes the skin of the elderly more vulnerable to damp conditions, redness and to breakdown. During the menarche (puberty in females), however, the secretion from sebaceous glands increases in response to an increase in adrenocortical hormones. The increasing output of sebum during the teenage years combined with hereditary factors can contribute to the development of acne vulgaris (common acne) (Wong et al 2003).

Decision making exercise

Sarah Woodford, a 14-year-old schoolgirl, has developed acne, which makes her very self-conscious about her appearance in front of her peer group, many of whom pass on their tips for cleaning her skin. Following repeated unsuccessful attempts to control the condition, Sarah finally goes to see the practice nurse at her local health centre.

- How would the practice nurse explain to Sarah the cause of her condition?
- What methods are available from which the practice nurse could choose a treatment for Sarah's individual needs?
- What other advice could be given to Sarah about her general health and hygiene at this time?

Hair

The hair follicle is situated in the dermis and is surrounded by its own nerve and blood supply (Fig. 13.1). Sebaceous glands and sweat gland ducts open directly into the hair follicle causing the scalp to become moist and oily, particularly in a hot environment (Bolander 1994). The cycle of hair growth comprises a period of growth for up to 2 years followed by a rest period and then atrophy. About 70–100 scalp hairs are normally lost each day (Hinchliff et al 1996).

Certain factors affect the rate of normal hair growth and loss. These include:

- nutrition
- hormones (puberty and the menopause)

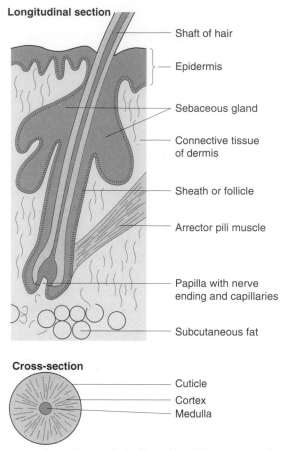

Figure 13.1   Structure of a hair. (From Hinchliff et al 1996.)

Table 13.1   Health risks to nails (after Bolander 1994)

Specific risks
   Biting and improper care
   Exposure to chemicals
   Frequent and prolonged immersion in water
   Ill-fitting shoes
   Ingrowing nails
   Bacterial and fungal infection of the feet

General health risks
   Poor nutrition
   Peripheral vascular disease
   Diabetes mellitus

- hereditary factors (baldness)
- age (decreased number of hairs with old age).

Most of the body is covered by hair, but it varies in type. Lanugo is the fine silky hair found on the fetus *in utero* and on premature babies, and which is lost from the body soon after birth. Vellus is colourless hair found on the female face. Terminal hair is found on the adult head and pubis and is the subject of hygiene care in relation to maintaining healthy hair covered later in this chapter.

Abnormal hair loss can occur in times of stress, trauma and poor nutrition, and as a result of drug therapies, especially cytotoxic drugs used in cancer cell treatment. Alopecia is the term given to hair loss of unknown cause.

Nails

Nails are keratinized plates resting on the highly vascular and sensitive nail bed (Hinchliff et al 1996). The external appearance of the nail bed is often used to indicate general health status as the shape, colour and condition of fingernails are easily observed. Toenails cause more problems for individuals than fingernails. Debilitated adults may have difficulties in maintaining adequate care and hygiene for their feet which will lead to their toenails becoming thick, brittle and prone to fungal infections (Table 13.1). Children may have problems with ingrowing toenails because of difficulties in maintaining well-fitting shoes, especially in times of rapid growth such as during adolescence. It may be necessary to resize children's feet every 3 months to maintain the correct shoe size.

The perineum

The perineum is the area located between the thighs, extending from the anus (posterior) through to the top of the pubic bone (anterior). Anatomical structures in this area are concerned with the expression of sexuality, reproduction and elimination (see Ch. 15 on sexuality and Ch. 18 on continence).

In the female, the external genitalia (vulva) consists of the mons pubis, clitoris, urethral and vaginal orifices, and the labia majora and minora. The normal moist environment around the vaginal orifice is maintained by secretions from Bartholin's glands, which are mucus-secreting glands in the lateral wall of the vagina. The slightly acid secretion varies in amount during the ovulation cycle, has a slight odour and helps to inhibit bacterial growth.

In the male, the perineal area includes the penis, the scrotum and the anus. The end of the penis (glans penis) through which the urethra opens in the centre is covered with a skin flap or foreskin in the uncircumcised male. Because the skin of both the penis and the scrotum is thin and hairless it is more easily irritated and injured than skin elsewhere.

The perineal areas of both men and women are prone to infections because they contain openings into the body and are also warm and moist environments. In both sexes, the urethral orifices lead to sterile bladders, but are in close proximity to the anus, which opens into the 'unclean' rectum. The main aim for hygiene care in this area is to prevent or eliminate infection. Prevention of odour is closely linked to the prevention of infection and is a cultural preoccupation in developed countries.

The mouth and teeth

The mouth has many physical and psychosocial functions that are important in supporting the health and well-being of an individual (Fig. 13.2). The nurse has an important role to play in helping patients and clients sustain their oral health through advice, support and delivery of oral hygiene.

The mouth or oral cavity forms the first part of the gastrointestinal tract (Fig. 13.3). It is lined by mucous membrane, which along with the three pairs of salivary glands – the parotid, sublingual and submandibular – secretes mucus and saliva to aid the mastication and digestion of food. The tongue is a large muscular organ involved in taste, speech and swallowing. There are numerous papillae and taste buds on the upper surface of the tongue. The teeth masticate food, help to shape the mouth and are involved in the formation of speech sounds. The deciduous teeth begin to erupt at between 5 and 8 months of age. In childhood there are normally 20 deciduous teeth. Gradual exfoliation of the deciduous teeth begins approximately from the age of 6. These teeth are replaced by 32 permanent teeth by the age of 18 to 25 years. A full complement of teeth has 16 in the lower and 16 in the upper jaw. Knowledge of the natural loss of teeth in childhood is important to the nurse caring for a child going for surgery under a general anaesthetic, as loose teeth may fall out and be inhaled during induction of anaesthesia.

The structure of the adult tooth contains three parts: the exposed section of the tooth is the crown (enamel), the root (dentine) which is held in place in the jaw bone by cementum, and the pulp cavity, which contains the blood vessels and nerves (Fig. 13.4).

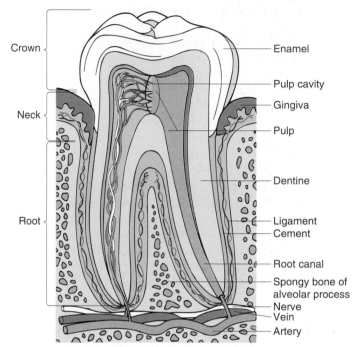

Figure 13.4   Structure of a tooth. (From Hinchliff et al 1996.)

- Ingestion and digestion of food
- Taste
- Speech
- Psychosexual – expression of intimacy
- Social interaction – non-verbal expressions

Figure 13.2   Functions of the mouth.

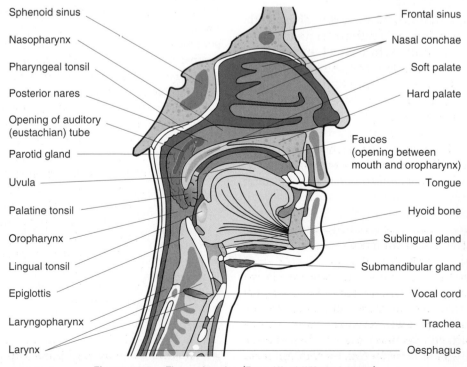

Figure 13.3   The oral cavity. (From Hinchliff et al 1996.)

Dental hygiene

The two major types of oral problems in the normally healthy individual are dental caries (cavities) and periodontal disease. The prevention of both these problems is necessary to prevent premature tooth loss throughout the lifespan. Particularly vulnerable times for tooth loss are during childhood and teenage years and the third age (over 50 years old). Pregnant woman have a higher susceptibility to gum disease (pregnancy gingivitis) due to the increase of hormonal activity and the effect this has on oral microorganisms.

Health promotion strategies addressed to all ages must take into account the interaction between the oral environment of the individual and dental plaque. As soon as food and drink are ingested, the acidity in the mouth increases. The pH is lowered considerably by foods containing sugar and until the acidity is buffered by saliva there is a risk of demineralization of the teeth with subsequent decay. The mouth contains many varieties of bacteria, which do not cause problems if suspended in saliva. However, once these organisms attach themselves to the teeth, gums or tongue surfaces via a mucopolysaccharide glue they become insoluble in water and problems begin. The bacterial deposits cannot be rinsed away and dental plaque forms. Plaque takes 24 hours to develop. It causes dental caries and periodontal disease, which may eventually lead to systemic disease (Taintor & Taintor 1997).

Saliva plays an essential role in maintaining a healthy mouth. Thin watery saliva flushes away some debris from around the gums and teeth and buffers any acids in the mouth. Thick sticky saliva will aid the formation of plaque and therefore increases the risk of periodontal disease and dental caries (Griffiths & Boyle 1993).

Dental caries involve the calcified structures of the tooth. Bacterial enzymes combined with dental plaque produce organic acids, which decalcify both enamel and dentine. Cavities or caries begin to develop once the bacteria have access to the central matrix of the tooth.

Gingivitis is a reversible prevalent disease of the gingivae (gums) and in some cases can lead on to periodontal disease. Periodontal disease is a chronic irreversible disease of the gingivae and supporting tissues of the tooth, i.e. the cementum, periodontal ligaments and underlying jawbone. Clinical features of gingivitis include red, swollen, bleeding gums. Clinical features of periodontal disease (periodontitis) include chronic and/or acute gingivitis, gingival recession, leading to the root (dentine) becoming exposed in the oral cavity, severe bone loss, tooth mobility and ultimately premature tooth loss.

Halitosis, also known as oral malodour or foetor oris, is a common complaint and has many causative factors which include strong spicy foods, coffee, smoking, alcohol, certain drugs and xerostomia (dry mouth). However, dental plaque is also a primary factor of halitosis due to its metabolic activity. Poor oral hygiene activity can lead to halitosis. People who stop cleaning their mouths will soon develop halitosis. Any form of oral sepsis such as gingivitis or periodontitis will produce a degree of halitosis. Rarer causes include diabetic ketoacidosis and severe renal or hepatic problems (Taintor & Taintor 1997).

Reflection and portfolio evidence

You are undertaking a practice placement with the primary healthcare team and have had experiences working alongside the health visitor, the practice nurse and a school nurse. Reflect on the health promotion advice given by each of these three nurses in their particular roles and with their particular client groups.

- Note the questions asked by clients related to those areas that deal with all aspects of hygiene care to include skin care, oral and dental care and hair care.
- Discuss the specific advice given by these health professionals and how it relates to your current knowledge base.
- What health promotion strategies were being used to encourage compliance with advice given?
- Record your learning in your portfolio.

The eyes

The eye is a delicate organ with its own built-in mechanisms for protection and hygiene. The conjunctiva covers the exposed surface of the eye and the inner surface of the eyelids and helps to prevent drying of the eye. The eye produces tear fluid, which is washed across the eye by the regular blinking action of the eyelashes. Tear fluid contains salt, protein, oil from sebaceous glands and a bactericidal enzyme called lysozyme, which helps protect the eye against infection. Tears are produced by the lacrimal and accessory glands, which respond to reflexes and the autonomic nervous system. Tears need a drainage system if the eye is not to become 'watery' (epiphora). Drainage is normally via canaliculi at the inner end of the lid margin into the lacrimal sac and duct and finally into the nasal cavity. Any condition that interferes with these three protective mechanisms may cause problems:

- People who wear contact lenses, particularly in a dry centrally heated building for long periods, may be at risk of excessive drying of the cornea and subsequent inflammation (Hinchliff et al 1996).
- The person who has had a stroke or is unconscious for any reason may be vulnerable to eye infections without adequate eye hygiene.
- Many elderly people suffer from 'watery eye' and may require surgery to prevent secondary infections (Hinchliff et al 1996).
- Neonates and young children are prone to get what is known as 'sticky eyes', and the condition may be due to

blockage or malformation of the lacrimal ducts and require surgery.

- *Chlamydia* infection passed from the mother to the baby during childbirth can cause serious eye infection in the neonate.
- Bacterial conjunctivitis can be a common problem in children's nurseries and schools, especially as children are prone to rub their eyes with dirty hands (Wong et al 2003).

PSYCHOSOCIAL

INDIVIDUAL ASPECTS OF HYGIENE CARE

Beliefs and attitudes to personal hygiene are developed during childhood and are strongly influenced by social and cultural norms. Nurses aware of the scientific principles on which they base their beliefs about hygiene care need to be sensitive to the family and cultural influences on their clients (Bolander 1994).

Historically, hygiene practices have been influenced by:

- social norms
- religious rituals
- the environment (accessibility of water for bathing)
- evolution of hygiene aids (e.g. showers, soaps, razors, electric toothbrushes, hair dryers).

Hygiene maintenance is a normal daily occupation and promotes a feeling of security and stability alongside well-being and self-esteem (Roper et al 1996). An important stage in the development of independence in hygiene self-care in childhood occurs during the toddler and preschool phase (i.e. at 1–6 years of age). During this time children develop physically, learn to gain self-control and mastery over body functions, and become increasingly aware of their own dependence and independence (Wong et al 2003). The social and cultural beliefs of the family are of great importance in this preschool period in influencing attitudes and practices in hygiene care and health promotion is usually directed through the parents and carers of the child. Peer influences become increasingly important through the school years and hygiene habits for both sexes may be influenced more by advertising, peer support and the wish to conform to group and sexual norms. Health promotion strategies by healthcare professionals during this phase of development need to consider these predominant social influences. During the late teenage years, values and attitudes become internalized and each individual justifies for themselves their choices in hygiene care.

CULTURAL AND SPIRITUAL ASPECTS OF HYGIENE

Historically, bathing was an important social activity and public baths were a feature of ancient Greek, Egyptian and Roman society (Encarta 2001). The ancient Roman facilities included exercise rooms, hot, warm and cold baths, steam rooms and dressing rooms. These facilities are again very evident in Western societies with the growth in numbers of modern health and fitness centres which include saunas, steam rooms and jacuzzis. Sociologists have argued that this recent trend is linked with treating 'the body' as a consumer commodity that must be maintained and groomed to achieve maximum market value (Lupton 1994). Body maintenance in the interest of good health is linked with the desire to appear sexually attractive for both sexes, but more especially for women (Bordo 1990). However, cultural habits in hygiene care still demonstrate links with past beliefs, which are often expressed culturally (Helman 2001).

The early Christian church considered physical cleanliness as less important than spiritual purity and after the decline of moral standards in the Roman Empire discouraged public bathing. Bathing, even in private, came to be regarded as unhealthy and was considered an indulgence. In the Middle Ages, the use of water to clean the body was rare and the only areas that needed to be cleansed were those visible to others. Even then, the 'dry wash', which involved rubbing one's face and hands with a cloth, was considered healthy right up to the 17th century (Vigarello 1988). The use of hot water was considered unhealthy as people believed that the pores of the skin would open and allow infection to penetrate the body, therefore being covered up meant that the body was protected from disease. Lay beliefs about how we become susceptible to colds can echo these earlier beliefs (e.g. 'allowing one's head to get wet', 'going outside after washing one's hair', 'getting one's feet wet', 'getting caught in the rain' (Helman 2001)).

The relationship between bathing, body hygiene and becoming healthy changed with the Industrial Revolution when the body could then be compared with a machine; the use of cold water was seen as invigorating and helping to firm up the body and also became associated with moral austerity. With the scientific discovery of microbes, washing became important to rid the body of disease, touching of certain body parts considered 'dirty' became prohibited and more frequent washing was encouraged (Vigarello 1988). At this time, buildings did not include bathing facilities and it was not until the level of dirt and disease increased after the Industrial Revolution that demand increased for good bathing facilities to reduce cross-infections such as cholera. By the late 19th century, private homes of the upper classes began to have separate rooms set aside for bathing, and municipal baths were built for the general public to use (Encarta 2001).

In developed countries today most private homes have their own bathroom facilities, which are often multiple as en suite bathrooms have become the norm in new housing at the end of the 20th century. There is now a more marked preoccupation with cleanliness and showers have become more commonplace, even in temperate climates. Cleansing products and deodorants are heavily marketed as body odour can be regarded as the ultimate 'social sin'. However, the preoccupation with 'smelling good' is being counterbalanced by a movement that accepts natural odours as normal and has antipathy to the use of 'chemicals' on the skin (Bolander 1994).

Bathing has also been an integral part of the ritual cleansing of religious practices over many centuries. Baptism in Christianity and the mikvah in Orthodox Judaism are derived from bathing rituals, while bathing is an important part of Muslim and Hindu religious ceremonies. Muslims perform ablutions before prayer and are very particular that all bodily excretions are removed.

Culturally certain hygiene habits may appear distasteful and noisy to nurses in developed countries. Internal cleansing rituals such as sniffing water up into the nose and blowing it out into a basin may provoke disgust, but this can be a normal practice among Muslims and Hindus, while colonic irrigations are a method of internal cleansing of the gut among those who practice yoga.

The 'short back and sides' image of hair hygiene in developed countries is not relevant to a Sikh, to whom the hair (kes) is sacred and should not be cut, but should instead be kept covered by a turban. Rastafarians do not like to wash their long hair.

Items of clothing are also sacred in certain cultures and should not be removed during hygiene care. These can include neck threads (marriage thread for Hindu women), bangles and comb (kara and kasngha for Sikhs), nose jewels (wedding symbols for Bangladeshi women), and a stone or medallion around the neck (protection for Muslims) (Sampson 1982). There are many other cultural and religious habits among different cultural and religious groups that have an important impact on the delivery of appropriate and sensitive hygiene care. It is important to be sensitive to any requests that may seem strange, but are in fact normal to the individual concerned.

Reflection and portfolio evidence

Review your own personal hygiene routines and practices over 1 week. Reflect on what or who have had the most influence on your current practices. What standard of hygiene care would you find intolerable for yourself? (Recall situations when you did not have access to hygiene facilities for whatever reason.)

In your practice placement in a healthcare institution:

- Review the quality of hygiene facilities and also access to them.
- Observe whether there are institutional patterns in the delivery of hygiene care.
- Analyse to what extent current facilities and patterns of care allow for the particular cultural and spiritual norms of the individuals who are experiencing health care.
- Record your findings in your portfolio.

CARE DELIVERY KNOWLEDGE

Knowledge for the assessment of needs and implementation of care is the main focus for this section. Although in most instances hygiene care is delivered to meet the total needs of the patient, in order to incorporate the specific knowledge underpinning practice, the material in this section is presented under four headings as follows:

- body hygiene care, including reference to foot and nail care and perineal hygiene
- oral and dental hygiene
- hair care
- eye care.

ASSESSMENT OF AN INDIVIDUAL'S HYGIENE NEEDS

Decision making around the delivery of hygiene care to a patient or client is dependent upon many factors, which include the patient's ability to self-care, the facilities available, including family members or informal carers, and the nurse's expertise and time. Accurate assessment of the individual patient's needs and level of participation should be encouraged wherever possible. Although there is still a need for the timing to be negotiated to fit organizational needs, the ritualization of bed bathing to the morning shift whether in hospital, hostel or community should become a thing of the past.

With children, infants and babies, bath times and routines in any healthcare facility should mimic as closely as possible the child's normal routine with the parents or significant carer being involved directly in providing care. Although the child may view hygiene rituals as unpleasant, they can be fun. There should be facilities both in time and the design of the environment that will maintain and encourage playtime for the infant and young child during the delivery of hygiene care. Children also need privacy, but there should be a balance between allowing them privacy and understanding how much help they require to be safe and to achieve the goals of good hygiene. A baby needs a warm environment and less exposure to prevent chilling. Teenagers will expect that facilities will allow them to maintain their privacy, while older adults may expect the nurse to respect their usual routines for bathing and not demand bathing as a daily ritual if their normal habit is to bath less frequently (Jones 1995).

The ability to care for one's own hygiene needs is important to all individuals and is a prime motivating factor in focusing the nurse on teaching self-care to children or adults with intellectual disabilities. Goals set should be commensurate with the individual's intellectual ability and may need to be frequently revised in order to allow feelings of achievement if progress is slow. Being sensitive to the intimate nature of care and the need for personal control is important in facilitating privacy and dignity (Cambridge &

Carnaby 2000). Perceptions of lack of control can lead to the client being agitated and aggressive (Hoeffer et al 1997, Kovach & Meyer-Arnold 1996).

Evidence based practice

Carnaby & Cambridge (2002) examined the provision of intimate and personal care for people with intellectual disability (ID), particularly those with profound and multiple ID. There is little research evidence or theoretical literature to inform this area of care. In a small descriptive exploratory study, the authors mapped the key management and practice issues and suggest ways forward for the providers of services for people with ID in relation to the quality and outcomes of intimate and personal care.

The motivation to maintain personal hygiene as part of a personal self-image can be lost when a person is depressed or disturbed mentally. The nursing role is then focused on encouraging self-care through specific behaviour modification techniques or other counselling approaches that aim to improve the individual's feeling of self-esteem. Equally, the individual may be confused or have a loss of short-term memory and need constant direction in order to be encouraged to maintain his or her independence in hygiene care (Roe et al 2001).

Decision making exercise

During your practice placement you are allocated on a morning shift to work with a registered nurse who has responsibility for the care of six elderly women with varying degrees of mental and physical disabilities. Your partner is keen that all hygiene care should be delivered by the end of the morning.

- Decide on what information you need to collect in order for you to make decisions on how to prioritize the care you give.
- Reflect on and discuss how you would cope with the wishes of your primary nurse to complete the care by lunchtime.

(In completing this exercise, cross-reference to any work you have done on assertiveness and dealing with potential conflicts of opinion.)

Overall goals for hygiene care will vary depending upon the particular circumstances and needs of the individual patient (Bolander 1994). These include some or all of the following:

- providing comfort and relaxation for the patient
- ensuring cleanliness through the removal of secretions, microorganisms and surface dirt

- improving self-image by removing odours and enhancing physical appearance
- improving skin and muscle condition by stimulating the circulation through massage.

If patients or clients need help from the nurse in meeting their hygiene needs, the following elements should be considered when making an assessment:

- psychosocial needs: the need for privacy and dignity, personal habits of the patient, cultural background of the patient
- physical needs: level of dependence or independence, temporary or long-term dependence, therapeutic value of hygiene care
- facilities and time available: choice of method to deliver care, time of day (patient choice where possible), aids required.

The activity of washing removes sweat, sebum, dried skin scales, dust and microorganisms from the skin's surface. If not removed, microorganisms multiply and lead to body odour and infection. When people are ill, increased anxiety can lead to increased sweating and therefore the need to wash more frequently. In surgical patients, prevention of wound infection and cross-infection is a paramount consideration in decisions about how often and by what method to deliver hygiene care. Patients who are incontinent may need more frequent and sensitive attention to their hygiene needs.

Aesthetically care should be given according to the norms of good taste and culturally specific values. The method selected should be effective in terms of the patient's and the nurse's time and energy. It should promote and maintain the patient's independence, enhance the nurse–patient relationship and provide an opportunity for two-way information processes such as health promotion activities. Body hygiene care may also be therapeutic if part of a treatment regimen that includes the need for exercise of joints and muscle relaxation while the individual is submersed in warm water. Perineal hygiene care post childbirth also promotes wound healing in the mother who has perineal sutures (Calvert & Fleming 2000).

Decision making around hygiene care is concerned with skilful adaptation of practice when the facilities within the context of care and the actual needs of the patient are incongruent.

Evidence based practice

Hancock et al (2000) collected the impressions of 200 patients (both medical and surgical) and 200 nursing staff (registered, enrolled and trainee enrolled nurses) in relation to two bed bathing methods. Data collection included questionnaires and semi-structured interviews. Data regarding costs were obtained from appropriate cost centre managers. The results of the study found the soft towel bathing method to be more cost effective and provide more patient and nurse satisfaction than the traditional bed bathing method.

- Shower
- Complete bed bath
- Towel bath
- Partial bed bath or 'top and tailing' in infants and small children
- Therapeutic baths

Figure 13.5   Methods for body hygiene.

Facilitating body hygiene care

There are many different ways of delivering body hygiene care (Fig. 13.5). Although nurses in multiple contexts use some or all of these methods on a daily basis, textbooks generally concentrate on the techniques of bed bathing the highly dependent patient. There has been a major shift in conventions around decision making in this area of total body hygiene as the emphasis is placed on patient independence in maintaining his or her own hygiene care.

Conventional methods of bed bathing are physically tiring for the patient and the nurse. To overcome some of the disadvantages of bed bathing, towel bathing has been used in the USA for some time and has been introduced elsewhere on a limited basis (Hancock et al 2000, Wright 1990). A 2-metre towel is soaked in a solution that contains a cleansing agent at a temperature of 43°C for which no rinsing is required. The patient is wrapped in the towel and massaged clean.

Although bathing is usually associated with the use of soap and water, various bath and shower gels containing an emollient have become increasingly popular as an alternative. Soap lowers skin surface tension by removing sebum (oily substance) from the skin, which facilitates cleaning. Care should be taken as some soaps remove too much sebum, and in the elderly with frail skin this may cause excessive drying of the skin. Special hypoallergenic soaps are available for people who experience allergic reactions. For babies and young children integral 'baby baths', which include bath cleanser and shampoo, for example Infacare, are readily available. People have individual preferences for the fragrance of the soap, the type of deodorant and other lotions and powders used following skin hygiene.

Decision making exercise

Find and read a copy of the article by Hancock et al (2000).

- Appraise the positive and negative points regarding towel and bed baths.
- If given the scope to change practice how would you decide between these two methods of delivering hygiene care?
- Debate the barriers to change that might occur in implementing a new method of delivering hygiene care based on evidence.

Special areas for care: the perineal area

In children care of the genitalia or perineum is important. For babies and young children who are not yet toilet trained, this area needs extra hygiene care and the application of water repellent creams to prevent skin damage. Children should generally be encouraged to self-care, but in the older child there is a tendency to avoid cleaning this area (Wong et al 2003). For boys over 3 years of age who are not circumcised, the foreskin should be retracted and the exposed surface cleaned (except in circumstances where cultural beliefs will not allow this). However, care must be taken to retract the foreskin very gently as it may be tight (phimosis) and overstretching can create scarring, leading to sexual and micturition (passing urine) difficulties in the future.

In adults of both sexes who cannot maintain their own hygiene, extra sensitivity is needed in dealing with perineal care because of cultural and spiritual taboos in exposing this area of the body. Perineal care in women following childbirth is managed differently, especially if there is a surgical wound in the area (Calvert & Fleming 2000).

Special areas for care: nails and feet

Although nails can be subjected to much abuse, especially fingernails, most people can maintain nail hygiene according to their own particular standards and values. In children, hygiene care to keep nails clean is particularly important after outdoor play, toileting and before meals as the eggs from intestinal parasites or helminths (roundworms, hookworms, pinworms, threadworms or *Toxocara* from dogs or cats) can be ingested and the child then becomes infected. Besides good hand and nail hygiene, children should be discouraged from biting their nails and from scratching the bare anal area (Wong et al 2003).

Foot care and good nail care are also important in the elderly, and especially in any person who has diabetes mellitus as poor peripheral circulation makes this group of people vulnerable to skin breakdown with subsequent delayed healing. Specialist foot nail care is required through the expert skills of the chiropodist/podiatrist and the nurse's role is primarily in recognizing the need to refer clients and in providing preliminary care and advice. Primary healthcare nurses and specialist diabetic nurses, however, will be expected to give additional health education and care to the diabetic client (George 1995).

Therapeutic baths

The temperature of the water in a bath can be used for therapeutic reasons as well as hygiene. Baths at skin temperature (37°C) are relaxing, those hotter or colder can be stimulating. Hot baths can help to relieve pain and discomfort and may control convulsions and induce sleep. Cold baths can be helpful in reducing fever and inflammation. All the body can be submerged or only a body part such as the perineum in a sitz bath or a foot bath. If any substance is added to the bath to have an effect on a disease, the bath can be termed as 'medicated'. Alkaline baths have been used extensively in the treatment of rheumatic conditions. Steam baths use medicated vapours to help lung conditions. Mineral baths are usually public baths that use the natural warm mineral springs of a certain region to aid in the recovery of numerous conditions. These are the fashionable spas of the 19th century and are still used today to promote general health (Encarta 2001). Alternative therapies, which include aromatherapy oils added to the bath water and therapeutic massage given during a bed bath, may be used as an adjunct to hygiene care to promote healing and a general feeling of well-being (Price & Price 1995, Tiran 1996).

Bathing aids

For the disabled patient or client, particularly if confined to a wheelchair, bathing is potentially a very important time. Warm water will help to relax stiff muscles, there is the opportunity to increase the range of muscle movement, and there is also a change of position and atmosphere, which promotes a general feeling of well-being. To be able to get in and out of the bath in comfort and to be able to remain in the bath is a much appreciated luxury and one that can be difficult in institutional care where time and staffing are in short supply. Special facilities for the disabled include the Parker bath (Fig. 13.6), with its unique design features, which allow the client to slide into the bath. It can be moved into several positions to aid both the client and the nurse. There are many different aids for bathing for the disabled

on the market (see Ch. 17 on mobility) that can be used in the home in an ordinary bath.

Principles of care

Whatever procedure is selected to deliver body hygiene, the principles of safety, prevention of cross-infection and promotion of privacy and dignity should be followed. Safety extends to promoting good back care and posture for the nurse or carer by encouraging the use of appropriate bathing aids. Parents of babies and infants, in preparation for bathing their baby, should be aware of the dangers in lifting baby baths when full of warm water and also when disposing of the water after bathing. Children should never be left alone in the bath as there is always a danger of drowning regardless of the water level.

The process of providing care should be methodical, logical and safe, taking into consideration the specific limits of the patient, whether temporary, for example post-surgery, or permanent, for example due to physical disability. If teaching or encouraging a child or adult with a learning disability or the frail elderly, goals should be set for what the patient can realistically do without causing undue discomfort and exposure during the bathing process. Being sensitive and not taking over is very important as most people are intrinsically motivated to participate in their own care and dislike any loss of dignity and freedom of action. Quality standards for the delivery of hygiene care can be audited using tools contained in the Department of Health document *Essence of Care* (Department of Health 2001).

Giving hygiene care also allows the nurse to undertake other activities that are necessary for the overall decision making about care for the clients (Table 13.2). This

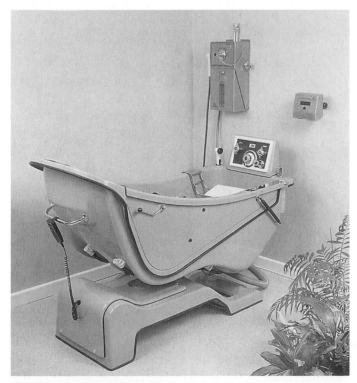

Figure 13.6 A Parker bath.

Table 13.2 Nursing activities that can be incorporated into the delivery of hygiene care (after Wilson 1986)

Type of activity	Details
Observations	Observe for signs and symptoms of physical problems Note any non-verbal expressions of anxiety and fear
Interpersonal communication	Encourage disclosure by patient (intimate procedure) Time for trusting and building relationships Opportunity to offer empathy and support
Health promotion	Information giving about the immediate condition and its treatment Advice and support for self-care strategies on discharge or in the long term
Social interaction	Recognition of the influence of family, life and work on the patient or client Growth and development of the nurse as a person and a practitioner

particular aspect is often overlooked in skill mix debates when it is argued that hygiene care does not need the skills of a registered nurse. The opportunity to make relevant observations, to initiate and sustain the nurse–patient relationship, to explore the patient's concerns and to promote a healthy lifestyle is a fundamental part of the delivery of body hygiene care.

Reflection and portfolio evidence

Obtain a copy of the Department of Health (2001) *Essence of Care: Patient-focused Benchmarking for Health Care Practitioners* and review the two sections personal and oral hygiene, and privacy and dignity. It might be helpful to also look at an article outlining the implementation of an audit tool (Field & Reid 2002). In your practice placement:

- Observe current practice in the delivery of personal and oral hygiene.
- Investigate how and when practices are currently audited for benchmarking 'best practice'.
- Undertake a reflective audit of your own practice in relation to a number of patients allocated to your care.
- Record your learning in your portfolio.

ORAL AND DENTAL HYGIENE

Assessment

The nurse's role in the maintenance of oral hygiene involves the use of general observation skills and specific assessment tools. Although it has been recognized that much of the responsibility for the delivery of oral care in an institutional setting has devolved to the junior or untrained nurse, the initial and ongoing assessment is the responsibility of the registered practitioner. Specific assessment tools should aid this process. However, to date, these tools are not yet in common use (Coleman 2002, Evans 2001) and reliability is dependent upon the same nurse carrying out the assessment in order to reduce the subjective nature of the decision making about oral care. It is important to encourage the use of an objective assessment tool that is valid, reliable and practical to use on a day-to-day basis.

The content of the various oral assessment tools include:

- direct observation of areas of the oral cavity
- assessment of the functions of the mouth
- risk factors that have the potential to create oral problems.

All tools include scoring systems that indicate the severity of the patient's oral condition. Jenkins (1989) developed a practical tool that acts as an 'at risk' calculator. Table 13.3 demonstrates the common features of the various assessment tools presented in the literature (Eilers et al 1988, Holmes & Mountain 1993). As it is important to use an

Table 13.3 Common features of different oral assessment tools

Feature	Details
Observation of areas within mouth	Lips: colour, moisture, texture Tongue: colour, moisture, texture Gingiva: colour, moisture, haemorrhage, ulceration, oedema Teeth: shine, debris Palate: moisture, colour, ulceration
Functions within the mouth	Saliva: thin, watery, hypersalivation, scanty, absent, thick, ropey Voice: normal, deep, raspy, difficult or painful speech Swallow: normal, difficult, pain on swallowing fluids or solids, diminished or no gag reflex
Predisposing stressors	Mouth breathing Oxygen therapy Mechanical ventilation Restricted oral intake Chemotherapy or radiotherapy Drugs and concurrent diseases
Subjective data from patients	Taste changes Pain profile

objective measure, especially where care is being delegated to many (including junior) staff, the registered nurse may need to assess which of the tools, if used, will provide the most valid and reliable information for the particular client group in his or her care.

Reflection and portfolio evidence

While on practice placement, observe the assessment and implementation of oral care for the specific patients in your care. Remember that age groups, certain conditions and drug treatments can have an impact on oral health.

- Review current practice in a specific practice placement.
- Compare your findings with those in Evans's (2001) article.
- Complete a search of the recent literature related to assessment tools for oral care.
- Record your findings and learning in your portfolio.

In the assessment of different client groups it is important to remember that specific predisposing factors may put them at considerable risk of developing oral problems. Children with Down syndrome and other disabling conditions tend to have thick, ropey, sticky saliva that fails to 'wash' food debris away and adheres to the tooth surface. This process encourages the early formation of plaque (Griffiths & Boyle 1993).

Teenagers wearing orthodontic appliances (braces) and those with an oral deformity such as a cleft lip or palate who have removable or fixed appliances will need special advice on how to maintain their oral hygiene, but may need encouragement from the nurse to sustain these practices (Griffiths & Boyle 1993, Taintor & Taintor 1997).

For the older client, the ageing process leads to a decreased salivary flow. Although an increasing number of elderly people retain their own teeth, if the client is wearing dentures, these should be checked for fit to prevent trauma to the palate and gums. If the individual client has diminished neuromuscular control he or she may have difficulty in maintaining oral care through lack of hand to mouth coordination. To maintain oral health comfort, dignity and adequate nutrition in the elderly, nursing care should be of a high standard (Fitzpatrick 2000, Frenkel & Newcombe 2001).

For the elderly mentally infirm, it may be the client's behaviour that needs to be targeted during rehabilitation so that the individual's coping strategies can be improved. This assessment will involve other members of the healthcare team in order to measure the client's progress against preset short- and long-term goals. The Simon Nursing Assessment for the elderly mentally infirm includes an assessment section for oral hygiene (O'Donnovan 1992). There are many risk factors to optimum oral health in the mentally ill. These arise from the condition itself (see Annotated Further Reading) or the drug treatment to control the symptoms of the illness (Table 13.4).

Table 13.4 Drug groups that cause xerostomia (after Sreebny 1997)

Drug group	Mechanism of action
Antihistamines Antispasmodics Anticholinergics Antidepressants Antipsychotics Tranquillizers Anticonvulsants Narcotic analgesics	Reduce salivary production
Antibiotics	Alter the balance of commensal organisms so that candidal organisms can invade the mouth
Cytotoxics and chemotherapeutics	Reduce the autoimmune response and therefore allow easy growth of invading organisms
Corticosteroids	Reduce the healing properties of tissues
Diuretics	Potential dehydration resulting in a reduction in salivary flow

Evidence based practice

Simons et al (1999) found that dental assessments were often not conducted when residents were first admitted to a random sample of residential homes ($n = 48$ of 110) in England. Care plans did not include oral care and dental care was sought only when residents or their relatives complained of acute dental problems.

In the same study Simons et al (1999) found that the majority (927 of 1041) of older people living in the sampled residential homes received medications known to produce xerostomia. A reduced salivary flow impairs debris removal and increases the risk of tissue ulceration and accumulation of dental caries.

Many other conditions, treatments and drugs can put the individual client at particular risk of developing oral problems. Some of these treatments are included in the risk assessment tools referred to earlier (see Table 13.3). Many drugs cause xerostomia (dry mouth) and damage the normal defence and healing processes of the oral cavity and are detailed in Table 13.4.

If an individual complains of halitosis there is a need to establish the cause and assess its severity. A subjective assessment of the degree of severity of the halitosis by the individual concerned has been shown to correlate well with measurements of the amount of sulphide in the mouth. A portable sulphide monitor is used and gas chromatography can provide an accurate assessment of the wider range of compounds that can be responsible for halitosis. Usually a dentist or periodontologist carries out such a full assessment. Treatment is aimed at reducing any oral flora and is best achieved by brushing the teeth and cleaning between the teeth.

Facilitating oral care

In the delivery of oral care to clients or patients the nurse has many decisions to make concerning the most appropriate tools and solutions to use in caring for the dependent patient. Likewise in the health promotion role, the advice and education given to the independent client needs to be specific to the individual client needs. It is therefore necessary to have knowledge of and experience in using the various tools and solutions available.

Methods for dental and oral care

The single most effective method of promoting dental health is the daily removal of dental plaque. In addition the reduction of refined sugars in the diet is essential to maintain dental health; however, plaque is the primary cause of tooth and gum disease and not sugar.

Oral hygiene itself aims to reduce dental caries and maintain a healthy mouth. Various tools and solutions are used to achieve these aims. For the individual, having clean 'white' teeth and fresh breath may be even more important social goals and the timing of care may vary according to the family and cultural norms.

The toothbrush is the most effective method for removing plaque. Ideally the design should include a small head with soft multitufted nylon bristles. Power brushes, that are battery operated or rechargeable devices, have an oscillating round brush head that is also efficient at removing plaque without causing damage to the gums (Heanue et al 2003). Manually, a good simple technique is to brush in small circles dividing the mouth up into sections and systematically brushing each section. Brushing gums is just as important as the area between the teeth and gums can trap plaque, which will lead to gingivitis. Single-tufted brushes with a pointed tip are useful for patients with trismus (limited mouth opening). The use of dental floss or tape is recommended to clean between the teeth. All the above tools are relatively easy to use when the client can understand how and can control their use. Problems arise when the client is dependent on the nurse for oral care.

Although toothbrushing is the method of choice, in the past, nurses have failed to use them with clients, particularly because they feared causing trauma and perceived them as unsuitable for an edentulous mouth. The choice of toothbrush and method for using it are of prime importance for different client groups.

> ### Evidence based practice
>
> A review by Moore (1995) found that there has been little change in oral care nursing practices over the previous 30 years. There has been neither enough research into oral care nor application of the research findings available in the assessment and decision making about oral care for specific client groups. Adams (1996) verified the lack of knowledge of qualified nurses related to oral health in her study completed on medical wards. Miller & Kearney's (2001) review comments that oral care continues to be carried out in a ritualistic way with conflicting advice based on subjective conclusions from sporadic research.

Young children need to have their teeth brushed for them and the nurse involved in giving advice to parents and carers should be able to provide the correct information. As flossing between teeth can potentially cause gum damage, it is important to avoid flossing for a child under 10 years of age and to get expert advice if the older child needs this doing for them. For the disabled child or adult, electric or specially adapted standard toothbrushes are necessary.

Toothpaste is the most common substance used to clean teeth and since the introduction of fluoride into toothpaste there has been a large reduction in dental decay, especially in children (Marinho et al 2003). The fluoridation of water has been widespread, although the ethical debates related to personal choice have prevented its implementation in some areas. Although special fluoride supplements (rinses, gels, tablets and drops) have been available for children,

there is concern that with the increasing amounts of fluoride in toothpaste, there may be a danger of the child developing fluorosis. Ensuring that children do not swallow toothpaste and rinse their mouths carefully is important in order to prevent fluorosis. Fluoride supplements should only be used on the advice of a dentist.

Other solutions in common use are listed in Table 13.5. Overall chlorhexidine is the most effective antiplaque agent. There is a need to research more fully the effectiveness of some of the solutions that are still in common use in institutional healthcare settings. Commercially available solutions may contain alcohol, which has no benefit. Ensuring regular appropriate care is essential to reduce the risk of halitosis and infection (Stiefel et al 2000, Xavier 2000).

Other tools used for giving oral care to the dependent patient include foam sponges, swab on forceps and the swab on the finger technique (Ransier et al 1995). Foam sponges have the advantage of causing little oral trauma, but are ineffective at removing debris from the surface or from in between teeth (Pearson 1996). The swab on a forceps technique can be difficult to manipulate and may be more prone to causing trauma. The swab on the gloved finger if used with a gentle sweeping action can be effective in removing debris without causing undue trauma (Griffiths & Boyle 1993). However, in any dependent person with facial muscle weakness that affects the mouth it is important that food and debris are not missed as the action of the swabbing may cause food to be compressed into one part of the mouth. Remember, the technique of the user is important in order to remove plaque regardless of tool used to deliver oral care (Pearson 1996).

> ### Evidence based practice
>
> Pearson (1996) completed a small experimental comparative study on the use of foam swabs and toothbrushes to remove dental plaque. Using herself and a volunteer, the researcher used either foam sticks or a toothbrush for 6 consecutive days as a method of cleaning the mouth and teeth. Total visible removal of plaque was more effective when using the toothbrush. The foam stick was not able to remove plaque from some sheltered areas of the teeth and the gingival crevices.

Denture care

Dentures, both full and partial, are the most common oral appliance, especially among the elderly population, and need regular rinsing and cleaning, particularly after eating. Dentures should be removed at night to prevent the development of oral candidiasis (thrush). As with teeth, the most effective method for removing plaque is through brushing and rinsing. Proprietary denture cleaners are available as

Table 13.5   Solutions in common use for oral hygiene: actions and limitations (after Griffiths & Boyle 1993)

Solution	Action	Limitations
Chlorhexidine gluconate (solution, gel, spray)	Effective antiplaque Well tolerated by most client groups	Reversible staining of teeth
Hexetidine and cetylpyridinium, (mouthwash, gargle)	Antiplaque	Not as effective as chlorhexidine
Hydrogen peroxide and sodium perborate (diluted as mouthwash at 3%)	Mucosolvent that breaks down thick and viscous saliva	Unpleasant taste Short-term use only Incorrect dilution leads to chemical burns Risk of borate absorption
Sodium bicarbonate (powder diluted in water)	Mucosolvent Cleansing	Unpleasant taste Further research needed to ascertain how useful in practice
Thymol (mouthwash)	Antibacterial at high concentrations Refreshing taste	Little to no antibacterial action at low concentrations
Sodium chloride (mouthwash, gargle)	Effective cleansing agent Well tolerated	None indicated
Lemon and glycerine (impregnated swabs on a stick)	Lemon is a salivary stimulant Glycerine for lubrication, but astringent	Overuse can lead to salivary gland exhaustion and increased xerostomia Low pH increases the risk of dental caries
Phenol (mouthwash, gargle, spray)	Cleansing	Epiglottic and laryngeal oedema Contraindicated in children Needs further research to test effects on plaque
Povidone–iodine 1% (mouthwash/gargle)	Cleansing	Mucosal irritation Hypersensitive reactions No antiplaque activity
Benzydamine hydrochloride (mouthwash, spray)	Relief of oral ulceration	Numbness or stinging

solutions, brush-on cleaners or pastes, but all have some disadvantages such as staining, bleaching and corrosion of metal. Regular brushing with unperfumed soap and water is considered one of the best methods of cleaning dentures (Griffiths & Boyle 1993). A common problem may be loose-fitting dentures, especially if the wearer is ill and poor nutrition leads to physical deterioration. A temporary method to overcome this problem is to insert a soft lining until a new set of dentures can be made. In residential or nursing home care many of the elderly residents have dentures, but loss of dentures can now be prevented by labelling dentures using a commercially available naming kit (i.e. Indenture).

HAIR CARE

Hair styling and grooming feature very highly in maintaining physical and psychological health and a positive body image. Most people can and wish to maintain their own hair according to their own choice. In institutions where individuals are unable to care for themselves it is often therapeutic if a member of the family or a friend provides this aspect of hygiene care. Self-care is a significant goal to achieve for those with physical and mental disability.

Hair care among different ethnic groups can be part of deeply embedded beliefs that are cultural as well as religious, and these need to be respected. Hair care for black children or adults, if dependent, may need specific combs and techniques (Joyner 1988). Hair loss from the head from whatever cause can be a significant source of worry, especially if it occurs for no known cause in children and adolescents (Clore & Corey 1991).

All of the above variations in hair care need to be taken into account in assessing and facilitating hygiene care. Resources, which include time, should be available to provide optimum hair care in any healthcare institution. Daily combing and brushing can usually be maintained through self-care, family support and nursing care. However, standards of care for shampooing can vary, and in the acute care setting may inevitably be given lower priority when resources are stretched. Many institutions for both acute and long-term care have back-up hairdressing services available, but often at a financial cost to clients.

Hair infestation

Head lice are endemic and although they are not responsible for the spread of any disease, they are responsible for considerable social distress. They are cosmopolitan in that they can infest anybody and do not discriminate between class or cleanliness. Infestation with head lice can be quite debilitating if left untreated. However, this rarely happens today. The term 'feeling lousy' originates from feeling weak and 'nitwit' refers to poor performance at work due to untreated infestation (Connolly et al 2002) .

Head lice eggs hatch after 7–10 days and the eggshell that remains is called the nit. New hatchings are about 1 mm long and females do not mate until fully grown (i.e. 6 days old) and about 3mm in length. Spread is through contact, and can be very quick as the two heads need only have direct contact for approximately 1 minute to allow the lice (usually fully grown lice) to move across from one hair to the other. Lice usually prefer short clean hair to long greasy hair.

School nurses, practice nurses and health visitors are key healthcare workers in dealing with head lice in children. Both education and public health acts make it mandatory for health professionals to monitor and diagnose the presence of head lice in schoolchildren, but it is then the responsibility of the parents to cleanse the head. Free prescriptions for head lice preparations are available for children under 16 years of age. Most health districts now use a rotational policy for the main chemical treatments for head lice as there is evidence that resistance has developed (Downs et al 2002). Table 13.6 shows the main lotions in use. All lotions used for treatments can cause undue irritation of the skin.

A non-chemical approach to the treatment of head lice, i.e. 'bug-busting', has been developed (Ibarra 1995, Plastow et al 2001). It involves removing the lice from the head before they are large enough to spread or reproduce. The method involves shampooing and conditioning the hair twice a week followed by combing with a fine-toothed plastic comb when the hair is wet. It was found through measuring the lice (1 mm long is newly hatched) that it was possible to clear the hair of lice within a fortnight by completing this

treatment twice weekly. Although it is effective and may be the method of choice for parents who do not wish to use chemicals because of non-compliance with the treatment regime, there is evidence that chemical removal remains more effective overall even in areas where there is intermediate resistance to the solution (Roberts et al 2000).

Decision making exercise

On a recent placement the school nurse has asked you to help her with a health promotion session on the control of head lice that she is about to do for parents in a local primary school.

- Find out about the rotational system of treatment of head lice by chemical means in your area.
- Check the advice being given in your local area by the Health Education Authority about non-chemical treatments for head lice.
- Discuss the evidence for both types of treatment with your school nurse.
- Decide with the school nurse on the best approach to the proposed health promotion session.

EYE CARE

In general, eye hygiene is part of the process of maintaining personal hygiene and practices from washing the area around the eyes with a clean face flannel through to using commercial products for cleansing lids and lashes (e.g. Lid-Care by CIBA Vision) and the removal of eye cosmetics is a matter for individual choice. The normal defence mechanisms of blinking and washing tears over the eye are sufficient to maintain healthy eyes. However, in health care particular groups of people can be at risk and need special eye hygiene care. These include:

- the newborn
- the unconscious person
- persons who have had an eye injury or surgery.

Although pupillary and corneal reflexes are present in the newborn infant, the tear glands do not begin to function properly until the infant is 2–4 weeks old. Particular risks for the newborn include ophthalmia neonatorum, an infectious conjunctivitis that needs specific treatment with antibiotic drops (guttae) or ointment (unguentum). The eyes are usually cleansed with sterile water before the insertion of drops or ointment. Conjunctivitis is common in infants and older children and the many different causes need specific treatments and eye hygiene measures (Wong et al 2003).

In the unconscious person, the corneal reflex is lost and the eyes may tend to remain open and become dry. Drying of the eyes can lead to corneal ulceration and subsequent loss of sight. Regular cleaning of the lids and lashes, the

---

Table 13.6 Lotion groups for treatment of head lice

Compound	Lotion	Limitations
Organochlorines	Lindane	Resistance is becoming widespread Not often used
Anticholinesterases	Malathion Carbaryl	Inactivated by heat, some hair products and chlorine from swimming pools Shampoos weaker than the lotions
Pyrethroids	Permethrin Phenothrin	Generally wide margin of safety Mild itching or burning Shampoos have been used successfully

installation of an eye lubricant, and keeping the eyes closed are necessary to prevent damage to the eyes.

Following eye surgery or eye injury specific hygiene practices are usually instigated by the specialist ophthalmic nurse, but a key role is in health promotion in order to prepare the patient for continuing self-care following discharge. As the eye is such a sensitive organ, self-care is often difficult to achieve, especially by the elderly and those who have difficulty in remembering instructions or in manipulating the dropper or the ointment tube. It is important to know and practice the correct technique and be able to educate relatives and friends to deliver the care (Marsden & Shaw 2003).

PROFESSIONAL AND ETHICAL KNOWLEDGE

The imagery and politics of hygiene care are important areas for discussion with a particular focus on the continuing role of nurses in decision making and controlling this area of their professional practice. Institutional care often removes choice and the patient's right to refuse care must be recognized despite creating ethical dilemmas in maintaining standards of care.

The words 'basic nursing care' have been adopted by nurses as synonymous with meeting the hygiene needs of patients. Dictionary meanings for the word 'basic' are given as 'forming the base or essence' or 'fundamental' (*Oxford English Dictionary* 1989). *The Essence of Care* is the title of the Department of Health's document outlining quality standards for care in core areas of nursing to include 'personal and oral hygiene' (Department of Health 2001). The dictionary also acknowledges a meaning for 'basic' which implies having relatively little value. Professionalization of nursing seems to have permitted the word 'basic' to become synonymous with the notion of being 'simple' or 'easy', thus implying a hierarchy of skills with 'technical' nursing skills where less body care is involved having greater importance and status (Lawlor 1991). Acceptance of the 'simple and easy' meaning allows this fundamental aspect of the professional nurse's role to be delegated to the most junior member of the nursing team or the unqualified nurse (Adams 1996, Pyle et al 1999). Hygiene care, however, remains a core activity for the development of knowledge and decision making within the domain of nursing practice.

Evidence based practice

Pyle et al (1999) found that most nursing staff considered oral hygiene an unpleasant activity and often delegated this task to untrained support workers or nursing assistants. They validated previous research carried out in Sweden by Wardh et al in 1997 where it was found that nursing assistants were most often involved in giving the care and they judged this activity to be repulsive.

THE RITUALIZATION OF HYGIENE CARE

The nursing profession has in the past been preoccupied with learning techniques for the delivery of hygiene care, in particular the bed bath. In the context of nursing within an institution there was a habit of giving hygiene care at a fixed time of the day (e.g. during the morning shift only) (Gibson et al 1997, Walsh & Ford 1990). These factors have led to the ritualization of hygiene care, particularly in an institutional context. Clients are often given little choice in how their individual preferences are met (Jones 1995) and nurses themselves accept hygiene care as a routine chore that requires little decision making.

Historically, Adams (1984) traces the obsessional concern of nurses for soap and water to aspects of institutional life bequeathed by the Poor Law. An immediate bath on admission was an institutional rule, part of an initiation ceremony. There were often 'bath teams', with each member of the team carrying out a specific task, for example one undresses, one baths and one dries. The general public regard 'frequency of bathing' as one of the main criteria for assessing standards of care for the elderly in community institutions. Being kept clean and looking clean is associated with being respectable. It may be that little has changed in long-term care for the elderly, as for this particular client group 'cleanliness is next to godliness'.

HYGIENE CARE AND THE IMAGE OF THE NURSE

According to Foucault (1975) when an individual becomes ill and enters an institution for care the boundaries of what might be considered normal in society are breached. This contention has particular implications for the breaking of the rules of privacy associated with the delivery of hygiene care. The body of the individual becomes 'objectified' in a way that allows healthcare professionals to observe and treat the individual without seemingly having to consider the emotions that body exposure may arouse both in the patient and in the nurse (Lawlor 1991, Seed 1995, Wolf 1997).

Nursing is also considered as 'dirty work' because it deals with the 'body' and body products. It is viewed as acceptable that people of low status should do this work and it has been argued historically that women are best suited to this type of care giving. Paradoxically the women (nurses) who administered body care were expected to be both morally and physically pure (Wolf 1986). The notion that nurses should be female is an extension of their roles as wives and mothers and this gives permission for intimate care.

However, sexual stereotypes of female nurses are perpetuated by the media and by film and TV dramas. These stereotypes can be selected by male patients and instigated as part of the banter with female nurses, especially when having to subject themselves to the intimacy of hygiene care. Wearing a uniform may be important not just for cross-infection protection, but also because it is symbolic in that it gives the nurse permission to administer intimate care (Edwards

1998, Seed 1995). In units where a uniform is not now worn, special garments such as plastic aprons may still be worn during the process of facilitating hygiene care.

There are equally powerful boundaries that the male nurse needs to cross in caring for female patients. The male nurse's role in giving hygiene care is more atypical of the accepted status quo in society in that nursing is seen in the context of 'motherhood', with a predominantly female profession giving intimate care. Therefore the need to seek permission may be more prominent when a male nurse seeks to give hygiene care to a female, especially if of a similar age. Seed (1995) found that male students were confronted with the feeling that they were doing something immoral in delivering intimate care to women.

According to Edwards (1998) age also has an impact with the older person submitting to intimate care as they no longer regard themselves as a symbol of sexual taboo. Edwards (1998) also found that staff of both genders felt uneasy when giving intimate care to the opposite gender of a similar age. This was reported to be the case whether staff were aged 20 or 50.

Evidence based practice

In Lawlor's (1991) classic study, she describes her research into body care by nurses. She shows from her interview data that nurses learn through experience to touch and handle other people's bodies in a way that is deemed non-sexual and minimizes embarrassment. Elements used to do this included defining the situation as a professional encounter, displaying a 'matter of fact' manner, careful use of language, avoiding overexposure of a body part, the use of humour to minimize embarrassment, and the expectation that the patient and the nurse will behave 'properly'.

CONSENT AND PRIVACY

Respect for privacy, dignity and patient autonomy is central to giving good quality hygiene care (Mattiasson & Hemberg 1998). The processes for obtaining informed consent for treatment are well established in law and in health care (see Ch. 2 on safety and risk and the Department of Health website). In accepting help with hygiene care, patients signify their implied consent through taking part in the process or submitting to the process (McHale et al 1998). However, in the confused or intellectually impaired, nurses may make decisions for patients based on what they believe is in their best interest. Behavioural problems can occur when patients are frightened by the bathing process and feel out of control (Hoeffer et al 1997). The dying patient may wish to be left alone and not be subjected to the daily traditional bath. In some cases nurses, instead of being the patient's advocate, may deliver hygiene care despite lack of implied consent or

even in the face of patient dissent in order to maintain the perceived professional standard of care (Lentz 2003).

Privacy and dignity are very important when giving intimate care especially with the sharing of facilities in an institution or even with interruptions of the process of giving hygiene care by other members of the multiprofessional team. Ensuring privacy is a key component in maintaining dignity. In a study on the meaning of dignity for patients and relatives, they indicated that being covered up and having the curtains drawn around during care activities is a very important example of ensuring individual respect and dignity (Gallagher & Seedhouse 2002).

Reflection and portfolio evidence

When in your practice placement in a healthcare institution reflect on the approaches taken to meet patients'/clients' hygiene needs.

- Note whether all hygiene care is delivered at a set time during the patients' day.
- Observe how nursing staff deal with the patient who is reluctant or refuses hygiene care when offered.
- Monitor your own behaviour and communication skills when approaching patients to offer assistance with hygiene.
- Record any interruptions to the process of giving hygiene care and note how this is handled in relation to maintaining patient privacy and dignity.
- Record your reflections and debate the issues with your peer group.

THE POLITICS OF HYGIENE CARE

Government policy for the past 30 years has focused on the premise that where at all possible the chronically sick, disabled and frail elderly should be cared for in their own homes. Although the burden for initial assessment of overall needs was transferred to the social worker through the Community Care Act 1990, since 1996 (under the Community Care Direct Payments Act 1996) control of finances to purchase services has become more patient/client and/or carer centred. The aim of the 1996 Act was to promote independence through encouraging partnership processes in the allocation and spending of funding on care packages. Clients should be able to make their own choices to meet their needs in innovative ways provided that these public funds are used effectively. Good partnership working between social services departments, local health and housing authorities and the client is vital in facilitating this scheme.

Although the initial assessment of care needs is completed by social workers with input from all members of the multiprofessional team, nurses are involved in the more detailed assessment and delivery of hygiene care needs.

There is an increase in day case surgery, early discharge from hospital policies and home treatment, even for acute illnesses. A large part of the overall workload of the professional nurse working in the community is the prioritization of patient needs often within a framework of diminishing resources. Generally, the actual delivery of hygiene care in the community, like institutions, is primarily undertaken by care assistants and is subject to strict budgetary limits. This leaves the biggest burden of care with relatives and friends or informal carers (Atkinson 1992). For informal carers there are major difficulties that need to be overcome. According to Atkinson (1992) these include:

- the physical cost of hygiene care – it can be heavy, time consuming and dangerous
- resouces (e.g. hoists and shower units) can be slow to arrive and suffer from cut-backs
- community nurse visits once a fortnight and then only if no relatives are available
- little instruction is given to carers about how best to manage – 'relatives have to rely on hints from neighbours'
- restricted entry into day centres, especially if in the middle of a 'career of disablement'
- carers are reluctant to ask for help outside the home even if experiencing considerable physical problems with giving care.

Attitudes to the importance of hygiene care are a factor in the allocation of resources. In order to rationalize resources, care assistants (CA) have been widely employed in various settings to help improve efficiency and reduce healthcare costs. This reflects the view that personal care tasks, such as bathing, dressing, and bed making, can be allocated to care assistants, leaving the registered nurse (RN) time to perform the more technical tasks such as assessment, drug administration and wound care. In practice, however, there is often overlap between the two roles, with CAs performing tasks deemed to be the domain of the RN and RNs continuing to engage in activities considered to be the responsibility of CAs (Thornley 2000). The nature of the RN role is all embracing and does not lend itself to being categorized into specific tasks (Perry et al 2003). However, in relation to the delivery of personal care, with current policy over costing in the UK there is a need to prioritize how RNs spend their time (Heath 2000). The delegation of 'the task' of the delivery of hygiene care should not detract from the accountability of the RN for the overall assessment of need and the quality of care delivered to patients/clients.

Decision making exercise

When making decisions about the allocation of nursing support for hygiene care within a system where resources are limited what should be the priority for the community nurse who has to make these decisions? Consider your answer by examining which of the following should take priority.

- Patient-defined needs.
- The nurse's perceptions of what the patient needs.
- The resources available.
- Debate your findings and also the political role of the nurse in advocating for resources.

The material presented in this chapter demonstrates the knowledge needed by the nurse in order to make decisions about hygiene care and work collaboratively with the multidisciplinary team.

PERSONAL AND REFLECTIVE KNOWLEDGE

The delivery of high standards of hygiene care requires the nurse to have detailed knowledge and skills and to be able to take appropriate and sensitive decisions in facilitating hygiene care for each individual client. Research based evidence is needed to set standards and the nurse should be actively engaged in reviewing and applying such evidence in daily practice. This chapter provides a starting point in the development of your knowledge, which needs to be constantly updated.

It is important to reflect, integrate and consolidate the knowledge gained from this chapter with the knowledge gained from your practice experience. This can be achieved through reflection on your own personal experiences and those of your peer group of students and through the case study work, which you can complete on your own or which may form the basis for a group seminar.

EXPERIENTIAL EXERCISES IN PRIVATE OR PRACTICUM

Learning about all aspects of hygiene care for all client groups is a fundamental part of any nursing course. Much of your practice experience is gained directly with patients or clients in partnership with an assigned clinical supervisor or mentor. Expert nurses forget how embarrassed a student may feel when they first have to deliver intimate hygiene care to a client and take for granted their own knowledge and skills in the delivery of hygiene care. Reflective notes made in a personal learning diary will be useful so that you can discuss your feelings later if you wish. Problems faced by students in the delivery of hygiene care are often not discussed (Seed 1995, Wolf 1997).

You may, however, get the opportunity to practice and reflect on your own personal feelings and reactions in the relatively safe environment of a 'practicum' or 'learning laboratory'. Experiential exercises in assessing 'the normal' in your fellow students and in providing hygiene advice and care to your fellow students under different circumstances will help you gain confidence in your own ability before being exposed to patients and clients.

These exercises are not so much concerned with the technique of delivery of hygiene care (although this can be included), but with issues surrounding the 'taken for granted' aspects of hygiene care delivery, especially in an institutional care setting. These exercises can form the basis for feedback within a group discussion session or for reflective notes in your journal or learning diary.

Examples of experiential exercises

1. Complete an oral assessment and give or facilitate oral care to your student partner who can 'role play' circumstances such as being confined to bed in the supine position, being paralysed, being blind, being non-cooperative and aggressive, being confused and unable to follow your instructions.
2. Reflect on your own needs while giving yourself a 'strip wash' at home. Consciously note the temperature of the water, how often you change it, how much soap and rinsing you like, what movements you use in washing, how much pressure you apply in drying your skin, and how you deal with cleansing your face, eyes and ears. Discuss your findings with your peers. Appraise how you may need to adapt personal habits to fit the needs of different client groups.
3. Experience the feeling of being helpless, dependent and embarrassed because someone else has to wash you through exercises in washing one another in the safe environment of a learning laboratory. Explore feelings around being washed by a member of the opposite sex.

CASE STUDIES IN GIVING HYGIENE CARE

The following case studies will help you consolidate knowledge gained through studying this chapter and completing any relevant reading outside the chapter content.

Case study: Learning disabilities

David Hargreaves, aged 25 years, has recently been discharged from a long stay hospital to the care of his ageing parents. He has been in institutional care for most of his life because of a severe learning disability. He is also physically disabled and requires much support and encouragement in maintaining his own hygiene care. He can wash his face and clean his teeth regularly, but it needs two people to give him full body hygiene care. His parents are finding it increasingly difficult to provide this care because of

their age and lack of strength. They had been waiting some years for a grant to make suitable alterations to their home that would allow them to have a purpose-designed shower unit built.

- What other information would you need in order to make decisions regarding responsibility for support and care for this family?
- How would you prioritize their needs?
- Who do you think has the ultimate responsibility for decisions about resourcing the needs of this family?

Case study: Mental health (and child)

Li is a second generation member of a Vietnamese family who have settled in England. She has married a fellow Vietnamese and has recently given birth to her second child, a daughter. Her son is 2 years old. Li had been depressed after the birth of her son and is beginning to show the same symptoms again. Her husband has become anxious as she is neglecting herself and the children. He has sought help from the health visitor (whom the family know) at the local health centre. Because her condition has deteriorated and it is difficult for her husband to cope with the newborn baby and his son, Li is admitted along with her two children to a special family unit that cares for women with postnatal depression.

- How might the needs of this family be assessed by the multidisciplinary team of the family unit?
- In relation to self-care, what strategies might be employed to encourage Li to care for her own hygiene needs initially?
- How much self-care might you expect Li's son to be able to perform for his stage of development?
- Are there any special cultural practices among Vietnamese people that the multidisciplinary team need to be sensitive to in relation to the hygiene practices of Li and her two children?
- On what basis might the multidisciplinary team make a decision that Li can return home with her two children?

Case study: Adult

John is a 75-year-old retired lecturer. He is married and has two sons who are also teachers. Three years ago he had a stroke, which has left him with weakness of the left arm and leg. He has been feeling weak and unwell for the past 3 months. He has lost his appetite and a considerable amount of weight. After a visit to his general practitioner he is admitted to an acute medical unit for investigation of his weight loss.

- What factors should be considered in assessing John's specific hygiene needs?
- When facilitating John's hygiene care, what other observations can be made by the nurse that will help with the overall assessment of John's problems?
- Because of weight loss, John's dentures are ill-fitting. Decide on the specific advice and care John may need in relation to his oral hygiene.

Case study: Child

Simon is 3 years old and has recently complained to his dad about pain on passing urine. He has not spoken at all about this to his mum and appeared acutely embarrassed when dad mentioned this problem. It is clear that Simon's mum will need to take him to see the family doctor since his dad will be unable to do this due to work commitments. Simon is diagnosed as having balinitis (infection under the foreskin). He is prescribed systemic antibiotics and his mother is advised to cleanse the area and apply an antiseptic cream. Simon is cared for by a childminder and his mum and dad.

- Initially what strategies could the mother be advised to use in order to introduce Simon to the idea of being seen and examined by the doctor? How would this advice relate to your role in dealing with children who need help with intimate hygiene care delivery in hospital?
- Consider the impact that this special hygiene care and treatment might have on Simon's privacy and dignity. How could he be helped to cope with the childminder administering this care?
- Simon becomes very interested in this 'new' aspect of hygiene and begins to retract his foreskin when using the toilet. How could his family manage this new habit?

Summary

This chapter has sought to draw together the knowledge and practice underpinning the delivery of high quality hygiene care. It has included:

1. An overview of applied biology related to the skin, the mouth, eyes and hair.
2. Insight into individual, cultural and spiritual norms related to personal hygiene habits and care.
3. An outline of issues in the assessment of hygiene needs with particular reference to total body care, oral and dental hygiene, hair infestation, and eye care.
4. A review of current methods for the delivery of hygiene care with discussion on their evidence base.
5. A discussion of the professional, ethical and political issues surrounding patterns for the delivery of hygiene care in institutions and in the community.
6. Raising awareness of the personal feelings that may arise when undertaking the intimate work involved in providing hygiene care.

Annotated further reading and websites

Bolander V 1994 Sorenson and Luckmann's basic nursing: a psychophysiologic approach, 3rd edn. Philadelphia, Saunders, Ch. 38
This chapter does not cover the actual techniques for delivering hygiene care. There are many textbooks on the market that will describe 'how to do it'. Sorenson and Luckmann's text is one that comprehensively covers all aspects of nursing care and is a very useful resource text, especially Chapter 38.

Griffiths J, Boyle S 1993 Colour guide to holistic oral care: a practical approach. Mosby, Aylesbury
Although this book was published in the early 1990s, overall it remains relevant and is a very good book for much more in-depth information on all aspects of oral and dental hygiene. Chapters focus on different client groups and their special needs and will be particularly useful when you move into your specialist branch of nursing.

Hinchliff S, Montague S, Watson R 1996 Physiology for nursing practice, 2nd edn. Baillière Tindall, London, Ch. 6.1
This well-produced second edition of a popular physiology book is a very good reference book for filling in the gaps on the biological basis of hygiene care and providing relevant material for most of the other chapters in this book.

Lawlor J 1991 Behind the screens: somology and the problems of the body. Churchill Livingstone, Edinburgh
Lawlor conducted her research in the Australian nursing context and her book is now a nursing classic. It is a very accessible, reflective and analytical account on all the rituals and practices that surround the personal and cultural management of the delivery of hygiene care in institutional settings.

Lupton D 1994 Medicine as culture: illness, disease and the body in western societies. Sage, London
For those interested in the sociology of health, disease and medicine this is an interesting book that provides many references for further reading for studying the sociology of health care in more depth. It includes chapters on power relations between medicine and nursing and also the feminist perspective on healthcare issues.

Wong D L, Hockenberry M J, Wilson D et al (eds) 2003 Whaley and Wong's Nursing care of infants and children, 7th edn. Mosby, St Louis
For students who wish to specialize in children's nursing, this book is a very comprehensive resource book for all aspects of infant, child and teenage care.

http://www.doh.gov.uk/essence of care/essence of care.pdf
The Department of Health site is useful as a key resource for all policy documents pertaining to health care in the UK. The Essence of Care document outlines the expected standards for quality practice. For this chapter refer to the two sections personal and oral hygiene, and privacy and dignity. You can obtain access to policy documents on community care through this site.

http://www.patient.co.uk/dental.htm
From this site you can access many key sites, for example: the British Dental Association Fact Files; British Dental Health Association; British Fluoridation Society; British Society for Disability and Oral Health. All these sites provide information to the public related to dental health and also provide access to policy reports related to the provision of dental care in the UK.

http://www.podiatryonline.com
This is a very useful resource site for information on foot care and conditions. Check in particular 'Best practice' portal to obtain access to 'Free patient handouts'. All conditions are explained in the same format with diagrams and photographs to illustrate the text.

http://www.hairscientists.org/index.htm
This site was set up by the Trichological Society formed in 1999 as 'the professional body for the advancement of hair sciences throughout the world'. It has a very helpful menu that covers basic information on 'hair' through to all the conditions associated with hair health.

http://www.patient.co.uk/eyecare.htm
This site provides a portal of entry to many Eye Health UK websites each site providing information on eye health care. Each address is annotated with the type of material found in that particular site.

Acknowledgement

Thanks to Beverley J. Smith, independent dental hygienist, for her specialist advice for the mouth and oral care section of this chapter.

References

Adams J 1984 Soap opera. Nursing Mirror 159(22):22, 31–32

Adams R 1996 Qualified nurses lack adequate knowledge related to oral health, resulting in inadequate oral care of patients on medical wards. Journal of Advanced Nursing 24:552–560

Atkinson F I 1992 Experience of informal carers providing nursing support for disabled dependents. Journal of Advanced Nursing 17:835–840

Bolander V 1994 Sorenson and Luckmann's Basic nursing: a psychophysiologic approach, 3rd edn. Saunders, Philadelphia

Bordo S 1990 Reading the slender body. In: Jacobus M, Keller E F, Shuttleworth S (eds) Body politics: women and the discourses of science. Routledge, London, pp 55–68

Calvert S, Fleming V 2000 Minimizing postpartum pain: a review of research pertaining to perineal care in childbearing women. Journal of Advanced Nursing 32(2):407–415

Cambridge P, Carnaby S 2000 Making it personal: providing intimate and personal care for people with intellectual disabilities. Pavilion, Brighton

Carnaby S, Cambridge P 2002 Getting personal: an exploratory study of intimate and personal care provision for people with profound and multiple intellectual disabilities. Journal of Intellectual Disability Research 46(2):120–132

Clore E R, Corey A 1991 Hair loss in children and adolescents. Journal of Pediatric Health Care 5(5):245–250

Coleman P 2002 Improving oral health care for the frail elderly: a review of widespread problems and best practices. Geriatric Nursing 23(4):189–199

Community Care Act 1990 HMSO, London

Community Care Direct Payments Act 1996. HMSO, London

Connolly M, Ross A M, Fleming D M et al 2002 Head lice infestation in the UK: is the incidence falling? British Journal of Dermatology 147 (Suppl. 62):49

Department of Health 2001 Essence of care: patient-focused benchmarking for health care practitioners. HMSO, London. Online. Available: http://www.doh.gov.uk 1 May 2003

Downs A M R, Stafford K A, Hunt L P et al 2002 Widespread insecticide resistance in head lice to the over-the-counter pediculocides in England, and the emergence of carbaryl resistance British Journal of Dermatology 146(1):88–93

Edwards S C 1998 An anthropological interpretation of nurses' and patients' perceptions of the use of space and touch. Journal of Advanced Nursing 28(4):809–817

Eilers J, Berger A M, Peterson M C 1988 Development, testing and application of the oral assessment guide. Oncology Nursing Forum 15(3):325–330

Encarta 2001 Microsoft Corporation, Seattle. CD-ROM. http://www.microsoft.com/encarta/eng

Evans G 2001 A rationale for oral care. Nursing Standard 15(43):33–36

Field A, Reid B 2002 An analysis of an audit tool of ward-based practice. Nursing Standard 16(40):37–39

Fitzpatrick J 2000 Oral health care needs of dependent older people: responsibilities of nurses and care staff. Journal of Advanced Nursing 32(6):1325–1332

Foucault M 1975 The birth of the clinic: an archeology of medical perception. Vintage, New York

Frenkel H, Newcombe R 2001 Improving oral health in institutionalized elderly people by educating caregivers: a randomized controlled trial. Community Dental and Oral Epidemiology 29:289–297

Gallagher A, Seedhouse D 2002 Dignity in care: the views of patients and relatives. Nursing Times 98(43):38–40

George M 1995 A feat for nursing? Nursing Standard 9(31):22

Gibson F, Horsford J, Nelson W 1997 Oral care: ritualistic practice reconsidered within a framework of action research. Journal of Cancer Nursing 1:183–190

Griffiths J, Boyle S 1993 Colour guide to holisitic oral care: a practical approach. Mosby, Aylesbury

Hancock I, Bowman A, Prater D 2000 The day of the soft towel? Comparison of the current bed bathing method with the soft towel bed bathing method. International Journal of Nursing Practice 6(4):207–213

Heanue M, Deacon S A, Deery C et al 2003 Manual versus powered toothbrushing for oral, health (Cochrane Review). Cochrane Library, Issue 2. Update Software, Oxford. Online. Available: http://www.cochrane.org

Heath H 2000 Defining nursing and personal care. Elderly Care 12:26–27

Helman C 2001 Culture, health and illness, 4th edn. Butterworth-Heinemann, Oxford

Hinchliff S, Montague S, Watson R 1996 Physiology for nursing practice, 2nd edn. Baillière Tindall, London

Hoeffer B, Rader J, McKenzie D et al 1997 Reducing aggressive behavior during bathing cognitively impaired nursing home residents. Journal of Gerontology Nursing 23(5):16–23

Holmes S, Mountain E 1993 Assessment of oral status: evaluation of three oral assessment guides. Journal of Clinical Nursing 2:35–40

Ibarra J 1995 A non-drug approach to treating head lice. Community Nurse (Nurse Prescriber) 1(25):25, 27

Jenkins D A 1989 Oral care in the ICU: an important nursing role. Nursing Standard 4(7):24–28

Jones A 1995 Reflective process in action: the uncovering of the ritual of washing in clinical nursing practice. Journal of Clinical Nursing 4(5):283–288

Joyner M 1988 Hair care in the black patient. Journal of Pediatric Health Care 2(6):281–287

Kovach C R, Meyer-Arnold E A 1996 Coping with conflicting agendas: the bathing experience of cognitively impaired older adults. Scholarly Inquiry for Nursing Practice 10(1):23–42

Lawlor J 1991 Behind the screens: somology and the problems of the body. Churchill Livingstone, Edinburgh

Lentz J 2003 Daily baths: torment or comfort at end of life? Journal of Hospice and Palliative Nursing 5(1):34–39

Lupton D 1994 Medicine as culture: illness, disease and the body in western societies. Sage, London

McHale J, Tingle J, Peysner J 1998 Law and nursing. Butterworth Heinemann, London

Marinho V C C, Higgins J P T, Logan S et al 2003 Fluoride toothpastes for preventing dental caries in children and adolescents (Cochrane Review). Cochrane Library, Issue 2. Update Software, Oxford. Online. Available: http://www.cochrane.org

Marsden J, Shaw M 2003 Correct administration of topical eye treatment. Nursing Standard 17(30):42–44

Mattiasson A, Hemberg M 1998 Intimacy: meeting needs and respecting privacy in the care of elderly people. Nursing Ethics 5(6):527–534

Miller M, Kearney N 2001 Oral care for patients with cancer: a review of the literature. Cancer Nursing 24(4):241–254

Moore J 1995 Assessment of nurse-administered oral hygiene. Nursing Times 91(9):40–41

O'Donnovan S 1992 Simon's nursing assessment. Nursing Times 88(2):30–33

Oxford English Dictionary 1989 2nd edn. Clarendon Press, Oxford

Pearson L 1996 A comparison of the ability of foam swabs and toothbrushes to remove dental plaque: implications for nursing practice. Journal of Advanced Nursing 23(1):62–69

Perry M, Carpenter I, Challis D et al 2003 Understanding the roles of registered general nurses and care assistants in UK nursing homes. Journal of Advanced Nursing 42(5):497–505

Plastow L, Luthra M, Powell R et al 2001 Head lice infestation: bug busting vs. traditional treatment. Journal of Clinical Nursing 10(6):775–782

Price S, Price L 1995 Aromatherapy for health professionals. Churchill Livingstone, Edinburgh

Pyle M A, Nelson S, Sawyer D R 1999 Nursing assistants' opinions of oral health care provision. Special Care in Dentistry 19:112–117

Roberts R J, Casey D, Morgan D A et al 2000 Comparison of wet combing with malathion for treatment of head lice in the UK: a pragmatic randomized controlled trial. Lancet 356:540–544

Roe B, Whattam M, Young H et al 2001 Elders' perceptions of formal and informal care: aspects of getting and receiving help for their activities of daily living. Journal of Clinical Nursing 10(3):398–405

Roper N, Logan W, Tierney A 1996 The elements of nursing, 4th edn. Churchill Livingstone, Edinburgh

Sampson A C 1982 The neglected ethic: cultural and religious factors in the care of patients. McGraw–Hill, London

Seed A 1995 Crossing the boundaries: experiences of neophyte nurses. Journal of Advanced Nursing 21:1136–1143

Simons D, Kidd E A M, Beighton D 1999 Oral health of elderly occupants in residential homes. Lancet 353:1761

Sreebny L M 1997 A reference guide to drugs and dry mouth. Gerodontology 14:33–47

Stiefel K, Damron S, Sowers N 2000 Improving oral hygiene for the seriously ill patient: implementing research-based practice. Medsurg Nursing 9:40–43, 46

Taintor J F, Taintor M J 1997 The complete guide to better dental care. Facts on File, New York

Thornley C 2000 A question of competence? Re-evaluating the roles of the nursing auxiliary and health care assistant in the NHS. Journal of Clinical Nursing 9:451–458

Tiran D 1996 Aromatherapy in midwifery practice. Baillière Tindall, London

Vigarello G 1988 Concepts of cleanliness: changing attitudes in France since the Middle Ages (transl J Birrell). Cambridge University Press, Cambridge

Walsh M, Ford P 1990 Nursing rituals, research and rational actions. Butterworth-Heinemann, London

Wardh I, Andersson L, Sorensen S 1997 Staff attitudes to oral health care: a comparative study of registered nurses, nursing assistants and home care aides. Gerodontology 14:28–32

Wilson M 1986 Personal cleanliness. Journal of Clinical Practice, Education and Management 3(2):80–82

Wolf Z R 1986 Nursing work: the sacred and profane. Holistic Nursing Practice 1(1):29–35

Wolf Z R 1997 Nursing students' experience bathing patients for the first time. Nurse Educator 22(2):41–46

Wong D L, Hockenberry M J, Wilson D et al (eds) 2003 Whaley and Wong's Nursing care of infants and children, 7th edn. Mosby, St Louis

Wright L 1990 Bathing by towel. Nursing Times 86(4):36–39

Xavier G 2000 The importance of mouth care in preventing infection. Nursing Standard 14(18):47–51

Chapter 14

Skin integrity

Kerry Lewis and Lorraine Roberts

KEY ISSUES

SUBJECT KNOWLEDGE
- Structure and function of the skin
- Ageing and the skin
- Wound healing processes
- Importance of appearance
- Cultural influences related to skin care and adornment

CARE DELIVERY KNOWLEDGE
- Assessment of the skin
- Assessment and management of a person with a wound
- Evaluation of the effectiveness of wound management
- Management of acute and chronic wounds

PROFESSIONAL AND ETHICAL KNOWLEDGE
- Nurse's role in promoting skin health
- Nurse's role in developing and maintaining quality systems of care
- The developing role of the nurse in skin integrity: clinical, educational, professional and ethical consideration for practice

PERSONAL AND REFLECTIVE KNOWLEDGE
- Reflective diary
- Case studies

INTRODUCTION

The skin or integument is a major organ of the body, providing a barrier between the internal and external environments. It is also an organ that is highly visible to others, and therefore any damage, alteration or deformity in its structure can cause not only physical, but also psychological, social and environmental problems. Skin integrity is concerned with the maintenance of this barrier in its optimum condition.

The aim of this chapter is to provide the requisite knowledge and decision making skills to enable the nurse, within the limitations of his or her role, to care for patients with skin problems. It also intends to help nurses to reflect on current practice relating to skin care and encourage the maintenance of their own skin health.

OVERVIEW

Subject knowledge

The biological section covers basic anatomy and physiology of the skin. The level addressed is related to the knowledge you need in order to understand and apply the information that appears in this chapter. A more in-depth knowledge can be gained by reading specific anatomy and physiology books. The process of skin healing will be explored.

The importance of appearance and its effect on self-image is highlighted in the psychosocial section. Cultural influences are included and you are encouraged to reflect on how your own self-image is at times affected by your appearance.

Care delivery knowledge

Assessment of the skin is discussed. The knowledge, skills and understanding required to assess, plan, implement and evaluate the care of patients with wounds are addressed in broad terms. This is followed by a more in-depth discussion of the management of three common types of wound.

Professional and ethical knowledge

The contribution of nurses to the development of quality systems of care relating to skin integrity is explored. The need for and opportunities available to nurses in the development of their knowledge and expertise in relation to different aspects of skin care are examined. Clinical, educational, professional and ethical considerations for practice regarding the evolving role of the nurse in tissue viability are highlighted.

Personal and reflective knowledge

In this section you are encouraged to learn from your practice experience through suggested portfolio activities related to the types of skin conditions and wounds you see in practice.

Consolidation of your learning from the chapter and from practice experience is achieved through completing decision making exercises based on four case studies.

On page 326 there are four case studies, each relating to one of the branch programmes. You may find it helpful to read one of them before you start the chapter, and use it as a focus for your reflections while reading.

SUBJECT KNOWLEDGE

BIOLOGICAL

STRUCTURE OF THE SKIN

The skin is one of the largest organs in the body. An adult's skin covers an area of about $2\,m^2$ and weighs approximately 4.5–5 kg. Every square centimetre of skin contains approximately 125 sweat glands, 25 sebaceous glands, 250 nerve endings, 50 sensors to pain, pressure, heat and cold, approximately 1 m of blood vessels, and millions of cells. Skin is made up of three main structures (Fig. 14.1):

- the epidermis or outer layer
- the dermis or base layer
- the skin appendages such as hairs, nails and glands.

These structures are also termed the integumentary system.

Epidermis

The epidermis is the outer or cuticle layer of the skin, and consists of several layers of cells. It contains no blood vessels or nerve endings and its main function is to protect the underlying dermis. It has four or five different layers of cells depending on its location. From the deepest to the most superficial these are:

- stratum basale (or germinating layer)
- stratum spinosum
- stratum granulosum
- stratum lucidum (not present on hairy skin)
- stratum corneum (or cornified layer).

The cells in the stratum basale undergo mitosis and reproduce themselves. This enables the skin to repair itself when injured, and ensures an effective barrier against infection. As new cells are produced, they migrate to the surface of the skin. During this movement the cells' normal cytoplasm is replaced by keratin, a waterproof substance which

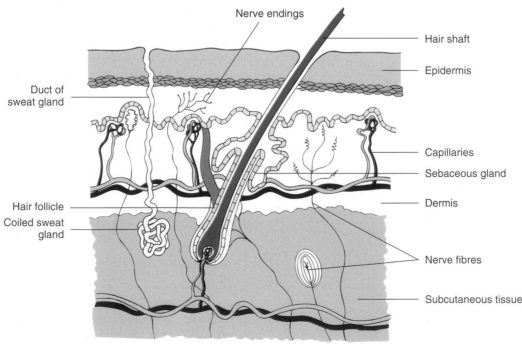

Figure 14.1 Section through the skin. (After Cull 1989.)

gives the external layer of skin, the stratum corneum, its tough protective quality.

The greater part of the epidermis is made up of keratinocytes, the cells that produce the outer surface of the skin. Scattered among these cells are two other types of cells known as melanocytes and Langerhans' cells.

Melanocytes are responsible for producing melanin, which produces the skin's pigmentation or colouring. White- and black-skinned people have the same number of melanocytes per unit of surface area, but in black-skinned people the melanocytes are more active and produce pigment at a faster rate. Melanin protects other cells of the skin against the damaging effects of strong sunlight. Exposure of the skin to the sun stimulates the melanocytes to produce more melanin. This reaction causes the characteristic darkening of the skin (suntanning). Black-skinned people are therefore better protected against the sun's ultraviolet rays.

Overexposure to sunlight can cause sunburn and skin cancers such as malignant melanomas and non-melanotic skin cancers (NMSC), primarily basal cell and squamous cell cancers. The number of people developing skin cancers in England has been rising rapidly in recent years. The Office for National Statistics (1996) has produced tables to highlight the increase in malignant melanomas since 1971. The figure shows an increase in males from 2 in 100 000 in 1971 to 7 in 100 000 in 1996. The increase in females over the corresponding years is from 3 in 100 000 to 9 in 100 000. The incidence has increased to a greater extent than mortality, mainly due to improvements in treatment and earlier detection.

Evidence based practice

The Office for National Statistics (1996) highlighted the rise in malignant melanomas. These cancers can generally be avoided if people protect their skin and avoid getting sunburn. The increase in incidence is thought to be due to intermittent sun exposure of untanned skin during holidays and other outside activities.

Langerhans' cells are thought to be important in the body's immune responses. They absorb small particles of foreign material such as nickel in jewellery and are responsible for setting up the allergic reaction common in contact allergic eczema (dermatitis). The resultant rash usually clears up within 1 week following removal of the irritant once it has been identified. The key to managing this condition in the long term lies in identifying and avoiding contact with the allergen.

Dermis

The dermis is the deepest layer of the skin. It is composed mainly of connective tissue and contains fewer cells than the epidermis, the main ones being fibroblasts, which produce collagen, a protein that attaches the skin layers to the rest of the body with tiny elastic fibres. These fibres give the skin its suppleness and ability to stretch. The upper part of the dermis contains rows of projections known as dermal papillae, which bind the two layers of skin together at the dermal–epidermal junction. The dermis contains a good blood supply and is responsible for nourishing and maintaining the epidermis, which does not have its own blood supply. The dermis also contains sensory receptors to heat, cold, touch and pain.

Glands

Three types of glands are present in the skin:

- Sebaceous or oil glands secrete an oily substance known as sebum, which lubricates and protects hair and skin.
- Sudoriferous or sweat glands assist in the regulation of body temperature through evaporation.
- Ceruminous glands produce cerumen or wax, which is found within the outer ear where it protects the ear by preventing the entry of foreign bodies.

Information on hair and nails can be found in Chapter 13 on hygiene care.

FUNCTIONS OF THE SKIN

The skin has five main functions.

Regulation of temperature

The production of sweat by the sudoriferous glands during hot weather helps reduce the body temperature through a process of evaporation. Changes in blood flow also occur. During hot weather peripheral blood vessels dilate, enabling heat loss by radiation. Conversely, in cold weather peripheral blood vessels constrict in order to maintain vital organs at an optimum temperature for functioning (see Ch. 6 on homeostasis).

Protection

The skin provides a physical barrier against harm, protecting the underlying tissues from abrasion and bacterial invasion. The melanin prevents damage from the sun's ultraviolet rays and the waterproof quality of the skin stops excessive loss of body fluid.

Excretion

Sweat contains water, salts, urea, ammonia and several other compounds. During sweating small amounts of these substances are excreted.

Stimuli reception

The skin contains many different types of receptors. The most common are receptors to temperature, pain and touch. These provide information about the external environment.

Synthesis of vitamin D

The skin aids in the synthesis of vitamin D. The precursor to vitamin D, 7-dehydrocholesterol, is present in the skin and is converted to cholecalciferol in the presence of ultraviolet light. After further conversion in the liver and then the kidneys, 1,25-dihydroxycalciferol is produced. This aids in the absorption of calcium from the dietary intake.

Tortora (1999) identifies two further functions of the skin: immunity, due to the action of the Langerhans' cells; and as a blood reservoir, due to the ability to divert blood to muscles during exercise through vasoconstriction.

AGEING AND THE SKIN

During an individual's lifespan, changes occur in the physical properties of the skin. In order to maintain healthy skin different requirements must be met at different stages of an individual's life. For instance, during infancy the skin is delicate and until the child is continent the skin requires protection from the damaging effects of urine and faeces. Similarly, during adolescence skin changes result in increased perspiration and oil production, sometimes leading to the development of acne.

During pregnancy there is an increase in activity of the sebaceous glands and melanocytes, resulting in increased oil production and patches of darker pigmentation on the skin – commonly linea nigra, which is a pigmented line down the abdomen, and chloasma, which are darker areas on the face often referred to as the 'mask of pregnancy'. Although the skin has the ability to stretch, during pregnancy the increase in size of the abdomen can be so great that the collagen fibres rupture, leaving visible scars. These are known as striae gravidarum or 'stretch marks'.

In old age, the production of cells slows down and they become smaller and thinner. The collagen and elastic fibres lose their shape and elasticity, and the amount of fat stored in the subcutaneous tissues lessens, resulting in skin wrinkles. There is a decrease in the number and an increase in the size of active melanocytes, producing concentrated areas of pigment commonly known as liver spots. There is also a reduction in the amount of intracellular fluid resulting in dry skin, which can lead to itching or 'senile pruritus', and increased skin fragility. The use of moisturizers or emollients can help to prevent excessive flakiness of skin.

For many people the desire to preserve a youthful complexion brings with it the necessity of a continued battle against the ageing process. There is, however, a marked difference in deterioration of skin through the normal ageing process and that caused by exposure to ultraviolet light (photoageing). Photoaged skin is lax in appearance and may have uneven pigmentation and generally is wrinkled with the appearance of leather (Fisher et al 1997). Although creams and lotions may result in a superficial improvement in skin texture altered by normal ageing, cosmetic surgery is becoming more and more popular. Protection of the skin against sun damage from an early age is the only way to combat photoageing. Prevention is better than a cure.

Decision making exercise

Liza Gordon is an 18-year-old student who enjoys holidays abroad with her friends. She has been admitted to the day care ward for a biopsy of a 'suspicious' mole, which turned out to be benign. Liza is very concerned about her appearance and is anxious to protect her skin against sun damage and the long-term effects of ageing.

- What skin care advice would you give to Liza before discharge?
- Read Chapter 5 of *Health Promotion: Foundations for Practice* (Naidoo & Wills 2000), in which the authors discuss the five approaches to health promotion (i.e. medical, behavioural change, educational, empowerment and social change). Which approach do you consider would be most effective in helping Liza to maintain skin health in the long term?

SKIN HEALING

Should the skin become cut or damaged, creating a wound, the process of healing has four distinct phases:

- coagulation
- inflammation
- regeneration
- maturation.

Skin heals by primary or secondary intention.

Primary intention

This type of healing occurs when the edges of the wound are opposed, as in a surgical incision. Healing tends to be rapid due to the close proximity of the wound edges (Fig. 14.2), and involves:

- coagulation – within 8 hours following surgery the cut surfaces become inflamed, a blood clot fills the incision track, and phagocytes and fibroblasts migrate into the area
- inflammation – phagocytes begin to break down the clot, and cell debris and collagen fibres are produced by the fibroblasts and begin to bind the two surfaces together
- regeneration – after 3–4 days epithelial cells spread across the incision track, the section of clot above the new

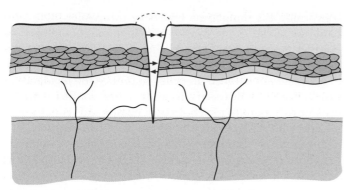

Figure 14.2 Wound healing by primary intention. The wound edges are in close proximity (often brought together by sutures). Healing occurs rapidly along the length of the wound.

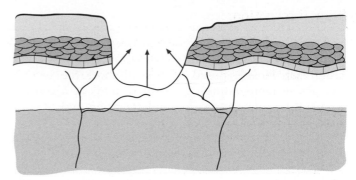

Figure 14.3 Wound healing by secondary intention. The wound edges are distanced due to crater formation. Healing is slower and begins at the bottom of the crater.

cells becomes a scab, the clot in the incision track is absorbed, and myofibroblasts draw the edges of the wound together by a process of contraction
* maturation – epithelial cells continue to be laid down until the full thickness of skin is restored.

Secondary intention

This type of healing occurs where there is a significant loss of tissue or where the skin edges are not opposed, as in an ulcer. Healing tends to be slower, but the exact time will depend on the extent of the damage (Fig. 14.3). It involves:

* coagulation – the surface of the wound becomes acutely inflamed and phagocytes start to break down the necrotic tissue
* inflammation – granulation tissue develops at the base of the wound and starts to grow up towards the wound surface
* regeneration – phagocytosis causes the necrotic tissue to separate, exposing a new layer of epidermal cells, and contraction occurs to reduce the size of the wound (as wound contraction is a normal process, it is important not to pack the wound with dressings unless specifically indicated, for example for a wound sinus, as it interferes with this process)
* maturation – when granulation tissue fills the wound cavity and reaches the level of the dermis, epithelial cells migrate across the wound towards the centre, forming a single layer of cells. Epithelialization continues until full-thickness skin is restored.

Benbow (2002) uses the term 'tertiary healing' to describe a wound where there is a significant delay between injury and wound closure; for example, extensive tissue loss or dehiscence. Bale & Jones (1997) use a similar term, 'healing by third intention', to identify a wound containing a foreign body or infection that is left open until the problem has been resolved. Whether this is truly a separate and distinctive type of healing is a matter of debate.

THE OPTIMUM ENVIRONMENT FOR WOUND HEALING

A variety of factors need to be present to create the optimum environment for wound healing to take place. These include:

* a good blood supply
* optimum temperature
* moisture
* oxygen
* freedom from contaminants and necrotic tissue.

Blood supply

Healing requires an integral blood supply to provide oxygen and nutrients to the developing cells. Reconstitution of the blood supply is termed angiogenesis and occurs during the regeneration phase of healing. Care must be taken not to disturb this process by the inappropriate use of dressings; for example dry dressings such as gauze can stick to wound beds, resulting in trauma when they are removed.

Evidence based practice

Thomas & Loveless (1997) present a comparison of the properties of 12 different hydrocolloid dressings that looks at:

* thickness
* fluid handling properties
* moisture vapour permeability
* conformability
* acidity/alkalinity of extract
* fluid retention/gel cohesion.

This comparison of data should help the nurse to choose the appropriate dressing from a range of similar items. Remember that patient choice and the availability of dressings will also be factors in providing evidence based care.

Temperature

The optimum temperature for human cell growth is 37°C. Wounds kept at a constant temperature of 37°C will heal faster than those exposed to thermal shock (i.e. extreme changes in temperature). To keep wounds at a constant temperature, unnecessary wound cleansing and dressing changes should be avoided.

Moisture

The exudate produced by a wound contains nutrients, enzymes and growth factors that can aid the healing process. Lytic enzymes found in the exudate autolyse (break down) any necrotic tissue present, and growth factors increase the development rate of cells and result in less scarring.

A moist wound environment facilitates wound healing, reduces the amount of tissue inflammation, produces less scarring and results in less pain for the patient. If the wound is allowed to dry out, a scab or eschar forms. This impedes cell migration and consequently slows down the healing process. Excessive exudate may indicate that the wound is still in the inflammatory stage, which may suggest the presence of infection. It needs to be contained to prevent damage to the surrounding skin.

Oxygen

All cells require oxygen in order to develop and mature. An integral blood supply is therefore essential to ensure that cells receive an adequate oxygen supply in order to remain viable. The external administration of oxygen to the wound site, for example via an oxygen mask and tubing, will not benefit tissue perfusion, but will dry the wound site and delay wound healing.

Freedom from contaminants and necrotic tissue

The presence of foreign bodies and dead or devitalized tissue delays wound healing and provides a focus for infection, which will in turn also delay wound healing.

PSYCHOSOCIAL

THE IMPORTANCE OF APPEARANCE

Physical appearance is important to most people. As the skin is visible to others, its condition often influences how an individual feels about him or herself. People who feel attractive often feel positive about themselves.

Images in the media of suntanned, high profile individuals such as fashion models may help to encourage the idea that a suntan is both healthy and desirable. Accordingly, suntanned skin can promote a sense of psychological well-being. As a consequence, despite current health education concerning the dangerous effects of ultraviolet light, sunbathing – either in natural or artificial sunlight – remains a popular pastime. The Department of Health (1993: 67) recognizes the need to 'secure an alteration in people's attitude to a tanned appearance' in order to reduce the incidence of skin cancer. It is necessary to address the conflict between the improvement to psychological health and its detrimental effect on an individual's physical health. Gross (1992: 532) examines Festinger's theory of cognitive dissonance. Cognitive dissonance is a state of 'psychological discomfort and tension' caused by a person knowing that an action may cause harm, but at the same time participating in that action. Gross puts forward a way of choosing between two activities that are equally attractive. This involves highlighting the undesirable features of each activity in order to help with the decision making process. Although this may help in deciding whether or not to sunbathe, it must be acknowledged that an individual may still decide that the psychological benefits of sunbathing are more important and therefore continue the activity.

Reflection and portfolio evidence

You may wish to extend your personal reflection here into a debate with your fellow students on the choices to be made.

- Is an individual's psychological or physical health more important?
- If it is necessary to make one dimension of health a priority, which would take priority for you at a personal level? Justify your decision.
- In your practice placement review the above debate in relation to one patient or client.
- Record key points in your debate and your conclusions in your portfolio.

Although the nurse should aim towards holistic care, there are times in a person's life when choices have to be made. The nurse has an important role in helping the individual decide whether the psychological or the physical dimension of health should take priority.

Just as a healthy skin can help to promote a positive self-image, a skin disorder can have a detrimental effect. For thousands of years skin disorders have often been regarded as unclean: lepers, for instance, have often been treated as social outcasts. It may be argued that certain more common skin disorders continue to evoke a less than compassionate reaction nowadays, particularly those that are visible, such as eczema or psoriasis. The impact of a skin disorder on a person's self-image can depend very much on the individual's ability to cope with it. If the disorder affects the person's ability to carry out and meet their self-care needs, or if it causes stress to the individual or the family, it can seriously undermine their self-regard. The disorder can come to be viewed in a way that is out of all proportion to the problem itself and overshadow the individual's entire life.

Self-image

It is important to understand that the nurse's approach can have a significant effect on how the client responds to a skin disorder. Any signs of disgust, alarm or even fear may encourage the client to view their condition as offensive to others. Furthermore, the nurse needs to be aware of any signals that may be conveyed to the client. With thought, the nurse can project and encourage a more positive self-image. If the skin disorder is not infectious and does not require the use of gloves when handling, the client's self-image can be enhanced if the nurse touches the affected area with unprotected hands. In addition, the client will benefit from being able to discuss any feelings about the condition with both relatives and the nurse. Moreover, a simple explanation of the aetiology (cause), and prognosis (probable course) of the condition may help the client to accept it. Some conditions of the skin, for example burns, ulceration and extensive surgery, can cause great distress to both the client and the nurse. In order to help the client accept the condition, the nurse will first need to come to terms with it him or herself.

Exposure therapy

There are two distinct ways to help a client come to terms with any bodily disfigurement: gradual exposure and confrontation (see the section on desensitization in Ch. 19 where the terms 'graded exposure' and 'flooding' are used).

Gradual exposure

This is a process by which a client is gradually exposed to a disfigurement over an extended period of time, in order to give him or her time to accept it. In the case of a patient who has undergone a mastectomy, for instance, the patient can first of all be shown the dressing so that she can get used to the size of the wound. The dressing can then be removed and the patient given time to come to terms with the appearance of the wound. This gradual exposure continues at a rate with which the patient can cope. It has been argued, however, that the gradual exposure of a disfigurement subconsciously compounds the view that it is offensive to others.

Confrontation

The confrontational approach proposes that the patient should be encouraged to come to terms with the disfigurement quickly and that such an approach is, in the long term, less traumatic. The confrontational approach aims to encourage a frank and open technique, with exposure taking place as quickly as the patient can tolerate (Marks 1987). It can be argued, however, that patients need more time to adapt to physical change. Moreover, nursing and medical

staff may be unable to provide the degree of support necessary if the patient has to adjust rapidly to a new body image.

CULTURE AND APPEARANCE

Different cultures have very different approaches to and ideas about physical appearance. What is considered to be attractive in one culture may be regarded as physically unattractive in another. While a suntanned appearance may be desirable in western culture, some eastern cultures, notably Japan, may favour an altogether paler complexion. The traditional 'geisha' look was originally achieved using face-whitening powder from dried nightingale droppings.

Some cultures use skin decoration to produce the opposite effect. The Tuareg paint their skin with turmeric to make themselves less desirable and therefore less vulnerable to evil spirits. In Ethiopia, the Surma women insert clay discs into their lower lip to cause it to protrude. It is thought that this was first done to make the women less desirable to slave traders.

Beauty is a matter of subjective judgement (i.e. 'beauty is in the eye of the beholder'). To some extent, the skin plays an important part in the perception of an individual's attractiveness, and for hundreds of years has been decorated in many ways to enhance or diminish its appeal.

Cosmetics

These are used to accentuate attractive facial features and disguise imperfections. In many cultures they have religious significance; for example, in Hindu society three stripes painted across the forehead signify a holy devotee of the Lord Shiva (Jacobson 1992).

Decorative tattoos

These have developed from ancient origins and are often related to religious ceremonies and marriage rites. Tattoos involve staining of the skin with coloured pigments, and should be considered permanent. They often result in stereotyping the wearer and several articles highlight the problems wearers come up against (Armstrong et al 2000, Cronin 2001, Stuppy et al 1998). In recent years the number of people with tattoos has risen sharply, as they have become a fashion accessory for both males and females. Most noticeable was the increase in the number of adolescents having tattoos (Chivers 2002). As a result there has been a corresponding increase in the number of people requesting tattoo removal as the novelty factor wore off.

Decision making exercise

During a trip to the seaside, Mandy, a student nurse aged 18, had a large tattoo put onto her right upper forearm. The tattoo is of a large red heart with the name of her current boyfriend etched through the centre. She did not tell anyone of her intention to do this. The tattooed area is very sore and Mandy is a little concerned about how she will cope on night duty that evening.

- Decide on the possible short- and long-term implications of Mandy's actions.
- The next morning Mandy is very tearful and regretful, and as you come on duty she takes you to one side and asks you what she can do about the tattoo. What advice would you give her?
- How do you think patients may react to Mandy given that they may have particular views of what is acceptable in the visual appearance of nurses?

Tribal markings

These are a form of tattooing where patterns are cut directly into the skin. They often hold religious significance or show membership of a particular tribe or group. They are deemed to be an essential feature of some cultures and are considered attractive in both males and females.

Piercing

There has been a huge increase in the popularity of body piercing. Ears, nose, navel, eyebrows and nipples have all been subject to this trend and have become fashion statements, particularly among teenagers and young adults (see section on annotated further reading: Chivers 2002).

Skin adornments, particularly tattoos and body piercing, have implications for healthcare workers.

CARE DELIVERY KNOWLEDGE

Problems affecting skin integrity are wide-ranging, varying for example from nappy rash to disfiguring wounds. Although core areas of knowledge and skills such as the prevention of cross-infection and asepsis are applicable in many instances, the management of specific skin conditions and disorders may demand more specific expertise. The role of the nurse will differ according to the type and extent of the skin problem. For instance, when caring for an adult with a chronic skin condition such as atopic eczema, the focus of the nurse's role will primarily be that of a health promoter, empowering the individual to manage and live with his or her condition.

The wide range of conditions and possible therapeutic interventions prohibit detailed discussion of every example. Instead, the following discussion focuses on a general assessment of skin, and then on one of the common problems of skin integrity, namely wounds. The many common skin

conditions cannot be dealt with in this chapter as they are numerous and demand a specialist knowledge base in dermatology nursing.

ASSESSMENT OF THE SKIN

Assessment of the skin not only gives an indication of the condition of the skin itself, but can also help in identifying the client's physical health, emotional state and lifestyle. As assessment is undertaken in circumstances other than those purely related to problems of skin integrity, it will be discussed as a separate entity. Assessment requires close observation of the skin and includes visual inspection, palpation and noting skin odour. In addition, it is important to ask the client questions about his or her skin. Good illumination is necessary, and if there is any discharge from skin lesions, the nurse should wear disposable examination gloves. Above all, it is important that the nurse employs a sensitive approach and respects the dignity and privacy of the client.

Assessment of the skin should include observation of each of the following aspects of the skin:

- colour
- temperature
- moisture
- texture
- thickness
- turgor
- the presence of blemishes and lesions.

Evidence based practice

Phillips (2001) discusses the opinion of a group of European experts on the role of natural rubber latex (NRL) in latex allergy. The European Commission requested the report by the Scientific Committee on Medicinal Products and Medical Devices, produced in 2000.

Key points arising from the report as Phillips (2001) highlights are:

- Medical devices made from NRL, such as latex gloves, can cause allergic reactions and have the potential in sensitive individuals to cause type 1 (life-threatening) reactions.
- Risk groups for latex allergy include individuals who are predisposed to allergy and those who are frequently in contact with latex gloves, such as healthcare professionals and patients requiring multiple surgery.
- Avoidance of latex allergy or latex allergic contact dermatitis can be facilitated by the use of products with low amounts of allergenic proteins and sensitizing chemicals.
- Latex sensitive individuals must avoid direct contact with NRL. Product information detailing ingredients/content should help with this process.

Colour and areas of discoloration

Skin colour varies between individuals, most obviously between people of different ethnic origins. There are also differences in skin colour in different parts of the body of each individual. For example, the nipples and areolae are darker than the rest of the skin, particularly in women during pregnancy. Similarly, areas that are exposed to sunlight, such as the face and the arms, tend to be darker due to increased melanin concentration. These differences aside, and with the exception of older people in whom pigmentation can increase unevenly, skin colour is usually uniform within an individual.

An assessment of skin colour should first of all involve looking at areas that are not generally exposed to sunlight, such as the palm of the hand. It should be noted, however, that for the first few days of life the hands and feet of newborn babies are a bluish colour, termed acrocyanosis, due to inadequate peripheral vasculature. Assessment thereafter should involve looking for specific changes in skin colour, for instance:

- cyanosis (a bluish colour)
- pallor (a decrease of colour)
- jaundice (a yellow–orange colour)
- erythema (redness).

These changes in colour are most obvious in certain parts of the body. For instance, cyanosis and pallor are particularly evident at the nail beds and buccal (mouth) mucosa. It is especially important to look at these areas in dark-skinned clients, as changes in general skin colour are less evident. Asian children may have Mongolian blue spots, which are very common and are normal. In addition, the nurse should note any bruising. Although bruising can be normal, extensive or fingertip-type bruising can be a sign of abuse and should be investigated further, following agreed protocols.

Decision making exercise

Carole, aged 28, is admitted to the mother and baby unit of a psychiatric hospital with her 3-week-old daughter Jasmine. Carole is suffering from postnatal depression and has for the past week been neglecting herself and has shown little interest in caring for Jasmine.

- What aspects of skin assessment would you focus on when determining Carole's and Jasmine's skin health?
- In what ways could the assessment of a patient's skin lead you to suspect underlying health problems?

Temperature

Feeling the client's skin with the back of your hand best assesses skin temperature. The temperature of the skin increases or decreases with an increase or decrease in the circulation of blood through the dermis. Although it is normal for hands and feet to be colder than the rest of the body when exposed to a cold environment because of reduced peripheral blood flow, localized areas of increased or decreased temperature may indicate a problem. For example, if the skin surrounding a wound is hot, inflamed, red and painful, a wound infection may be present. Similarly, if a limb is cold and pale, there may be circulatory impairment. When clients have had vascular surgery or a plaster cast or bandages applied to a limb, it is therefore important to assess for skin changes that may indicate impaired blood flow.

Moisture

Moisture refers to the wetness and oiliness of skin. It is related to the level of hydration and general condition of the skin. Normally the skin is smooth and dry except in the folds of the skin where it is moist. An increase in skin temperature arising from a hot environment or exercise is accompanied by perspiration, and is a normal phenomenon. However, when a client has a fever resulting from, for example, an infection, the skin may initially feel dry and hot, but become damp from perspiration as the fever breaks. In older people dry skin, which is often accompanied by itchiness, may be a problem.

Texture

Usually the skin is smooth, soft and flexible, although in older people it sometimes becomes wrinkled and leathery. Skin thickness varies in different parts of the body: for example, skin is thickest on the palms of the hands and soles of the feet. Stroking and palpating the skin with the fingertips, which enable the nurse to gauge smoothness, thickness, suppleness and softness, can assess skin texture. Localized areas of changes to skin texture may indicate previous trauma or lesions. Should such changes be apparent, the nurse should ask the client about them. Rough and dry skin may result from exposure to cold weather or overwashing.

Turgor

Turgor refers to the elasticity of the skin, which is normally elastic and taut. It can be assessed by gentle pinching, lifting and letting go of an area of skin, usually on the back of the hand. Normally, the skin should quickly return to its former position. If it does not, it may indicate that the client is dehydrated. However, some loss of skin elasticity is normal in older individuals. Excessive accumulation of fluid in the tissue – termed oedema – gives the skin a taut shiny appearance. It results from either direct trauma to the skin or an underlying condition. The presence of oedema increases susceptibility to further skin damage and delays wound healing.

Blemishes and lesions

Many skin blemishes and lesions are normal, for instance birthmarks, moles and freckles, and minor cuts, abrasions and blisters. Equally, nappy rash and heat rash are common among babies and children and mild acne is not uncommon in adults. Other blemishes and lesions, however, may require further investigation and it may be necessary to refer the client to a doctor. For example, changes in an existing mole may indicate the development of a malignant melanoma.

Rashes may be caused by infection, such as a postviral rash, chickenpox, meningitis and shingles, or an allergic response, for example to particular chemicals, food products or medication. Other lesions may arise from skin infestations such as scabies, as a result of accidental or intentional trauma to the skin, or as a result of skin disease such as psoriasis or eczema. When abnormal blemishes, including scars or lesions, are detected, their colour, size, location and specific characteristics, and, where appropriate, distribution and grouping, should be noted. Clients should be asked about such blemishes, in particular to determine their cause.

Evidence based practice

According to McHenry et al (1995), the prevalence of atopic eczema (or dermatitis) has increased substantially over the past 30 years. It affects 5–15% of children and 2–10% of adults. The condition appears to develop from a complex interplay between genetic, immunological and environmental factors. The two most commonly cited environmental factors are house dust mites and certain foods, particularly milk, dairy products and eggs.

Where individuals have existing skin conditions or diseases that cannot be completely cured, effective assessment and management will focus on minimizing the effects of the skin problem and maximizing health potential and quality of life. The effect of such chronic conditions can have a profound effect on the individual and his or her family (Fig. 14.4).

Scratching affects concentration and may cause bleeding
Disrupted sleep results in tiredness and irritability
Social and intimate relationships may be affected
Embarrassment
Poor self-image
Reduced self-esteem
Lack of confidence
Reduced socialization
Reduced participation in certain social activities (e.g. swimming)
Teasing and taunting by others
Self-disgust
Restrictions on career and occupational opportunities
Anger, frustration and despair resulting from lack of control of
    eczema
Increased washing of clothing and bedding
Time-consuming management
Restricted choice of some products (to avoid exacerbating eczema)
Increased expenditure on treatments and some products
    (to improve management of eczema)

Figure 14.4 Effects of atopic eczema on the individual and his or her family.

CLASSIFICATION OF WOUNDS

Wounds can be classified in a variety of different ways. They can be classified according to:

- cause (e.g. stab wound)
- status of skin integrity (e.g. open or closed wound)
- cleanliness of wound (e.g. presence or absence of infection or foreign bodies)
- the characteristics of the wound bed of open wounds
- extent of skin damage (e.g. full-thickness burn).

However, Westaby (1985) suggests that there are really only two types of wound:

- wounds characterized by skin loss
- wounds where there is no skin loss.

In practice, wound classification systems are often incomplete and overlap; for example, a surgically closed infected wound and an open, chronic, sloughy, bacterially contaminated wound. A simple wound classification system is given in Figure 14.5.

Acute wounds result from surgery or accidents. However, in some instances acute wounds progress to chronic wounds as a result of complications. Acute surgical wounds tend to be surgically closed and clean, while accidental wounds may be either clean or infected, and can also be open or closed. Chronic wounds usually result from underlying diseases and tend to be open, as in the case of pressure sores and leg ulcers. Chronic wounds are more likely to be colonized or infected.

Open wounds can be further classified according to the observable characteristics of the wound bed:

- epithelializing (pink)
- granulating (red)

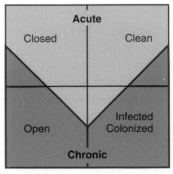

Figure 14.5 Wound classification diagram.

- infected (green)
- sloughy (yellow)
- necrotic (black).

Severity of skin damage

It is not always easy to determine the extent of skin damage: that is, whether there is superficial, partial or full-thickness damage, but it is sometimes useful to do so. For instance, burns and pressure sores are often graded and described in such terms (Table 14.1). The European Pressure Ulcer Advisory Panel (1999) suggests grading damage by tissue type.

Despite the limitations of wound classification, it is nonetheless useful as it helps to identify both the potential complications of a given wound and the implications for wound care in each case, and this can guide decision making when planning wound care. Algorithms or flow charts based on the classification of wounds aid in identifying priorities in wound care, and have been devised to guide nursing decisions and actions in wound management.

Reflection and portfolio evidence

During your next practice placement select one patient who has been allocated to you who has sustained a wound of any type. Reflect on the need for a holistic assessment of the care needed for that person. Involve the patient as a partner in your assessment.

- Using Morison's (1992) four levels of patient assessment, decide what aspects you would focus on during assessment to enable you to provide appropriate holistic care to meet that patient's immediate and long-term health needs.
- Record a summary of your experiences and a commentary on your learning in your portfolio.

Table 14.1 Classification of pressure sores (Benbow 1994)

Grade	Features
I	Discoloration, persistent erythema of intact skin
II	Partial-thickness skin loss involving the epidermis and/or dermis. Abrasion, blister or shallow crater
III	Full-thickness skin loss involving damage or necrosis of subcutaneous tissue; a deep crater without undermining of adjacent tissue
IV	Full-thickness tissue loss with extensive destruction, tissue necrosis or damage to muscle, bone or supporting structures

WOUND MANAGEMENT

The management of wounds will be discussed in general terms, followed by a more in-depth discussion of three specific types of wounds, namely accidental wounds, closed surgical wounds and chronic wounds.

Assessment of a person with a wound

When undertaking an assessment of a person with a wound, it is necessary to consider the person as a whole and not just to focus attention on the wound itself. Morison (1992: 22) states that assessment can be thought of on four levels, namely assessment of:

- general patient factors that could delay wound healing
- immediate causes of the wound and any underlying pathophysiology
- local conditions at the wound site
- potential consequences of the wound for the individual.

Morison's (1992) approach allows the nurse to:

- determine whether any health promotion activity is necessary to prevent a recurrence of the wound (e.g. advice on how to prevent sunburn)
- consider any factors that may retard wound healing and take measures to overcome these (e.g. inadequate nutrition)
- plan and provide holistic care that meets the needs of a person with a wound, rather than just treating a wound per se.

Dealey (1999) stresses the need to consider the environment in which care is to be given.

The immediate and longer-term care of a patient with a wound requires an assessment and understanding of the psychological effects, and of the functional, social and economic consequences of a wound for the patient, if holistic care is to be provided. It is likely that apart from nurses, several other members of the multidisciplinary team will be involved in the care of a patient with a wound. Good communication between team members to facilitate the sharing of information is essential for achieving agreed goals.

Assessment of the wound site

When assessing the wound site itself, the following should be noted:

- the location of the wound
- the size and shape of the wound
- the characteristics of the wound bed (in open wounds) and wound margin
- the degree of exudate
- the presence of infection (Fig. 14.6)
- odour from the wound
- pain
- the condition of the surrounding skin

Localized pain
Localized erythema
Localized rise in skin temperature
Local oedema
Excess exudate
Pus
Offensive odour
Pyrexia

Figure 14.6   Signs of clinical wound infection.

- signs of other specific complications such as a haematoma
- where appropriate, the presence of foreign bodies, the type of skin closure and the presence of drains and details of drainage.

Open wounds can be traced onto plastic film to obtain a visual record of the wound size. These films can be annotated to show areas of the wound bed with different characteristics. Maximum wound dimensions can be taken from the tracing. Wound depth can be measured using sterile probes. Serial photographs can also be taken to show wound changes over time, which will give some indication of the effectiveness or otherwise of treatment regimens.

If patients have existing wounds or have received wound care in the past, it is important during assessment to establish whether the patient has had any allergies to wound care products. Details of existing wound care should be recorded. Patch testing for allergies to any proposed wound care products is useful, particularly if large areas require dressing, as in the case of an extensive venous leg ulcer.

Reflection and portfolio evidence

Find a copy of other wound assessment charts that may be in use in practice areas you have visited, or appear in the literature. Examples are provided by Benbow (2001) and Bennett & Moody (1995).

- Compare these other assessment tools with Morison's (1992) tool (Fig. 14.7), and from your present experience and knowledge of wound care decide which tool would be the most valid to use and why. (Validity is the extent to which the tool measures what it is supposed to measure.)
- Test your chosen tool for reliability when two or more students observe the same wound, either in reality or using slides or computer simulation, and then compare any statements or scores for similarities and differences. (Reliability is the extent to which the tool measures consistently.)
- How would a tool help you in your decision making about wound management?
- Record your findings and learning in your portfolio.

Wound assessment charts can be useful tools when undertaking and recording the findings of wound assessments. Figure 14.7 shows an example of an open wound assessment chart developed by Morison (1992).

Facilitating wound healing

The general aim of wound management is to provide optimum conditions for facilitating natural wound healing as quickly and comfortably as possible with minimum scarring. This includes identifying and addressing factors that may affect wound healing. These can be divided into three broad categories as follows:

- local factors relating to the wound environment (e.g. presence of necrotic tissue, oedema)
- general client factors (e.g. nutritional status, compliance with treatment)
- treatment – nursing and medical factors (e.g. radiotherapy, dressing choice).

Successful wound healing is dependent on the body's ability to heal. Wound care can only help to facilitate this process. Some wounds will not heal, for example inoperable fungating carcinoma, and here the aim of wound management is to contribute to an optimum quality of life for the client by containing wound odour and discharge, protecting the wound and controlling any pain.

The aims of local wound management are to provide an optimum environment to enable natural wound healing processes, to remove causes of delayed healing and to protect the wound from further damage (see Subject Knowledge).

If a wound is necrotic, one of the first priorities is to remove the necrotic tissue. Devitalized tissue, as Benbow (2002) states, not only hinders healing and increases the risk of infection, but also masks the extent of the injury. Removal of necrotic tissue can be achieved by mechanical means, chemical means, biosurgical means (maggot/larval therapy), or by providing the right local conditions for autolysis to take place (see section on annotated further reading: Vowden & Vowden 1999).

Evidence based practice

Thomas et al (2001) cite that approximately 50 articles have been published over the past 4 years that describe the use of maggots. Although many are anecdotal reports, three studies and preliminary results of a large randomized controlled trial involving 140 patients are included. Maggot therapy appears to be cost-effective in a variety of wound types, has the ability to combat infection, including methicillin resistant *Staphylococcus aureus*, and has no significant risk of adverse events, although pain, particularly in ischaemic limbs, appears to increase with larval therapy.

OPEN WOUND ASSESSMENT CHART

Type of wound (e.g. pressure sore, fungating carcinoma, etc.) ....

Location ....

How long has wound been open? ....

General patient factors which may delay healing (e.g. malnourished, diabetic, chronic infection) ....

Allergies to wound care products ....

Previous treatments tried (comment on success/problems) ....

Special aids in current use (e.g. pressure-relieving bed, cushion) ....

....

....

TRACE THE WOUND WEEKLY, ANNOTATING TRACING WITH NATURE OF WOUND BED, ORIENTATION OF WOUND, POSITION/EXTENT OF SINUSES, AND UNDERMINING OF SURROUNDING SKIN

All other parameters should be assessed at every dressing change.

Wound factors/Date								

1. NATURE OF WOUND BED
  a. healthy granulation
  b. epithelialization
  c. slough
  d. black/brown necrotic tissue
  e. other (specify)								

2. EXUDATE
  a. colour
  b. type
  c. approximate amount								

3. ODOUR Offensive/some/none								

4. PAIN (SITE)
  a. at wound site
  b. elsewhere (specify)								

5. PAIN (FREQUENCY) Continuous/intermittent/ only at dressing changes/none								
6. PAIN (SEVERITY) Patient's score (0–10)								

7. WOUND MARGIN
  a. colour
  b. oedematous								

8. ERYTHEMA OF SURROUNDING SKIN
  a. present
  b. maximum distance from wound (mm)								

9. GENERAL CONDITION OF SURROUNDING SKIN (e.g. dry eczema)								

10. INFECTION
  a. suspected
  b. wound swab sent
  c. confined (specify organism)								

WOUND ASSESSED BY:

Figure 14.7 Open wound assessment chart. (Reproduced by kind permission of Mosby International, from Morison M 1997 A color guide to the nursing management of chronic wounds 2nd edn.)

Wound sites also need to be free of clinical infection. If a clinical wound infection is suspected (see Fig. 14.6) a wound swab should be taken before wound cleaning and sent for microscopy, culture and sensitivity. An appropriate systemic antibiotic may be prescribed. The use of topical antibiotics is rarely indicated because of the risk of contact sensitivity and bacterial resistance (Podmore 1994). Chronic wounds in particular may be colonized by microorganisms that do not cause clinical infections and do not appear to affect wound healing.

Consideration should be given to whether the wound needs to be cleansed or redressed as unnecessary intervention delays wound healing. Wounds should be cleaned if there is superficial slough, pus, excessive exudate or visible debris such as grit or residue from previous dressings.

Reflection and portfolio evidence

Under the Subject Knowledge section, you were given a list of conditions for optimum wound healing (p. 309). Referring to this list, decide why unnecessary wound cleansing or redressing delays wound healing.

Reflect on the wound care activities you have observed during practice placement.

- How were the wounds cleaned and how often?
- What reasons were given for the choice of wound cleansing agent and the method of cleaning in each case?
- In wounds described as necrotic, what means were used to remove the necrotic tissue – mechanical, chemical, biosurgical or promoting autolysis? Why was the particular method chosen in each particular case you have seen?
- Record your findings in your portfolio.

Generally, if wounds require cleansing aseptically, they should be cleaned with warm sterile sodium chloride 0.9% solution. Unlike antiseptics, sodium chloride 0.9% solution does not have a toxic effect on skin tissue. Although antiseptics may be used in specific circumstances, such as heavily contaminated wounds, it is necessary to weigh the benefits against the possible tissue damage they may cause. Preference should be given to irrigating wounds under moderate pressure (8 psi) rather than using cotton wool or gauze, which shed fibres into the wound, thereby delaying wound healing and providing a focus for infection. In addition, such mechanical cleansing can damage newly formed tissue.

The choice of dressing, if required, depends on a variety of factors. These include:

- the local conditions of the wound site and surrounding skin
- other requirements arising from the individual patient's needs, wishes and lifestyle
- cost-effectiveness and product availability.

Although it is not possible to determine the ideal characteristics of a wound dressing to suit all wounds, there are some features that the 'ideal' dressing should possess (Fig. 14.8).

In many instances, a single dressing will not suffice. For example, a primary dressing may meet the requirements of the wound–dressing interface, but may not possess the absorptive qualities needed to contain exudate and a secondary absorbent dressing will need to be applied. Secondary dressings, including bandages, have the following functions:

- to protect and support the wound and surrounding skin
- to maintain the position of primary dressings
- to absorb moisture
- to control bleeding or oedema (as a result of pressure exerted by secondary dressings).

Vacuum assisted closure (VAC), which exerts a negative pressure on the wound, may be appropriate for high exudating wounds. Apart from removing exudate, the system, as Collier (1997) describes, reduces localized oedema, increases localized blood flow, enhances epithelial migration, promotes new granulation tissue and reduces bacterial colonization of the wounds.

In selecting a dressing the nurse needs to understand the properties, actions, indications and contraindications for the use of each dressing being considered, and match this information to the specific requirements of the patient and the wound. The use of an algorithm and a dressing formulary will help nurses in decision making in this area of wound management (see section on annotated further reading: Eyers 2001).

When undertaking wound care, it is essential that the nurse understands and adheres to the principles of asepsis to promote the prevention of cross-infection (see Ch. 4 on infection control). If the client has several wounds that require redressing, the cleanest wounds should be dressed first.

Maintains a moist wound environment
Provides thermal insulation
Provides a barrier to microorganisms
Protects from trauma
Is non-toxic and non-allergenic
Is absorptive and removes excess exudate
Is sterile
Will not shed fibres into the wound
Is non-adherent and easily removed
Is flexible and conforming
Is comfortable
Controls odour
Is acceptable to the patient
Is easy to use
Requires infrequent dressing change
Is cost-effective
Has a reasonable shelf life and storage requirement
Is available

Figure 14.8 Features of an ideal dressing.

There are occasions where wounds can be cleaned and dressed using a clean technique rather than an aseptic technique. A clean technique, as Hollingworth & Kingston (1998) describe, adheres to the same principles of preventing cross-infection, but clean single-use gloves and/or safe-to-drink tap water are used rather than sterile alternatives. A clean technique rather than an aseptic technique has been used, for example, in minor traumatic wounds until all gross contaminants have been removed (Morison 1992), and in the treatment of leg ulcers in the community (Moffatt & Oldroyd 1994). More recently, Hollingworth & Kingston (1998) cite evidence to support the use of a clean technique in a wide range of wounds. However, they stress that it is necessary to risk assess each individual with a wound in order to determine whether a clean or aseptic technique is more appropriate.

Decision making exercise

Mr Heron, a 60-year-old farmer, has a venous leg ulcer, which is shallow, clean, granulating and 5 cm × 5 cm. There is a moderate amount of exudate. He has no known allergies to specific dressing products. In the role of the community nurse:

- Select an appropriate dressing for the wound.
- Justify your choice in terms of promotion of wound healing, patient comfort and cost-effectiveness.
- Did you give consideration as to whether or not your choice of dressing would be available?
- Do you think you had enough information on which to base your decision? If not, what other information would you require before making a decision?

EVALUATION OF THE EFFECTIVENESS OF WOUND MANAGEMENT

The evaluation of wound management may take place at two levels:

- An organization may wish to keep a record of specific wounds and evaluate the effectiveness of the measures taken to deal with and minimize the incidence of these wounds.
- At the level of individual wounds, an evaluation should be made each time the dressings are changed by observing and measuring to see if the wound is healing as expected.

Evaluating individual wounds is important for two reasons. First, as wound healing progresses and the characteristics of the wound change, different dressings may be required. Second, if there is no change or the wound has deteriorated, it is necessary to reflect on the factors that may be responsible for delayed healing. The dressing choice may

need to be changed or othe... However, unless the woun... ficient time must be given... effective before changing... of the multidisciplinary... the discussion and reapp... evaluate patients' progr... views on the progress... eration to their quality of life, ... addressed.

Evidence based practice

Bux & Malhi (1996) carried out an audit into the use of dressings in practice. The correct choice of dressing was made for only 48% of the 50 wounds observed. The correct choice and use of dressings was observed for only 20% of the wounds. The importance of training and information related to wound care was highlighted, and the development of wound care guidelines and a hospital wound product formulary were encouraged.

MANAGEMENT OF ACUTE AND CHRONIC WOUNDS

Accidental wounds

An accidental wound is defined here as an acute wound that has occurred as a result of an accident or a specific non-medical incident. They are sometimes referred to as traumatic wounds. Accidental wounds involving the skin can range from minor cuts and abrasions to major wounds such as the loss of limb or crush injuries. Also included are burns, scalds, bites and stings.

Although the focus of this discussion is on the management of patients with accidental wounds in the Accident and Emergency department, the principles of first aid care are applicable in all situations. In all cases, it is necessary to assess the patient, and if possible to obtain a history of the wound. This includes the cause, circumstances, time of accident, estimate of blood loss and any other information relevant to the management of the patient. Psychological care of the patient – and any accompanying relatives or friends – is extremely important, as the suddenness of the situation can cause considerable distress and anxiety. It is also important to identify and address any pain the patient is experiencing.

The management of major accidental wounds is decided and directed by the casualty officer. Rapid accurate assessment of the client's condition and underlying pathology is essential. Priority must be given to the re-establishment and maintenance of the airway, breathing and circulation, and the control of bleeding before dealing with the wound itself.

examination must then be conducted to
[th]ere are no other injuries that need to take pri-
[the] management of the wound (see Ch. 3). The
management of the wound, as Wijetunge (1992)
[stat]es, should only commence once the patient's condi-
[tion] is stable.

In the case of minor wounds, such as slight cuts and abrasions, an initial assessment of the patient is still necessary,
but attention can quickly be focused on wound care to minimize the risk of infection. Other measures may, however, be
necessary; for example, depending upon the circumstances,
it may be appropriate to take the opportunity to offer health
education or the patient may require a tetanus injection.

The cause of the wound will give an indication of the
likely damage and complications, and will help to guide
wound management decisions. For instance, puncture
wounds caused by stabbing have only a small entry site, but
cut a deep track and may damage internal tissue and organs.
As such a wound goes deep into the body, the risk of infection is high. Abrasions, on the other hand, can result in large
tender areas where the superficial layers of skin have been
removed. They often contain foreign particles such as grit,
which can cause infection and tattooing if not effectively
removed. If a large foreign body is embedded in the patient
it must be removed in theatre as there is a risk of major
haemorrhage when it is removed (see section on annotated
further reading: Walsh & Kent 2001).

Accurate documentation is essential. In cases of criminal
or civil prosecution or claims for industrial injury compensation, the patient's records may be used as evidence.
Where a patient is a victim of a non-accidental injury that
warrants police investigation, such as a stabbing or a road
traffic accident, particular care must be taken with the
patient's property, including clothing, as it may be required
for further examination and used as evidence. Where child
abuse is suspected, for example if a child appears to have
cigarette burns on its buttocks, it is essential to follow the
local hospital policy regarding the management and reporting of such cases, so that further action can be taken as
appropriate. The nurse must use considerable tact when
dealing with such situations.

Surgical wounds

Surgical wounds may be open or closed depending upon
the reasons for surgery. In this section the role of the nurse
in the promotion of wound healing by primary intention is
discussed. The role of the nurse is to:

- prevent infection
- monitor the wound to detect the onset of any
  complications
- prevent trauma to the wound site
- promote nutritional and fluid intake.

To prevent infection the nurse must prevent the chain of
infection from completing all the links (Walsh 1997). The
nurse will need to consider his or her own health: a nurse
with a cold or sore throat will be a reservoir for infective
organisms and should not be involved in wound care.
Following surgery, wounds may be dressed with an island
dressing which can be removed after 24–48 hours, or
covered with a film dressing which is usually left *in situ*
until the sutures are removed. Dealey (1999) suggests that
whichever method is used, the patient can resume normal
hygiene activities.

Skin closing sutures pierce the skin and enter the subdermal layers and are therefore a potential route of entry for
infection. Unless there is exudate, wound cleansing should
not be undertaken, as the introduction of moisture to the
sutures facilitates the passage of microorganisms by capillary action along the sutures into the subdermal layers.
However, should wound care be required, Bale & Jones
(1997) advocate strict asepsis. When removing sutures, the
nurse must ensure that when the suture is cut and then
drawn from the wound, the part of the suture that is above
the surface of the skin is not allowed to pass beneath the surface of the skin. This prevents microorganisms from being
drawn into the track left by the suture in the subdermal
layers. If drainage tubes are used, they should be secured to
prevent the shunting of the tubes in and out of the wound,
thus reducing the risk of bacteria entering the drainage
incision.

The wound should be assessed as previously described
(see pp. 315–316). A specific assessment tool for surgically
closed wounds may be used, for example the tool developed
by Morison (1992). The use of a clear dressing allows the
nurse to observe the wound without removing the dressing,
and so reduces the risk of contaminating the wound. In addition, the nurse must observe the drainage for colour and
consistency and, in open drainage systems, odour.

To prevent trauma the nurse must ensure that there is no
rubbing or pulling on the wound closures and drainage
tubes. This can be achieved by applying a light dry dressing
to the incision site. Wound drainage tubes should be
secured and supported.

Evidence based practice

Tritle et al (2001) undertook an aesthetic comparison of
commonly used closure techniques in a porcine model.
Nylon sutures, absorbable monofilament sutures, tissue
glue and adhesive tape were compared. Results indicated
that the adhesive tape with underlying deep (subdermal)
closure gave good cosmetic results, was convenient and
saved time and material costs. They recommend adhesive
tape closure as an alternative for closure of neck incisions.

Surgical patients require an increased calorie and protein
intake to aid wound healing. Vitamins C, A and B, and
zinc, manganese, copper and magnesium are also vital.

The nurse should help the patient select appropriate food to meet these requirements. Liaison with a dietician is helpful in some instances. Assistance with feeding may be necessary.

Chronic wounds

The management of a patient with a chronic wound requires a different approach from that for someone with an acute or surgical wound. This is due to the longstanding nature of the problem and the prolonged time it takes, subsequently, for healing to occur. The two most prevalent open chronic wounds are leg ulcers and pressure sores, both of which can affect the patient's whole life. In order to provide a framework for discussion, the management of pressure sores is used as an example. However, the principles of pressure sore management can be applied to any chronic wound. Holistic care is important when nursing patients with pressure sores. The effects of the sore can be wide ranging, causing the patient to suffer not only physical, but also psychological, social and economic problems.

Pressure sores, bed sores, decubitus ulcers and pressure ulcers are some of the many terms used to describe the sores, and each has been criticized for its inaccuracy. Sores are not only caused by pressure, and do not only occur in people who are in bed or lying down. No one term covers all the possible causes and situations in which sores can occur. For the purpose of discussion, the term pressure sore is used, as it is a widely used term that is recognized by all healthcare professionals.

Chapman & Chapman (1986: 106) define a pressure sore as 'a localized area of cellular damage resulting either from direct pressure on the skin, causing pressure ischaemia, or from shearing forces … causing mechanical stress to the tissues'. It is the ischaemic changes in the tissues that cause the damage rather than the pressure itself. When direct pressure is exerted on the skin at a level greater than the mean capillary pressure of 25 mmHg, the capillaries are occluded and the blood supply to the tissues is restricted. This causes tissue ischaemia, and eventually, if the blood supply is not re-established, tissue necrosis. With shearing force the tissues are stretched to such an extent that capillaries rupture, resulting in a marked reduction in the amount of blood reaching the tissues and tissue necrosis.

Assessment of a patient with a pressure sore

A thorough assessment of the patient can assist in the identification of both internal and external factors relating to the patient's condition and ability that may affect wound healing. The pressure sore assessment wheel (Fig. 14.9) incorporates many areas of patient assessment and some areas specific to the assessment of pressure sores, giving an overall assessment framework. Each of these is explained in turn as you progress around the wheel.

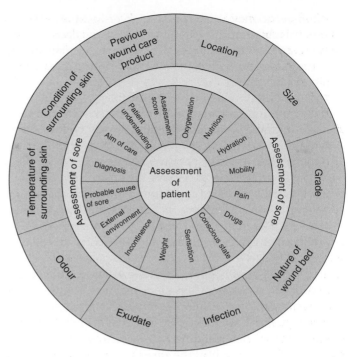

Figure 14.9   Pressure sore assessment wheel.

The 'inner wheel' highlights the many 'patient' factors that have an indirect effect on healing, namely:

- The importance of adequate 'oxygenation', 'nutrition' and 'hydration', which have been discussed previously (see Subject Knowledge).
- Anything that modifies the patient's ability or desire to move about ('mobility') may affect the wound.
- 'Pain' can prevent a patient from changing his or her position as often as required.
- 'Drugs' can have varying influences on healing, depending upon their effects – some drugs such as glucocorticosteroids may alter the texture of the skin, while others such as sedatives may reduce the patient's level of alertness, resulting in the associated problems of reduced movement and decreased awareness of risk.
- Reduced 'consciousness' can lead to a patient being unable to identify the need to move, and can prevent him or her from doing so.
- Loss of 'sensation' can result in a patient being unaware of the position he or she is in and the need to change it.
- Extremes of weight, i.e. body mass index of above 30 or below 20, could compromise healing and increase the risk of further sore development.
- Faecal and urinary 'incontinence' can cause contamination of wound sites, excess moisture in the wound area and problems with adherence with certain dressings, particularly in relation to pressure sores on the buttocks, sacrum or hips.
- 'External environment' covers a large area relating to resources – the general environment in which the patient is being nursed (e.g. own home, hospital single room or

multi-occupancy room, nursing or residential care) can affect the type of dressing or treatment available or possible, as can the amount of assistance the patient can expect from nursing staff, other carers and relatives or significant others.

- It is important to identify the 'probable cause of the sore' developing as this may influence the care required – if shearing force is suspected attention may be focused on handling and positioning patients to prevent further damage, but if direct pressure has caused the problem the main objective is to remove the pressure.
- The patient's 'diagnosis' can sometimes affect the wound healing – conditions such as diabetes mellitus, vascular disease, malignancy and anaemia can alter the cellular environment and therefore interfere with the healing process.
- The 'aim of care' is not always apparent – for patients in the terminal stages of illness, it may not be possible to heal the pressure sore in the time the patient has left to live; in which case the aim of care may be to prevent the wound from deteriorating and to increase patient comfort, rather than to heal the sore.
- 'Patient understanding' of his or her condition and treatments and the patient's ability to comply with regimens may also affect the overall choice of treatment.
- A current assessment score using a risk calculator, such as that produced by Norton in the early 1960s or Waterlow in 1985, help to identify future risks and allow the

implementation of preventive treatment for the prevention of the development of sores.

The 'outer ring' of the assessment wheel consists of the factors you should consider when dealing with the wound itself. These factors have been covered earlier (see p. 315).

In addition to the points above, it is important to assess and manage the psychological impact of living with a chronic wound.

Any plan of care relating to pressure sore management needs to contain a core of information:

- an up-to-date assessment of the wound
- current at-risk assessment score and review dates
- cleansing solution to be used
- primary dressing requirements
- secondary dressing requirements – padding, bandaging
- method of carrying out dressing
- frequency of dressing changes
- referrals made and advice received
- associated factors – use of pressure relieving aids and mattresses, mobility programme and turning regimen
- patient and relative involvement
- patient and relative educational needs.

Pressure sores should not be seen as a nursing problem, but rather as a challenge to the full multidisciplinary team, in which each member has a role to play. The flowchart showing multidisciplinary involvement (Fig. 14.10) is not

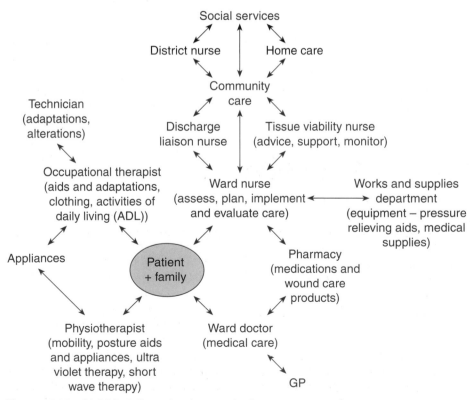

Figure 14.10 Multidisciplinary involvement in the management of pressure sores.

exhaustive, but serves to highlight the level of integration that may be required. Care should be implemented in accordance with the written patient care plan. It is advised that a limited number of nurses are involved in implementing the wound care. Continuity and consistency are important if the pressure sore is to be given the best chance of healing. Different nurses may use slightly different techniques; dressings may therefore be applied in a different manner. This may affect the rate and amount of wound healing; for instance, one nurse may pack a wound tighter than another or one nurse may irrigate a wound where another nurse would keep the wound dry. Continuity of care also helps evaluation, as the nurse becomes familiar with the wound and is better able to detect changes in its size, shape and general condition.

Decision making exercise

Steven is 45 years old and suffers from cerebral palsy. He is cared for by his 67-year-old mother in a purpose-built ground floor flat and has two care assistants who attend him in the morning and at night to get him up and put him to bed. Steven attends a day centre 5 days a week. He is unable to walk and is confined to a wheelchair. He is difficult to feed and faecally incontinent. He has been catheterized for the past 2 years. During a visit to the day centre you notice a small broken area on his left buttock.

- Decide which factors you need to assess in order to plan the care Steven will require to heal the present sore.
- Draw a spider diagram showing which members of the multidisciplinary team can assist in the management of the present sore.
- Given the amount of support Steven already has, what other preventive measures may be necessary to prevent any further deterioration of Steven's skin?

Evidence based practice

The impact of pressure sores on a patient's quality of life is an area that is largely unexplored by research. Douglas (2001) addressed the issue of quality of life in relation to the other major type of chronic wound, leg ulcers. The article provides an insight into the physical and psychological effects of having a leg ulcer and explores the patient/nurse relationship.

If a pressure sore does not heal, further intervention may be an option. This could entail debridement or skin grafting. Debridement is discussed earlier in the chapter. The aim of debridement is to leave the wound bed clean and

bleeding, so that granulation can take place (David 1986). This may be required prior to skin grafting.

Skin grafting has developed rapidly since the advent of genetic engineering. As well as the more established types of grafting, i.e autografting (taking skin from one site to a second site on the same person), and pedicle or flap grafts, there are now many new techniques available. Ballard & Baxter (2000) describe a variety of innovations within tissue engineering. These include the development of keratinocytes in a laboratory; the ability to produce, within a 1-month time period, an epithelial tissue graft, from an initial sample of 8 mm, which is large enough to cover an adult body, and several new bio-engineered human dermal replacements, e.g Dermagraft™, Intergra™ and Apligraf™.

PROFESSIONAL AND ETHICAL KNOWLEDGE

This section focuses on professional and ethical issues that are relevant to the quality of care provision relating to skin integrity. Examples are given to illustrate how nurses can influence the development of quality systems of care at an organizational level. The responsibility of the nurse to provide safe effective care – either by developing his or her professional competence or by acknowledging his or her limitations and seeking appropriate expert help – is explored.

Reflection and portfolio evidence

Reflect on the practice areas where you have worked in all fields of nursing.

- List examples of health promotion activities relating to skin integrity that you have observed.
- Reflect on the number of areas and occasions in which there was an opportunity to provide health promotion in relation to skin care and integrity.
- Record one incident where you took an active part in health promotion related to skin care and comment critically on what you learned through undertaking this activity.

THE NURSE'S ROLE IN PROMOTING SKIN HEALTH

The nurse has an important role to play in promoting health and there is considerable potential for nurses in all care settings to promote skin health. Health promotion activities can range from teaching parents the necessary skin care for their newborn babies, to empowering individuals to manage their own chronic skin conditions, such as psoriasis and eczema.

How nurses fulfil a role in promoting skin health in part depends on individual situations and circumstances. The knowledge base provided in this chapter, along with a more in-depth understanding of health promotion (see Naidoo &

Wills 2000), will enable the nurse to select the appropriate health promotion activity to assist specific individuals to achieve and maintain optimum skin health. To be effective it is essential that such activities are planned, in order to achieve identified health goals. It is also important that the nurse recognizes individual limitations, and where necessary ensures that patients receive specific expert help. In addition, where longer-term interventions are needed and input from other healthcare professionals or agencies is required, as is often the case with chronic skin problems, consideration must be given to how continuity can be ensured.

The nurse also has a responsibility to maintain his or her own skin health. This is not only important with respect to the nurse's health, but also to that of the patients in his or her care, particularly in respect of the prevention of cross-infection.

THE NURSE'S ROLE IN DEVELOPING AND MAINTAINING QUALITY SYSTEMS OF CARE

There is considerable scope for nurses, along with other healthcare professionals, to be involved in the development and maintenance of quality systems of care relating to skin integrity. Examples of this include involvement in the development of standards of care, benchmarking, clinical guidelines and protocols, procedures, policies, integrated care pathways and auditing clinical practice. In the development of quality systems of care, cognizance should be given to nationally produced guidelines as appropriate; for example the guidelines produced by the National Institute for Clinical Excellence, such as the clinical guidelines for pressure ulcer risk assessment and prevention (National Institute for Clinical Excellence 2001), and National Service Frameworks.

The development of clinical guidelines and protocols, for example, help to maintain standards and the continuity of care, by providing an agreed framework for decision making for the treatment and management of specific aspects of care. Integrated care pathways for the prevention of pressure sores and wound management are two examples relating to skin integrity. Eyers (2001) discusses the role of the multidisciplinary wound management policy group at the Queen's Medical Centre (Nottingham, UK) in developing and evaluating evidence based policies and procedures with the aim of providing high-quality care related to the detection and management of wounds. Among their achievements has been the development of a wound formulary and wound management guidelines. These are reviewed annually and ensure that staff have access to current evidence based information on which they can base wound management. In addition, group protocols, alongside a learning package, have been developed to ensure that appropriately qualified healthcare professionals use wound management products in an appropriate and cost-effective way.

A relatively recent development in the UK healthcare system, in which nurses are able to make an important contribution, is the development and implementation of integrated care pathways (Walsh 1998). Nurses also have a significant role in developing, undertaking and participating in the audit of clinical practice. As an example which relates to skin integrity, a hospital may keep records of the incidence of pressure sores, and may wish to investigate what measures were taken to prevent the development of pressure sores and what care was given when pressure sores developed. Auditing may be undertaken to see if the agreed standard for the assessment and prevention of pressure sores was being met through the correct implementation of a pressure sore prevention protocol. Equally, the management of existing pressure sores may be audited to see if the actual management reflects the agreed wound care protocol, and whether specific aspects of care follow established procedures. The document *Essence of Care* (Department of Health 2001) contains benchmarking tools related to eight fundamental aspects of care, one of which is pressure ulcers. These tools provide benchmarks of best practice against which nurses can measure the quality of practice in their own clinical areas.

THE DEVELOPING ROLE OF THE NURSE IN SKIN INTEGRITY: CLINICAL, EDUCATIONAL, PROFESSIONAL AND ETHICAL CONSIDERATIONS FOR PRACTICE

The role of the nurse in relation to skin integrity has developed greatly over the past decade. The Riverside Community Leg Ulcer Clinic was an innovation in its time (Moffatt & Oldroyd 1994), but such nurse-led clinics are now more commonplace. As well as link nurses and clinical specialists in tissue viability, there are now nurse consultants who have a greater ability to carry out an extended range of wound care procedures. In addition, new methods of communication have affected the environment of care. Telemedicine allows the practitioner to seek specialist advice from a distance, with the use of video conferencing, digital imaging and the NHS intranet (see section on annotated further reading: Newton et al 2000). Due to the increasing role development and the advancements in technology it is necessary to explore the clinical, educational, professional and ethical implications for practice. Some of the more salient issues are discussed below.

Extended practice

With ever-growing technological development, nurses are taking on additional roles. This makes a higher level of skill and knowledge necessary. The UK Central Council (1992) produced guidelines on the extended role of the nurse in its document *Scope of Professional Practice*. To date, there has been no corresponding publication from the Nursing and Midwifery Council to guide extended practice, although clause 6 of its *Code of Professional Conduct* (Nursing and Midwifery Council 2002) does address professional knowledge and competence. The UK Central Council (1994) *Standards for Specialist Education and Practice*, which have been adopted by the Nursing and Midwifery Council, differentiate between advanced practice and specialist practice. While stating that no standards will be set for advanced practice, they do, however, give some guidance regarding the requirements of specialist practice. As nurses are responsible and accountable for their own practice, the following framework raises several professional issues that the nurse needs to address before taking on an extended role:

- Is it within my role as a nurse?
- Will the nursing profession support me if I carry out this extended role?
- Is the practice evidence based?
- Do I have the knowledge, expertise and time to carry out this extended role?
- What are the risks and benefits to the patients/clients?
- Am I willing to take responsibility for carrying out this extended role, or would it be better carried out by another healthcare professional?

The nurse should only consider taking on an extended role when he or she is satisfied that these issues have been addressed appropriately.

Record keeping

As Culley (2001) discusses, the Health Service Commissioner has highlighted inadequate record keeping in tissue viability as an issue in a number of related legal proceedings, professional misconduct cases and investigations. The need to produce accurate and effective records in all aspects of the expanding role of the tissue viability nurse has been stressed. Although Culley's (2001) discussion focus on the role of the tissue viability nurse, it can be argued that the same applies to any nurse who is involved in the management and record keeping of patients who require care in respect of tissue viability. The utilization, for example, of agreed evidence based wound care assessment documentation, care pathways and protocols, will facilitate this process. The effective clinical audit of record keeping will, as Culley (2001) suggests, monitor the effectiveness of the systems that are currently in place, and inform improvements towards best practice.

Consent

The Nursing and Midwifery Council (2002) stress the necessity of obtaining consent prior to giving any treatment or care. Although in many instances implied consent (Montgomery 1997) has been adequate, one needs to consider, with the expanding role of the specialist nurse,

alongside advancements in wound care technology, whether documented verbal or written consent may be required for some interventions. For example, should implied, verbal or written consent be obtained, and from whom, for larval treatment or allografting (replacing epidermal loss with genetically unrelated cells), particularly given the ethical considerations? These issues need to be addressed to ensure that clear lines of accountability are drawn, that informed consent is obtained at an appropriate level and that clinical practice and documentation reflect professional, legal and ethically acceptable practice.

In any care setting nurses will meet patients or clients with a variety of problems and needs relating to skin care. This chapter provides the knowledge and decision making skills that nurses will need (within the limitations of their roles) to make informed decisions about and provide appropriate, effective, evidence based care for patients or clients and their families, in order that they might achieve and maintain optimum skin health. The importance of a holistic problem solving approach to care is stressed, as is the need for effective communication between healthcare professionals.

Decision making exercise

Larval therapy involves the placement of live, sterile greenbottle larvae (maggots) onto a necrotic wound where they will digest the devitalized tissue and defaecate into the wound. The faecal material contains enzymes that are beneficial to wound healing. Having done their job the larvae are incinerated in the clinical waste.

- What information do you think a patient would require in order to give informed consent for the treatment to be used?
- Debate the legal and ethical requirements for informed consent and discuss the difficulties that may arise in providing this treatment for wound care.

As the scope of professional nursing practice extends, there will be greater opportunities for nurses who are caring for patients with a variety of skin-related problems and needs to become involved in the nurse-led care initiatives. It is therefore imperative that nurses develop specific research and evidence based expertise so that they are able to assume responsibility and accountability for their future roles. The portfolio activities will help you to reflect on current nursing practice, and to consider the knowledge base underpinning nursing decisions and the appropriateness and effectiveness of the nursing care of clients or patients with skin problems. Developing an enquiring approach to care will also help you question your own decision making and nursing practice.

PERSONAL AND REFLECTIVE KNOWLEDGE

PORTFOLIO ACTIVITIES

Reflection assists in making links between theory and practice, and helps to address the affective aspects of practice. In relation to affective aspects, reflection on observed practice, both in respect of others and one's self, as well as the response/reaction of the patient and significant others, enables you to consider the appropriateness of actions, alternative approaches to care, and to take forward new learning, as well as identifying areas for further development. Reflective activities, such as keeping a reflective diary and undertaking critical incident analysis, using for example Gibbs's (1988) reflective model, will assist in this process. The activities suggested below aim to help you to relate theory to practice, consider affective perspectives, identify areas that need to be developed and consider the transfer of learning to future practice – all of which contribute to portfolio development.

Keep a diary of the nursing care of patients with problems and needs relating to skin integrity. Make sure you maintain confidentiality by omitting information that would make patients identifiable. For each case, address the following questions:

- What was the nature of the skin problem?
- How was it assessed?
- What specific care was proposed?
- What was the rationale for the proposed care?
- What specific skills were needed to implement the proposed care?
- What other healthcare professionals were involved in the patient's care?
- Was the care appropriate and effective? How was this determined?
- Were there any other care options that might have been more effective?

CASE STUDIES IN NURSING PATIENTS WITH SKIN PROBLEMS

The following case studies will help you bring together the knowledge and decision making skills required to address the needs of specific individuals with a variety of different skin problems.

Case study: Adult

Miss Green is 75 years old and lives alone in a one-bedroom ground floor flat. One morning, after the arrival of the district nurse, Miss Green slips on the kitchen mat and falls, sustaining a deep laceration to her head. The hot tea she is carrying splashes onto her arm causing a large but superficial burn.

- Decide what first aid treatment the district nurse should administer for the two skin injuries.

- On arrival at the Accident and Emergency department the doctor examines Miss Green and finds that during the fall she has sustained a fractured neck of femur. Miss Green subsequently requires a hip replacement. Decide what care Miss Green will require in respect of her hip wound for the first 10 postoperative days.

Case study: Child

Margaret and David MacDonnell take their 5-year-old son Robert on holiday to a well-known seaside resort. As it is an overcast day Margaret has not applied any sun protection to Robert. Robert spends the whole day in just a pair of trunks playing on the beach. That evening Robert complains that his skin hurts and when David examines Robert he finds that his back is badly sunburnt.

- Decide what immediate measures should be taken to treat the effects of Robert's sunburn?
- Given the opportunity, how would you help Mr and Mrs MacDonnell ensure effective sun protection for Robert in the future?

Case study: Mental health

Josie is 28 years old and single. She is attending a day unit for the adult mentally ill for treatment of anxiety–depression. During the post lunch rest period Josie shouts for you to come to the female toilet where she says she requires your help. When you arrive you find that Josie has inflicted several superficial lacerations to her wrists and forearms using the broken handle of a teaspoon from her lunch tray.

- What immediate first aid measures are needed?
- Decide what measures the nurse will need to take to ensure that Josie receives appropriate wound care until her lacerations heal.
- Decide what actions the nurse should take to ensure appropriate reporting and recording of the incident and to minimize the risk of Josie repeating the behaviour.

Case study: Learning disabilities

Joseph is 40 years of age, has Down syndrome and lives in residential care. He has developed the habit of picking the skin on the back of his hand, which has resulted in a small but deep wound. Although the wound has been covered with a plaster, Joseph continues to pick at the wound site and the nurse thinks that the present dressing is inadequate.

- Decide what factors should be taken into account when choosing an appropriate dressing for Joseph?
- What nursing knowledge and skills would the nurse require to facilitate wound healing in Joseph's case?

Summary

This chapter has focused on the knowledge and decision making needed to provide high-quality skin care for patients/clients and ourselves. It has included:

1. Information to understand the biological basis underpinning tissue viability, and also the psychological, social, cultural, environmental and economic factors involved.
2. An appreciation of the importance of conducting a thorough and appropriate assessment of the skin disorder/wound and of the patient as a whole, prior to the implementation of care.
3. Knowledge for the management of wounds/skin disorders based on current evidence based protocols, care procedures and outcome measures to evaluate effective wound/skin care.
4. Health promotion strategies to encourage a healthy skin.
5. Acknowledgement of the vital role of specialist nurses and the multidisciplinary team in ensuring consistent quality care especially for patients with chronic skin conditions/wounds.
6. Legal and ethical issues in skin care with particular reference to consent to treatment.

Acknowledgement

We would like to thank Mrs D. E. Cotrel-Gibbons, Health Lecturer, for her contribution to the surgical wound section.

Annotated further reading and websites

Ballard K, Baxter H 2000 Developments in wound care for difficult to manage wounds. British Journal of Nursing 9:405–412
This article discusses some of the latest developments in wound care, including vacuum assisted closure, tissue engineering and the use of growth factors.

Chivers L 2002 Body adornment: piercing and tattoos. Nursing Standard 16:41–45
This article explores the different types of, and sites for, body piercing. It also highlights the adverse side effects.

Cullum N, Deeks J, Sheldon T A et al 2003 Beds, mattresses and cushions for pressure sore prevention and treatment (Cochrane review). In: The Cochrane Library, Issue 1. Update Software, Oxford
A review of 35 randomized controlled trials of the use of support surfaces for treatment and prevention of pressure sores. Although it is unable to determine the most effective surface it does provide a wide range of information on different support surfaces.

Eyers G 2001 Prevention of pressure damage at the Queen's Medical Centre. British Journal of Nursing 10:(Suppl.):s50–s56
This is a useful article, which discusses the role of a multidisciplinary wound management policy group in ensuring the provision of high-quality, evidence based care in wound management.

Fernandez R, Griffiths R, Ussia C 2003 Water for wound cleansing (Cochrane review) In: The Cochrane Library, Issue 1. Update Software, Oxford
This review, although limited, compares the use of tap water, normal saline and non-cleansing in acute and chronic wounds.

McHenry P M, Williams H C, Bingham E A 1995 Management of atopic eczema. British Medical Journal 310:843–847
This article offers a comprehensive framework for good practice in the management of atopic eczema based on the consensus of opinion of the participants of a joint workshop of the British Association of Dermatologists and the Research Unit of the Royal College of Physicians of London.

Murphy A 1995 Cleansing solutions. Nursing Times 91:78, 80
This article provides a concise guide to wound cleansing agents.

Newton H, Trudgian J, Gould D 2000 Expanding tissue viability practice through telemedicine. British Journal of Nursing 9(Suppl.): s42–s48
This article discusses the use of telemedicine for patients with complex tissue viability needs, from the perspective of the authors' experience.

Vowden K R, Vowden P 1999 Wound debridement. Part 1: non-sharp techniques. Journal of Wound Care 8:237–240
The article focuses on non-sharp techniques for wound debridement and is well illustrated with photographs. It is the first of a two-part update on wound debridement.

Walsh M, Kent A 2001 Accident and emergency nursing, 4th edn. Butterworth-Heinemann, Oxford, Ch 8
This chapter gives a useful overview of the management of soft tissue injury and wound care in an A and E setting.

http://www.epuap.org/
The European Pressure Ulcer Advisory Panel was formed in 1996 to provide guidance across the EU countries. The website contains information on the panel and guidelines for practice.

http://www.worldwidewounds.com/
This is the Electronic Journal of Wound Management Practice produced by the Surgical Materials Testing Laboratory, Bridgend, South Wales, in association with the Medical Education Partnership.

http://www.lasg.co.uk
The Latex Allergy Support Group provides a quarterly newsletter, a guide to products that contain natural latex and information for sufferers.

http://www.nice.org.uk
Home page for the National Institute for Clinical Excellence (NICE). It provides links for both professionals and the public into a variety of pages that give guidance for best practice. See technical appraisal guidance no. 24 related to debridement and specialist wound care.

http://www.eczema.org/navif.shtml
The National Eczema Society is dedicated to the needs of people with eczema, dermatitis and sensitive skin. A wide range of literature on skin conditions is provided on this website.

http://www.tvs.org.uk/
The Tissue Viability Society runs this useful website providing information for professionals, patients and carers. It contains some patient information leaflets that can be downloaded. Also provides information on forthcoming events and access to the Journal of Tissue Viability.

References

Armstrong M L, Masten Y, Martin R 2000 Adolescent pregnancy, tattooing and risk taking. American Journal of Maternal Child Nursing 25:258–261

Bale S, Jones V 1997 Wound care nursing: a patient-centred approach. Baillière Tindall, London

Ballard K, Baxter H 2000 Developments in wound care for difficult to manage wounds. British Journal of Nursing 9:405–412

Benbow M 1994 Improving wound management. Community Outlook January:21, 22, 24

Benbow M 2001 Assessing wounds. Practice Nurse 21:44, 46, 48

Benbow M 2002 The skin. 2: Skin and wound assessment. Nursing Times 98:41–44

Bennett G, Moody M 1995 Wound care for health professionals. Chapman & Hall, London

Bux N, Malhi J S 1996 Assessing the use of dressings in practice. Journal of Wound Care 5:305–308

Chapman E J, Chapman R 1986 Treatment of pressure sores: the state of the art. In: Tierney A J (ed) Clinical nursing practice. Churchill Livingstone, Edinburgh, pp 105–124

Chivers L 2002 Body adornments: piercing and tattoos. Nursing Standard 16:41–45

Collier M 1997 Know how: vacuum assisted closure (VAC). Nursing Times 93:137–138

Cronin T A 2001 Tattoos, piercing and skin adornments. Dermatological Nursing 13:380–383

Cull P (ed) 1989 The sourcebook of medical illustration. Parthenon, Carnforth

Culley F 2001 The tissue viability nurse and effective documentation. British Journal of Nursing 10:(Suppl.):s30 s39

David J A 1986 Wound management: a comprehensive guide to dressing and healing. Martin Dunitz, London

Dealey C 1999 The care of wounds, 2nd edn. Blackwell Science, Oxford

Department of Health 1993 The health of the nation: One year on … A report on the progress of the health of the nation. HMSO, London

Department of Health 2001 The essence of care: Pressure ulcer risk assessment and prevention. HMSO, London. Online. Available: http://www.doh.gov.uk/essenceofcare/contents.htm 3 Mar 2003

Douglas V 2001 Living with a chronic leg ulcer: an insight into patients' experiences and feelings. Journal of Wound Care 10:355–360

European Pressure Ulcer Advisory Panel 1999 Guidelines. Online. Available: http://www.epuap.org/ 3 Mar 2003

Eyers G 2001 Prevention of pressure damage at the Queen's Medical Centre. British Journal of Nursing 10(Suppl.):s50–s56

Fisher G J, Wang Z-Q, Datta S C et al 1997 Pathophysiology of premature skin ageing induced by ultraviolet light. New England Journal of Medicine 337:1419–1428

Gibbs G 1988 Learning by doing: a guide to teaching and learning methods. Oxford Polytechnic, Oxford

Gross R D 1992 Psychology: the science of mind and behaviour, 2nd edn. Hodder & Stoughton, London

Hollingworth H, Kingston J E 1998 Using a non-sterile technique of wound care. Professional Nurse 13:226–229

Jacobson D 1992 India: land of dreams and fantasy. Todtri, New York

McHenry P M, Williams H C, Bingham E A 1995 Management of atopic eczema. British Medical Journal 310:843–847

Marks I M 1987 Fears, phobias and rituals. Oxford University Press, Oxford

Moffatt C J, Oldroyd M I 1994 A pioneering service to the community: the Riverside Community Leg Ulcer Project. Professional Nurse 9:486, 488, 490, 492, 494, 497

Montgomery J 1997 Health care law. Oxford Polytechnic, Oxford

Morison M 1997 A color guide to the nursing management of chronic wounds, 2nd edn. Mosby, St Louis, p25

Naidoo J, Wills J 2000 Health promotion: foundations for practice, 2nd edn. Baillière Tindall, London

National Institute for Clinical Excellence 2001 Pressure sore risk assessment and prevention. National Institute for Clinical Excellence, London. Online. Available: http://www.nice.org.uk

Nursing and Midwifery Council 2002 Code of professional conduct. Nursing and Midwifery Council, London

Office for National Statistics 1996 www.statistics.gov.uk/ then search: skin cancer

Phillips P 2001 A review of the expert opinion on latex allergy. Electronic Journal of Wound Management Practice. Online. Available: http://www.worldwidewounds.com/

Podmore J 1994 Leg ulcer: weighing up the evidence. Nursing Standard 8:25, 27

Stuppy D, Armstrong M L, Casals-Ariet C 1998 Attitudes of healthcare providers and students towards tattooed people. Journal of Advanced Nursing 27:1165–1170

Thomas S, Loveless P 1997 A comparative study of the properties of twelve hydrocolloid dressings. Electronic Journal of Wound Management Practice. Online. Available: http://www.worldwidewounds.com/

Thomas S, Jones M, Wynn K et al 2001 The current status of maggot therapy in wound healing. British Journal of Nursing 10:(Suppl.):s5–s12

Tritle N M, Haller J R, Gray S D 2001 Aesthetic comparison of wound closure techniques in a porcine model. Laryngoscope 111:1949–1951

Tortora G J 1999 Principles of human anatomy, 8th edn. John Wiley, Chichester

UK Central Council 1992 The scope of professional practice. UK Central Council, London

UK Central Council 1994 Standards for specialist education and practice. UK Central Council, London

Walsh M (ed) 1997 Watson's Clinical nursing and related sciences, 5th edn. Baillière Tindall, London

Walsh M 1998 Models and critical pathways in clinical nursing: conceptual frameworks for care planning, 2nd edn. Baillière Tindall, London

Westaby S (ed) 1985 Wound care. Heinemann, London

Wijetunge D 1992 An A and E approach. Nursing Times 88:70, 72, 73, 76

Chapter 15

Sexuality

Steve Eastburn

KEY ISSUES

SUBJECT KNOWLEDGE
- Defining sexuality
- Sexuality: the historical context
- Masculinity and femininity
- Sexual development
- The sexual response
- Sexual behaviour

CARE DELIVERY KNOWLEDGE
- Sexuality and nursing models
- Assessment and sexuality
- Discussing sexuality with clients
- Problems related to clients' sexuality
- Nursing actions

PROFESSIONAL AND ETHICAL KNOWLEDGE
- Nursing as a female profession
- Key issues in the four branches of nursing
- The law and sexuality
- Sexuality and current policy

PERSONAL AND REFLECTIVE KNOWLEDGE
- Case studies
- Suggestions for portfolio evidence

INTRODUCTION

The concept of sexuality is important for nursing practice because it is an essential element of people's lives and people's health. This chapter explores the nature of sexuality and suggests how nurses can incorporate it into their day-to-day work with clients. Nursing theory has acknowledged the significance of human sexuality, but it is an aspect of practice that nurses have great difficulty with. This is probably due to two factors:

- firstly, sexuality is not easy to define
- secondly, it includes aspects of people's lives that usually remain private.

Sexuality is a delicate subject surrounded by mystery and misunderstandings. Consequently it can be easily avoided by nurses and clients. The aim of this chapter is to explore the meaning of sexuality and identify the relevance of the concept for nurses in practice.

OVERVIEW

Subject knowledge

The chapter begins with an exploration of definitions and meanings of sexuality. It includes an overview of the historical context, and identifies some of the problems associated with understanding images of sexuality in the past. Masculinity, femininity and gender roles are then addressed, leading into an outline of the processes involved in the development of an individual's sexuality. This includes information on the male and female reproductive systems and the biological control of human sexual development and the human sexual response. It also includes psychosocial theory related to the development of sexual identity and gender roles.

Following this is an overview of sexual norms and a summary of key research on sexual behaviour in Britain. This ends with a consideration of the relationship between emotion and sexual behaviour.

Care delivery knowledge

Care delivery knowledge begins with an outline of sexuality as an aspect of nursing models and moves on to discuss the assessment of an individual's sexual health and sexuality related problems. It includes guidance on how to discuss sensitive issues with clients. To conclude this section, types of sexuality related problems are identified with appropriate nursing actions.

Professional and ethical knowledge

This section discusses the importance of nursing as a mainly female profession and identifies issues specific to the four branches of nursing. It includes an overview of legal issues and health policy related to sexuality.

Personal and reflective knowledge

This section comprises four case studies (pp. 348–349), one for each branch of nursing. The case studies help to raise important issues for clinical practice and there are a number of questions to stimulate debate. You may like to read one of these before beginning this chapter, to use as a focus for reflection. After the case studies there are a number of exercises to help you develop your personal portfolio. The exercises encourage you to reflect on and learn from practice.

SUBJECT KNOWLEDGE

DEFINING SEXUALITY

Defining sexuality is not an easy task. Sexual activity, including feelings, thoughts and actions, is central to such a definition, and the concepts of masculinity and femininity are also significant. Writers who have grappled with the nature of sexuality have often included these ideas, but the need to take a broad view has been emphasized. These views are perhaps best summarized by Byers (1989: 312) who states that:

> Sexuality is the expression and experience of the self as a sexual being. It is, therefore, a state of both the body and mind and a crucial part of the personality. Sexuality is not limited to overt sexual activity, such as sexual intercourse, but includes solitary activities like studying, walking and relaxing. Sexuality is part of every relationship, whether it is primarily a sexual relationship or not; it is the rapport that is established between the self and body.

Although this definition emphasizes the broad nature of sexuality as a component of people's lives, its generality may still leave people asking '… but what does it really involve?' There is no simple answer, but in the literature the common elements shown in Figure 15.1 can be identified.

These elements attempt to expand on the concept of sexuality; however, they are not exhaustive. Because sexuality is

```
Sex
Sexual orientation
Gender and associated roles
Relationships
Self-image
Self-esteem
Human attraction
Love
```

Figure 15.1 Elements of sexuality.

a social construct, and is open to change and interpretation, complete and accurate definitions cannot exist. They are also surrounded by the notions of normality, what is right, and what is wrong. In coming to an understanding of sexuality it is therefore essential to take into account its changing nature and the social and historical forces that shape it.

Studies on the history of sexuality emphasize how people's attitudes and behaviour have changed (Foucault 1979). Van Ooijen & Charnock (1994) summarize this by focusing on a range of issues, for example common sexual practices, forbidden sexual activities, the relationships between men and women, religious influence on social norms and the portrayal of sexual symbols in art and language. These changes are difficult to appreciate, however, because the language and concepts used to compare sexuality throughout the ages are based on the understanding of the sexuality norms of today. For example, the popular image of Roman times is one in which sexual activity had a high public profile. Behaviours that would not be accepted today were seen as normal practice. Victorian times on the other hand have been characterized by repressive attitudes towards sex. These attitudes manifested themselves in the language of the day, and the delicate subject of sex was surrounded by taboos and managed through strict social etiquette. More recently, the 1960s are famous for 'free love' and the liberated youth.

Although there may be some truth in these stereotypes they are nevertheless generalizations and tend to concentrate on sexual activity rather than a broader understanding of sexuality. In turn, these views of previous generations have inherent dangers.

Firstly, they may be inaccurate. Secondly, there is an assumption that a person's sexuality develops during his or her 'formative' years and then remains stable. For example the 1930s and 1940s may conjure up images of marriage for life, sexual faithfulness in the nuclear family setting, and sex as a taboo subject in day-to-day conversation. These images are arguably more myth than reality, but they can influence the way a nurse views an older person in the early 21st century. It is easy to see how the subject of safe sex may not be considered appropriate by a nurse working with a 75-year-old person if the nurse believes that people from that generation think and behave according to the popular images.

An important development in the recent history of sexuality is the increasing acceptance of sexual activity as a valid topic for scientific study. This has perhaps resulted from more openness in society and also from the need to focus attention on human immunodeficiency virus (HIV) and acquired immunodeficiency syndrome (AIDS). Sexual problems and the impact of ill health on sexuality are recognized as issues that may require professional help. Also nursing and other professions are incorporating a holistic model of health into their practice that views sexuality as an important dimension of human life.

MASCULINITY AND FEMININITY

Sexuality is a broad term referring to a central part of people's lives. It is reflected by what they do, say and feel, and especially in the way that people interact with each other. A traditional way of interpreting sexuality is through their understanding of masculinity and femininity and the roles associated with being a man or woman. Although this may be blurred in today's society, gender-specific roles are still influential. In starting to explore sexuality then, the ideas of masculinity and femininity are important.

Descriptions of masculinity and femininity are associated with stereotypical images of men and women. These images can be seen in films, cartoons and popular magazines and although they can be the butt of jokes, they can also be ideals, or sources of aspiration.

It could be argued that these images are outdated and that to be masculine today the characteristics of the so-called 'new man' have to be taken into account. Many would disagree, though, suggesting that the emergence of the new man is a myth and that many traditional gender differences and inequalities still exist (Hudson & Williams 1995). Others suggest that the experience of being a woman has changed as many more women take on paid employment and the nature of family life has altered (Giddens 1993). Whatever the case, images of masculinity and femininity influence people in their day-to-day lives through their choice of jobs, the clothes they wear and the types of interests they develop.

Gender roles

In society there is a distinction between men's and women's roles. This can clearly be seen by the type of employment that men and women take, and the social pressures influencing the decisions around their selection. From an early age children have ideas about what they would like to be when they 'grow up'. With responses like 'I want to be a train driver' or 'I want to be a nurse' you can guess with some confidence the gender of the child. Although children's aspirations differ from one society to the next, and from one generation to the other, boys' views of their future will clearly contrast with those of girls. Of course these childhood wishes are not likely to come true for many, but nevertheless adult roles are largely gender-specific and comply with general expectations. There are exceptions, but being exceptions, they tend to reinforce the rule. For example, a female bricklayer and a male

secretary will probably be seen as unusual, and may even acquire local celebrity status.

It has been argued that with the changing employment market and the disappearance of traditional heavy jobs through automation and computer technology, men's and women's roles are less distinct (Beechey 1987). This could be the case, but gender role differences are not the sole province of paid employment. They are also evident in leisure interests, household tasks and the relationships and interactions within a family. Some of these differences may be seen as inequalities, with some roles having greater accessibility to those activities generally viewed as rewarding or stimulating. Men living in family settings in some social groups may have access to a greater proportion of these activities, for example, leisure time, careers, or peer group interaction. Although the research is becoming dated, there has been evidence that marriage affected men's health more positively than women's. In simple terms married men were healthier than single men whereas married women were less healthy than single women. Although this does not demonstrate cause and effect, the associations between family life and a number of indicators of health for men and women consistently suggested that marriage was 'healthy' for men and 'unhealthy' for women (Gove & Tudor 1972). Family structures and employment patterns have changed significantly since the early 1970s and the evidence on the links between marital status and health is less clear.

Roles people take in society, particularly those in paid employment and those within a family, express something about them as individuals. They enable people to express sexuality to those around them and enable them to develop a positive self-image. Sometimes these roles are associated with pressures, however. Role strain occurs when the duties or expectations associated with a person's roles become a burden. The individual finds it difficult to wear many hats. Role conflict occurs when a person's roles show signs of incompatibility. For example, a woman can be a mother and be expected to make decisions regarding her children. She can also be a daughter and be expected to take advice from and listen to the wisdom of her parents. Such pressures can make the fulfilment of these roles difficult or impossible at times.

Reflection and portfolio evidence

Make a list of the different roles you currently take.

- Are there any competing pressures between these roles?
- How might these roles change in the future?
- What would happen if you suddenly had a big, unexpected demand from one of your role obligations?
- Devise a plan to balance between your obligations for each role with your available resources.

(You might find the time planning exercise in Ch. 8 on relaxation and stress useful here.)

DEVELOPMENT OF AN INDIVIDUAL'S SEXUALITY

The reproductive system

For the first few weeks after fertilization the embryonic internal and external genitalia for males and females are the same. At about the seventh week hormonal changes lead to sex differentiation and the male reproductive system develops under the influence of increased androgen levels.

In childhood, the greatest time of physical change related to sexuality occurs during puberty. These changes are hormonally controlled and the process begins at around 11–12 years of age for girls and 12–13 years of age for boys. It involves the development of fully functioning reproductive systems and the body changes that result in the characteristic adult male and female physiques (Fig. 15.2).

Adult male reproductive system (Fig. 15.3)

Testes

The testes have two functions:

- production of sperm
- secretion of testosterone.

The testes are made up of a fine network of convoluted seminiferous tubules. Under the influence of hormones, stem cells in the convoluted seminiferous tubules undergo a series of changes. These result in the production of spermatozoa, which pass into the epididymis to mature before ejaculation. During ejaculation the sperm pass out of the tail of the epididymis and into the vas deferens. As the sperm pass along the vas deferens and ejaculatory duct, the seminal vesicle, prostate gland and bulbourethral gland secrete fluid containing chemicals and nutrients. This mixture is called semen and its purpose is to allow the sperm to survive and move along the female reproductive tract.

Testosterone is a hormone needed for spermatogenesis and the sex drive. It is also responsible for the development of the following male secondary sex characteristics:

- enlargement of the penis and testes
- enlargement of the larynx producing a deeper voice
- growth of facial hair and pubic hair
- increased sebaceous gland activity
- muscle development.

Penis

The penis contains three cylindrical masses of erectile tissue: two corpora cavernosa running along the top and sides, and a smaller corpus cavernosum on the underside, which contains the urethra. The glans penis at the end of the shaft of the penis is normally covered by a fold of skin, the prepuce

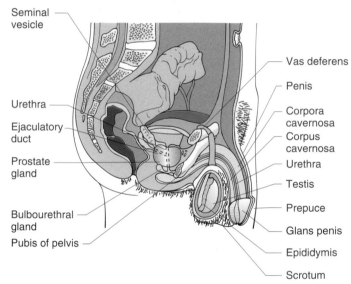

Figure 15.3 Anatomy of the male reproductive system. (From Hinchliff et al 1996.)

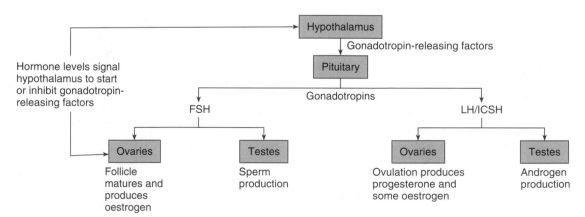

Figure 15.2 Hormonal control of sexual development. FSH, follicle-stimulating hormone; ICSH, interstitial-cell-stimulating hormone; LH, luteinizing hormone. (After Offir 1982.)

or foreskin, which is sometimes removed surgically (circumcision). During sexual arousal the erectile tissue fills with blood and the penis enlarges and becomes firm.

Adult female reproductive system

Internal genitalia

The ovaries (see Fig. 15.4) have two functions:

- production of ova
- secretion of progesterone and oestrogen.

Each ovary contains many oocytes. These are the cells that undergo a series of changes to develop into mature graafian follicles. Ovulation occurs when a follicle ruptures and releases an oocyte into the fallopian tube. This happens once a month during the menstrual cycle.

The hormone progesterone 'prepares' the woman's body for pregnancy. It increases the growth of the endometrium and breasts and influences cervical mucus production and uterine muscle activity. Another hormone, oestrogen, influences oogenesis and follicle maturation, the onset of puberty and the development of female secondary sex characteristics, and the growth and maintenance of reproductive organs. Female secondary sex characteristics include:

- growth and development of breasts
- body hair, e.g. pubic hair
- changes in fat distribution to produce the female physique
- vaginal secretions.

The fallopian tubes extend from the uterus towards the ovaries. They open into the peritoneal cavity with funnel-like projections. The oocyte moves into the first part of the fallopian tube and is fertilized in the ampulla partway along its length. Peristalsis and ciliated cells help the oocyte move to the uterus, which is a hollow, thick-walled muscular structure that assists in the implantation of the embryo, nurtures the developing fetus and moves the baby out

through the vagina at birth. The epithelial layer is the endometrium and this changes in thickness and structure under hormonal control during the menstrual cycle. The cervix is at the lower end of the uterus.

The vagina is a canal connecting the cervix to the external genitalia. It expands during childbirth and intercourse and has an acidic environment to protect it from pathogenic organisms. It becomes lubricated during sexual arousal with secretions from the vestibular glands and with some fluid leakage from the vaginal walls. The distal end of the vaginal orifice is partially occluded by the hymen. This usually ruptures during first intercourse, but it can also be ruptured by tampons or exercise.

External genitalia (Fig. 15.5)

The mons pubis is a fatty pad over the pubic bone. The labia majora are covered in skin and have many sebaceous glands and the labia minora meet at the anterior end at the clitoris. The clitoris is rich in nerve endings and plays an important part in the sexual response. The vestibular glands secrete a fluid which lubricates the vagina during sexual arousal.

The menstrual cycle

This is controlled by circulating hormones, but can be influenced by emotional factors. It has the following three phases:

1. The proliferative phase (oestrogen causes cell proliferation in the uterus, the endometrium thickens and the cervical mucus becomes thinner and more profuse), which ends with ovulation.
2. The secretory phase (vascularity of the endometrium increases under the influence of progesterone and cervical mucus thickens to block the cervical canal; hormonal secretion from the corpus luteum declines if fertilization does not take place and the endometrium begins to degenerate).

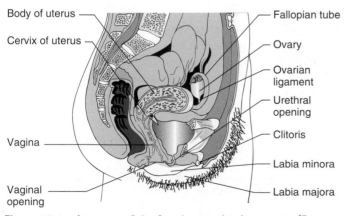

Figure 15.4 Anatomy of the female reproductive system. (From Hinchliff et al 1996.)

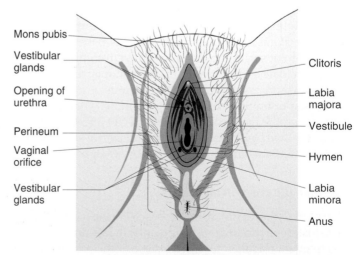

Figure 15.5 The female external genitalia. (From Hinchliff et al 1996.)

3. The menstrual phase (the flow of blood and endometrial tissue, which lasts 3–6 days); prostaglandins stimulate the uterus to contract and this causes the characteristic pain (dysmenorrhoea).

Premenstrual syndrome

Before the menstrual phase some women experience a range of symptoms. Pelvic congestion and overall body water retention can give a feeling of distension. Also tiredness, irritability, depression and loss of concentration are not uncommon. The increase in body weight alongside these symptoms can lead to body image changes and feelings of low self-esteem. The reasons for these symptoms are unclear. Some theories suggest fluid retention is the cause, others that a vitamin deficiency (vitamin B_6) resulting from hormonal variations affects the functioning of the brain leading to mood changes.

The intensity of the premenstrual syndrome varies from individual to individual, but these variations do not seem to be linked to the degree of hormonal change. Also the significance and character of premenstrual changes have varied throughout history. This suggests that the premenstrual syndrome is influenced by social and psychological as well as biological factors (Webb 1985).

Menopause

Some of the changes in sexual response for women are associated with the menopause. This usually happens between the ages of 45 and 55. It is the time when the ovaries cease to function and a woman's reproductive life ends. The hormonal changes are sometimes associated with a range of symptoms, and the pattern of symptoms can vary. Sweating, hot flushes, insomnia, depression, fatigue and headaches are sometimes experienced at this time of life. Webb (1985) believes that the evidence to link these symptoms with hormonal changes is far from conclusive. Coming to terms with the end of a reproductive life plus other stressful life events commonly experienced at this age might be the causes of such symptoms. She cites the variations between women from different social classes and women from different societies as evidence to suggest that the menopause has significant social and psychological determinants.

It is important to stress that the hormonal changes occurring during the menopause do not directly affect a women's interest in sex. Oestrogen levels do not control sex drive nor do they affect a woman's ability to enjoy sex or have orgasms.

The 'mid-life crisis' in men

Men at this time of life might be experiencing a slow decline in testosterone production. This results in less firm erections, less frequent ejaculations and a longer refractory period (see below). Men can also experience social and psychological pressures leading to a 'mid-life crisis' (Atkinson et al 1990).

In the same way that it is difficult to attribute menopause purely to biological factors, any changes in a man's sexual activity at this time of life cannot always be associated with decreasing androgen levels.

THE SEXUAL RESPONSE

The sexual response in men and women is controlled by complex interactions between the central nervous system, the peripheral nervous system, neurotransmitters, hormones and the circulatory system (Boone 1995). It has four stages:

1. Arousal, which in men results in penile erection, testicular elevation and flattening of the scrotal skin, and in women results in vaginal lubrication, clitoral enlargement, upper vaginal dilation, vaginal constriction of the lower third, uterine elevation and breast and nipple enlargement.
2. Plateau, which in men is associated with an increase in secretions from the urethral Cowper's glands and an increase in blood pressure, heart rate, respiratory rate and muscle tone, and in women is associated with retraction of the clitoris against the pubic bone and increases in blood pressure, heart rate, respiratory rate and muscle tone.
3. Orgasm, which in men is characterized by a rhythmical contraction of the perineal muscles, closure of the bladder neck and ejaculation, while in women may be single or multiple and involves contractions of the perineal muscles, uterus and fallopian tubes, although not all women experience orgasm.
4. Resolution, when the physiological changes are reversed. There is also a refractory period, which is the resting time that must elapse before the next sexual response can be initiated, and this may be shorter for women (Masters & Johnson 1966).

The impact of age-related physiological changes on the sexual response

For men

Men may experience the following age-related changes:

- arousal: erections may occur less frequently and more and longer direct stimulation of the penis is required to establish and maintain an erection
- plateau: may be prolonged and ejaculation more easily controlled
- orgasm: the number and force of contractions decrease, but the sensation may be equally satisfying
- resolution: the length of time between orgasm and the next possible erection increases.

For women

Reduced oestrogen levels result in thinning of the vaginal mucosa, replacement of breast tissue by fat and shrinking of the uterus. These may affect the sexual response in older women as follows:

- arousal: longer direct clitoral stimulation may be required, the vaginal opening expands less and vaginal lubrication may be reduced
- plateau: sensation may alter due to a decrease in vaso-congestion and a reduced tenting of the vagina
- orgasm: contractions may be fewer
- resolution: the clitoris loses its erection more rapidly, but the refractory period after orgasm does not seem to lengthen for women as it does for men.

Decision making exercise

From the information on the effects of ageing on the sexual response:

- Can you see any physiological reasons why sexual activity might have to stop for older people?
- Can you see any physiological reasons why older people might not enjoy sexual activity?
- What implications do your answers have for nurses working with older people?

SEXUAL IDENTITY

A number of sociologists and psychologists have attempted to explain how people develop a sexual identity. There is agreement among many that relationships and interactions with those close to us play an important part. Others emphasize the biological factors and believe that our genetic make-up determines our sexual identity. The key theories are outlined below.

Freud's psychoanalytical theory

Freud's (1923) psychoanalytical theory offered an explanation of why boys and girls grow up differently, and has since been developed by many psychologists. Freud focused on five stages of development. At each stage he identified the way in which individuals learned to balance the satisfaction of the 'libidinal' or pleasure drive of Id against Ego and Superego. The effectiveness of resolution at each stage, Freud contended, had lasting ramifications on the subsequent personality development.

Oral stage: 0–18 months of age

Newborn infants are unable to do little more than suck and drink and the libidinal drive finds its outlet in this activity. The infant derives its gratification orally, both for food and for pleasure. In early life sucking is passive to gain nourishment, although as the infant develops this occasionally turns to aggressive biting. During this stage of life only Id is present in the personality. Superego and Ego have not yet developed. Consequently the infant becomes frustrated if his demands are not met immediately.

Anal stage: 18 months to 3 years of age

During this period restrictions are placed upon the child's life for the first time. Initially the child discovers that the breast is no longer available immediately when it is wanted. Then potty training begins, restricting bowel evacuation and urination to specific times. These constraints frustrate Id and result in temper tantrums. Eventually, with the development of Ego, the child learns to exert some control over Id and uses the potty. It is at this time that the libidinal drive passes to the anus and the child finds the control of bowel movements to be pleasurable, both from expelling the bowel contents and by retaining them.

During these first two stages of development the infant is unaware of gender differences. All children are seen as 'little males'.

Phallic stage: 3–5 years of age

The child becomes aware of its gender and discovers that pleasure can be derived from the penis or clitoris. The libidinal drive then centres on this body area and the child derives satisfaction from playing with its sexual organ. This continues until the behaviour is shamed into stopping by the child's parents. During this phase the child forms an incestuous desire for the parent of the opposite sex. In the male child this is called the Oedipus complex. The boy's love for his mother becomes very intense and this leads him to become very jealous of anyone who competes for his mother's attention. Consequently conflict arises with his father. The child wishes to replace his father as the object of his mother's attention; however, he fears that if he does so then he will be punished. He has noticed that girls and his mother do not have a penis. This, he suspects, is because they were castrated as a punishment when they were younger. He fears that if he continues with the feelings he has for his mother then his father will also castrate him. To protect his penis he represses the feelings he holds for his mother and identifies with his father. This way he both retains his penis and by identifying with his father he also fulfils his desire for his mother.

In the female child a different process, the Electra complex, occurs. Initially the female child is drawn towards her mother. She discovers, however, that unlike her father and boys, she does not possess a penis. She assumes that she has been castrated, for which she blames her mother and feels inferior. Freud called this phenomenon 'penis envy'. The girl realizes that she will not get a replacement penis and consequently sublimates the desire for a penis with the desire for a baby. She looks to her father to provide her with this and transfers her affections to him. This also brings problems, though. If the girl looks to her father to provide affection then she will be in direct competition with her mother.

In consequence she fears that her mother may withdraw her love for her. To prevent this she internalizes the images of her mother as carer, so that her mother will continue to love her. This is the final part of the Electra complex, where the girl identifies again with her mother, and is called anaclytic identification.

The phallic stage is a very ambivalent period for a child of either gender and parental attitudes during this stage have profound ramifications on the child's development.

Latency stage: 5 years of age to puberty

Following the traumas of the phallic stage, this period is relatively quiet. The child's sexual interests are replaced by interests at school, playtimes, sports and a range of new activities. Possibly for the first time the child meets people from outside the family and with whom new relationships are formed. Children who were unsuccessful in passing through the earlier stages can find the world outside the family confusing and threatening and they often have difficulty forming new relationships in this period.

Genital stage: puberty to adulthood

With the onset of puberty the individual experiences a jolt from the sexual dormancy of the latency stage. Individuals have intense libidinal drives to engage in full sexual activity. The capacity for full physiological sexual responses has also developed by this stage and in turn, individuals are able to experience themselves as complete sexual beings. At this stage boys lose sexual attachment for their mother. Similarly girls lose their attachment for their father. This allows them to make sexual attachment to members of the opposite sex; however, during this stage, the individual has to learn to express sexual energy in socially acceptable ways.

Despite criticisms, Freud's theory highlights the importance of relationships and interactions between children and the adults around them. It also identified the importance of sexuality in many aspects of life, and stimulated a wealth of research in this area. The nature and quality of relationships during these formative years seem to be significant in the development of an individual's sexuality. The difficulties people have in forming relationships with others result in part from early childhood experiences with parents. In certain settings nurses will work with people who have problems with their identity. Crises with an individual's identity, in particular their sense of sexuality, are likely to have their origins in childhood development, and advanced nursing practice may involve the exploration of clients' relationships with their parents.

Neoanalytical theory

Some writers modified Freud's ideas, basing their explanations of gender identity on other experiences in early childhood. Chodorow (1978) emphasizes the importance of the early maternal bond that exists apparently in all societies.

Girls never completely break this bond and their consequent identity incorporates a significant relational element. Boys on the other hand have to break this bond in order to develop a masculine identity. This masculine identity is characterized by independence, individuality and a rejection of the feminine. Girls grow up being able to relate closely to others whereas boys take a more analytical view of the world and value achievement rather than caring or compassion. As a result, women require a close relationship in order to maintain their self-esteem, but men feel threatened by such close emotional attachments.

This theory is based on the primary role of the woman as the main carer of children, especially in the early years, and has been criticized for assuming a straightforward female psychological make-up that fails to take into account other feelings, for example aggression and assertiveness (Sayers 1986). On the other hand it may help to make sense of some men's apparent inability to express their emotions.

Sociobiological theories

Sociobiologists use ideas from evolutionary biology to explain human behaviour and sexual identity. Symons (1979) argues that sexual behaviour is influenced by the biological need to reproduce. People strive to be successful in reproduction so that genetic information can be passed on to the next generation and sexuality concerns those activities that help to achieve this success.

Men have many sperm and it makes sense for men to seek to use as many as they can. This has been given as an explanation for men being more promiscuous than women. Women have relatively few ova, and these being precious, their owners need to make sure that they are used carefully. It is in the interests of women therefore to be selective in whom they choose as a mate. They need to make sure that their genes are amalgamated with others of a high quality. This theory has implications for the development of attitudes. Men should approve of casual sex and have many partners, whereas women should be less approving of casual sex and should seek long-term commitment from a small number of partners. Related to this is the explanation of men's jealousy and desire to control women's sexuality. Because a man provides for the mother and child he needs to make sure that his work is being used to rear his own offspring and not anyone else's. For this reason men would be disapproving of their wives engaging in extramarital sex.

This sociobiological theory has its critics. Travis & Yeager (1991) argue that society is more complex than the picture painted here and sexual behaviour has meanings other than the purely reproductive. For example, the theory does not take into account the developing nature of sex and sexuality throughout an individual's lifespan. Also it attempts to legitimize inequalities between men and women by suggesting that they are natural and normal. This fails to explore the importance of socialization and the use of power in establishing and maintaining gender inequalities.

Social learning theory

This is concerned with the processes through which boys and girls learn their gender-related roles (Mischel 1966). It does not see biology as particularly important in determining behaviour, but emphasizes the association and interactions between children and others. This is, in the first place, the communication that takes place with parents. Behaviour consistent with gender is reinforced through rewards. So when parents and others react in a positive way towards a girl in a pretty dress playing with dolls and an urchin of a boy climbing trees, this behaviour is likely to be repeated. Initially children look to others for models of behaviour and these can include parents, siblings, teachers and people in the media. This means that learning how to behave as a woman or a man is partly influenced by parental upbringing, but the influence of people and images outside the family explain why children can differ from their parents. This theory is dynamic in that it takes account of an individual's changing nature and incorporates such things as trends and fashions. However, it tends to see people as initially shapeless, waiting to be moulded by the environment and those around them. In this sense, self-will, motivation and the ability to manipulate the environment and other people are ignored.

Social learning theory attempts to explain how culture is learned, that is how individuals acquire certain patterns of beliefs, values, attitudes and norms. In turn, culture has a strong impact on sexuality and, of course, different cultures assign different meanings to sexuality. Some cultures emphasize equality between partners, including goals of mutual pleasure and psychological disclosure. Others believe that the exchange of pleasure or communication of affection through sexual touching plays no major role in the expression of sexuality (Monga & Lefebvre 1995). Some cultures permit premarital sex, while others condemn it. Culturally determined formal rituals can also play an important part in the development of a sexual identity, for example the circumcision of Jewish boys and the practice of female circumcision in some African countries. Nurses need an understanding of these cultural differences so that they can give culture-specific care (Lavee 1991).

NORMS

By learning from others, as well as the forces and pressures that exist in society, individuals acquire an understanding of what is 'normal', 'right' and 'good'. People need to know what they 'ought' to be doing and thinking in their relationships with others. These social rules are learned during observations and interactions with others in the process of socialization. However, the same process may help some people acquire prejudicial attitudes towards individuals or groups.

Norms are behaviours seen as socially acceptable and help to define what is morally right. There are two problems with this, though. Firstly, the existence of a commonly held view or norm does not in itself make it morally right. Homosexual behaviour has been seen as unacceptable by many people but this is not the same as saying it is morally wrong. Secondly, as discovered by Kinsey et al (1948) and Kinsey & Gebhard (1953) in the USA, the so-called norms of sexual behaviour do not necessarily match up with the lived experience of a large proportion of the population. People do not always live by these social norms. This might be a case of people not acting according to their public beliefs. Turned the other way round, it may mean that people feel unable to display attitudes that are faithful to their private and innermost thoughts for fear of powerful social sanctions such as ridicule or social isolation.

In addition, public attitudes vary so that groups in society have their own associated norms and appropriate forms of behaviour. This introduces further potential for conflict. For example the norms of sexual behaviour held by the youth culture could be very different from those held by parents or by professionals. There is a possibility that parents, teachers, doctors and nurses will see their own 'standards' as right and begin to impose them on those who they feel they are responsible for. For nurses working in the area of sexual health promotion with teenagers this creates an ethical problem. Should they try and persuade young teenagers not to have sex or should they accept this as a fact and offer advice on safe sex? The former might frighten the teenager off and prevent them using services or seeking help. The latter might expose the teenager to a range of physical and psychological risks.

There are also inequalities in the way that norms are applied to groups within society. Certain behaviours may be viewed as acceptable for men, but not for women or acceptable for adults but not for teenagers. Similarly attitudes towards a stable heterosexual couple may differ from that towards a stable homosexual couple.

Differences between norms and actual behaviour are beginning to be uncovered as knowledge about the sexual behaviour and practices people are involved in develops. There are difficulties with this type of research though. For example the words used to describe sexual activity may not have common meaning. Also respondents may be unwilling to tell the truth. It might be argued, however, that with sophisticated research methods and with the increasing social acceptance of the subject of sex, people are more open to discussions of sexual behaviour. Nevertheless it is worth bearing in mind that the accuracy of research in this area is always open to question because of people's unwillingness or inability to discuss such issues.

Homosexuality

The idea of a homosexual identity, in which people attracted to others of the same gender have their own culture and their own lifestyle, is a relatively new phenomenon. Gay bars and clubs, newspapers, associations and holidays have not existed in an organized and overt way for very long. In past centuries individuals were not clearly labelled with a sexual identity that described them as either heterosexual or homosexual. Homosexual activity has always existed, but it was not necessarily seen as exclusive to a specific group of people. In Roman times, for example, it formed part of a range of experiences for some people. Bancroft (1989) describes the development of a gay culture through history, noting varying periods of acceptance and repression of homosexual activity.

In the recent history of developed countries homosexuality has been characterized by rejection. This has been seen in public attitudes and the prejudice and institutionalized inequalities within the legal frameworks of many countries. Minority groups are used as scapegoats for things going wrong in society and throughout history homosexuals have been perceived as the minority group responsible for many ills within society, from the downfall of the Greek empire to the spread of the AIDS virus.

The high incidence of homosexual activity in single-sex restrictive institutions such as prisons, monastic orders and boarding schools, and the numbers of people reporting homosexual experiences, are viewed as examples of the flexibility of the human sexual nature or the fact that individuals cannot be pigeonholed into clearly definable orientations. The hostility towards homosexuality may be a denial of the 'naturalness' of a mixed sexual identity. Similarly the 'laws of nature' have been used to support hostility towards homosexuality. 'Our bodies are not made for it' is the sort of argument put forward. This relates sexual activity to procreation, and homosexuality therefore has no function. A further explanation for the non-acceptance of homosexuality is its association in history with other types of antisocial behaviour, for example witchcraft and heresy.

The medical profession in the 19th century gave a different interpretation of homosexuality from that of the church. Rather than it being a sin, it was seen as a sickness that individuals were either born with or acquired. Treatments were developed to 'cure' homosexuality. The 20th century saw some ambivalence in medicine's attitude towards homosexuality, but the idea that it was something to treat predominated and it was not until 1974 that the American Psychiatric Association removed homosexuality from its list of pathological diagnoses.

Female homosexuality is written about less frequently and has had a lower profile throughout history. This may not mean that women have been less likely than men to be involved in homosexual activity, but could be a reflection of the domination of women by men across a range of social institutions.

Although biological and behavioural sciences tell something about the development of sexual identity, sexuality seems to be a complex mix of biological, psychological and social factors. After exploring the nature of sexuality and how it develops it is important to know how it manifests itself. One of the obvious ways in which sexuality is expressed is through sexual relationships and sexual activities. How people do this and what activities they participate in is the focus of the next section of this chapter.

SEXUAL BEHAVIOUR

Compared with other aspects of people's lives, sexual behaviour has received little academic attention. *The National Survey on Sexual Behaviour in Britain* (Wellings et al 1994) had a difficult start because the Department of Health withdrew its backing at the last minute and the researchers had to find alternative support. The impetus for the work came from the need to find out more about the relationships between sexual practices and the spread of HIV and AIDS, but the social and political sensitivity of the subject meant that the researchers had problems in starting. Similarly Kinsey in the 1940s in the USA (Kinsey et al 1948) and Lanval (1950) at about the same time in Belgium suffered in their attempts to discover more about sexual behaviour. This type of research was seen as pornographic and not worthy of academic attention. Despite these problems Kinsey persisted, and his findings have been seen as highly significant in developing our understanding of sexual behaviour. Essentially he tried to discover through interviewing over 10 000 people what sexual practices were common, for example how many people masturbated and how many had experienced homosexual activities. It was apparent from the findings that individuals' experiences were very different from the official social norms at the time. The reported incidence of homosexuality, masturbation and premarital intercourse, and the active role of women in sexuality differed from what might have been expected, and caused some social and political disquiet (Gagnon 1988).

Wellings et al (1994) is the most extensive study on sexual behaviour in Britain. It was initiated to discover how the spread of AIDS and HIV might be related to certain sexual practices and it therefore concentrated on issues like unprotected sex, number of partners and activities involving risks. Because of its broad quantitative nature it tells little about the meaning of sexual experiences to individuals. It does, however, give details of who does what with whom, at what age and how often, and relates these sorts of things to class and educational level. One of its major drawbacks is its failure to include people over 60 years of age. This perhaps reflects the commonly held view that 'old people don't do that sort of thing'.

Some of the findings are given below.

Heterosexual behaviour

- Over the last 40 years the median age of first heterosexual intercourse has fallen from 21 to 17 years of age for women and from 20 to 17 years of age for men.
- Fewer than 1% of women who were 55 years of age in 1991 reported that it happened before they were 16, compared with nearly 20% of women in their late teens.
- Early sexual intercourse is linked with lower social class and educational attainment, but this association is much weaker than it used to be.
- First intercourse is now more likely to involve contraceptive equipment (usually the condom) than for previous

generations, but the younger first timers are less likely to use contraception than those in their late teens.

- First heterosexual intercourse tends to be associated with more planning and less spontaneity than previously, and for the majority this is within an established relationship.
- Women tend to have older partners for this experience whereas men have age peers. It rarely occurs for the first time during marriage and it is very rare for a man's first intercourse to be with a prostitute.

Heterosexual partnerships

- There are extreme variations in the numbers of partners reported. Young people, divorced people and single people reported the highest numbers and there was a significant trend towards increasing partner change with higher social class.
- In general, people appear to be having more partners these days, but this may be clouded by older people's memory difficulties, and their unwillingness to report the facts.
- Men tend to have partners younger than themselves, but more than 50% of men were found to have partners within 2 years of their age.

Heterosexual practices

- The frequency of heterosexual sex (oral, anal and vaginal intercourse) varies considerably, with the peak activity occurring in the mid-twenties and then a gradual decline, which is more marked for women.
- People in longer relationships reported a lower frequency of heterosexual sex and the decline in activity with age seemed to be associated with this factor rather than other age-related changes.
- Vaginal intercourse was the most frequently practised activity.
- 70% of people had experienced oral sex (cunnilingus or fellatio) and the evidence suggests an increasing popularity of orogenital contact especially in the younger age group.
- An experience of anal intercourse was reported by 13.9% of men and 12.9% of women, and those reporting recent experience tended to be in the younger age groups.
- Manual classes were more likely to report anal sex and non-manual classes were more likely to report oral and non-penetrative sex, although these associations are weak.

Homosexual behaviour

- 6.1% of men and 3.4% of women reported a homosexual experience in their lifetime and 1.1% of men and 0.4% of women reported having had a homosexual partner that year.
- It appeared that a homosexual experience was transitory for many and was reported across a wide cross-section of society.

- A minority of men reported larger numbers of male partners than those reporting female partners. Also men regularly participating in homosexual anal intercourse did so both as a receptive partner and as a penetrative partner. There was no evidence to suggest that men exclusively adopted one or other role in homosexual practices.
- An important finding supported by other studies is the high prevalence of bisexual behaviour. This means that the popular image of being either heterosexual or homosexual is inappropriate and that the classification of people's sexuality is complex.

Evidence based practice

A similar survey was carried out in the UK to try and help understand the trends in the incidence of sexually transmitted diseases and teenage pregnancies. *The National Survey of Sexual Attitudes and Lifestyles* took place between 1999 and 2001 and was reported in three articles in the *Lancet* (Johnson et al 2001).

A sample of 4762 men and 6399 women aged between 16 and 44 were interviewed. The following is a selection of the findings:

- In the last 5 years the mean number of heterosexual partners was 3.8 for men and 2.4 for women.
- 4.3% of men reported paying for sex.
- 2.6% of respondents reported homosexual partnerships
- Condom use has increased since 1990.
- There has been an increase in the number of sexual partners since 1990.
- The proportion of women reporting first intercourse before the age of 16 increased up to the mid-1990s and has now levelled off.
- A small minority of teenagers have unprotected first intercourse.
- Early motherhood is more strongly associated with educational level than family background.

Surveys on sexual behaviour are fraught with problems because of the sensitive and private nature of the topic. The findings from such surveys must be treated with caution because their accuracy and reliability may be influenced by individuals' honesty and openness in their responses. Nevertheless, this kind of research provides professionals with important information.

EMOTIONS AND THE SEXUAL RESPONSE

Webb (1985) believes that many studies into sexual behaviour emphasize the physical aspects and do not provide insight into the social and psychological factors involved. For example what is it that makes certain phenomena sexually arousing to some people but not to others, and how are desires and attractions between people explained?

The human sexual response is a complex process and sexual attraction towards others is not easily explained. Emotions are central to these experiences and they can influence and be influenced by the physical aspects of sexual activity. Bancroft (1989) describes the psychosomatic circle of sex, which emphasizes the importance of social and psychological factors in sexual activity and their ability to influence the physiological processes involved.

The evidence on how anxiety influences the sexual response is unclear, perhaps because of the difficulty in defining anxiety. Also it may be important to distinguish between anxiety generated by the sexual activity itself and anxiety resulting from other sources. Anxiety influences sexual responses through a number of mechanisms as follows.

1. It excites the peripheral autonomic nervous system, which controls important physiological changes associated with sex. As a result the neurological control of vasocongestion of the genitals, and of orgasm, may be affected, preventing these changes from occurring, slowing them down or speeding them up.
2. It may disrupt thought processes so that erotic stimuli are not perceived. This is equivalent to having something on your mind, making it difficult to concentrate on anything else.
3. Anxiety and the sexual response become associated through past experiences and the individual may subconsciously inhibit sexual responses in order to avoid anxiety, thereby reinforcing the initial anxiety.
4. Anxiety occurs as a reaction to a failure of sexual response.

Bancroft (1989) also discusses the role of anger and mood in influencing the sexual response. Anger can stimulate the sexual response or it may impair it, and this seems to be difficult to explain. Some people are able to be sexually aroused and angry at the same time, but others are not. Sexual response may facilitate anger, but on the other hand a sexual interaction may have a calming affect. Also a failure to respond sexually could generate an angry reaction and an individual's avoidance of sex may be a way of expressing anger.

The relationship between mood and sexual response appears less complex, but it has received relatively little investigation. It is easy to appreciate how feeling low or depressed could influence a person's sexual desire or interest in sexual activity. Feeling low leads to more negative thoughts, particularly about oneself, and generates low self-esteem. What is not easy to determine is the role sexual dysfunction has in creating depression in the first place. Also sexual problems and depression may be related to other underlying causes, for example biochemical or hormonal changes.

CARE DELIVERY KNOWLEDGE

This section focuses on the inclusion of sexuality in nursing models, communication issues as part of the assessment process, the types of sexuality problems and frameworks for nursing actions.

MODELS OF NURSING

Some models of nursing include explicit definitions of health, and identify the nature of the problems people experience that require nursing assistance. For example, Roper et al (1996) focus on the activities of living and the difficulties people may have in carrying them out. Within this model 'expressing sexuality' is seen as an important activity, and one that ought to be considered by nurses in all settings with all clients. The activity is very broad and includes sexual activity, gender identity and relationship issues. The model describes the nurse's role in helping people express their sexuality and there is an emphasis on the impact of health conditions and illnesses on this part of people's lives.

Orem's (1995) model has self-care as its central concept and nursing is a helping activity introduced when individuals are having difficulty managing their own self-care. Life is seen as the meeting of a range of needs. Health conditions and illnesses have a direct impact on the types of needs and the skills and knowledge an individual requires to meet them. One of the universal needs relates to 'being normal'. This is obviously a broad concept and it includes ideas on reaching one's potential and living according to social norms and values. Although being less specific than the Roper et al (1996) model, Orem (1995) sees sexual activity and gender identity as important areas of concern for nurses because they are part of 'being normal'.

Other models of nursing tend to be more process orientated. This means that they do not try and define the nature of human problems requiring help. They concentrate on the nature of the activity of nursing and what nurses have to do to help people. Peplau (1988) focuses on the relationship between the nurse and the client and how this is used to help the client to develop. Together the client and nurse identify and explore the client's problems. They move on to discuss methods for coping with the problems, and end by evaluating what they have both learned, and how they have both developed. The nurse relies on the client's perceptions, experiences and feelings to identify the nature of the problems to be managed. This model therefore does not explicitly include sexuality as a relevant area of nursing concern. Implicit, though, is the importance of this aspect of people's lives and how there may be particular problems for some individuals.

Decision making exercise

List common life events for men and for women between the ages of 45 and 55.
How might these events affect peoples' intimate relationships with those close to them?

ASSESSMENT OF SEXUALITY AND SEXUAL HEALTH

The World Health Organization (1975: 6) defines sexual health as:

> ... the integration of the somatic, emotional, intellectual, and social aspects of sexual being, in ways that are positively enriching and that enhance personality, communication and love.

This is a positive definition, but being very broad it helps little when working directly with clients. Early UK government policy (Department of Health 1992) emphasized the negative aspects of sexual health – the incidence of sexually transmitted diseases and teenage pregnancies – as indicators of a community's poor sexual health. In this way the policy tended to focus on prevention of problems rather the promotion of positive health. The Department of Health (2002: 5) in *The National Strategy for Sexual Health and HIV* is more specific and gives professionals a clearer understanding of the nature of sexual health and the ways in which sexual health can be promoted. It identifies sexual health as:

> ... an important part of physical and mental health. It is a key part of our identity as human beings together with the fundamental human rights to privacy, a family life and living free from discrimination. Essential elements of good sexual health are equitable relationships and sexual fulfilment with access to information and services to avoid the risk of unintended pregnancy, illness and disease.

Reflection and portfolio evidence

During a clinical placement, make a point of looking at a written assessment of a client.

- What aspects of sexuality have been included in the written assessment?
- What aspects could have been included?
- How does the plan of care address any sexuality related issues?

DISCUSSING SEXUALITY WITH CLIENTS

Sexuality is a sensitive subject and it may be for this reason that nurses regularly fail to address it with clients (Gamel et al 1993, Gregory 2000, Lewis & Bor 1994, Matocha & Waterhouse 1993, Smook 1992, Webb 1988). Like many aspects of human interpersonal activity there is no easy guide to instruct nurses on how to manage conversations about sexuality. It has been argued that nurses face serious ethical issues by even considering that such conversations are theirs to be managed (Batcup & Thomas 1994). Take for example a client who has a health problem that the nurse feels could be seriously affecting his or her sexuality. If the client says nothing about the way he or she feels about him or herself or does not admit to any such sexuality problem does the

Decision making exercise

The questions that you ask during an assessment can contain implicit assumptions. Because of this, questions might be inappropriate or offensive to some patients.

Read the following statements and then answer the questions listed.

'I see from your records that your next of kin is your partner. Is she fit and well?'
'What method of contraception do you use?'
'Does the pain prevent you from having sexual intercourse?'
'Does this restlessness that you have at night in bed disturb your partner?'

- What are the possible assumptions in the questions?
- How might a client react if the assumptions are incorrect?
- How might this error of judgement affect your relationship with the client?

nurse have a duty to dig deeper on the assumption that it may be the client's embarrassment that prevents him or her from telling the truth? If the nurse does this is the nurse in danger of setting the agenda and putting ideas into the client's mind? By asking specific questions the nurse can demonstrate to the client that it is legitimate to talk about issues related to sexuality or sexual activity. On the other hand, the questions could lead the client to consider aspects of their lives in detail, and begin to see 'new' problems. For example 'Does the pain affect your sex life?' implies that the client ought to have a sex life and suggests that a sex life might normally be affected by such pain. This type of question could lead the client along a line of discussion they had not previously considered. Sociologists have described this management of the conversation as a form of professional control, with the nurse exerting power over the client (Foucault 1973).

Language

Reflection and portfolio evidence

Look at the following statements and identify the possible meanings for each.

'We no longer sleep together'
'I can't stand her anywhere near me now'
'I haven't had a relationship since it happened'
'Since the operation I can't stand him to see my bits and pieces'
'I'm not the man I used to be'
'I got around a bit in my younger days'
'The tablets have stopped me from getting it up'

- Would you assume one particular meaning?
- How would you find out exactly what was meant?

One of the difficulties in conversations on delicate or sensitive subjects is deciphering the true meaning. The nurse will sometimes need to take the lead and make sure that there is a mutual understanding. This will involve exploration and clarification.

Using the client's language and terminology may help the nurse and client feel at ease with some of these delicate subjects. However, there is still a danger that, despite using the same words, there is not a mutual understanding. The use of 'proper' or medical terms can also be misunderstood and can act as a barrier in the conversation. Using slang or colloquial terms may be at odds with the client's perception of a professional nurse and can present as patronizing or condescending. The way to proceed is to be open with the client about the difficulties with terminology and to agree to use words you are comfortable with and ones that you both understand. Essential communication skills in assessing problems related to client's sexuality thus include:

- using silence to allow the client to talk
- listening to what the client says and does not say, being aware of and sensitive to the way he or she expresses ideas, picking up clues and hints
- reflecting the client's ideas by repeating and paraphrasing their words
- clarifying the meaning behind statements, making sure that you both understand things in the same way
- interpreting the client's words to uncover the significance of events and explore the hidden feelings and meanings in the conversation
- focusing on certain topics as a way of encouraging and guiding clients to discuss areas of their concern.

Reflection and portfolio exercise

Some questions for initiating conversations on sexuality with clients might include:

- 'Has anything (e.g. a recent experience, illness, operation) affected your relationships with people close to you?'
- 'Tell me about your partnership/relationship/marriage.'
- 'How do you feel about yourself as a woman/man/ wife/husband/ partner/mother/father?'
- 'Has your illness/operation/being in hospital changed the way you feel about yourself?'
- 'Has your illness/operation/being in hospital affected your sex life?'
- 'How are things between you and your partner?'
- 'Some of the tablets you are taking can affect aspects of your sex life. Have you noticed anything?'

POTENTIAL PROBLEMS RELATED TO CLIENTS' SEXUALITY

Nurses need to consider clients' sexuality across the spectrum of healthcare settings. This means that the way sexuality becomes part of an assessment will depend upon the nature of the client's presenting health conditions.

Sexuality can be an issue as:

- the client's primary reason for referral
- a problem secondary to another health condition
- a problem arising from difficulties coping with normal developmental changes.

Sexuality as a primary problem

Primary problems with sexuality include:

- difficulties with sexual activities or relationships
- unfulfilling sexual activity
- antisocial or inappropriate sexual behaviour
- fertility problems
- contraceptive difficulties.

These kinds of problems usually require the input of a specialist nurse. In some cases clients will raise these problems with generic nurses, for example practice nurses, health visitors or community psychiatric nurses. It is important for these staff to be aware of the specialist services available, for example sex therapists, psychosexual counsellors, fertility clinics and family planning clinics.

Reflection and portfolio exercise

What aspects of sexuality might you need to consider in an assessment of clients in the following settings?

- An adult surgical ward.
- A small residential placement for people with learning disabilities.
- A ward for older people with long-term mental health problems.
- A children's medical ward.

Sexuality problems secondary to other health conditions

Most nurses will be concerned with these types of sexuality problems. Since there are many diseases, illnesses and health conditions that can affect an individual's sexuality, the potential for nurses in this area is massive. Sexuality is a complex blend of physical, psychological and social factors. It is not always possible to identify the cause and effect relationship between illness and sexuality problems. For example a client with diabetes mellitus might have a low self-esteem. He might also have difficulties obtaining and maintaining an erection. It would be difficult to judge just how the diabetes mellitus, the low self-esteem and the erectile dysfunction interrelate in terms of cause and effect. Physiological changes could cause the erectile dysfunction, which in turn could cause a low self-esteem. On the other hand the diagnosis of diabetes mellitus could induce feelings of poor self-worth,

Table 15.1 Sexuality related problems sometimes associated with certain types of health conditions

Type of health condition	Sexuality related problems
Musculoskeletal conditions	Sexual activity Body image Work and leisure activities Dressing and hygiene
Cardiovascular and respiratory conditions	Energy levels Breathing Body image Emotional state Male and female sexual response
Neurological conditions	Sensations Movement and coordination Male and female sexual response Libido
Endocrine and hormonal conditions	Body image Growth and development Libido Male and female sexual response Onset of puberty
Skin conditions	Body image Emotional state Sensations
Genitourinary conditions	Body image Choice of clothing Libido Male and female sexual response
Mental health problems	Body image Interpersonal relationships Libido Male and female sexual response Self-concept Work and leisure activities
Learning disabilities	Emotional state Relationship skills Self-concept Development of socially acceptable sexual behaviour Vulnerability to sexual abuse Work and leisure activities

Table 15.2 Potential side effects of medications on sexual activity

Type of medication	Drug	Side effects on sexual activity
Diuretics (e.g. used for clients with heart failure)	Thiazides	Erectile dysfunction Decreased libido
	Spironolactone	Erectile dysfunction Decreased libido Gynaecomastia (enlargement of male breast)
Beta-blockers (e.g. used for clients with high blood pressure and clients with anxiety)		Erectile dysfunction
Sympatholytics (e.g. used for clients with high blood pressure)	Methyldopa	Erectile dysfunction Ejaculatory failure
	Prazosin	Erectile dysfunction Retrograde ejaculation in clients with benign prostatic enlargement
Antidepressants	Tricyclics and monoamine oxidase inhibitors	Erectile dysfunction Ejaculatory failure
Antipsychotics	Phenothiazines	Erectile dysfunction
Anxiolytics	Benzodiazepines	Erectile dysfunction
Cytotoxics		Amenorrhoea Decreased sperm count
Antihistamines		Decreased vaginal lubrication Erectile dysfunction
Glucocorticosteroids		Weight gain Changed fat distribution

which in turn could generate erectile dysfunction. Sexuality problems that coexist alongside physical ill health can therefore be difficult to understand.

Table 15.1 lists the sexuality related problems that are sometimes associated with types of health conditions. The list is not exhaustive, but gives an indication of some of the problems to consider when working with clients.

Medications and sexual function

A number of medications have potential side effects on sexual activity and some of these are listed in Table 15.2.

Reflection and portfolio exercise

On a clinical placement make a point of talking to a client about aspects of his or her sexuality that might be affected by current health status, illness, physical and mental abilities, etc. Using your knowledge of the client and any written information, consult with your mentor to decide on appropriate topics to discuss .

- What did you decide to ask about and why?
- How did you feel?
- How did the client feel?
- What did you learn about your ability to discuss sexuality with clients?
- Could you use these skills in other settings?
- What other skills/knowledge do you need to develop?

Nurses assessing clients' problems need to be aware of these side effects and will need to give advice on them when helping clients develop regimens for managing their medications. This advice will enable clients to make fully informed decisions about the benefits and disadvantages of medications (Burns-Cox & Gingell 1995, Holzapfel 1994).

The list given in Table 15.2 is not exhaustive. It is possible that many clients taking prescribed medications experience side effects that affect their sexuality and sexual activity. As well as this, alcohol and nicotine are known to contribute to impotence. It is therefore important to find out about clients' medications and their use of leisure drugs.

Decision making exercise

Think about a patient you have worked with recently who has been taking a range of prescribed medications. Identify the possible side effects of these drugs on the patient's sexuality (you may wish to look in the *British National Formulary* (British Medical Association and the Royal Pharmaceutical Society 2003) for this).

- Did the care staff know whether the patient was experiencing any of these side effects?
- If not, why was this the case?
- Did the patient know about these possible side effects?
- So that the patient could give proper consent to taking these medications, how much do you think he or she should have been told?

Sexuality and normal developmental changes

People can experience difficulties in managing and coming to terms with normal developmental changes. Nurses have an important role in helping individuals to understand these changes and also in offering support and practical advice on how these changes can be managed. For example, school nurses are in an ideal position to help children understand the changes experienced during puberty and adolescence. These changes are physical, psychological and social, and nurses can explore issues such as menstruation, nocturnal emissions ('wet dreams'), masturbation, sexual relationships, safe sex, contraception, social roles and becoming an adult. Because these subjects are still surrounded by myth and taboo, there is a risk that children can grow up misinformed. This misinformation can result in a lack of awareness in the practical management of some of these changes. Also it can lead to the acquisition of uncomfortable and unhealthy attitudes and behaviours such as guilt and repression, and these can affect individuals for the rest of their lives.

Other developmental changes require individuals to adapt and readjust. In many cases these changes have an impact on sexual identity and sexual activity. For example, the menopause can be associated with dryness of the vagina and women can experience problems coping with this physical change. Also around this time, children leave home and middle-aged adults might be involved in caring for ageing parents. As a result of decreasing androgen production in the late forties or early fifties, men experience less firm erections and an increased refractory period. At the same time men and women can be involved in important career decisions and planning retirement. These physical and social changes require psychological and behavioural adjustment. People having difficulties making the necessary adjustments can develop a low self-esteem and a negative body image. Again, these can have a direct impact on the quality of relationships, sexual identity and sexual activity.

NURSING ACTIONS

Clients present with a wide range of problems related to sexuality. Also, clients are individuals and their experiences of these problems will all be unique. Consequently, it is impossible to describe appropriate nursing actions in detail since a full assessment is required in order to plan care. Nevertheless there are guidelines to help nurses plan appropriate care. Annon (1974) describes levels of intervention using the P-LI-SS-IT model:

> P – permission
> LI – limited information
> SS – specific suggestions
> IT – intensive therapy.

Permission

This is when the nurse openly acknowledges to the client that sexuality is a legitimate issue for discussion. This means that the nurse must be seen to be willing to discuss sexuality, either by asking specific questions or by allowing and encouraging clients to raise the issue themselves. This says to the client that it is within the nurse's role to discuss sexuality and also that it is 'normal', usual and acceptable for clients to have concerns or problems related to their sexuality.

Limited information

This next stage requires the nurse to give explanations, facts or reasons about why the client might be having the sexuality problem. Obviously the nurse must have sufficient knowledge and experience to understand and interpret sexuality problems. Also this demands communication and teaching skills so that explanations can be understood and remembered. This level of intervention enables the client to make sense of the problems, and gives him or her the opportunity to consider ways of resolving or improving the situation. This stage might involve the nurse helping the client to correct any misconceptions or dispel any myths surrounding sexuality.

Specific suggestions

A client having difficulty resolving his or her own problems is likely to need specific guidance or advice. This means that the nurse must draw on research and previous experience to make practical, acceptable and realistic suggestions. The nurse must assess the client's abilities, knowledge and attitudes so that appropriate suggestions are made. Some suggestions could involve referral to other agencies. Therefore the nurse must be aware of the range of specialist services available, the nature of the services provided and the appropriate reasons for referral so that the client can decide how to proceed.

Intensive therapy

This level is usually beyond the skills of the generic nurse. Clients and partners can be involved in a programme of sessions to instruct, coach and demonstrate ways of overcoming the particular sexual problem. This could focus for example on relationship and communication difficulties between partners on alternative ways of 'pleasuring' or sexual expression between partners or on medical and surgical interventions to treat or improve the sexual response.

Like Annon's (1974) model, Webb (1985) outlines a number of roles for nurses in their work with clients' sexuality problems. These are as:

- facilitator – the nurse encourages the client to open up and discuss sexuality using a non-judgemental approach
- validator – the nurse helps to dispel misunderstandings about sexual activity and perceptions of 'normality' and it is emphasized that acceptable sexual practices are those that participants enjoy and freely consent to
- teacher – the nurse uses a range of teaching skills to pass on information
- counsellor – the nurse uses listening and counselling skills to enable the client to explore his or her own sexuality
- advocate – the nurse supports and encourages clients to make their own fully informed decisions about treatment and care
- referral agent – the nurse gives advice on other services available and discusses appropriate referrals with the client
- specialist therapist – the specialist nurse is experienced in assessing complex sexual problems and can provide a range of specific interventions to solve these problems.

PROFESSIONAL AND ETHICAL KNOWLEDGE

In this section the following four aspects are discussed: nursing as a female profession, information specific to the four branches of nursing, key legal issues related to nursing and clients' sexuality, and sexuality and health policy.

NURSING AS A FEMALE PROFESSION

The concepts of masculinity and femininity are especially important for nursing because the profession itself is associated very strongly with being female. This has implications for men in nursing, and also for women in nursing wanting to move into areas traditionally associated with masculine characteristics, for example management and positions of leadership. In a broader context the feminine characteristics have been used to explain the subservient role of nursing in the political hierarchy of healthcare professions (Versluysen 1980). Because nursing is viewed by many as a female profession and women are often seen as subservient, nurses as a group command little political power (Salvage 1995). What is beginning to be touched upon here is the political nature of gender and sexuality. The descriptions of femininity and masculinity indicate the traditional views of the differences between men and women. These views are arguably not neutral because some characteristics are seen as more important for society and consequently attract higher social prestige and status. This is evident in the health service where medicine maintains power and prestige and is still seen as a male profession. Male nurses and female doctors as exceptions to these stereotypical images might be viewed with suspicion in some clinical areas. Also the day-to-day working relationships between doctors and nurses can be influenced by these gender politics (Stein 1967, Stein et al 1990).

Nurses must also be aware of the potential effects of their own gender on clients. Nursing often involves intimate activities. Clients are required to expose their bodies and to be touched in sensitive, sometimes erogenous zones. Many of these activities are normally only associated with sexual encounters. This can result in embarrassing situations for the client and the nurse, and both can use a range of strategies to diffuse or cope with this embarrassment (Lawler 1991, Meerabeau 1999). These situations can be compounded by the gender mix between the client and the nurse. For example, a male nurse washing the genitals of a male client could generate a range of thoughts and feelings for both parties, some of which might be uncomfortable and difficult to deal with.

INFORMATION SPECIFIC TO THE FOUR BRANCHES OF NURSING

Adult nursing

Staff working within this branch need to be aware of the relationship between sexuality and ageing. The degenerative changes associated with ageing can affect self-esteem, body image, sexual desire and sexual response. A decrease in circulating androgens will lower libido, and changes in neurological and vascular systems can affect sensation and response. These changes may not be important for some people, but many of these potential problems can be overcome by practical advice and medical intervention. These physiological changes do not in themselves prevent older people from having an active and pleasurable sex life and research suggests that sexual activity plays an important part in people's lives well into old age (Bretschneider & McCoy 1988).

Decline in sexual activity in older people is perhaps more to do with demographic and social factors than a decrease in ability or desire (Diokno et al 1990). Many older people are widows or widowers. They have fewer social contacts and their chances of meeting a new partner are reduced. Also the attitudes that youth is beautiful and that older people should not be sexually active may force older people to believe that they are no longer sexually attractive and that it is not right for them to have sexual desires. Comfort & Dial (1991) suggest that 'most of our aged stop having sex for reasons similar to those why they stop riding a bicycle: general infirmity, fear that it would expose them to ridicule, and for most, lack of a bicycle.'

Learning disabilities nursing

A key concept to consider in caring for clients with learning disabilities is consent. If there are doubts about an individual's knowledge or level of understanding, then any relationships or sexual activities he or she is involved in could constitute abuse. This judgement of the ability to consent is difficult, but rests on a consideration of the individual's cognitive functioning and ability to assert his or her wishes in pressured situations (Gunn 1996). This will have implications for nurses, in particular how such a judgement is reached and how clients can be helped to gain the appropriate knowledge and skills (Sundram & Stavis 1994).

A central issue here is deciding what is meant by appropriate knowledge and skills. For example, if a client expresses a desire to wear clothes normally worn by the opposite sex should nurses discourage this or should nurses help the client to understand, promote and actively enjoy his or her chosen cross-dressing identity? On the one hand nurses might aim to encourage client decision making and choice, but on the other hand aim to help clients develop attitudes and behaviour that allows for a degree of integration in the community. The difficulty in this case is that such an expression of sexuality may prevent what is usually understood as social integration. There may, however, be a cross-dressing community into which the client can integrate, but this may prove difficult because of the client's level of social skills or the stigma associated with learning disabilities. With regard to consent and choice nurses may have to consider whether it is appropriate for clients to make decisions about some aspects of their lives, but not others. Like many other aspects of learning disabilities nursing there is a danger that nurses might impose their norms of sexuality, overtly or covertly, and restrict the client's potential.

McCarthy & Thompson (1995) identify how staff's norms and attitudes have led to restrictive practices in relation to the sexuality of people with learning disabilities, to the extent that help and guidance has failed to take into account recent changes in attitudes towards sexuality in the community at large. For example same-sex relationships are 'pathologized'

and discouraged, women are seen to have a passive role in sexual activity, and cross-dressing can be prevented by promoting heterosexual relationships. Carr (1995) suggests the following important points for nurses dealing with the sexuality of adults with learning disabilities:

- Sociosexual education is vital because of people's vulnerability in the community.
- A sociosexual educator needs to liaise closely with parents and other professionals as a way of sharing knowledge and reducing unnecessary anxiety.
- A sociosexual educator needs to understand the legal implications of carrying out this role to protect all individuals concerned – this relates in particular to the teaching methods used to help people develop appropriate skills and how practical demonstrations and client participation for subjects like masturbation and the management of menstruation might be interpreted as assault.

Reflection and portfolio exercise

Ager & Little (1998) proposed the following rights for people with learning disabilities:

- The right to be informed about sexuality and its place in human life, at times and at a level that allows this area of human being and experience to be as positive as possible.
- The same right as everyone else to enjoy sexual activity. The concomitant right to remain celibate and to refrain from sexual activity of any kind.
- The right to contraceptive advice and services, both to avoid pregnancy and to avoid the risk of sexually transmitted diseases.
- The same right as any other citizen to marry or form ongoing relationships.
- The same right to choose parenthood as that enjoyed by everyone else.
- The right not to be sexually abused and to be protected from sexual abuse.

How are these rights implemented in practice, in both learning disabilities and in other areas of care?

Children's nursing

Illness can intrude in the development of a child's sexuality. A variety of endocrine conditions as well as some chronic illnesses can directly affect growth and physiological development to the extent that puberty is delayed or absent. Similarly chronic illness in childhood can influence exposure to the social and psychological experiences that seem to be important in the development of sexual identity. Smith (1993) and Haka-Ikse & Mian (1993) identify a number of factors influencing normal sexual development in children as follows:

- the involvement of an adult same-sex role model in the child's immediate environment

- witnessing displays of affection between others (touch and language)
- receiving comforting touch and praise that result in feelings of trust and security
- exploring one's own body and being allowed to gain pleasure from it (e.g. through masturbation)
- learning that your body is your property and that others need your permission to touch it
- learning appropriate levels of privacy related to the body, in a way that prevents a feeling of guilt
- learning about other's needs for privacy
- having curiosity encouraged about gender and sexuality, receiving open and honest answers appropriate to the child's level of understanding
- having opportunities for play with peers of the same and of the opposite sex
- being free to participate in gender-based play
- being free to participate in mutually agreed private sexual play with peers
- learning about physical changes during puberty
- learning that sex is 'good, natural and healthy'.

Adolescence is characterized by experimentation, rebellion and risk taking behaviour. There are obvious risks in relation to unwanted pregnancies, sexually transmitted diseases and emotional trauma during this stage of development. A healthy sexual development should include an understanding of rights, responsibilities and relationships as well as the mechanics of sexual activity. This has implications for nurses in many areas, particularly those in primary health care, school nursing, and health education and promotion.

Mental health nursing

Mental health problems may have an impact on expressing sexuality and nurses are likely to be working with clients' unmet needs in this aspect of their lives (McCann 2000). The interrelationship between sexuality and mental health is complex. There is a two-way relationship in which problems in expressing sexuality can seriously affect an individual's self-concept. Also, low self-esteem and anxiety can intrude into personal relationships affecting libido and sexual function. This relationship can become a vicious circle, with low self-esteem limiting sexual expression, which further reduces self-esteem. In this situation the client can feel out of control.

Ferguson (1994) discusses the relationship between sexuality and mental health and stresses the significance of social, political and financial forces as determinants of this relationship. Sexuality incorporates the idea of social roles and social norms, and in order to express 'masculinity' or 'femininity' within our society there is an expectation of people to adopt gender-specific attitudes and behaviour. This is where the nurse can be caught in a trap because he or she might see it as valuable to help the client fit back into these social roles as a way of regaining self-esteem and

control. On the other hand it could be argued that the roles in themselves are 'pathological' because of the associated stresses and inequalities. Does the nurse in these types of cases strive to help the client conform or challenge these social roles to help the client adopt a new perspective? There is a problem when the origins of mental ill health are located not so much in the individual, but in the organization and structure of society. As an example, Ferguson (1994) outlines how differences in the patterns and types of mental illness experienced by men and women are more a product of social forces than genetic make-up. This has implications for the role of the nurse and suggests that as well as having an individual focus, nursing should be involved in social and community action as a way of addressing social forces and social inequalities.

Other important issues in this relationship between sexuality and mental health are:

- the function of assertiveness and communication within personal relationships and how inability in these areas may lead to feelings of low self-esteem
- the impact mental illness can have on personal relationships, in particular on the expression of intimacy within relationships
- the function of the psychiatric services in defining, monitoring and treating sexual deviance, and their social role in maintaining the stigmas surrounding certain sexual practices
- the potential for therapeutic relationships between clients and professionals to develop into relationships involving inappropriate sexual expression – this can create difficulties for clients and staff and needs to be handled openly and sensitively
- the balance required between the client's right to sexual expression and the need to protect vulnerable clients from exploitation – this will be an important issue for nursing and care staff working in homes for people with long-term serious mental health problems.

KEY LEGAL ISSUES

Sexuality is an important aspect of all branches of nursing. If nursing claims to be holistic in its outlook then it needs to take into account the links between health and all areas of people's lives. When people are unable to meet their own needs, nurses play an important role in assisting, guiding or advising. In cases of extreme disability and dependence the nurse may have to take over and act on the client's behalf, for example washing a client who is unconscious, or feeding a person with a severe learning disability. An ethical issue arises for nurses in the area of sexual need. If a client is having severe difficulties meeting sexual needs what can or should a nurse do? Earle (2001) raises the issue of facilitated sex and explains this as a continuum ranging from giving information to sexual surrogacy. Giving information to a client or creating a climate which allows for intimacy between client and

Evidence based practice

Sexuality is central to an individual's life. It influences a wide range of thoughts, feelings and behaviours. Because of this, the relationship between the law and sexuality is wide ranging. It is beyond the scope of this chapter to cover the legal aspects of sexuality in detail. It is, however, important to be aware of the areas of law that might need to be considered by nurses across a range of settings. These include laws related to: sex discrimination, families, child care, reproduction, abortion, sexual deviance, sexual abuse, rape, indecency, consent, confidentiality, privacy. This is not exhaustive. For a more detailed introduction to these areas see Dimond (1995).

partner may seem unproblematic whereas arranging paid-for sexual services or facilitated masturbation may raise legal and ethical dilemmas. Earle argues, though, that all levels of help on this continuum of facilitated sex could be seen as potentially problematic. Buying pornography for a client may be seen as acceptable by some professionals and not by others. Similarly escorting a client to a gay club to help him or her meet sexual partners may be interpreted as positive or negative depending on your perspective.

POLICY AND SEXUALITY

Sexual health has become an important issue for policy makers over the last decade. The Department of Health (2002) published the report *National Strategy for Sexual Health and HIV* with the following aims:

- to reduce the transmission of HIV and sexually transmitted infections (STIs)
- to reduce the prevalence of undiagnosed HIV and STIs
- to reduce unintended pregnancy rates
- to improve health and social care of people living with HIV
- to reduce the stigma associated with HIV and STIs.

A criticism of these aims might be that they are disease focused and tend to ignore many other aspects of sexuality and positive sexual health. The Royal College of Nursing produced in 2000 a guidance document *Sexuality and Sexual Health in Nursing Practice* (Royal College of Nursing 2000). Whilst it incorporates a disease focus, it does emphasize a broader nature of sexual health and makes important suggestions on how sexuality can become an aspect of clinical work for nurses. This report acknowledges the difficulties nurses may have in discussing sexuality based problems with clients but goes some way in trying to break down the barriers and stigma. Organizations like the Department of Health and the Royal College of Nursing are beginning to place sexuality on the policy and practice agenda.

PERSONAL AND REFLECTIVE KNOWLEDGE

This final section now finishes with four case studies based on clients with sexuality related problems. There are a number of questions after each case study to help you consider the issues. After these are a number of exercises to help you reflect on your practice and develop your portfolio evidence.

CASE STUDIES RELATING TO SEXUALITY

Case study: Adult

Mrs Ellis is a resident in a private nursing home. She is 75 years old and has been a widow for 10 years. Despite having severe osteoarthritis in her knees and hips she sees herself as relatively fit. She is mentally alert and enjoys mixing with other residents, especially during meal times and organized social events. She has early signs of heart failure, which prevents her from having surgery for her arthritis and also makes her feel tired and out of sorts at times. She requires assistance with dressing, personal hygiene and going to the toilet, but is able to move around the home independently in her wheelchair. She has made a close association with a man in the home and they spend time together most afternoons.

- How might Mrs Ellis's age and disability affect the way she sees herself as a woman?

- What would your reaction be if you were Mrs Ellis's primary nurse and she said she would like to develop the relationship with her friend into a sexual one?
- What are the potential problems with confidentiality and what should Mrs Ellis's primary nurse do to maintain confidentiality?

Case study: Learning disabilities

John Brown is 26 years of age and has moderate learning disabilities. He lives at home with his parents and visits a day centre every day where he participates in a social skills training programme, which is partly organized by a community nurse. The nurse discovers from the day centre staff that John regularly visits a local public toilet to participate in homosexual activities. This emerged at a day centre group meeting when another of the service users, who openly admits to visiting the same toilets, said he had seen John there.

John is usually withdrawn and initiates little conversation or interaction with people at the day centre. He has a close relationship with the nurse, but is reluctant to talk about his sexual activities with anyone. John is not used to making decisions in his life and has everything organized for him by his parents. Generally the staff see John as an inoffensive young man who creates no fuss in the day centre because on the whole he does as he is told.

- Supposing the claim about John's sexual behaviour is true, is this behaviour 'normal' in society?
- Should the nurse be concerned about this behaviour? Why or why not?
- Do you think the nurse should do anything and if so, what?
- How do you think John's parents might react if they discovered what he was doing?
- Do you think John's parents have a right to know?

Case study: Child

Susan Jones is 15 years old and has cystic fibrosis. This is a hereditary condition affecting a number of body systems. The respiratory system produces large amounts of thick, sticky sputum, breathlessness can be particularly disabling, and the illness is likely to lead to a premature death. Susan needs oxygen therapy much of the time and requires regular physiotherapy to keep her chest clear. Like other children with this condition, Susan's physical development has been retarded and she is short for her age and underweight.

Susan lives at home with her parents and 12-year-old sister. She has missed a lot of school over the last year and although a couple of friends visit on occasions she has lost touch with her peer group. Her parents are very caring and worry about her repeated chest infections. They believe that the infections flare up after Susan has had friends around and as a result they discourage too many visitors.

- How might Susan's ill health have affected her self-concept?
- Adolescence is a crucial time for the development of a sexual identity. What important aspects of adolescence might Susan have missed out on?
- How could a community nurse promote the development of Susan's sexual identity?

Case study: Mental health

David Anderson is a 35-year-old single man who lives alone in his new four-bedroom detached house on the outskirts of a large city. He has been admitted to an acute admission ward in a psychiatric hospital suffering from severe depression. He has recently split up from his partner of 6 months and the advertising business he owns is struggling, to the extent that he is considering laying off staff. His career has been all-consuming and David has never been one for 'getting married and settling down'. He has had a number of short-term relationships over the last 10 years and he explains the breakdown of his recent relationship as mainly his fault. He has not been interested in sex and 'found it difficult to perform these days'.

- How might recent events be contributing to the way David feels about himself?
- Describe the possible relationship between David's lifestyle and his sexual difficulties.
- As David's primary nurse what could you do to help him regain his ability to express his sexuality?

Summary

This chapter has focused on developing knowledge and insight into human sexuality and the implications for practice. It has included:

1. Defining sexuality and examining how the concept has evolved to become integrated into self-concept and within society.
2. Expression of sexuality was examined in gender identification and development.
3. Examining the human sexual response and sexual behaviour throughout the lifespan.
4. The implications for practice were considered, beginning with an examination of approaches for discussing and assessing sexuality with clients.
5. To be comfortable in assessing clients; however, nurses need to be comfortable with their own sexuality. Consequently, exercises were included to help to raise self-awareness.
6. Potential areas of difficulty that clients might experience were highlighted and some actions that nurses could use to help to address them were suggested, particularly by incorporating the use of Annon's (1974) P-LI-SS-IT model.
7. The implication of nursing being predominantly a female profession was considered. Nursing practice often involves intimate activities and the juxtaposition of delivering care with the potential effects of gender was also discussed.
8. Finally, in a brief overview of contemporary policy, the *National Strategy for Sexual Health and HIV* (Department of Health 2002) and *Sexuality and Sexual Health in Nursing Practice* (Royal College of Nursing 2000) were highlighted. Although they were criticized for being disease focused, it was recognized that sexuality is, at last, being addressed by policy makers.

Annotated further reading and websites

Aggleton P 1996 A compendium of family planning service provision for young people. Health Education Authority, London
This short text provides a regional breakdown of services for young people. It is a useful resource for discovering what is available in your area (in the UK). The services included are advice and counselling on contraception, termination of pregnancy, sexually transmitted diseases and a full range of sexual issues likely to affect young people.

English National Board for Nursing and Midwifery 1996 Caring for people with sexually transmitted diseases including HIV disease. English National Board for Nursing and Midwifery, London
This open learning pack is designed to help nurses, midwives and health visitors involved in the care, management and education of people with sexually transmitted disease. The first four sections are general in approach and are useful for all nurses caring for clients with sexuality related problems. These sections include discussions of sexuality and health and ways of working with clients.

Heath H, White I 2001 The challenge of sexuality in health care. Blackwell, Oxford
This book gives a comprehensive overview of issues in sexuality and health care. It describes the normal processes and issues that arise at different stages of a person's life connected with sexuality. It goes on to discuss sexuality in relation to illness, disfigurement, physical and mental disability.

Tallmer M 1996 Questions and answers about sex in later life. Charles, Philadelphia
A short but readable text that attempts to dispel some of the myths surrounding sexuality and older people. It is based on the author's counselling experience and uses case histories and research to illustrate the importance of sexuality in later life. Its question-and-answer format gives the text a practical and matter of fact approach. It would be useful for anyone working with older people.

Wells D (ed) 2000 Caring for sexuality in health and illness. Churchill Livingstone, Edinburgh
This book is an introduction to the theory and practice of psychosexual care. It focuses on the role of the healthcare professional in promoting sexual health and includes exercises to help reflect on practice.

http://www.sexualityandu.ca
This Canadian website is a useful source of information on sexuality education including topics such as sexually transmitted diseases, contraception and lifestyle choices. It has sections for health professionals, parents, teachers, adults and teenagers.

http://www.sexualhealth.com
This site provides a range of information on and links to sexuality education, counselling and therapy.

http://www.bbc.co.uk/health/sex/
This site covers a number of factsheets and articles on sex and sexual health. It has particularly good links to UK organizations related to sexuality.

http://www.engenderhealth.org
This site covers men's and women's health. It has a worldwide perspective and includes a selection of online courses and professional material for people wanting to learn about sexuality.

References

Ager J, Little J 1998 Sexual health for people with learning disabilities. Nursing Standard 13(2):34–39

Annon J S 1974 The behavioural treatment of sexual problems. Enabling Systems, Honolulu

Atkinson R L, Atkinson R C, Smith E E et al 1990 Introduction to psychology, 10th edn. Harcourt Brace Jovanovich, Orlando

Bancroft J 1989 Human sexuality and its problems. Churchill Livingstone, Edinburgh

Batcup D, Thomas B 1994 Mixing the genders, an ethical dilemma: how nursing theory has dealt with sexuality and gender. Nursing Ethics 1(1):43–52

Beechey V 1987 Unequal work. Verso, London

Boone T B 1995 The physiology of sexual function in normal adults. Physical Medicine and Rehabilitation: State of the Art Reviews 9(2):313–322

Bretschneider J, McCoy N 1988 Sexual interest and behaviour in healthy 80- to 102-year-olds. Archives of Sexual Behaviour 17:109–129

British Medical Association and the Royal Pharmaceutical Society 2003 British National Formulary no. 45. British Medical Association, London

Burns-Cox N, Gingell C 1995 Drugs and sexual dysfunction. Practice Nursing 6(19):32–34

Byers S 1989 Sexuality and sexual concerns. In: Schoen Johnson B (ed) Psychiatric–mental health nursing: adaptaion and growth, 2nd edn. Lippincott, Philadelphia, pp 310–325

Carr L 1995 Sexuality and people with learning disabilities. British Journal of Nursing 4(19):1135–1141

Chodorow N 1978 The reproduction of mothering. University of California Press, Berkeley

Comfort A, Dial L 1991 Sexuality and aging: an overview. Clinical Geriatric Medicine 7(1):1–7

Department of Health 1992 The health of the nation. HMSO, London

Department of Health 2002 The national strategy for sexual health and HIV. HMSO, London

Dimond B 1995 Legal aspects of nursing, 2nd edn. Prentice-Hall, London

Diokno A, Brown M, Herzog R 1990 Sexual function in the elderly. Archives of International Medicine 150:197–200

Earle S 2001 Disability, facilitated sex and the role of the nurse. Journal of Advanced Nursing 36(3):433–440

Ferguson K 1994 Mental health and sexuality. In: Webb C (ed) Living sexuality: issues for nursing and health. Scutari, London, pp 99–119

Foucault M 1973 The birth of the clinic. Tavistock, London

Foucault M 1979 The history of sexuality, vol. 1, An introduction. Allen Lane, London

Freud S 1923 The Ego and the Id. Hogarth, London

Gagnon J H 1988 Sex research and sexual conduct in the era of AIDS. Journal of AIDS 1:593–601

Gamel C, Davis B D, Hengeveld M 1993 Nurses' provision of teaching and counselling on sexuality: a review of the literature. Journal of Advanced Nursing 18:1219–1227

Giddens A 1993 Sociology. Blackwell, Oxford

Gove W R, Tudor J F 1972 Adult sex roles and mental illness. American Journal of Sociology 78:812–835

Gregory P 2000 Patient assessment and care planning: sexuality. Nursing Standard 15(9):38–41

Gunn M 1991 Sex and the law: a brief guide for staff working with people with learning difficulties. Family Planning Association, London

Haka-Ikse K, Mian M 1993 Sexuality in children. Pediatrics in Review 14(10):401–407

Hinchliff S, Montague S, Watson R 1996 Physiology for nursing practice, 2nd edn. Baillière Tindall, London

Holzapfel S 1994 Aging and sexuality. Canadian Family Physician 40:748–766

Hudson R, Williams A M 1995 Divided Britain. John Wiley, Chichester

Johnson M A, Mercer C H, Erens B et al 2001 Sexual behaviour in Britain: partnerships, practices, and HIV risk behaviours. Lancet 358:1835–1854

Kinsey A C, Gebhard P H 1953 Sexual behaviour in the human female. Saunders, Philadelphia

Kinsey A C, Pomeroy W B, Martin C E 1948 Sexual behaviour in the human male. Saunders, Philadelphia

Lanval M 1950 An inquiry into the intimate lives of women. Cadillac, New York

Lavee Y 1991 Western and non-western sexuality: implications for clinical practice. Journal of Sex and Marital Therapy 17(3):203–213

Lawler J 1991 Behind the screens. Nursing: somology and the problem of the body. Churchill Livingstone, Edinburgh

Lewis S, Bor R 1994 Nurses' knowledge of and attitudes towards sexuality and the relationship of these with nursing practice. Journal of Advanced Nursing 20:251–259

McCann J 2000 The expression of sexuality in people with psychosis: breaking taboos. Journal of Advanced Nursing 32:132–138

McCarthy M, Thompson D 1995 No more double standards: sexuality and people with learning difficulties. In: Philpot T, Ward L (eds) Values and visions: changing ideas in services for people with learning difficulties. Butterworth-Heinemann, Oxford, pp 278–289

Masters W, Johnson V 1966 Human sexual response. Churchill, London

Matocha L K, Waterhouse J K 1993 Current nursing practice related to sexuality. Research in Nursing and Health 16:371–378

Meerabeau L 1999 The management of embarrassment and sexuality in health care. Journal of Advanced Nursing 29(6):1507–1513

Mischel W 1966 A social-learning view of sex differences in behaviour. In: Maccoby E E (ed) The development of sex differences. Stanford University Press, Stanford, pp 195–254

Monga T N, Lefebvre K A 1995 Sexuality: an overview. Physical Medicine and Rehabilitation: State of the Art Reviews 9(2):299–311

Offir C 1982 Human sexuality. Harcourt Brace, San Diego

Orem D 1995 Nursing: concepts of practice. Mosby, London

Peplau H 1988 Interpersonal relations in nursing. Macmillan, London

Royal College of Nursing 2000 Sexuality and sexual health in nursing practice. Royal College of Nursing, London

Roper N, Logan W, Tierney A 1996 The elements of nursing. Churchill Livingstone, Edinburgh

Salvage J 1995 The politics of nursing. Heinemann, London

Sayers J 1986 Sexual contradiction: psychology, psychoanalysis and feminism. Tavistock, London

Smith M 1993 Pediatric sexuality: promoting normal sexual development in children. Nurse Practitioner 18(8):37–44

Smook K 1992 Nurses' attitudes towards the sexuality of older people: an investigative study. Nursing Practice 6(1):15–17

Stein L 1967 The doctor–nurse game. Archives of General Psychiatry 16:699–703

Stein L, Watts D, Howell T 1990 The doctor–nurse game revisited. New England Journal of Medicine 322(8):546–549

Sundram C J, Stavis P F 1994 Sexuality and retardation: unmet challenges. Mental Retardation 32(4):255–264

Symons D 1979 The evolution of human sexuality. Oxford University Press, Oxford

Travis R, Yeager C 1991 Sexual selection, parental investment and sexism. Journal of Social Issues 47(3):117–130

Van Ooijen E, Charnock A 1994 Sexuality and patient care: a guide for nurses and teachers. Chapman & Hall, London

Versluysen M C 1980 Old wives' tales? Women healers in English history. In: Davies C (ed) Rewriting nursing history. Croom Helm, London, pp 175–199

Webb C 1985 Sexuality, nursing and health. John Wiley, Chichester

Webb C 1988 A study of nurses' knowledge and attitudes about sexuality in health care. International Journal of Nursing Studies 25(3):235–244

Wellings K, Field J, Johnson A M et al 1994 Sexual behaviour in Britain: the national survey of sexual attitudes and lifestyles. Penguin, Hamondsworth

World Health Organization 1975 Education and treatment in human sexuality: the training of health professionals. World Health Organization, Geneva

Chapter 16

Confusion

Moonee Gungaphul

KEY ISSUES

SUBJECT KNOWLEDGE
- Physiological factors that may lead to clients becoming confused
- Psychological factors that may lead to clients becoming confused
- Environmental factors that may lead to clients becoming confused
- Attitudes towards people who are confused

CARE DELIVERY KNOWLEDGE
- Nursing assessment of confused clients
- Risk assessment
- Planning nursing care for clients who are confused
- Specific strategies to help clients with chronic confusion

PROFESSIONAL AND ETHICAL KNOWLEDGE
- Ageism and stereotyping
- Advantages and disadvantages of caring for confused clients in the community
- Supporting carers in the community

PERSONAL AND REFLECTIVE KNOWLEDGE
- Application of the knowledge gained from this chapter to all branches of nursing
- Case studies

INTRODUCTION

Confusion is a negative characteristic of mental health. It is marked by poor attention and thinking, which lead to difficulties in comprehension, loss of short-term memory and often, irritability alternating with drowsiness. It is also a word which, when used in everyday language, can mean different things to different people. For healthcare staff, therefore, the clinical meaning of confusion must be specific to prevent inappropriate care and support.

OVERVIEW

This chapter explores the various causes of confusion. From this base the rationale for strategies to help clients who are confused is explained.

Subject knowledge

In Subject Knowledge the physiological factors that may lead to individuals becoming confused are identified. This is followed by an exploration of the psychological and environmental factors that also may lead to or worsen confusion.

Care delivery knowledge

Care Delivery Knowledge addresses the assessment of confused clients and how care may be planned. The specific therapies of reality orientation, reminiscence therapy and validation therapy are outlined and appraised.

Professional and ethical knowledge

In Professional and Ethical Knowledge, common attitudes held towards people who are confused are considered. With more care being delivered within the community, the advantages and disadvantages of this policy, and ways of supporting carers, are discussed. The focus is mainly on the elderly confused as it is this group who are likely to suffer long-term irreversible confusion.

Personal and reflective knowledge

Finally, Personal and Reflective Knowledge summarizes the main points of the chapter to help consolidate your knowledge of confusion. On pages 363–364 there are four case studies, each one relating to one of the branch programmes. You may find it helpful to read one of them before you start the chapter and use it as a focus for your reflections while reading. These are followed by activities that you can use to develop your learning portfolio.

SUBJECT KNOWLEDGE

BIOLOGICAL

As a term used within health and social care, confusion can be difficult to define. It is not easily distinguished from other terminology such as disorientation or delirium, with which it is sometimes used synonymously, and it is generally associated with negative mental health status. As defined by the American Psychiatric Association (1994), confusion includes cognitive and behavioural characteristics. Although observed as behaviour, it results from adverse physiological, psychological or environmental factors, which in turn interfere with the functioning of the nervous system. Therefore confusion on its own is not a condition, but is a symptom of an underlying pathology.

Some of the factors that may lead to confusion are listed in Table 16.1. Although these can cause confusion in individuals of all ages, it is, however, far more likely to be observed among elderly people.

TYPES OF CONFUSION

There are two types of confusion: short-term and long-term. Short-term or acute confusion has a sudden onset, is reversible and involves no destruction of brain cells. In the older age group, almost any severe physical illness can cause an acute state of confusion (Lipowski 1983, Liston 1982). Younger people can also develop acute confusion, though,

Table 16.1 Factors that can lead to confusion

Physical	Psychological	Environmental
Constipation	Anxiety states	Translocation
Diabetes mellitus	Depression	Stressful environment
Drugs or alcohol	Fear	Isolation or loneliness
Fatigue		External or internal
Hormonal disturbance		stimuli
Hypothermia		
Infection		
Neoplasm		
Vascular disorders		
Vitamin deficiencies		
Urinary retention		

and factors that may lead to it include epilepsy (especially following a seizure), hyperpyrexia, post electroconvulsive therapy and poisoning.

In contrast, long-term or chronic confusion occurs due to degenerative changes in the brain. This is called dementia. It is slow in onset, is usually irreversible and involves substantial destruction of brain cells.

PHYSIOLOGICAL CAUSES OF CONFUSION

There are six major physiological factors that can lead to confusion developing:

- infections
- endocrine disturbances
- electrolyte imbalance
- poisons
- trauma
- dementia.

Infections

Infections causing a fever can lead to confusion, often referred to in this instance as delirium. Infections arise due to pathogens invading the body systems, commonly via the urinary or respiratory tracts. Additionally, a chest infection may cause hypoxia, preventing adequate oxygenated blood reaching the brain, and worsening the confusion. Pathogens may also be transported from the primary site of infection, via the circulatory system, to infect the nervous system directly, again, worsening the confusion. Angus (1989) noted over 50% of cases of meningitis in older people were due to bacteria that usually infect the lungs.

Endocrine disorders

Disorders of the endocrine system can interfere with the operation of the nervous system resulting in confusion. For example, a malfunction of the thyroid gland can lead to hypothyroidism, one of the symptoms of which can be confusion (Tortora & Grabowski 1993). Similarly, if diabetes mellitus has not been stabilized, or if food has not been taken after the administration of insulin, hypoglycaemia and associated confusion can develop.

Electrolyte imbalance

Sodium is an important element in maintaining osmotic stability within body tissues. In cases of chronic renal failure, congestive heart disease, cirrhosis of the liver, inappropriate intake of water or secretion of antidiuretic hormone, the resulting sodium deficiency leads to the electrolyte abnormality of hyponatraemia, often shown by tiredness and confusion (Sheridan et al 1985). Although relatively uncommon, it can be induced iatrogenically in the elderly who are often prescribed diuretics that can cause excessive sodium to be excreted. In turn, this leads to electrolyte disturbances which manifest as confusion. Furthermore, the habitual use of laxatives, a common practice by the elderly (Conn 1992), can lead to problems of hydration, electrolyte imbalance and eventual confusion.

Electrolyte disturbances can also result from an inadequate intake of food and drink, i.e. malnutrition. In addition, malnutrition can result in the body lacking essential vitamins such as vitamin B_{12}. The deficiency of this vitamin leads to changes in mental health observed by characteristics such as forgetfulness, depression, irritability and confusion (see Ch. 7 on nutrition).

The elderly are the group to suffer poverty and are often unable to obtain an adequate diet (Barr & Coulter 1990). In turn, many older people are likely to be undernourished and develop syndromes associated with malnutrition and other metabolic disorders. Indeed, Fralic & Griffin (2001) identified a generally accepted myth that malnutrition was part of the ageing process. In an institutional environment such as a hospital, nursing home or other such place managed by professional staff, this should not be difficult to remedy with appropriate changes to diet and dietary supplements. Increasingly, institutional care is becoming unavailable for the elderly however, who are being supported to live in their own homes (Department of Health 1999a, 2001, 2002a; Knapp & Lawson 1995). Therefore difficulties can arise when individuals remain in their home, and are unable to change their dietary regimen.

Reflection and portfolio evidence

On your next clinical placement find out the following:

- What blood test is undertaken to determine whether an individual has an electrolyte imbalance?
- Why would individuals be prescribed diuretic medication over a prolonged period?
- How do diuretics work?
- In people who are prescribed long-term diuretic medication such as furosemide (frusemide), how is the electrolyte balance maintained?
- Why is this information important to the nurse working in the community with elderly people who are confused?

You will need to be familiar with the physiology of the kidney before attempting this exercise. You may find your pharmacist and the *British National Formulary* (British Medical Association and the Royal Pharmaceutical Society 2003) useful points of reference.

Poisons

In addition to environmental toxins, poisons that cause confusion include alcohol and drugs.

Alcohol

Intoxication with alcohol can lead to short-term confusion and, sometimes, memory lapses associated with brain damage (Roberts 1996). In turn, this can result in physical, psychological and social problems. In the long term, prolonged excessive consumption of alcohol can cause vitamin B_{12} deficiency, causing irreversible damage to the brain, and leading to Korsakoff syndrome of which chronic confusion is one of the main features.

Drugs

Drug-related confusion may result from:

- an overdose
- the drug's cumulative effect
- an interaction between different drugs
- the individual's reaction to the drug.

In particular, confusion can be induced by the use of certain neuroleptic drugs and compound analgesics. Some stimulants and sedatives can also lead to disorientation and confusion if they are stopped suddenly. In people who have particularly abused illicit drugs or alcohol, sudden withdrawal often produces a delirious state with associated confusion.

Being the greatest users of the health service, elderly people are more likely to be prescribed long-term medication (Blane 1991). Occasionally, due to the side effects of the drugs, or due to the interaction of a combination of drugs, confusion in the form of an iatrogenic dementia can develop (Strickland et al 1999).

Ghodse (1995) noted that a wide range of psychoactive drugs can impair an individual's general awareness and ability to concentrate. In particular, lysergic acid diethylamide (LSD or acid) results in altered perception and confusion. The illicit use of 3,4-methylenedioxymethamphetamine (MDMA, better known as ecstasy) has always been a public concern. MDMA, banned in the UK since 1971 as a class A drug, has been popularized as a recreational drug among contemporary youth culture arising from the mistaken belief that it has relatively harmless properties (Henry 1992). MDMA inhibits the reuptake of serotonin leading to an accumulation of excessive amounts of the neurotransmitter within the neural synapses. This in turn gives the euphoric feelings associated with taking the drug.

Excessive serotonin also raises the body temperature, which can result in dehydration, inappropriate blood clotting, convulsions and coma (Cook 1995, Jones & Owens 1996). Following publicity of this fact, many users attempted to compensate for the dehydration by drinking copious amounts of water. Again, this strategy is potentially dangerous. Day (1996) found that some users of MDMA drank so much water that they severely disturbed their electrolyte balance.

In the long term, exposure to MDMA damages the neuroreceptors and reduces the secretion of serotonin (Kish et al 2000), which is associated with depression (Cook 1995,

Day 1996), memory impairment (Reneman et al 2000) and, subsequently, confusion.

Trauma

Physical damage to the brain can result in confusion. The nature of the confusion will be governed by the part of the brain affected and the nature of the injury. If the injury is minor and reversible then the probability that the confusion will lessen is high. For example, confusion arising from concussion reduces as the concussion resolves. On the other hand, if the confusion arises from trauma that has caused permanent damage to the brain, recovery is unlikely.

Dementia

Irreversible destruction of brain cells is the major feature of dementia. The most common type is Alzheimer disease, which accounts for approximately 65% of all dementias (Kaplan & Sadock 1991, Strickland et al 1999). Multi-infarct dementia is also common and results from many 'mini strokes' over a period of time: the brain cells supplied by the damaged blood vessels are deprived of nutrients and oxygen and they subsequently die, leading to the onset of dementia and confusion. A new, thankfully rare, form of dementia has been identified that effects young people. Variant Creutzfeldt–Jakob disease (vCJD) is transmitted via infection by a prion found primarily in the carcasses of cattle suffering from bovine spongiform encephalitis (Nixon 1999). The infection within the UK herd was highest during the 1980s following the relaxation of animal feedstuff regulations. Since the early 1990s, known infected cattle have been excluded from the human food chain. As the incubation period of this disease is thought to be up to 25 years, however, people are still being newly diagnosed with the condition. Unfortunately, by the time that symptoms have appeared, the prognosis is poor and deterioration to death is rapid.

PSYCHOSOCIAL

PSYCHOLOGICAL CAUSES OF CONFUSION

Confusion arising from psychological sources may be due to either an organic or a functional illness. With organic illnesses such as Alzheimer disease, confusion has a slow insidious onset and during the early stage of the illness there may be lucid periods or 'flashbacks'. Confusion from organic illness is also accompanied by a deterioration of intellect, memory loss, sensory disturbances and disruption of the personality.

Confusion may also be experienced by a person with a functional illness. For example, an individual suffering a panic attack may also feel confused (Kaplan et al 1994). Functional disorders that give rise to perceptual dysfunctions, such as delusions or hallucinations, can also lead to confusion as the individual loses touch with reality.

ENVIRONMENTAL INFLUENCES ON CONFUSION

A variety of environmental factors can exacerbate confusion. They include:

- increased noise levels
- lack of personal space
- poor lighting
- distortion of light and darkness
- a lack of familiar faces.

The environment is particularly important in the care of individuals suffering from chronic confusion, such as those with Alzheimer disease, who are able to function in their usual environment, but will deteriorate rapidly if moved to a new unfamiliar environment. This is because the nature of the disease makes their short-term memory ineffective. Long-term memory is preserved though, and individuals are able to function when using this information (i.e. the familiar environment). Because they are unable to use short-term memory, however, when they encounter a new environment, they consequently become confused.

Attention to the immediate environment forms the basis of reality orientation therapy – a strategy that can be used to help individuals who are confused.

CARE DELIVERY KNOWLEDGE

NURSING ASSESSMENT OF CONFUSED CLIENTS

It must be remembered that confusion is a symptom of an underlying pathological condition rather than a condition in its own right. Consequently, the purpose of assessment is to identify the condition causing the confusion as, until this is addressed, strategies to help manage the confusion are of limited value. When assessing individuals who are confused it is therefore important to consider them as a whole rather than dwelling only on the confusion. In addition to a physiological assessment and a recent psychosocial history, a comprehensive biographical assessment should be made to record the individual's 'life review'. This can help to identify their needs or problems, lifestyle and circumstances (Butler 1974). Additionally, the life review can be used as the basis of therapies such as reminiscence therapy to promote positive experiences in elderly people with confusion (Haight 1992).

The individual who is confused will probably have difficulty in comprehending and communicating, so it is essential that the assessor has good interpersonal skills. This is facilitated by the active listening and observation outlined in Chapters 1 (Communication) and 19 (Rehabilitation). Three major areas should form the focus of assessment: physiological, psychological and environmental.

Physiological assessment

This part of the assessment is to exclude underlying physiological factors that may be contributing to the confusion. It begins by recording the vital signs of temperature, pulse, respiration and blood pressure. An overall visual impression of the client should also be recorded. In particular, observing the condition of the skin will indicate the level of hydration and nutritional state whereas cyanosis may indicate a poorly oxygenated blood supply to the brain.

The individual's ability to communicate and comprehend should be also determined. It may be that the client uses aids to communication such as spectacles or a hearing aid. If so it should be verified that these are worn correctly and are effective as sensory deficits may manifest as confused behaviour. Hearing deficits should always be investigated as a stereotyped myth of old age is that old people become deaf. Often, when investigated, a build-up of earwax can be found and, once this is addressed, the client's hearing is restored and their 'confusion' disappears.

Psychological assessment

The term confusion is frequently used to describe a wide variety of other behaviours. Confusion may also be misdiagnosed for other mental health problems, especially in the elderly, the most common of which is depression. It is therefore essential that this is eliminated, which can be achieved through taking a comprehensive history of the pattern of confusion and the use of instruments such as the Hospital Anxiety and Depression Scale (Zigmond & Snaith 1983) and the Clifton Assessment (Pattie & Gilleard 1979).

Hospital Anxiety and Depression Scale

This comprises a 14-item questionnaire, each question being rated from 1 to 4 according to the level of agreement. Seven of the questions measure aspects of anxiety, with the remainder indicating the severity of depression. This is a generally accepted, standardized instrument and can be used to identify depression in the elderly.

Clifton Assessment

The Clifton Assessment Procedures for the Elderly (CAPE) assesses:

- psychomotor activity
- cognition
- behaviour.

Psychomotor assessment is carried out using the Gibson Spiral Maze (Gibson 1961) (Fig. 16.1). The client is required to trace a line from the centre of the spiral outwards, avoiding the obstructions and to complete this as quickly as possible. The time taken to complete the maze and the number of errors form the basis of the score – the lower the score the better.

For the cognitive assessment, the client answers 12 set questions relating to personal data, orientation and mental ability. These are scored out of the possible 12 items. Patients with depression are expected to score 8 or more,

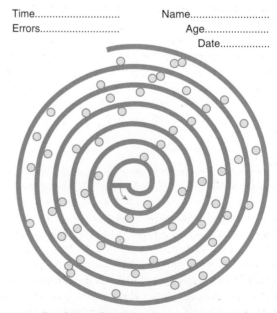

Figure 16.1 The Gibson Spiral Maze, reproduced at about 45% of its actual size. (From Gibson 1961, with kind permission of Hodder Arnold.)

while those with dementia are likely to score 7 or less (Pattie & Gilleard 1979).

Behavioural assessment is carried out using the Behaviour Rating Scale, which measures the level of dependence or independence based on 18 items, including bathing, dressing, mobility, eliminating and socializing. This scale identifies dependency with the highest scores. Therefore the fewer activities individuals can achieve, the higher their score.

By using the CAPE it is possible to make reliable judgements about an individual's confusion and mental impairment. The score can be used immediately; however, it is usual to record several scores obtained over a period of time to monitor any improvement or deterioration. Although a helpful instrument, CAPE should be used with caution. Some people with mild confusion may be unable to carry out the activities or only partially achieve them. Others may have a different ethnic origin and a limited ability to understand the questions due to a limited knowledge of the language or cultural differences. Others may have sensory deficits or failings. Furthermore, considering the frail people involved, the assessment must not be rushed since inaccurate conclusions may result (Goodwin 1991).

Reflection and portfolio evidence

You will require a personal stereo and two to five colleagues to complete this exercise. It will take approximately 20 minutes to complete the task plus time for reflection on the questions at the end.

Obtain a pre-recorded cassette of someone speaking. I would advise you to obtain Alan Bennett narrating his diaries *Writing Home* (Bennett 1994) if you can as he also gives his account of his mother's progression into Alzheimer disease.

Put on the headphones and join your colleagues for a conversation on any topics that occur as the conversation develops. Aim for the conversation to last for around 20 minutes. Switch on the cassette player and set the volume level so that you can clearly hear the tape at a level just below ordinary conversation level. At the end of 20 minutes, switch off the personal stereo and discuss the following with your colleagues:

- Could you participate in the conversation?
- Did your colleagues think you participated in the conversation?
- What difficulties (including difficulties with memory, non-verbal communication and verbal communication) did you encounter?
- What difficulties (including difficulties with memory, non-verbal communication and verbal communication) did your colleagues encounter?
- How might this experience help you when working with clients suffering from perceptual dysfunctions?

Environmental assessment

It is important to include environmental factors in an assessment. Confusion worsens in unfamiliar surroundings. For example, when clients are admitted to a new unit staffed with unfamiliar people their state of health may deteriorate with a consequent loss of sleep and increased distress. This is the 'translocation syndrome' (Smith 1986). Therefore, when assessing clients in a new environment it must also be considered whether they can function to their fullest abilities in their usual surroundings.

Evidence based practice

Following publication of *A First Class Service: Quality in the New NHS* (Department of Health 1998), clear national standards were set and implemented via the National Service Frameworks for Mental Health (Department of Health 1999b) and for Older People (Department of Health 2001). These contributed towards a commitment to support clients/patients with mental health needs, either in the home, residential setting or in hospital. The National Service Frameworks are 10-year programmes aimed at ensuring clients and their carers are treated with respect, dignity and fairness. As part of the key interventions, there should therefore be early recognition and management of mental health needs in primary care with support from specialist mental health teams for the elderly. Consequently, for people with confusion, early assessment and prompt management should result in a more positive outcome.

RISK ASSESSMENT

The government stated its ambition to assist the care for individuals in their homes in the document *Caring about Carers* (Department of Health 1999a). Although the motives behind this document are debatable, the outcome is that informal carers are expected to provide care for their relatives, and the role of health and social care workers is to assist in this process. The advantage of this policy is that it discourages moving clients with short-term memory loss to a new unfamiliar environment, so minimizing their confusion. This must be balanced against the clients' risks to themselves and to others, their risks to and from their carers, and the availability of adequate home support. Therefore, a risk assessment should identify whether it is possible to support the client to remain safely in their own environment or whether they should be admitted to an appropriate care facility.

PLANNING NURSING CARE FOR CLIENTS WHO ARE CONFUSED

Whenever possible, the plan of care should be made with the cooperation of all involved in the care, for example informal carers, relatives and members of the multidisciplinary team (Department of Health 2000, 2002b). The care plan should involve the client; however, with a severely confused individual, this may be beyond their ability.

Plans must also incorporate strategies to assist informal carers to cope with the needs of the confused individual. They are likely to include providing information about the pattern of the illness, promoting their involvement in the care process, providing information about accessing support agencies, co-ordinating health and social care services and monitoring for signs of fatigue. These are discussed in more detail later in this chapter.

Evidence based practice

Carers of people with demanding illness are subject to intense physical, psychological and social pressures. The effects are particularly severe if carers are frail themselves. Schulz & Beach (1999) found an association between mortality and those who experienced intense mental or emotional strain in elderly caregivers. Similarly Chan & Chang (1999) found carers at risk of developing physical and psychological symptoms as a result of the stress of caring. This reinforces the need to involve carers in formulating care plans and ensuring that they receive adequate support.

Short-term confusion

The assessment should ideally identify the causes of the confusion, and the difficulties they create. In the planning stage strategies to address these are developed. Physiological causes must be addressed as a priority and in most instances this will lead to a rapid reduction in the level of confusion. If the confusion arises from a mental illness it is important that an accurate medical diagnosis is made, as different pathways of treatment are required. In a functional mental illness, such as depression with accompanying confusion, the symptoms become less severe and the confusion will improve as the underlying illness is treated. In contrast, if there is an organic cause of confusion, such as Alzheimer disease, the pattern of care is likely to be a progressive increase in care and support as the condition worsens. An incorrect diagnosis will consequently lead to inappropriate care and perpetuate the confused state.

Long-term confusion

If the underlying cause of confusion cannot be treated, as in dementia, there are three main types of therapy that can help to address the symptoms. These are:

- reality orientation
- reminiscence therapy
- validation therapy.

Reality orientation

Confusion is accompanied by disorientation in which the concepts of time, place and person become disturbed. These cause difficulties for the individual regarding self, others, the environment and the relationship between them. Reality orientation attempts to address this by helping the individual to refocus on the world about them (Birchenall & Streight 1993). It uses a variety of cues, stimuli and tips to help remember time, place and names. Continued use of reality orientation reduces the need for the client to ask staff the time or the date or the location of places, such as the toilet or bedroom, and it decreases the chance that the client will be labelled confused or disorientated (Perko & Kreigh 1988). It also helps to maintain a safe environment, and promotes a sense of security, dignity, independence and self-esteem (Holden & Woods 1982).

In practice, reality orientation confronts the individual with facts such as the day, date, names and news. For example, a carer may say 'Hello Mr Smith. My name is Geoff. What is my name?' and repeat the greeting every time he meets the client throughout the day. Each correct response is given positive reinforcement, but it is important not to react negatively should an incorrect response be given.

There are two modes of reality orientation:

- intensively in group sessions
- ongoing 24-hour reality orientation relying on the use of cues, signs and colours placed at strategic points around the unit or in the client's house. For example, the client may have a colour coded bed area, the toilet may have an iconic picture of a toilet on the door, and the living area may have a large clock, a calendar and weather description in a prominent area.

Critics of reality orientation argue that it distresses clients and their carers if expectations are not achieved. It is also criticized for its repetitive nature. Reality orientation is unlikely to help individuals suffering from severe dementia; however, if the deterioration is not so advanced, it may slow the pace of deterioration and it often improves the client's mental state.

Reminiscence therapy

Reminiscence is an activity that everyone engages in. It is a common notion that older people live in the past and always talk about the 'good old days'. When considering Erikson's eighth stage of development 'ego integrity vs. despair' (Erikson 1980) it can be assumed that people in their later years look back over their life and accept its meaning. Older people, according to Klein et al (1985), may hesitate to talk about their past, however, because they do not want to meet with rejection (think of the reaction of Del and Rodney in the television series *Only Fools and Horses* when Uncle Albert reminisces about his experiences during the war) and may actually need help and encouragement to reminisce.

Reminiscence as a form of therapy is used to help elderly people with chronic confusion by focusing on times when they were in full possession of their skills and abilities (Norris & Eileh 1982). Thus, in individuals suffering from dementia, reminiscence therapy exploits the phenomenon that long-term memory remains relatively intact even when short-term memory does not function. If short-term memory is not working it then becomes very difficult to engage in day-to-day social interactions. Reminiscence therapy therefore provides a means of using the functioning long-term memory to allow a conversation to develop. This, in turn, improves the individual's self-esteem.

To enhance the process of reminiscing, a comprehensive life review should be developed, which can then be used as a focus for reflection (Butler 1974). Here, help from friends and relatives is invaluable. Norris (1986) uses the following criteria to ensure appropriate material is obtained:

- it is relevant to the past experiences of the individual
- it involves the stimulation of as many senses as possible
- it is used sparingly so as not to overwhelm the individual who is confused.

Care must be taken when selecting members of the reminiscence group that all members have similar life experiences. For example, clients from different ethnic backgrounds may have totally different experiences of the 1939–1945 war and this can lead to further confusion or even conflict.

People with confusion have the same feelings and needs as other people. Reminiscing can be a valuable form of therapy that brings the person with confusion into meaningful and enjoyable interactions. Reminiscing may also create feelings that are difficult to cope with, either by the client, or the carer, or both, and appropriate support strategies to enable these issues to be resolved must be arranged before the group begins. For health professionals this will be through debriefing and clinical supervision. Clients must be monitored for distress, however, and time must be allocated following the group to allow one-to-one support should it be required.

Validation therapy

It should be acknowledged that in the later stages of dementia, no effective treatment is available to prevent the progressive intellectual deterioration. Time spent promoting a reality orientation programme is then frustrating as no progress will be made and the process can become distressing for all concerned. An alternative is provided in validation therapy (Feil 1982). Like 24-hour reality orientation, it is an ongoing process; however, unlike reality orientation, it does not confront the behaviour but seeks to find the underlying meanings. It involves not allowing any factual errors to interrupt the meaningful dialogue on topics of interest to the individual. Therefore, when a client aged 80 years says something like 'My father is waiting for me, I must go home' the nurse does not confront the client with reality by replying 'Your father is dead and ….' In validation therapy, the nurse cultivates the statement to find the underlying meanings. Using this mode of therapy, interaction with the client who is confused should be on their ground, on their terms, and on the subjects that they raise and choose to discuss (Morton & Bleathman 1988). Consequently, in validation therapy communication and subject matter are matched to the stage of confusion. Often, it will be found that individuals who fail to respond to reality orientation will show a significant improvement if validation therapy is used instead (Fine & Rouse-Bane 1995).

Decision making exercise

Jack Greaves looks after his wife Edna, who has advanced Alzheimer disease. Unfortunately, Jack has a benign prostatic hypertrophy and is to be admitted to hospital for a prostatectomy. Although Edna is able to live at home with Jack, her illness is so advanced that she would be unable to stay in the house alone and arrangements have been made for her to be admitted to a local nursing home until Jack is well enough to look after her again.

Following admission to the nursing home, Edna was unable to settle. She became very distressed, restless and confused. She refused to eat her meals and continually asked where her Jack was.

Jack was advised not to visit on the day of admission so did not visit until the following day. By this time, Edna's mental state had deteriorated considerably. Jack became extremely distressed at his wife's condition and stated that he would cancel his surgery to take her home and look after her.

- How would you explain the change in Edna's condition to Jack?
- What advice could you offer Jack?
- What actions could have been taken to minimize Edna's distress?
- What are the advantages and disadvantages of respite care?

PROFESSIONAL AND ETHICAL KNOWLEDGE

ATTITUDES TOWARDS PEOPLE WHO ARE CONFUSED

The passive acceptance of confusion and the notion that it is an inevitable characteristic of a particular condition or disorder promotes complacency, adding to the burden of the individual's low self-esteem, dependence and isolation. It is therefore important to look positively and objectively at the issues and to conduct a comprehensive assessment to help identify the cause(s) of the confusion and endeavour to promote a realistic programme of care or management. Promoting a relationship with an individual who is confused is not easy, though, especially when their behaviour is disturbing. To establish a relationship, attitudes of respect and a willingness to work with the individual must be imparted. In other words, it should not be seen as part of a job. Professional engagement is positive in outlook, non-judgemental, and seeks to promote the potential of the client (Egan 1994).

ATTITUDES TOWARDS ELDERLY PEOPLE

In the past, dependent elderly people have been treated very badly. Robb (1967) found their treatment particularly distressing, documenting rudeness, rough handling and neglect. Even when she brought this to the attention of those with ultimate responsibility, the matters were brushed aside. Fifteen years later, according to Holden & Woods (1982), attitudes towards elderly people remained discriminatory, rejecting and negative. Recently, in examining the health care provision for the elderly, it was reported in *Adding Life to Years* (Department of Health 2002c) that although 17% of elderly people felt that they had received an inferior service to younger people, evidence to substantiate these claims was not found. The report cautions, however, that because no evidence was found, it does not follow that ageism is absent from the National Health Service. Indeed, Age Concern found that within contemporary society, ageism remains a major problem, particularly in health care (Age Concern 2002), while it is also claimed that some employers discriminate against people for no other reason but their age (BBC 2002).

Stereotypes, myths and ageism are reinforced in a society that values the younger generation more than the old. To return to health, this is reflected in the dilemma of whether or not to give aggressive life-saving treatments. Were it a younger person, the question would not arise since they 'have a lot of life left'. When rationing of resources occurs there are perhaps ethical arguments that help to understand this dilemma; however, it must always be remembered that elderly people are not a homogeneous group. Just like other age groups, elderly people have differing abilities, skills and other attributes. Stereotyping them all as being frail, cantankerous or confused is therefore a cardinal mistake, and is addressed in the National Service Framework for Older People (Department of Health 2001) within which standard one is to identify and stop age discrimination.

ADVANTAGES AND DISADVANTAGES OF CARING FOR CONFUSED CLIENTS IN THE COMMUNITY

Most elderly people prefer to live in their own homes and, in the UK, the majority do so. Because of the effects of dementia on short-term memory, moving an individual from familiar surroundings to a new environment often results in a deterioration in their condition. It could therefore be argued that strategies to enable individuals to stay in the community are in the clients' best interests. What then are the disadvantages to this policy?

The elderly are the largest users of the NHS and their numbers in proportion to the working population are growing (Central Statistics Office 2002). When the Conservative government was elected into power in 1979, most elderly care services were provided within NHS inpatient beds. These were very expensive to maintain and the demographic evidence revealed that because people were living longer, and because of a falling birth rate, the proportion of elderly within the country, and the cost of maintaining the health services to support them, would rise dramatically. Community care was seen as the way forward as it would be a much cheaper option than providing institutional care.

In the community, care is provided using informal (unpaid) carers, rather than statutory (paid for) services and this doctrine was promoted through emphasizing a return to 'family values' and taking responsibility for your own family's needs. Therefore the government was able to reduce expenditure on services for the elderly, making for sounder, cost-effective, financial management while at the same time promoting their policy of sound family values. The Griffiths Report (1988), forerunner of the NHS and Community Care Act 1990, further endorsed this position. Griffiths argued that care should be delivered in the community by using voluntary and commercial sectors instead of the existing statutory services. He argued that this strategy would 'widen the individual's choice and increase flexibility and innovation'. Of course, it really paved the way for less investment in statutory services and made more demands upon voluntary and informal carers. Added emphasis was given to the strategy by the reduction of the NHS and local authority beds and the growth in the number of private nursing beds (Department of Health 2003a,b; Evandrou et al 1990).

This initiative was compounded following the full implementation of the NHS and Community Care Act 1990 on 1 April 1993. On this date the responsibility for funding private nursing beds was transferred from the Department of Social Security to local authorities, who received an increase in their central support grant to compensate. This money was not ring-fenced, however, and since then many local authorities have chosen to invest more on (means-tested) domiciliary services to keep individuals who would previously have received residential or nursing home care in the community, and to benefit from the associated financial savings (Knapp & Lawson 1995).

As private nursing beds were also means-tested, elderly people with over £8000 of assets (assets includes the value of their house and its contents), and who required full-time nursing or residential care, were obliged to fund themselves, selling their assets if necessary to raise the money. Only elderly people with assets under this amount received funding from the local authority. Presently, apart from in Scotland where private nursing beds are not means-tested, assets over £18 500 are considered when elderly people require private nursing and personal care. In response to this disparity, and to counter the claims of erosion of elderly peoples' savings, the Health and Social Care Act 2001 introduced free nursing care for people who, where the local authority agree, need it. It is important to understand what is meant by nursing care, however. This is only a small percentage of the fee paid to private nursing homes. Charges for accommodation (hotel services) and social care are exempt from funding under this Act. Therefore, in England and Wales, residential care (including the residential component of nursing home fees) remains means-tested. This alone may prevent some elderly people receiving the care that they need.

Decision making exercise

Since her divorce 5 years ago, Jennifer Soames and her son Jason have lived with Jennifer's mother in the family home. Over the last couple of years, however, Jennifer's mother has become increasingly forgetful and restless, to the extent that she is becoming a danger to herself. She wanders aimlessly during the day and often gets up in the middle of the night believing it is daytime. Occasionally she has wandered away from the house and got lost, the most recent time being found walking down the centre of a busy road by the local policeman. She also forgets where the toilet is and, if Jennifer does not take her regularly, she is likely to 'have an accident' in the lounge.

Jennifer has cared for her mother but she is becoming very tired and feels that it is getting too much for her. She would like to have her mother admitted to a local nursing home; however, her divorce settlement has almost run out and she has no other income. She is worried that as the house in which she lives belongs to her mother, she would be evicted to pay the nursing home fees.

- Are Jennifer's fears of eviction valid?
- What support services are available to help Jennifer to care for her mother?
- How would you contact these services in your area?

PROBLEMS EXPERIENCED BY INFORMAL CARERS

Informal carers comprise families, friends and neighbours. At the present time around 6 million people in Great Britain have some informal caring responsibilities (Department of Health 1999a). Around half of these are within the working age range of 45–65 years, with the majority of the remainder being over the age of 65 (Department of Health 2002c). However, some informal carers are of school age (Department of Health 1999a).

Informal carers play an important part in meeting the needs of their dependent relatives. They are often placed under great strain, though, and have to carry out their tasks without the resources, space and purpose-built environments that are available to formal (paid) carers. Additionally, unlike formal carers, they cannot remain detached from their role of caring. They are unable to leave and go home at the end of the day and have little opportunity to switch off. To make matters worse, some informal carers become ill themselves as a result of the stress of caring for their relative (Braithwaite 1990, Lichtenstein et al 1998). For some carers, particularly those caring for people with dementia, sleep is often disturbed due to the dependent person waking up during the night. Indeed, caring for a relative suffering from dementia is, according to Levin et al (1989), the most stressful type of care.

In practical terms it is a matter of concern when carers experience high distress levels since they are less likely to continue caring, or, if they do, the quality of care that they give is likely to decline (Levin et al 1989). Unsupported, informal carers can actually worsen the condition by generating extreme distress for themselves and the dependent person (Lo & Brown 2000). Much of this distress can be avoided, however, if carers are provided with adequate support (Mitchell 2000).

SUPPORTING CARERS

Reflection and portfolio evidence

Imagine you have to look after your elderly dependent mother who is disorientated for time and place in your home. She is incontinent of urine and regularly gets up in the middle of the night, wanders outside, and if you do not catch her, quickly wanders off and gets lost. Recently she has also started to switch on the cooker, but forgets to light the gas.

Your mother is so dependent that you are unable to leave her for any length of time and you consequently have to give up your job. Your teenage children are too embarrassed to bring their friends home as they are ashamed of your mother's behaviour and complain that the furniture smells from where your mother has been incontinent.

- What social problems are you likely to experience?
- What financial problems are you likely to experience?
- What psychological problems are you likely to experience?
- How will looking after your mother affect your health and well-being?

Within contemporary society, the care of dependent elderly people relies on the contribution made by informal carers. Consequently, it is important that informal carers, as well as the client, are included within the care plan. This is recognized within mental health services, being an integral part of the National Service Framework for Mental Health (Department of Health 1999b) and the Revised Care Programme Approach (Department of Health 2000). Unfortunately, however, this was not extended to the National Service Framework for Older People, which only requires the client to be involved in care planning (Department of Health 2001).

With adequate support, informal carers can maintain a reasonable level of social activities, which may take the form of leisure, holidays and relationships with friends. The document *Caring about Carers* (Department of Health 1999a) emphasizes the government's commitment to supporting 6 million carers within the UK, by examining flexible work patterns and committing £140 million over 3 years to help carers take a break. As this works out at £7.78 per carer each year, though, other methods of support clearly need to be identified.

Support for informal carers may take the form of practical help such as taking the client out, helping with dressing, bathing and toileting, and simply keeping an eye on the client to check that they are alright. Support schemes, in terms of family-based respite care schemes such as befriending and home care, are useful adjuncts to promoting care in the community. Twigg & Atkin (1993) found in particular that carers of individuals with dementia valued day care both for the relief it brought and for the opportunities it gave them to maintain social contacts.

Support groups run by social workers and psychiatric nurses have been less well evaluated. Not all carers enjoy group activities, according to Twigg (1992). She found that some informal carers were not interested in hearing about other people's problems and felt that they had enough problems of their own. Other problems that informal carers face when attending support groups are transport difficulties, particularly in rural areas, and arranging care for the dependent relative, especially if the meeting times are inflexible.

Evidence based practice

Like yourself, many carers now have access to the internet, either from within their own home, from a local library or through internet cafes. There are many useful resources available on the internet that the practitioner, or increasingly carers, can access; they include:

- Age Concern (http://www.ageconcern.org.uk/)
- Alzheimer's Association (http://www.alz.org/)
- Crossroads (http://www.crossroads.org.uk/English/carers.htm#how)
- Help the Aged (http://www.helptheaged.org.uk/)
- Saga (http://www.saga.co.uk/)

Visit each site regularly and familiarize yourself with their content so that you can supply carers with up-to-date information and support.

With the finite resources, reduction of services and the strong emphasis on community care, it is likely that unless their symptoms are severely debilitating, dependent elderly people will be cared for in their own homes by informal carers, with the help and support of the statutory, voluntary and private sector services. The nurse's role has consequently evolved from providing to facilitating care, in partnership with other carers, to attempt to ensure that informal carers have sufficient support.

PERSONAL AND REFLECTIVE KNOWLEDGE

APPLYING THE KNOWLEDGE IN THIS CHAPTER TO ALL BRANCHES OF NURSING

You can develop your portfolio on working with people who are confused by collecting information gathered from any aspect of your work (activities and projects you have been involved as well as day-to-day practice), clinical supervision, research, websites and articles. To complete your portfolio you need to provide evidence of insight into personal and professional growth (Stuart 1998). This is achieved by reflecting on how your knowledge, feelings and skills have developed over time, again using clinical supervision where necessary to assist this process.

Examples that you could include within your portfolio are:

- evidence of any activity, project and papers/articles that you used when dealing with a person who was confused
- a reflective diary of your experiences of caring with a person with confusion
- identifying your level/experience/personal ability in caring for a person with confusion

- identifying transferable skills you have developed when caring for people who are confused, that you can use in future practice.

CASE STUDIES IN THE CARE OF CONFUSED CLIENTS

Four case studies now follow, one from each branch of nursing. You should work through each and answer the questions to consolidate the knowledge you have gained from this chapter.

Case study: Mental health

George Ferguson has been referred to the community mental health team. George has lived in the same house since his marriage to Ida 58 years ago. Unfortunately, last year Ida died and since that time there has been a progressive deterioration in George's behaviour. He has lost weight, and has often been found wandering aimlessly around his village. Recently he has taken to sleeping during the day and leaving his house, with the doors open, at night. He has also become very forgetful and caused concern to his neighbours last week when he put a saucepan of beans on a lighted gas ring and then left the house. Fortunately no one was injured but substantial smoke damage was caused to his kitchen.

- What are the possible causes for George's current problems?
- What information should the community psychiatric nurse obtain in the assessment and why?
- What support services are available to help George to remain at home for as long as possible?
- At what stage would George require admission to a hospital or nursing home?

Case study: Adult

Matthew Jones is a 63-year-old retired dentist. He is admitted to the Accident and Emergency department and smells strongly of alcohol. He is very agitated and restless, and appears disorientated of time, date and place. He is also very distressed, and his mood fluctuates from being tearful to being angry and verbally aggressive. When you are attending to him he keeps mistaking you for one of his friends and calls you 'Georgie'. You notice in your assessment that his chest sounds congested, and his extremities are cyanosed. You also think that you can smell acetone on his breath, but this is strongly masked by the smell of alcohol.

- What are the possible reasons for Matthew's confusion?
- What immediate actions should be taken?
- How long would you expect to wait before Matthew's confusion resolved?

Case study: Child

Kimberley Kingston, aged 8 years, was cycling when she hit the kerb and fell off her bike, hitting her head on the ground as she landed. She is reported to have lost consciousness briefly and was brought into the Accident and Emergency department. A skull X-ray shows no sign of a fracture, but she is to be kept in hospital overnight for observation. Kimberley is frightened and does not appear to know where she is or why she is there. She has no recollection of the accident.

- Why has Kimberley's confusion arisen?
- What immediate actions should be taken to help reduce Kimberley's confusion?
- How long would you expect Kimberley's confusion to last?

Case study: Learning disabilities

Pravin Dutt is a 34-year-old man who suffered brain damage at birth. Since the death of his mother, 9 years ago, he has been cared for in a group bungalow. Using the continued support from his carers Pravin has coped well with day-to-day activities of living. Along with three other residents he has also benefited from an active behaviour modification programme.

Recent changes in management and organization have resulted in Pravin becoming much more dependent upon others, in particular with elimination, and he has developed faecal incontinence. This has been followed by changes in his mental state manifesting as disorientation of time, date and place, restlessness and challenging behaviour.

- Identify the most probable cause for Pravin's change in behaviour.
- What actions should the carers take to relieve Pravin's distress?
- What actions could be taken to minimize Pravin's faecal incontinence?
- What are the likely outcomes of the actions taken and when would you expect them to be achieved by?

Summary

This chapter has explored how physiological, psychological and environmental factors can lead to the development of confusion. It has included:

1. Confusion is symptomatic of an underlying pathology and the focus of the initial nursing assessment must be to identify and exclude this.
2. Short-term confusion was seen to be treatable once the underlying cause was identified.
3. Long-term confusion, however, is usually as a result of an untreatable organic pathology and only amenable to symptomatic management.
4. The elderly are the group most likely to suffer long-term confusion.
5. There are many stereotyped views on both confusion and the elderly and it is important to be aware of these in order to give appropriate assistance to clients and their carers. This is particularly important as confusion in the elderly may have a physical or a iatrogenic cause, or it may be a symptom of depression.
6. Various strategies to help manage confusion within its different contexts were explored and the indicative criteria for each identified.
7. Currently, a large part of caring falls to informal carers within the community.
8. In view of the demographic trends within the population, the current pattern of higher percentages of elderly will continue. This suggests that the pattern of care is likely to remain unchanged, with the role of professionals working in the community being to assist informal carers to care, rather than providing care themselves.
9. The advantages and disadvantages of this policy were debated and the importance of adequate support for carers in the community was demonstrated.

Annotated further reading and websites

Mace N L, Rabins P V, Castleton B A et al 1992 The 36-hour day. Hodder & Stoughton, Sevenoaks
This is identified as a 'family guide' to caring for people at home with Alzheimer disease and other confusional illnesses. This is a useful text with comprehensive information on caring issues. It is suitable for both formal and informal carers.

BBC Video 1983 Where's the key? BBC Enterprises, London
An insightful film lasting about 1 hour that looks at the
effect of Alzheimer disease on the individual and her informal
carer. Although the setting of the film is the early 1970s
most of the issues raised remain unresolved in the
present day.

http://www.alzheimers.org.uk
This is the Alzheimer's Society website. This is an excellent,
comprehensive website that contains resources for practitioners,
carers and sufferers, not only of Alzheimer disease but also for
CJD sufferers. The library section also contains an excellent
resource of downloadable papers for professional use.

References

Age Concern 2002 Breaking barriers: health. Online. Available:
http://www.ageconcern.org.uk/ageconcern/news_578.htm

American Psychiatric Association 1994 Diagnostic and statistical
manual V. American Psychiatric Association, Washington

Angus R 1989 Infectious diseases of the nervous system. In:
Tallis R (ed) The clinical neurology of old age. John Wiley,
Chichester, pp 297–308

Barr N, Coulter F 1990 Social security: solution or problem? In: Hills J
(ed) The state of welfare in Britain: the welfare state in Britain since
1974. Clarendon Press, Oxford, pp 274–333

BBC 2002 Ageism at work 'still rife'. Online. Available: http://news.
bbc.co.uk/1/hi/business/1759955.stm

Bennett A 1994 Writing home: Alan Bennett's diaries 1980–90. BBC
Radio Collection, London

Birchenall J M, Streight M E 1993 Care of the older adult. Lippincott,
Philadelphia

Blane D 1991 Elderly people and health. In: Scambler G (ed) Sociology
as applied to medicine. Baillière Tindall, London, pp 160–172

Braithwaite V A 1990 Bound to care. Allen & Unwin, Sydney

British Medical Association and the Royal Pharmaceutical Society of
Great Britain 2003 British National Formulary, No. 45. British
Medical Association, London

Butler R N 1974 Successful ageing and the role of the life review.
Journal of the American Geriatrics Society 22(12):529–537

Central Statistics Office 2002 Social trends, No. 32. HMSO, London

Chan C W H, Chang A M 1999 Stress associated with tasks for family
caregivers of patients with cancer in Hong Kong. Nursing Research
22(4):260–265

Conn V S 1992 Self-management of over the counter medicines by older
adults. Public Health Nursing 9(1):29–36

Cook A 1995 Ecstasy (MDMA): alerting users to the dangers. Nursing
Times 91(16):32–33

Day M 1996 The bitterest pill: the drug ecstasy. Nursing Times 92(7):4–20

Department of Health 1998 A first class service: quality in the new NHS.
HMSO, London

Department of Health 1999a Caring about carers: a national strategy for
carers. HMSO, London

Department of Health 1999b National service framework (mental
health). HMSO, London

Department of Health 2000 Effective care co-ordination in mental health
services: modernizing the care programme approach. HMSO, London

Department of Health 2001 National service framework for older
people. HMSO, London

Department of Health 2002a National statistics: social trends. HMSO,
London

Department of Health 2002b Mental health policy implementation
guide: adult acute in-patient care provision. HMSO, London

Department of Health 2002c Adding life to years: report of the Expert
Group on healthcare of older people. HMSO, London

Department of Health 2003a Health and personal social services statistics.
Online. Available: http://www.doh.gov.uk/HPSSS/TBL_B16.HTM

Department of Health 2003b Health and personal social services statistics.
Online. Available: http://www.doh.gov.uk/HPSSS/TBL_B23.HTM

Egan G 1994 The skilled helper: a problem-management approach to
helping, 5th edn. Brooks/Cole, Pacific Grove

Erikson E H 1980, Identity and the life cycle. Norton, New York

Evandrou M, Falkingham J, Glennerster H 1990 The personal social
services: everyone's poor relation but nobody's baby. In: Hills J (ed)
The state of welfare in Britain: the welfare state in Britain since 1974.
Clarendon Press, Oxford, pp 206–269

Feil N 1982 Validation: the Feil method. Edward Feil Productions,
Cleveland

Fine J I, Rouse–Bane S 1995 Using validation techniques to improve
communication with cognitively impaired older adults. Journal of
Gerontological Nursing 21(6):39–45

Fralic J, Griffin C 2001 Nutrition and the elderly: a case manager's
guide. Lippincott's Case Management 64(4):177–182

Ghodse H 1995 Drugs and addictive behaviour: a guide to treatment.
Blackwell Science, Oxford

Gibson H B 1961 The Gibson spiral maze. Hodder & Stoughton,
Sevenoaks

Goodwin S E 1991 Planning care: from admission onwards. In: Benson
S, Carr P (eds) The care assistant's guide to working with elderly
mentally infirm. Hawker, London, pp 29–39

Griffiths R 1988 Community care: agenda for action – a report to the
Secretary of State for social services. HMSO, London

Haight B 1992 The structured life-review process: community approach
to the ageing client. In: Jones G, Miesen B M L (eds) Care-giving in
dementia: research and applications. Routledge, London

Health and Social Care Act 2001 HMSO, London

Henry J 1992 Ecstasy and the dance of death. British Medical Journal
305(6844):5–6

Holden U P, Woods R T, 1982 Reality orientation: psychological
approaches to the 'confused' elderly. Churchill Livingstone, Edinburgh

Jones C, Owens D 1996 The recreational drug user in the intensive care
unit: a review. Intensive and Critical Care Nursing 12(3):126–130

Kaplan H I, Sadock B J 1991 Synopsis of psychiatry. Williams & Wilkins,
Baltimore

Kaplan H I, Sadock B J, Grebb J A 1994 Kaplan's and Sadock's Synopsis
of psychiatry, behavioural sciences and clinical psychiatry.
Williams & Wilkins, Baltimore

Kish S J, Furukwa Y, Ang L et al 2000 Striatal serotonin is depleted in
brain of a human MDMA (ecstasy) user. Neurology 55(2):294–296

Klein W H, LeShan E J, Furman S S 1985 Promoting mental health of
older people through group methods. Manhattan Society for Mental
Health, New York

Knapp M, Lawson R 1995 Community care and the health service. In:
Glynn J J, Perkins D A (eds) Managing health care: challenges for the
90s. Saunders, London

Levin E, Sinclair I, Gorbach P 1989 Families, services and confusion in
old age. Gower, Aldershot

Lipowski Z J 1983 Transient cognitive disorders: delirium and acute
confusional states in the elderly. American Journal of Psychiatry
140(11):1426–1436

Liston E H 1982 Delirium in the aged. In: Jarvik L F, Small G W (eds) The
psychiatric clinic of North America. Saunders, Philadelphia

Lichtenstein P, Gatz M, Berg S 1998 A twin study of mortality after
spousal bereavement. Psychological Medicine 28(3):635–643

Lo R, Brown R 2000 Caring for family carers and people with dementia.
International Journal of Psychiatric Nursing Research 6(2):684–694

Mitchell E 2000 Managing carer stress: an evaluation of a stress management programme for carers of people with dementia. British Journal of Occupational Therapy 63(4):179–184

Morton I, Bleathman C 1988 Does it matter whether it's Thursday or Friday? Nursing Times 84(6):27

NHS and Community Care Act 1990 HMSO, London

Nixon R R 1999 CE update: microbiology. II. Prions and prion diseases. Laboratory Medicine 30(5):335–338

Norris A D 1986 Reminiscence with elderly people. Winslow Press, London

Norris A D, Eileh A E 1982 Reminiscence groups. Nursing Times 78(32):68–69

Pattie A H, Gilleard C J 1979 Manual of the Clifton Assessment Procedures for the Elderly (CAPE). Hodder & Stoughton, London

Perko J E, Kreigh H Z 1988 Psychiatric and mental health nursing: a commitment to care and concern. Prentice-Hall, New York

Reneman L, Booij J, Scmand B 2000 Memory disturbances in 'ecstacy' users are correlated with an altered brain serotonin neurotransmission. Pharmocology 148:322–324

Robb B 1967 Sans everything. Nelson, Thames Ditton

Roberts C 1996 The physiological effects of alcohol misuse. Professional Nurse 11(10):646–648

Schulz R, Beach S R 1999 Caregiving as a risk factor for mortality: the caregiver health effects study. Journal of the American Medical Association 282(23):2215–2219

Sheridan E, Patterson H R, Gustafson E A 1985 The drug, the nurse, the patient. Saunders, Philadelphia

Smith B A 1986 When is confusion translocation syndrome? American Journal of Nursing 86(11):1280–1281

Strickland T L, Longobardi P, Gray G E 1999 Health issues of minority elderly: dementia in minority elderly. Clinical Geriatrics 7(11):83–93

Stuart G M 1998 Therapeutic nurse–patient relationship. In: Stuart G M, Laraia M T (eds) Principles and practice of psychiatric nursing. Mosby, St Louis, pp 17–53

Tortora G J, Grabowski S R 1993 Principles of anatomy and physiology, 7th edn. HarperCollins, New York

Twigg J 1992 Carers in the service system. In: Twigg J (ed) Carers: research and practice. HMSO, London

Twigg J, Atkin K 1993 Policy and practice in informal care. Open University, Milton Keynes

Wake D 1995 Ecstasy overdose: a case study. Intensive and Critical Care Nursing 11(1):6–9

Zigmond A S, Snaith R P 1983 The Hospital Anxiety and Depression Scale. Acta Psychiatrica Scandinavica 67:361–370

Chapter 17

Mobility

David Nichol and Sam Annasamy

KEY ISSUES

SUBJECT KNOWLEDGE
- Mobility and its meaning
- Biological aspects of human mobility
- Movement and activity
- Developmental changes in mobility
- Physical effects of immobility
- Psychological and social effects of immobility

CARE DELIVERY KNOWLEDGE
- Assessment of mobility
- Planning mobility care
- Implementing mobility care
- Evaluation of care delivery

PROFESSIONAL AND ETHICAL KNOWLEDGE
- Nursing responsibilities in mobility care
- Implications of the Disability Discrimination Act 1995 and Disability Rights Commission Act 1999
- Facilities for mobility care
- Ethical issues in mobility care

PERSONAL AND REFLECTIVE KNOWLEDGE
- Using mobility aids and appliances
- Experiencing and understanding the difficulties of mobility impairment
- Case studies in decision making related to the immobile client in all branches of nursing
- Personal reflection of experience

INTRODUCTION

Mobility is a term often used by health professionals to denote functional capacity of patients or clients. Most people take this for granted and yet everyone is dependent upon movement for essential activities in life. Further, there is a tendency to be interested in mobility purely in physical or mechanical terms, though it is important to consider the physiological, psychological, sociological and environmental impact upon the individual. Mobility is vital for normal human development and well-being. Any degree of immobility will undoubtedly affect a person's quality of life, for example self-reliance, self-sufficiency, self-support, self-care, self-respect, self-esteem and self-confidence. Most individuals get up in the morning without restrictions or limitations and expect to have full mobility. For some, however, mobility requires great effort, getting out of bed or walking to the toilet becomes a major task, and for others it is only possible with help or even impossible with assistance. This chapter will focus on the groups of people who have difficulty mobilizing, with the intention of providing a deeper understanding and appreciation of the impact immobility has on the lifestyles and mental state of those affected. Assisting or encouraging patients/clients to mobilize and maintain mobility is an essential part of nursing care, whatever the branch of nursing.

OVERVIEW

Subject knowledge

The relevant anatomy and physiology of the musculoskeletal and nervous systems including the physical effects of exercise and immobility are discussed in the biology section. The psychological/sociological section will examine the developmental aspects of mobility, the psychosocial effects of immobility and attitudes towards the physically impaired both at societal and individual level.

Care delivery knowledge

This area includes examination of assessment tools/scales and use of appropriate aids for different situations and environments. Strategies in planning, implementing and evaluating interventions in mobility care are discussed.

Professional and ethical knowledge

This section will look at issues such as the nurse's accountability and responsibilities in mobility care, and ethical issues. Relevant policies are discussed such as the National Service Framework for Older People (Department of Health 2001) as well as those aimed at supporting the disabled and eliminating discrimination such as the Disability Discrimination Act 1995, the Disability Rights Commission Act 1999 and the Special Educational Needs and Disability Act 2001.

Personal and reflective knowledge

In this section exercises and case studies are included and provide an opportunity to examine the problems faced by patients/clients who have difficulties mobilizing and to consider appropriate nursing interventions. Linking theory with practice is part of a nurse's reflective practice and is essential for personal and professional development. You are encouraged to reflect on aspects of mobility care encountered during your clinical visits. You are also advised to keep records of practical experience and achievements in your portfolio.

On pages 386–387 there are four case studies, each one relating to one of the branch programmes. You may find it helpful to read one of them before you start the chapter and use it as a focus for your reflections while reading as part of your portfolio development.

SUBJECT KNOWLEDGE

BIOLOGICAL

This section will look at different definitions of mobility and demographic trends with regard to immobility, but the main focus of this section will be on an overview of anatomy and physiology of the musculoskeletal system including microscopic structure of bone, joints and muscles and how they function in mobility. Effects and complications of immobility are also discussed.

MOBILITY AND ITS MEANING

Chambers Dictionary defines mobility as 'Quality or power of being mobile; freedom or ease of movement' (Schwarz 1995) and *Collins English Dictionary* defines it as 'The ability to move physically: a handicapped person's mobility may be limited' (Makin 1991). Mobility as a lay consideration means being able to move, bend down, stand, sit down, get up, walk, run, dance, etc. and to perform any activities associated with movements without any assistance. Physical definitions, however, have more than physical effects and consequences. Immobility,

in a world where the environment caters primarily for those with full mobility, can affect not only physical health, but also psychological and social health. The concept of an optimum level of mobility changes over time and is not necessarily the same in all cultures at the same point in time. Increasingly in developed countries, full mobility is assumed to be the norm and this may have consequences for those that are affected by varying degree of immobility. Under such circumstances, it is not surprising that anything less than full mobility is regarded as a disability which may have devastating effects upon a person's well-being.

Disability means different thing to different people. The Department of Social Security (1998) regards disability as the inability to carry out 'a particular activity or task' to meet 'certain level of need'. Part 1 of the Disability Discrimination Act 1995 defines a disabled individual as a person who has 'a physical or mental impairment which has a substantial and long-term effect on his ability to carry out normal day-to-day activities'.

Reflection and portfolio evidence

- Write down your definition of 'disability'.
- Find out the definitions of 'impairment' and 'handicap'.

Compare and contrast the definitions.

Evidence based practice

The General Household Survey (Office of Population Censuses and Surveys 1999), using questionnaires investigating mobility difficulties in Britain, found that 8% of those who replied indicated having difficulties moving about, both indoors and outdoors; 7% suffered permanent immobility while only 1% were temporarily immobile as a result of trauma or illness. This figure tends to increase with age and gender, for example 4% of men and women with mobility difficulties were aged between 16 and 64 years, but for people aged 85 years and over the figures rise to 67% for women and 42% for men. It was also found that twice the number of men aged 65 and over than women of similar age group were able to perform certain tasks (mobility related) without assistance.

With demographic changes, as the elderly population (men aged 65 and over and women aged 60 and over) reaches 10.8 million (Office of Population Censuses and Surveys 2001), it can be suggested that mobility problems will continue to rise in future years. This could be considered from two perspectives. A negative perspective view is that there will need to be an increase in government funding thus making more demands on the already stretched National Health Service. On the positive side, as the number of immobile people increases, and they become more visible, changes may come about in mainstream society thus providing people with disability a greater say in policy making. Webb & Tossell (1991: 95) suggest that people can experience multiple marginalization and disadvantage through being elderly, disabled, and from an ethnic minority group. We can see, therefore, that mobility is reliant upon many factors; however, it is essential that the musculoskeletal system is functional.

THE MUSCULOSKELETAL SYSTEM

Movements of the body require the coordination of bones, muscles, tendons, ligaments, joints and nerves. Affection or impairment of any one of these will interfere or prevent normal mobility. Immobility over a long period of time can lead to specific and general complications of the body.

The skeleton has many functions (Table 17.1) and the skeletal system comprises two types of connective tissue, bone and cartilage. It is made up of 206 bones and microscopically consists of two types of bone: compact and cancellous (Hinchliff et al 1996, Tortora & Grabowski 1996).

Microscopic structure of bone

Compact bone

Compact bone (Fig. 17.1) is also referred to as Haversian bone in which nerves and blood vessels enter through the structure of Volkmann's canals, leading to the central canals within the compact structure, called Haversian canals. These canals are surrounded by concentric rings of lamellae, a hard calcified substance. Between these lamellae are small spaces known as lacunae, which contain osteocytes, the mature bone cells. Leading from the lacunae, in all directions, are tiny canals called canaliculi. Together these components are known as an osteon and they serve to ensure that each part of the bone receives nutrients and that waste products are disposed of.

Reflection and portfolio evidence

Examine the gross structure of the bony matrix of cancellous bone and note the regular pattern that is formed.

- Why do you think it is arranged in this way?
- How do you think this knowledge might help with your decision making in nursing practice?

Cancellous bone

Cancellous bone or non-osteon bone is sponge-like in appearance due to its internal meshwork structure of trabeculae (Fig. 17.1). Between the spaces of this arrangement lies red bone marrow in which blood cells are produced. Two types of cells lie on opposite surfaces of the trabeculae:

- osteoblasts, which are responsible for laying down new bone
- osteoclasts, which incorporate a phagocytic action to absorb bone.

This particular arrangement is designed rather like the external scaffolding of a new building.

The skeletal system consists of five types of bone:

- long bones
- short bones
- irregular bones
- flat bones
- sesamoid bones.

Table 17.1 Functions of the skeleton (from Tortora & Grabowski 1996 by kind permission of John Wiley & Sons)

Support	Provides a framework for soft tissue and attachment of muscles
Protection	Internal organs are protected from external injury by the bony structure (e.g. the heart and lungs are protected by the ribcage or thorax)
Assist in movement	Movement is produced by muscle contraction thus causing the bones to move
Minerals homeostasis	Minerals such as calcium and phosphorus are stored in bone, which acts as a reservoir, ready for mineral distribution when required
Site of blood cell production	Red marrow in cancellous bone produces blood cells in the process production known as haemopoiesis – mainly red blood cells, but some white cells and platelets are also produced
Storage of energy	Yellow bone marrow (fatty substance/lipid) is found in long bones. The lipids act as energy reserve

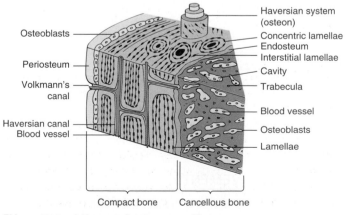

Figure 17.1 Microscopic structure of bone.

Decision making exercise

1. Consult your biology textbook and identify the location of the five types of bone.
   - Why do you think they are arranged into such shapes and structures?
   - When these different bones are fractured, why do they heal at different rates and why is it important for the nurse to know this?
   - What effect does age have on the healing rates of bone?
2. A child sustains a fracture of the distal (lower) part of the humerus following a fall while playing:
   - What knowledge do you as a nurse need to know about the structure, function and movement of this bone and surrounding bones and joints?
   - What advice would you give to the parents in relation to their child's joint movement and bone healing?

Joints

A joint is defined as the junction where two or more bones meet. The articular surfaces at the end of bones allow smooth movement. Other functions of joints include providing stability during movement as well as maintaining body posture.

There are many different types of joints in the body and not all are movable or concerned with movement. In order to concentrate upon our main concern of mobility, only synovial joints will be considered. (For a full description of bones and joints see McLaren 1996: 302–304.)

Synovial joints

These joints are fundamental to full mobility and are termed 'freely movable' or 'diarthroses'. They are enclosed within a fibrous capsule of connective tissue. Articular or hyaline cartilage lines the ends of the bones. The stability of these joints is enhanced by the presence of ligaments, which are attached between one bone and the other. Joint stability is also aided by the adjacent muscles, which are attached via tendons to bones. The nerve supply to joints comes from the surrounding muscles.

The joint capsule is lined with synovial membrane containing microscopic villi, which secrete synovial fluid to lubricate and nourish the articular surfaces. All synovial joints have a similar structure to one another, but they vary in terms of their shape and range of movement.

RANGE OF MOVEMENTS

To be effective in care and protect our patients we need to know the extent of movement and the limitations that exist.

Therefore it is important to know the normal range of movements (Fig. 17.2) as given below:

- flexion
- extension
- circumduction
- eversion
- pronation and supination
- abduction and adduction
- dorsiflexion and plantar flexion
- rotation
- protraction and retraction
- opposition.

Movement at synovial joints is limited by the shape of the articulating bones and the structure of extracapsular (and sometimes intracapsular) ligaments. Other limiting factors are the strength and tension of adjacent muscles. There are basically six types of synovial joints:

- ball and socket joint
- hinge joint
- pivot joint
- gliding joint
- saddle joint
- ellipsoid joint.

It is important that nurses learn about synovial joints so that they can identify normal movement and the range that exists.

Reflection and portfolio evidence

Gain access to a skeleton within your school or department and attempt the movements identified above on the skeleton. Attempt some of the common movements yourself.

- Make a note of the range that you may go through in a gym or exercise class when doing a 'warm up' or 'cool down' stretch.

Sit on a chair and then flex and extend your knee; the movement created is that of a hinge. Now stand with your foot firmly fixed to the floor, try (within your limitations) to rotate at the knee joint. Notice how there is some rotational movement, but bear in mind that the ankle joint is also rotating.

Further information can be found in McLaren (1996: 309–319).

It is important to note that classification of joints is not always comprehensive. For example the knee joint is referred to as a hinge joint, but this classification is not always a full and accurate description as the knee joint also responds to rotational forces. This led to the problem of loosening with the older varieties of artificial knee joints that were inserted in the past. They were designed to act

Circumduction:
A combination of movements that makes the body part describe a circle.

Rotation:
The pivoting of the body part around its axis, as in shaking the head. No rotation of any body part is complete (i.e. 360 degrees).

Protraction:
The protrusion of some body part, e.g. the lower jaw.

Retraction:
The opposite of protraction.

Abduction:
A movement of a bone or limb away from the median plane of the body. Abduction in the hands and feet is the movement of a digit away from the central axis of the limb. One abducts the fingers by spreading them apart.

Adduction:
The opposite of abduction, involving approach to the median plane of the body or, in the case of the limbs, to the central axis of a limb.

Inversion:
An ankle movement that turns the sole of the foot medially. Applies only to the foot.

Eversion:
The opposite of inversion. It turns the sole of the foot laterally.

Supination:
The opposite of pronation. When the forearm is in the extended position, this movement brings the palm of the hand upward.

Pronation:
A movement of the forearm that in the extended position brings the palm of the hand to a downward position. Applies only to the forearm.

Extension:
The opposite of flexion, it increases the angle between two movably articulated bones, usually to a 180degree maximum. If the angle of extension exceeds 180 degrees (as is possible when throwing back the head), this action is termed hyperextension.

Flexion:
The bending of a joint; usually a movement that reduces the angle that two movably activated bones make with each other. When one crouches, the knees are flexed.

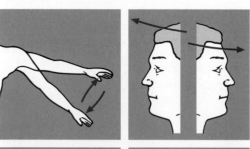
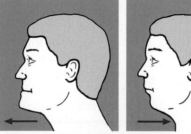
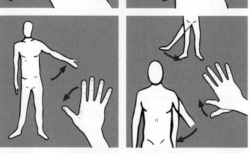
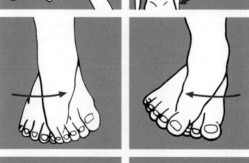
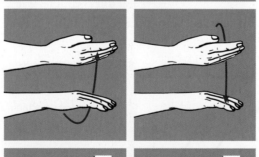
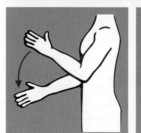
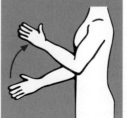

Figure 17.2   Types of movement of synovial joints. (From Hinchliff et al 1996.)

only in a hinge movement and did not take into account the rotational forces exerted on the knee.

Muscles

Skeletal muscles are responsible for voluntary movements and they are so called because of their attachment to bones. They are striated (striped) in appearance and have specialized cells that allow contraction. For stability to be maintained and movement to occur, muscles need to work effectively. Muscle contractions not only allow movement, but also maintain body posture. Another function of skeletal muscle is to produce heat thus contributing to the body temperature.

Active skeletal muscles require a great deal of energy. The nutritional aspects, especially sugar and carbohydrate intakes, are therefore of paramount importance. The full potential of mobility improvement or maintenance cannot be reached if there are nutritional deficits.

To aid movement, skeletal muscles are arranged around an origin and an insertion (Fig. 17.3). The origin is usually the least movable end of the muscle and the insertion the most movable. The ends of muscles terminate in a cord of connective tissue, a tendon. This is inserted into the periosteum (covering) of the underlying bone. As a general rule, the nearest (or proximal) tendon is the origin and the one furthest away (distal) is the insertion.

Sheets of fibrous connective tissue known as fascia surround skeletal muscles. Free movement is facilitated by the deep fascia, which carries blood vessels and nerves. The deep fascia also fills the spaces between muscle layers and sometimes provides the origins of muscles (Tortora & Grabowski 1996: 239).

Blood and nerve supply of muscles

There is a rich blood and nerve supply to the skeletal muscles. Each muscle is supplied by at least one nerve that contains motor and sensory fibres. Information is relayed from the cerebral cortex of the brain via the pyramidal tracts to the anterior horn of the spinal cord (the upper motor neurone) and impulses then travel from the anterior horn of the spinal cord to the muscle fibres (lower motor neurone).

Neuromuscular junction is the point where muscles and nerve meet. The end of the lower motor neurone is flattened and referred to as the motor end-plate. Acetylcholine is a chemical transmitter which is released when a nerve impulse reaches the motor end-plate. Impulses are allowed to move across the gap between the muscle and nerve thus producing body movement. This is due to acetylcholine becoming attached to the muscle receptors. Vesicles are found near the end-plate receptors and these release cholinesterase which in turn ceases the the action of acetylcholine.

There are sensory nerve fibres in these muscles and tendons and some are referred to as proprioceptors. These detect information about body movement and position and relay this information to the central nervous system. Some sensory nerve fibres respond to the stimuli of inflammation, ischaemia (lack of blood supply), compression and necrosis (death of tissue).

A great deal of energy is required during muscle stimulation and a good blood supply is needed to provide oxygen and nutrients and to remove waste products. A vast network of blood capillaries is therefore distributed within the muscle fibres for this purpose.

You may have noticed how marathon runners are given regular supplies of glucose drinks; this is not only to prevent dehydration, but also to combat the effects of muscle fatigue. This is a condition in which there is diminished availability of oxygen and it results from the toxic effects of waste products such as carbon dioxide and lactic acid.

Nurses should be able to understand the anatomical components involved and the physiological processes that occur when a patient's mobility is affected by paralysis, stiffness or fatigue or any other condition. Effective decisions and nursing interventions will depend on a good level of knowledge and understanding of the changes taking place.

Reflection and portfolio evidence

Exercise your fingers or grip something tightly with your dominant hand until you feel fatigued. At this point attempt to write neatly.

- When you are able, note down your observations.

Body levers

In order for movement to take place a system of levers is used incorporating the structures of muscles, bones and joints. Muscles cross at least one joint between the origin and insertion and movement is produced through a system of levers.

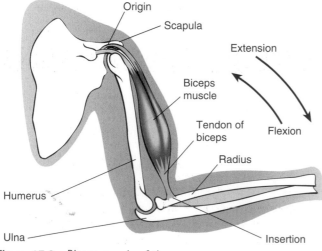

Figure 17.3   Biceps muscle of the arm.

These levers are the means of transmitting energy through muscular contraction to move different parts of the body. All levers have a fulcrum, an effort arm and a resistance arm, and are classified according to the differing arrangement of these. What is also important in the application of nursing is that by shortening the resistance arm, less effort is required to lift a large weight (i.e. bringing the patient closer to your body reduces the muscular effort required by you to move him or her). (For a full description and explanation of the different body levers, see McLaren (1996: 302–304) and see also Ch. 5 on handling and moving.)

Exercise and its effects

To maintain or improve our health, we all need to exercise. It has been stated (Herbert & Alison 1996) that physical performance and fitness are determined by:

- an individual's capacity for energy output
- neuromuscular function
- joint mobility
- psychological factors (e.g. motivation).

The capacity and extent of physical fitness is determined mainly by the above. The integrity of the involved systems such as the respiratory and cardiovascular systems is vital, therefore, to the overall result. Oxygen and nutrients are needed during exercise to maintain muscular activity. There is also a need to increase the removal rate of carbon dioxide, heat, water and metabolic waste products. It follows, then, that increased cardiac output is required via the coordination of the autonomic nervous system.

Vasodilation and increased blood flow occur during exercise and peripheral resistance in muscles falls as a result. To maintain total peripheral resistance at adequate levels there is therefore a compensatory vasoconstriction, especially in the gastrointestinal tract and kidneys. Venous return to the heart increases, which results in an increased stroke volume. This in turn leads to an increased systolic blood pressure. Excess heat generated through muscular activity during exercise is removed via the blood and causes sweating and flushing of the skin to facilitate heat loss through convection and evaporation (Herbert & Alison 1996).

Some of the benefits obtained through regular exercise are:

- an increased metabolic rate and prevention of obesity
- improved muscular and ligament strength
- prevention of disuse osteoporosis
- improved cardiovascular function
- maintenance of normal blood glucose levels
- reduction of stress and anxiety
- increased feeling of well-being.

For a full discussion of the physiological effects and benefits of exercise on the body, see Hinchliff et al (1996: Sections 3 and 4).

Evidence based practice

Exercise is clearly beneficial; however, how much exercise an individual takes depends upon many factors. The *National Time Use Survey* (Office of Population Censuses and Surveys 2000) identified that:

- men are more likely to do sport than women
- sporting activity decreases with age
- the higher the household income the more likely people are to participate in sport.

THE PHYSICAL EFFECTS OF IMMOBILITY

Immobility occurs when specific structures involved in facilitating movements are affected, for example:

- bony injury or disease
- joint problems
- muscle conditions
- disorders of the nervous system.

Restricted mobility or immobility can also result from other illness such as cardiac or respiratory conditions.

As nurses we must consider that immobility, whether partial or full, temporary or permanent, will in turn affect other body systems which may lead to complications.

Evidence based practice

The trend towards reduced activity in childhood was identified in research by the director of the Coronary Prevention in Children Project. A worrying low level of physical activity among British schoolchildren was revealed and suggests that there may be long-term effects such as high blood pressure, elevated blood cholesterol levels and coronary heart disease (Armstrong 1993). Further supportive evidence has led the Scottish government to develop a Physical Activity Task Force which has published a strategy to make Scotland more active (Scottish Executive 2003).

Decision making exercise

Reflect on your practice placements and using the above broad classifications:

- Review the reasons why some of your clients had difficulty with mobility.
- Decide whether the degree of immobility was temporary or permanent.
- From knowledge of the anatomy and physiology of movement, review the rationale for the patterns of care and treatment you have seen to improve mobility or overcome the effects of immobility.

Cardiovascular changes

There can be a shift in fluid and electrolyte balance with a resulting loss of potassium and sodium. Also, confinement to bed for periods longer than a week results in a breakdown of fibrin and a shortened blood clotting time. This increases the risk of thrombosis, especially in the lower limbs. The immobile person can also be more susceptible to infections, which may possibly be due to muscular inactivity interfering with transportation of lymph.

Respiratory changes

If, through immobility, recumbency (lying down) is increased, then the pressure of the abdominal contents pushing on the diaphragm can reduce lung volume. Stress is placed upon the muscles of inspiration, leading to inefficient respiratory muscular action. A decrease in the efficiency of the muscles of respiration can lead to an inability to cough effectively. This can result in an accumulation of mucus, creating the perfect medium for the growth and multiplication of bacteria.

Metabolic and hormonal changes

There is some disruption in the cyclic rhythm when immobilization and bed rest last over approximately 4 weeks. This leads to changes in the peak times for insulin (i.e. peaking of serum insulin in the evening despite food taken at meal times). The activity of the pancreas and the ability to take sugar is also reduced. Adrenaline peaks in the afternoon instead of early morning before awakening.

Aldosterone normally peaks at midday, but following long periods of bed rest, it ceases to peak at this time and instead the morning levels remain the same or slightly elevated.

Because the energy required through inactivity is decreased, the basal metabolic rate decreases unless an infection is present. One result of a reduced basal metabolic rate is an increase in the amount of body fat, which also results from the loss in body mass through protein breakdown.

There is an increased excretion of calcium via the kidneys after approximately 4 days' immobilization due to bone reabsorption giving rise to osteoporosis. This can result in increased blood levels of calcium (hypercalcaemia) because the kidneys are unable to cope with such large amounts.

Long periods of immobility can also result in increased nitrogen excretion because nitrogen breakdown exceeds nitrogen intake.

Gastrointestinal changes

There is a decrease in gastrointestinal activity following a 3-day period of bed rest when the stomach tends to secrete less gastric juice. A decreased intake of food due to inactivity and lowered basal metabolic rate can result in constipation. Diarrhoea can also result from faecal overflow due to the impaction of faeces. This, in turn, can lead to further electrolyte imbalance and dehydration.

Muscular changes

Muscular mass and strength can be affected by inactivity. This can be identified through girth measurements of the limbs. Tolerance to exercise is decreased leading to fatigue. There is therefore greater likelihood of falling, injury and further immobility.

Skeletal changes

Calcium metabolism is affected by impaired mobility. Bone reabsorption occurs, with a resulting decrease in bone density and disuse osteoporosis. When joints remain immobilized or if there is limited mobility for long periods of time contractures and stiffening of those joints can ensue. One common and severely debilitating contracture is seen in the ankle and referred to as a foot drop. The abnormalities of muscles, tendons and ligaments around an inactive joint can lead to structural joint abnormality, stiffness and pain.

Other changes

Other effects of immobilization can also be devastating. These include effects on the skin and the urinary system as well as effects upon sleep patterns. A final consideration relates to mental and developmental well-being as considered within the next section.

PSYCHOSOCIAL

THE PSYCHOLOGICAL AND SOCIAL ASPECTS OF MOBILITY

It is important to consider mobility from different perspectives and not simply the physical aspects. The factors which affect the way the subject of mobility is valued thought and felt about must be examined.

Childhood and adolescence

From the moment babies are born they are assessed against the criteria of normality. Various observations and recordings are undertaken, and comparisons made on the basis of present day knowledge and ideals. Tests to assess motor skills may have an inherent bias toward Westernized medicine. Children from other cultural backgrounds may be regarded as abnormal if similar criteria were applied. This is not to say that they have delayed motor development or abnormal development, but simply that they are being judged using irrelevant or inappropriate criteria. However, if mobility is not restricted or discouraged, infants will gain voluntary control of their movements at approximately 4 months of age, although accurate and deliberate fine movements can take up to 3 years to develop.

Humans differ from other species in the fact that they have the ability to walk in an upright position as well as having the capability to grip. By the age of 3 or 4 years, most children can balance on one foot for a second or so and can hop, run and jump. By the time they reach the age of 5 years they are able to use advanced motor skills that enable them with practice, to dance, dress themselves and use the fine motor movements that will improve with age to equip them for adulthood.

Adolescence brings the same body changes for the disabled as for anyone else. It brings the same sexual urges, yet young people who are disabled may feel frustrated and inadequate because they are mentally alert, but physically trapped. If the physical, psychological and social environment is deficient these milestones may be delayed or not achieved and lead to immobility. But even in health, the ageing process of later life can result in a decreased range of joint movements. Muscular strength and mass may be reduced and coordination diminished. This can lead to an unstable balance and an increased risk of falling (Masterson 1995).

Evidence based practice

Each year there are about 2.7 million accidents in the home which necessitate a visit to hospital. Of these accidents almost 4000 are fatal. By far the biggest cause of these accidents are falls, which account for 40% of the non-fatal injuries and 46% of all deaths. Most deaths from falls involve the older age groups with nearly 80% of the victims aged over 65 and only 5% under the age of 40 (Department of Trade and Industry 2002, Dowswell et al 1999).

Mobility in public places

Mobility is an important part of everyone's life. We live in a society of able-bodied people and conduct our daily activities surrounded by people who are fully mobile. As nurses we need to appreciate what effects immobility has on individuals in mainstream society and to consider what can be done to make society more inclusive for all people whatever their background.

At the outset of this chapter it was stated that we live in a world built around assumption of full mobility – a world in which immobility or impaired mobility is seen as abnormal and undesirable. This is particularly true in developed countries. Mobility problems can affect anyone from any social class or background or age group. The elderly (aged 65 years and over) tend to experience significantly more mobility problems than younger people (Office of Population Censuses and Surveys 1995: 82). The changes that take place in the musculoskeletal system tend to cause elderly people to

walk at a slower pace, take short steps and become unsteady. This leads to elderly people with mobility problems being labelled as disabled, hence stigmatized and stereotyped. Children are also expected to achieve certain goals as part of normal development in relation to mobility. From birth to adulthood these goals are stressed not only by health professionals, but also by the community. We need only to look at our own community to see what an alien environment it is for the disabled and the immobile. Public perception or image of immobility as a disability creates social, psychological and physical barriers. Steps, narrow doorways and cramped workplaces, for example, create boundaries for the immobile person. They limit access, further restrict movement in public places and reduce employment opportunities. As a result of the Disability Discrimination Act 1995 there has been a number of changes in some public places and amenities. Employers have begun to recognize their legal responsibilities by initiating structural change and providing equal opportunities for employment. Business organizations in UK can no longer afford to ignore the spending power, with regard to domestic consumption, of the 8.7 million disabled people. However, one may argue there is still a long way to go to integrate those with disability within the mainstream society.

Schools

Schools were designed with the expectation that the child was fully mobile. The disabled child was therefore expected to attend a special school. Progress has been made in some educational establishments to ensure the provision of access and facilities for children with disability. The introduction of the Special Education Needs and Disability Act 2001 makes it illegal for educational establishments, in particular higher and further education, to discriminate against students with disability. There are arguments that attempts to integrate those affected within the normal schools are failing because of inadequate or lack of resources. Where segregation occurs, the notion of normality is brought about through experience and socialization. In today's society where people have the choice to have therapeutic abortions, there is suggestion that the incidence of physical and mental abnormalities will eventually decline.

In the past, and to an extent today, institutions for the immobile were designed to house disabled people for most of their lives. This served to increase the marginalization and, as French (1994) states, 'By the 1950s and 1960s disabled people, whether they were in institutions or not, were so separated from the community that they were practically invisible.'

Bureaucracy and mobility

Bureaucrats and professionals, historically, have been the voice of the disabled in the way they make decisions. In the past researchers in the field and studies of disability have no personal experience of being disabled. There has also been a tendency for health professionals to make decisions on the assumption that they know what is best for their clients or patients. This top-down approach excludes clients from taking an active role in the decision making process, thus making them unable to make meaningful contribution in the management and control of their own lives.

Most health professionals require full mobility to be able to train and most have little practical experience of the physical and emotional effects of disability on the disabled person. We all have thoughts, ideas and personal views about those who are physically disabled. Our perception of a person can be influenced by social stereotypes, ethnocentrism and prejudice. A person with mobility impairment is usually identified as having a disability and as such is expected to behave in a particular way or to have socially inferior attributes. The meaning of disability is socially constructed. Hence it is important for nurses to examine critically their personal attitudes, beliefs and understanding regarding disability. Theories of attitudes, attribution and perceptions can provide nurses with a good basis for developing an understanding and insight of their clients' psychosocial needs.

It is difficult or inescapable to avoid associating mobility problems or disability with old people. The population of people aged 60 years old plus is 21% of the population in the UK, more than the population of children (Office of Population Census and Surveys 2001). Since industrialization there has been the notion that this group of people on reaching a certain chronological age (presently 65 years) become unproductive and dependent on welfare services. Contrary to popular belief the majority, however, do not require hospitalization or residential care and in fact 93% live in private households (Jones 1994). Family and informal carers are caring for them. Nevertheless a significant proportion of people over the age of 75 years require some assistance to aid their mobility.

There is the belief among health professionals that elderly people who suffer from chronic illnesses and have reduced activities or less active lives are unsuitable for therapy. This can be based on the false belief that the elderly are inflexible, rigid and unable or unwilling to change. Recent research has shown otherwise. Stereotyping of elderly or people with disability tends to strengthen and perpetuate negative attitudes towards their treatment and management. Policy such as the National Service Framework for Care of the Elderly will undoubtedly help professionals in making decisions based on clinical judgement and not on ageism.

Stigmatization

What we term 'mobilism' is based on the now widely quoted reference of Comfort (1977) in which ageism is identified as 'The notion that people cease to be people, cease to be the same people or become people of a distinct and inferior kind, by virtue of having lived a specific number of years.' So mobilism can be seen as 'The notion whereby people are seen as different and inferior simply through having a permanent or temporary, partial or complete, loss of physical mobility.'

Stigmatization can therefore occur because of people's fears, ignorance or embarrassment. It is based upon a simplistic stereotypical view that involves perceived negative attributes about other people. This results in the labelling of such people (Taylor & Field 1993). These labels are not a true reflection of reality, for example those with mobility problems can also be perceived as having mental problems or learning difficulties.

Reflection and portfolio evidence

Next time you have an opportunity to observe a carer assisting a disabled person or pushing a disabled person in a wheelchair in a public setting:

- Notice their interactions with others.
- Do others concentrate upon the carer or the disabled?
- Notice if there is any lack of interaction.
- Notice if there is any inappropriate interaction such as staring.
- Recall, honestly, how you feel and react when you meet a disabled person, particularly of your own age, in a social setting.
- How could knowledge gained from this chapter affect your attitude and feelings in future?

The effects of inappropriate interactions on the disabled can be devastating and the mass media plays its part in enhancing this negative image. It can lead to a loss of self-esteem and result in withdrawal from social life (Fig. 17.4) (Taylor & Field 1993).

Social exclusion results from inability to carry on normal social life such as visiting relatives, friends, interacting with other people, accessing services and other social or domestic activities. Anxiety, fear and depression may lead to loneliness.

Society in many respects assists in withdrawal by encouraging the permanently immobile to seek refuge in specific centres and homes. The point here is not to denigrate the valuable work done in such places, but to increase awareness of the consequences of such actions and policies.

Most of us have little appreciation of what is involved in any disability – the frustration of a lifetime of hardship and inequalities that many disabled people have to face, of having to depend upon others for what may be seen by the able-bodied as a natural right or ability. Immobility and ill health in general can have major consequences and effects on patients. By examining the psychological and sociological aspects of mobility or immobility we can gain a much greater insight into the associated problems.

There has been a gradual shift in nursing care philosophy and approach, from emphasis on providers to client-centred care and family centred in child. This has been supported

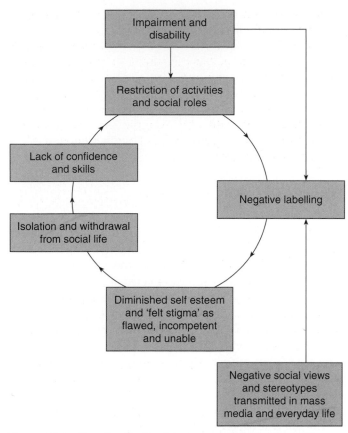

Figure **17.4** Negative feedback between stigmatization, self-esteem and participation in social activities. (From Taylor & Field 1993.)

Range of movement
Gait
Tolerance to exercise and activity
Body alignment
Balance

Figure **17.5** Elements within an assessment of mobility. (After Masterson 1995.)

daily activities of living or who may be more likely to sustain falls (Abbruzzese 1998). In 2002 the Department of Health introduced the Single Assessment Process in the National Service Framework for Older People (Department of Health 2001) to ensure effective assessment of needs and management of care.

Risk assessment and using tools and scales have become increasingly important in helping nurses to manage individual care more effectively. For example pain may affect the level of mobility and immobility which in turn can lead to skin breakdown, such as pressure sores. In these instances tools such as pain scales and risk calculators for pressure areas would be useful in the overall assessment (see Ch. 10 on pain and Ch. 14 on skin integrity, for full descriptions).

Decision making exercise

Make a list of those professionals and non-professionals who may directly or indirectly make a positive contribution towards the care of the immobile. From this list identify:

- Their different priorities in caring for an adult.
- Their different priorities in caring for a child.

How could the nurse contribute to the decision making process of this team?

by the introduction of the Partnership Act 1999, involvement of users and carers and move to empower clients/patients to be actively involved in the management of their health and care.

CARE DELIVERY KNOWLEDGE

MULTIDISCIPLINARY ASSESSMENT OF MOBILITY

The care surrounding immobile patients in hospital and community environment involves more than nursing care. Managing patients or clients with mobility problems requires a coordinated multidisciplinary approach to assessment, including the use of single documentation for all. Nurses play an important part in this coordinated approach because of their close regular contact with the patients. There are various tools available to assess levels of mobility, the most common element being a focus on the client being able to achieve the activities of daily living (ADL). One example is the Barthel ADL scale (Mahoney & Barthel 1965) measuring level of dependency on a 0 to 20 point scale. The Tinetti Performance Orientated Mobility Assessment Tool is another method used in assessing elderly who find it difficult to manage their

A number of elements of mobility must be incorporated within the assessment process (Fig. 17.5).

Batehup & Squires (1991) suggested that an assessment should include gait, initiation of mobility, turning and stopping. In hospital we are inclined to make such assessments on non-slip, non-carpeted floors. When considering discharge it is useful and beneficial to make such an assessment under conditions similar to those at home or better still in the patient's own home. To provide an overall picture specific mobility assessment should also be made in various positions (i.e. sitting down, standing and in recumbency) if possible. One must remember, however, that other factors such as personal differences, person's beliefs or perception and motivation for mobilizing may affect assessment. Similarly when assessing children and individuals with learning disabilities or mental illness we need to consider different developmental stages since they operate at different levels of understanding.

MANAGEMENT OF MOBILITY CARE

Mobility difficulties can result from a number of conditions, such as osteoarthritis, cerebral palsy, Parkinson disease, cerebral vascular accident, spinal injury and many more. In order to plan the care and rehabilitation effectively, we need to have not only a good level of knowledge and understanding of the aetiology but also being able to identify the following specific musculoskeletal problem(s) when carrying out nursing diagnosis:

● joint pain
● impaired physical mobility
● activity intolerance
● 'limited strength' or 'limited muscle power'
● paralysis.

Individuals cope with their mobility problems or disability in different ways, depending whether the onset is sudden such as an injury or insidious, for example a chronic condition. The former is more likely to cause denial or anger whereas a person who has been gradually experiencing mobility difficulty may have come to terms with some functional incapacity. Coping mechanism and readjustment will depend on acceptance by the individual of his or her physical limitation. It is crucial not to take a victim-blaming approach but

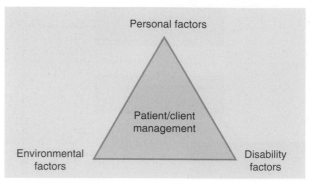

Figure 17.6   The mobility triad.

to look at the primary cause of the immobility. Planning care will involve the multidisciplinary team including the client/patient and the family or significant others as far as possible. Information and observations collected and recorded during assessment will be examined to identify general and specific problems or needs of the individual client. Depending on the nature, degree and cause of immobility and in consultation and negotiation with the client (if possible) short-term or long-term goals are set. These must be realistic and achievable to enable the client to carry on with his/her activities of daily living as independently as possible in order to provide an acceptable quality of life.

The main purpose of any management strategy is to enable the individual to function independently as far as possible either in hospital or in the community. This requires a coordinated and holistic approach in the planning, implementation and evaluation of the care programme, taking into consideration a number relevant factors. These factors are classified under three main areas – *personal, environmental* and *disability* – which we would refer to as the 'mobility triad' (Fig. 17.6). The factors are listed in Table 17.2.

For the client/patient to benefit from any informed choices, therapy, care and rehabilitation nurses must also ensure that the individual's psychological, emotional, social and cultural needs are met. In this section only the specific factors relating to functional capacity will be addressed. These include:

● range of movement
● gait and body alignment
● balance
● exercise and activity.

Range of movement

Muscles with full strength will have little benefit to patients if their joints are stiff from lack of movement. In certain instances such as joint replacement or ligament repair, flexion or extension may have to be limited for a time, but on the whole if a joint is allowed to be moved then this should be encouraged. Active joint movements not only increase and maintain the range, but also help maintain muscle strength and joint stability. These elements are essential for mobility.

Table 17.2

Personal factors	Environmental factors	Disability factors
Age and gender	Hospital and primary care settings	Causes – primary or secondary
Social and cultural background	Services in community	Nature of immobility – sudden or insidious onset
Personal values, attitudes and beliefs	Social security and welfare	Degree of immobility – partial or full
Denial or acceptance of mobility problem	Family and support networks	Types of immobility – temporary or permanent
Ability to cope, self-efficacy and personal coping mechanism	Self-help groups	Functional capacity – range of movement, gait/body alignment, balance and
Willingness to participate in care management and motivation	Users' and carers' associations	exercise/activity tolerance
Health status and level of dependency	Statutory and voluntary groups	
Personal care deficits	Policies – local, national and international	
Anger, fear and anxiety	Public and work places, leisure facilities – amenities and access	
Level of knowledge and understanding of condition	Equipment, aids and assistive technology	
Confidence, self-esteem, helplessness or despair	Health professionals and significant others	
	Transport facilities – personal and public	
	Accommodation and housing	
	Public attitudes	

If a joint is not moved then a fixed flexion deformity can occur. This is abnormal shortening of muscle tissue that becomes resistant to stretching and can lead to permanent disability due to fibrosis of the muscle or joint. The aim in mobility therefore is to prevent such an occurrence, as this will severely hamper the rehabilitation process. It takes only a few seconds to remind patients to move their knees, ankles or hips, whether they are confined to bed or not. Remember, though, that a part of the patient's limb may need support to achieve a full range of movements comfortably.

Gait and body alignment

Gait is the style and manner of walking and an observation of the patient's gait can be made at any time while he or she is walking. Normal walking consists of two basic movements:

- the stance, in which one leg bears most of the body weight at one point in the movement
- the swing, in which the foot does not touch the ground and the weight is taken on the opposite side.

There can be many styles of walking, most of which present no problem. Problems, however, can occur when the style of gait and alignment gives rise to or arises from instability. When an unstable gait or alignment has been diagnosed, it should be corrected. Occasionally it may not be possible to correct an unstable gait, for example for a client with spina bifida or cerebral palsy. Care should focus on preventing further damage and maintaining maximum function for as long as possible.

The age of a person is important; for example, a normal child's gait is not the same as that of an adult. However, abnormal gaits can be similar in both the child and the adult.

Although there are many different types of gait, body alignment and balance, the cause of instability can be multifactorial. The programme of implementation may involve, for example, the reduction of a patient's pain through the administration of analgesia or the application of local heat or cold substances. Programmes may also need to take poor eyesight into account. This is especially relevant in the elderly as some deterioration of eyesight is a natural part of growing old. In fact longsightedness (presbyopia) may begin to develop around the age of 40, so it is important therefore to initiate checks on a patient's eyesight if there is any doubt. Rooms that may seem adequately lit to a person with normal eyesight may be inadequate for those with some visual impairment.

Balance

Balance, or the state in which the body is in equilibrium, is an important factor in mobility (Galley & Forster 1987). Balance is a very complex area and depends upon the integrity of:

- the central nervous system
- the musculoskeletal system.

It relies upon the adequate functioning of:

- vision
- the vestibule (the cavity in the middle of the bony labyrinth or inner ear)
- proprioceptive efficiency
- tactile input, especially to the feet and hands
- integration of all stimuli by the central nervous system
- visuospatial perception
- effective muscle tone
- muscle strength
- joint flexibility.

Any damage to one or all of the above factors needs be taken into account before, during and after mobilization. The ear, for example, is the organ of balance, so any deterioration in function can lead to an increased number of falls (Windmill 1990). In such circumstances hearing tests and appropriate aids can improve and maintain a person's balance, thus preventing further falls and immobility.

Thapa et al (1994) assessed the balance of 303 community nursing home residents as a means of identifying the risk factors involved in falling. Although predictions were accurate, the researchers suggested that further studies should be undertaken because of the difficulties in measuring the balance of all the elderly frail clients in the study.

Mobility aids (assistive technology)

Ogden (1992) has identified five points for consideration when using walking aids. These are:

- Is there space available for the aid?
- Does the person have the ability to use the aid appropriately?
- Is the aid to be used indoors, outdoors or both?
- Is public or private transport required to accommodate the aid?
- Do stairs or steps need to be negotiated?

Most mobility aids such as walking frames, sticks or crutches (Fig. 17.7) are initially ordered by the physiotherapist and mobility commenced with their assistance. This is especially so for hospitalized patients, but nurses in the community are frequently the care workers who evaluate progress following a patient's discharge. There are community physiotherapists and occupational therapists, but because of resourcing difficulties they are often unable to evaluate all patients discharged with a mobility aid. Nurses may then undertake a formal or informal assessment of mobility. Although nurses may not have the relevant expertise to make the necessary adjustments or changes to equipment, a referral can be made to the appropriate person or department.

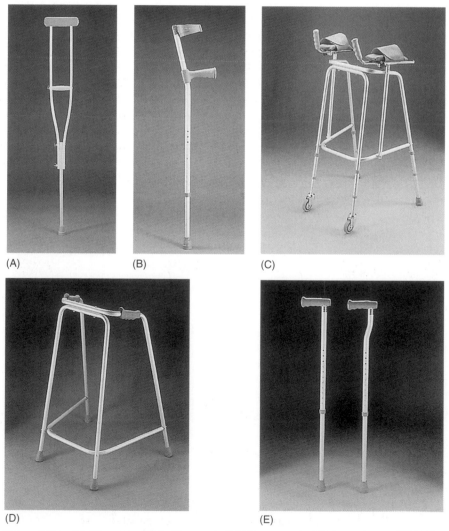

(A)   (B)   (C)

(D)   (E)

Figure 17.7   Walking aids. (A) Axilla crutch. (B) Elbow crutch. (C) Gutter frame. (D) Waist high frame. (E) Sticks. (Courtesy of Coopers Healthcare plc.)

Walking aids need to be in good working order. For example walking aids have a ferrule or ferrules at their base, which are usually made of rubber and add to the stability of the equipment by providing a larger point of contact with the ground or floor. Ferrules also help prevent slipping on shiny or wet surfaces. If mobility aids are required for long periods, these ferrules need to be regularly checked for wear.

If aids incorporate screws or bolts, these may have to be tightened for safe operation. If patients are able they or their carers can be taught how to make regular safety checks and how to make any necessary adjustments to their equipment. While evaluating the patient's overall mobility problem, the nurse may also need to evaluate the patient's dexterity and their effectiveness in checking all aspects of appliance safety.

If nurses prescribe, administer and initiate walking with mobility aids then they should ensure that the correct size has been ascertained, and be aware of their responsibilities under the Consumer Protection Act 1987. Crutches, for example, cannot be given to patients without proper advice on their use and maintenance. In the absence of physiotherapists, if nurses continue to mobilize patients with mobility aids they need not only a working knowledge of the equipment, but also an understanding of some of the basic principles involved to provide accurate and effective care. Judd (1989: 166) has identified two such principles as:

- the wider the base and weightbearing area of the aid, the greater the stability
- the higher the patient takes their weight, the more stable they will be.

It is seen, therefore, that patients using gutter frames are more stable than those using the more common waist high frames, and those using axillary crutches are more stable than those using elbow crutches. To enable appropriate assessment, evaluation and documentation there is also a need to be aware of the different gait patterns associated with such mobility aids (Fig. 17.8). The different points of the frame, footsteps and crutches shown in Figure 17.8 refer to the number of weightbearing areas that touch the ground or floor. It is important that in the absence of the physiotherapist the nurse can recognize when the equipment is used correctly and incorrectly. Axillary crutches, for example, are not designed so that the patient's weight is taken through the axilla. The crutches serve to stabilize the body by giving added support

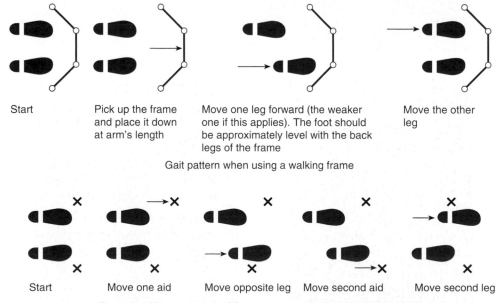

| Start | Pick up the frame and place it down at arm's length | Move one leg forward (the weaker one if this applies). The foot should be approximately level with the back legs of the frame | Move the other leg |

Gait pattern when using a walking frame

| Start | Move one aid | Move opposite leg | Move second aid | Move second leg |

Example of four-point gait. ✗ represents an axillary or elbow crutch in the early stages of recovery, or a stick in the later stages

Figure 17.8 Gait patterns with a walking frame and with crutches. (From Judd 1989, with permission.)

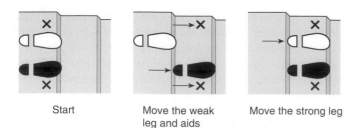

Start   Move the weak   Move the strong leg
         leg and aids

Descending stairs using crutches. The black area represents either the weak or non-weightbearing leg

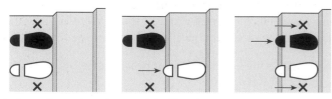

Ascending stairs using crutches. The black area represents either the weak or non-weightbearing leg

Figure 17.9 Ascending and descending stairs using crutches. (From Judd 1989, with permission.)

to the sides, while the weight is taken through the hands, wrists and arms. Using the axilla to take weight would only encourage a crutch palsy, which is caused by pressure on the brachial plexus. Crutches, therefore, need to rest two or three fingerwidths below the axilla. Patients should continue to maintain a proper and safe technique while ascending and descending stairs (Fig. 17.9).

Besides walking with or without aids, another part of managing poor balance is to ensure safety to and from the sitting position. Batehup & Squires (1991) see the prerequisites for this as a suitable chair (i.e. one that is at an appropriate height with appropriate arms and with a correct angle of the back and seat) and good technique, which can be facilitated by the carer. One such technique, used in the rehabilitation of stroke patients, is the Bobath method. The main principle is that the damaged body should be retrained in natural patterns of movement that are symmetrical. The aim is also to break the automatic patterns of spasticity associated with these patients (Holmes 1988). If we concentrate upon the stronger side of the body to compensate for the weaker side then we may inadvertently encourage further weakness and loss of mobility to the affected side.

Exercise and activity

Exercise is the undertaking of physical exertion with the main aim of improving fitness and health. Exercise and activity are fundamental to mobility and there are many different types of exercise. These have been described by Brunner & Suddarth (1989) as:

- passive – exercises that are usually carried out by the physiotherapist or the nurse without the assistance of the patient
- active assisted – exercises performed by the patient, but with assistance from the physiotherapist or nurse

- active – exercises undertaken by the patient without any assistance
- resisted – exercises performed against manual or physical resistance
- isometric or static – exercises carried out by the patient where muscles are alternately contracted and relaxed while that part of the body remains in a fixed position.

The reason for undertaking a particular exercise will depend on the diagnosis and the intended outcome. The patient, for example, may have a knee injury immobilized in a splint and have developed muscle wasting and weakness. In this case, static exercise of the quadriceps muscles may be required to regain muscular strength to achieve stability upon walking.

It is not always the case that passive movements are undertaken because the patient cannot perform active movements themselves; sometimes they are undertaken to prevent damage through overexertion. However, the nurse or physiotherapist needs to be aware that their efforts can be too vigorous during passive movement and can cause damage that will hinder progress.

If a programme of exercise and mobility is implemented, this should be agreed between the health care team and the patient, and the patient should be capable of the initial activity of standing and balancing. To achieve the latter, as discussed in the previous section, some mobility aid may be required.

Many of the aids you may have identified will be those that promote or extend one's ability to exercise and increase activity. Exercise tolerance, though, should not only imply the extent to which exercise can be undertaken without a mobility aid as frequently patients are unable to exercise effectively without such aids.

Exercise may be promoted for reasons other than simply physical well-being. Research by Adams (1995) describes a 12-week exercise programme undertaken by a young schizophrenic patient in which it was identified that this not only improved physical fitness, but also reinforced self-confidence and a positive body image and nurtured emotional and psychosocial skills.

It has been suggested by Banyard & Hayes (1994: 298), in relation to successful skills training, that there are two key features:

- guidance – which tells us what to do
- feedback – which tells us how successful we have been.

When planning an exercise programme, it is important to ensure that patients, whatever their age, are able to understand what is required, and what is about to be performed. Feedback will involve different means for different people and for different ages. Galley & Forster (1987) identify the aims in planning any exercise programme as:

- to motivate to improve morale
- to relieve symptoms, particularly the presence of pain and oedema

- to regain all possible function
- to provide a foundation for forward planning
- to set up a programme for independent working to note any restrictions and special precautions, whether local or general
- if possible, to prevent further disability
- to maintain or improve all unaffected functions
- to maintain or gain any physical fitness.

Patients are individuals and need to be considered as such. Implementing any exercise programme will involve unique demands on a patient's body: demands upon their muscles, ligaments, joints and other body systems. An ill child will not be able to tolerate exercise in the same way or to the same extent as a fit child, nor will a fit child tolerate the same programme as a fit adult. Different methods and ways to motivate different people are often required in conducting exercise programmes. Remember that exercise can also be used as a form of relaxation and psychotherapy and be beneficial to patients with severe mental health problems.

All decision making for nursing practice knowledge requires a thorough assessment and an ongoing evaluation of the progress of the client in maintaining his or her mobility within the nursing process cycle.

Decision making exercise

Imagine that you are about to conduct an exercise programme for a client group from within each of the branches of nursing (adult, child, learning disabilities and mental health).

- Reflecting on the specific needs of clients within your selected branch, decide what you would do to encourage, maintain or improve function and mobility.
- With fellow students and workplace colleagues, compare approaches that will be needed for different client groups in differing contexts of care.

PROFESSIONAL AND ETHICAL KNOWLEDGE

NURSING RESPONSIBILITIES IN MOBILITY CARE

The section that follows will concentrate upon the increased responsibilities placed upon nurses in recent years. It looks at our own knowledge base, and the political and societal changes in relation to mobility. With these in mind, it also suggests ways forward that may benefit our clients and patients.

As registered nurses, we are responsible professionals and as such are accountable to our clients. If we are working in areas that involve a great deal of assisted patient mobility or the use of mobility aids then we have a duty to maintain our expertise and update our knowledge in the field. If we are unsure of our responsibilities or our skills, then we need

to ascertain who is responsible, or ensure updating takes place. If the responsibility for mobility lies with others such as the community physiotherapist then we must ensure that patients are referred to the appropriate person or department. We must also ensure that local and national policies and procedures are adhered to, therefore enabling effective patient safety and comfort.

Nurses also need to become more proactive in the fight for greater patient rights. We may need to pinpoint, for example, inadequacies of the National Health Service and Community Care Act 1990 or the Chronically Sick and Disabled Persons Act 1970. This latter legislation has been said to encourage the medicalization of disability, with an over-reliance on the expert medical assessor or doctor. The social security system also forces the disabled to emphasize their inabilities to obtain benefit (Morris 1993).

However, disabled people are usually legislated for by the able-bodied and the legislators cannot wholly appreciate the problems that exist for the disabled or immobile.

Reflection and portfolio evidence

Much has been discussed and written over the past few years about the positive aspects of promoting exercise for health. What we also see though, in a system of limited NHS resources, is the increased cost of treatment for individuals who have sustained injuries due to inaccurate or over-exercising.

- Where do you think the nurse's responsibilities lie if this trend continues?

DISABILITY DISCRIMINATION ACT 1995

The aim of Disability Discrimination Act 1995 is to end discrimination within the area of disability.

The Act introduces rights in relation to:

- employment
- access to services and goods
- buying and renting of land or property
- education
- public transport.

Schools and further and higher education establishments, for example, have to take into consideration the needs of disabled students. However, certain exemptions apply to Northern Ireland and Scotland, as provision had already been made in other Acts.

Public transport regulations, within the Act, are designed to ensure safety, comfort and accessibility for the disabled, although again exceptions can apply to taxis if it is considered inappropriate or that the numbers of taxis would substantially diminish as a result of alterations. Trains and trams, too, can also be exempt in some circumstances.

Other areas such as access to goods, facilities, services and employment also go some way to improve the present situation. It is argued that even with the introduction of this Act, there has been a failure on the part of the government to deliver in many areas of needs. Disabled people still feel excluded from mainstream society. Unlike in the case of the Race Relations Act 1976 and the Equal Opportunities Commission, it has been stated that there are no powers to police the Disability Discrimination Act 1995 and that individuals with a grievance can only turn to industrial tribunals or small claims courts (Taylor 1995). This may lead to criticism that the Act lacks teeth for effective change. The Disability Rights Commission Act 1999 was introduced to oversee the working of the Disability Discrimination Act 1995 by making proposals or giving advice to the government. As nurses, and patient/client advocates, we have a duty and responsibility to protect the interests of those in our care. We need to be proactive to ensure improvements, even if this means legitimate pressure brought to bear upon central and local government so that the present law is made effective and future amendments can be made.

FACILITIES FOR MOBILITY CARE

As health promoters, nurses need to be aware of what facilities are available in the community and where they and their patients can obtain expert help and advice. Disabled Living Centres are examples of such facilities. These are situated in towns and cities throughout England, Wales and Scotland. They are financed through different means such as charities, health authorities, social services, donations or a combination of these. They can be accessed by anyone, for example patients, relatives, significant others, voluntary carers, voluntary organizations and health professionals. The centres give expert physiotherapy and occupational therapy advice on a wide range of disability equipment. This advice is unbiased and the equipment is available for trial. Assessments are also made as to the suitability of the equipment for individual patient or client use. The staff are also an invaluable source of information about the many different aspects of mobility and mobility aids. They can facilitate negotiations between patients and the relevant mobility or disability departments. They can also give patients the appropriate contact address or telephone number for financial aid or physical or psychological care.

These centres also assess new equipment and provide training and advice for professional and non-professional carers. They can also advise patients or carers about where or from whom to obtain equipment. Overall, the centres are an invaluable facility for people with permanent or temporary mobility problems, yet many people, including health professionals, are not aware of their existence.

ETHICAL ISSUES AND DILEMMAS

Historically, nursing practice could be said to have been paternalistic in its approach and endeavours to help patients who are disabled. This was done in a number of ways, consciously or subconsciously, by coercion, persuasion, control of information, limitation of options and choices, victim blaming, top-down approach, imposition of professional values and value-laden advice. But one may argue that tremendous strides have been made in the shift from a professionally centred approach to a more individual client and family-centred approach, though in some aspects of nursing practice much more could be done to involve the family of the patient or client.

Decision making exercise

Imagine that you are nursing Mr Singh, who is a 68-year-old patient on a very busy medical ward, admitted for investigations. He has difficulty mobilizing, but is able to walk slowly with assistance. The nurses have been taking him to the toilet using a wheelchair as he takes too much time to walk.

- Discuss the ethical issues or dilemmas of the scenario, using the four ethical principles mentioned in the text.
- What other ethical conflicts may arise with a patient who holds different cultural beliefs and values?
- What is meant by a 'utilitarian approach' and to what extent can it be applied to above scenario?

Today, nurses are accountable for their actions and practice and must take into account the role/contribution of patients or clients as 'partners in their care', as advised by the Nursing and Midwifery Council (2002) *Code of Professional Conduct*. In addition to adherence to the laws of the land, nurses need to have knowledge of the underlying principles of ethics to inform decision taking. Only a brief account of the ethical concepts will be examined here; the reader is advised to consult relevant books and websites on healthcare ethics for more detailed explanations or descriptions. Beauchamp & Childress (1995) provide some basic underpinning principles relevant to nursing and medicine. Firstly, the nurse is expected to *respect the autonomy* of the client, that is for individual patient or client to have rights and the capacity to make choices with regard to treatment and care. Secondly, to do no harm to the client (*non-maleficence*), in other words to avoid causing actual or potential harm to the individual either by negligence or by act of omission. Thirdly, to do good (*beneficence*) by promoting wellness and health. And fourthly, to treat every client with fairness and equity (*justice*), ensuring that care and treatment are carried out according to patient's interests and needs whatever the individual's background, social and cultural beliefs. Apart from legal obligations nurses have moral obligations and in practice are sometimes faced by ethical dilemmas in decision making.

Another important ethical principle to consider when making decisions is referred to as 'utilitarianism'. This suggests the nurse should act in a way that any benefits outweigh the disadvantages, offering the greatest good to the greatest number (Jones & Cribb 1997).

The following are examples of difficult situations for you to reflect upon:

- What would you do if the client made the wrong decision regarding choice of treatment or refused to comply with a mobilization or rehabilitation regime? To what extent can nurses intervene without being seen as infringing client's rights as an individual?
- What would be your response when a patient refuses your help and wants to die when he has become totally dependent on others for his activities of daily living?
- What might be your reaction when being told by a 40-year-old client that she wants an abortion because she is afraid of having a baby with learning/physical disability? What other issues might be involved?
- A 60-year-old client has been in a mental hospital for nearly 20 years and has no next of kin. He likes walking but is having difficulty mobilizing because of pain in his right hip. He has been diagnosed as having osteoarthritis and is being treated with drugs. Staff have decided not to seek the advice of the orthopaedic consultant.

What are the issues involved here and what ethical principles might be applied?

At the beginning of this chapter the meaning of mobility was explored. It was seen mainly from a physical perspective, especially since most people take full mobility for granted. To understand the full scope of this area of nursing practice, not only the anatomical, physiological and developmental functioning of mobility was examined, but also the psychological, social and environmental effects of immobility.

Nurses deal with mobility problems 24 hours a day and need to maintain their knowledge and skills in this area of nursing practice in order to make informed and effective decisions in the administration of quality care for their clients.

PERSONAL AND REFLECTIVE KNOWLEDGE

You were advised to carry out exercises at different points of this chapter. These were aimed at increasing your knowledge and awareness of mobility, immobility, and the problems that exist. This section now focuses on a variety of practical exercises that are designed to be undertaken in or around the formal classroom environment and care settings.

USING MOBILITY AIDS AND APPLIANCES

It is important that the person conducting these exercises is fully trained in the use of all the appliances used so that the correct advice about and practice of the techniques can be taught before the students embark on them.

At the outset the facilitator should stress that safety is of paramount importance in the exercises described below and should not be compromised. Students should also make the most of these experiences, which may therefore involve:

- asking for directions
- obtaining money from a bank or cashpoint
- making a purchase at a shop
- having refreshments in a café
- sitting in a public area.

Elbow crutches and axillary crutches

Once proper instruction has been given, and the students have been assessed as competent, they should be asked to venture into both the hospital and town or city to:

- experience what practical difficulties exist
- identify whether planners and architects have made adequate or inadequate provision for anyone using crutches

- experience how users of crutches are perceived and treated by the general public.

Two students will need to work together. One student will use the crutches and the other will identify (in writing) the findings. This demonstrates the first problem; the difficulty of using crutches and writing at the same time! Both students should have equal opportunity to practise both skills. To gain a better appreciation this should ideally be conducted over one day and group discussion take place the following day.

Wheelchairs

The process of this exercise is undertaken in the same way as the previous one, with the same three questions to be answered. However, there are two methods here:

- the three-student method – one student sits in the wheelchair, one assists and the third student observes and records any interactions with the public, and the difficulties encountered
- the two-student method – one student uses the wheelchair independently and the other student records the interactions and difficulties.

With both methods, each team should discuss between them the whole experience so that additional points can be made before feeding back to the whole group.

Obstacle audit

One simpler but less effective method is where students work in pairs and are initially given guidance about what obstacles to effective mobility might be. Each pair then goes out into the community and hospital where they identify, in writing, a list of obstacles to effective mobility. If facilities are available, a video camera is a useful aid to this exercise.

When the practical exercise is complete, the students return to the classroom setting where a full discussion takes place. This should include:

- the items identified
- the difficulties that may be encountered
- suggested reasons why changes or adaptations have not been made.

One might expect that the hospital planners and managers would have looked closely at such difficulties. They may have rectified the situation according to the needs of their clients and patients with mobility problems. However, this is not always the case, so again, we need to ask why and what is being done?

CASE STUDIES RELATED TO THE IMMOBILE CLIENT

The following case studies are included to help you consolidate knowledge gained from the chapter and your practice experience.

Case study: Adult

Mrs Mary Reed is an 87-year-old widow, lives alone and claims to be independent. She is finding it increasingly difficult to climb the stairs because of arthritis in both hips. Her daughter is concerned that she will fall and sustain serious harm and has tried to persuade Mrs Reed to move into a rest home, without much success. Mrs Reed is able, with difficulty, to visit the local shops for her daily needs but, with winter approaching, there is greater risk of her sustaining a fall. Mrs Reed's daughter has contacted her mother's general practitioner for help and so the district nurse is asked to assess the situation.

- What facilities and personnel are available to alleviate the situation?
- If, as the district nurse, you are called in to make an assessment, how would you approach it?
- How would you deal with the conflict of interests between the mother and the daughter?
- What options are open to the nurse?
- Can the nurse deal with all eventualities that may result from the assessment?
- We are obliged to act in the best interests of our patients (Nursing and Midwifery Council 2002) but there is the aspect of safety, and on the other hand, the patient's psychological well-being. Would a compromise be in order, and if so, what would it be?

Case study: Mental health

Mr Winston Brown lives in a bungalow with his wife. He came to England in 1960 from the West Indies. He is a 65-year-old man who has suffered from bouts of depression for the last 10 years. Mr Brown's problem is compounded by the fact that he suffered a stroke 6 years ago, which has left him with a permanent weakness down the left side of his body. However, he does manage to walk short distances with the aid of a stick, but requires help to get in and out of his chair. His long illness has taken its toll on his wife's physical and psychological condition and well-being. Mr Brown attends a psychiatric day centre three times a week, but his depression and mobility have not improved.

- Do you think that the patient's mobility problems have any bearing on his state of mind?
- Would it mean that if Mr Brown's mobility improved his mental health would do likewise?
- If it is identified that Mr Brown lacks the motivation to improve his mobility and state of mind, what can be done?
- What other issues should the nurse take into consideration when dealing with the family?
- Student nurses today undergo a shared Common Foundation Programme for the first 12 months of the course, regardless of the chosen branch. Does this overall experience equip a qualified mental health nurse to undertake this patient's full mobility care?

Case study: Learning disabilities

Stephen White is an 11-year-old boy who suffers from severe brain damage following a road traffic accident 2 years ago. He lives with his parents and his 15-year-old sister. Steven is now unable to talk coherently or walk. His arms and legs have developed flexion contractures over the last year. Stephen's mother, Margaret, is the main carer in the family and she is worried that what little mobility Stephen has, he is about to lose. He is attending the local physiotherapy department twice a week. Margaret does not want Stephen to be placed in a permanent care facility.

- Is it inevitable that full mobility will be lost?
- How do you think the family can help?
- Who else can help them, and how?
- It has been suggested that significant improvements have been made as a result of research findings surrounding the care of the severely disabled child (Beresford 1994). What is your experience in practice?
- Should the severely mentally and physically disabled be encouraged to mix with the able-bodied? What are the reasons for your answer?

Case study: Child

Mandy Roberts is a 7-year-old girl who fell and fractured her right tibia while climbing a tree. She was taken to the Accident and Emergency department and immobilized initially in a plaster slab then later a long leg plaster of paris was applied. She was taught how to use crutches and she and her parents returned home with instructions not to take any weight on her right leg. Two days later, Mandy's leg felt pain free and so she began to take her full weight upon it. Despite her parent's efforts to prevent this, Mandy continues to defy their instructions and says her leg is better and does not need crutches. They return to the hospital for a routine check, where Mandy's mother explains this to the nurse.

- It is evident that Mandy still requires full weight relief on her right leg. What can you do to encourage this?
- What advice can be given to Mandy's parents?
- What skills would you use to ensure compliance/concordance?
- In most cases we as nurses would encourage full mobility, yet here we are expected to limit this. Ensuring compliance or concordance, and limiting mobility at this stage will probably result in Mandy's full mobility in the future. If all patients with mobility problems who do not comply were to be admitted into hospital, extra resources would be required. Discuss whether hospital admission is the solution or not.

Summary

This chapter has drawn together theoretical concepts of mobility and applied this knowledge in relation to the practice of caring for individuals. It has included:

1. A consideration of mobility and its meaning to individuals and to society. This consideration examined mobility from a biological and developmental perspective. The physical and psychosocial effects of immobility upon individuals have also been explored.
2. Factors influencing nurse decision making in mobility assessment and management and issues in planning, implementing and evaluating care for those whose mobility may be restricted.
3. The professional role of the nurse in providing mobility care, and the implications of the Disability Discrimination Act 1995 and the Disability Rights Commission Act 1999.
4. Ethical issues in mobility care, and in the provision of facilities for those in need, have been presented.
5. Knowledge illuminated within this chapter has been combined with evidence from other referenced sources and applied within a range of situations. Suggestions have been made for portfolio development in relation to mobility care, to enable understanding of the difficulties of mobility impairment.

Annotated further reading and websites

Davis P S 1994 Nursing the orthopaedic patient. Churchill Livingstone, Edinburgh, pp 69–101
An excellent chapter entitled 'Why move?', which encompasses the practical problems of immobility.

Hunt G 1994 Ethical issues in nursing. Routledge, London
Invaluable text in which to incorporate the relationship of mobility.

Jones L 1994 The social context of health and health work. Macmillan, London
These five chapters include material that bears an important relationship to mobility, immobility and nursing care. Topics such as ageing, disability, differing health beliefs, professional power and control, and the politics of health care are discussed.

Judd M 1989 Mobility: patient problems and nursing care. Heinemann Nursing, Oxford
Few textbooks solely concentrate on the subject of mobility in nursing. This does, and is therefore a valuable reference.

Masterson A 1995 Mobility and immobility. In: Heath H B M (ed) Potter and Perry's Foundations in nursing theory and practice. Mosby, London, pp 481–584
This chapter includes many concise details on mobility related to nursing theory and practice.

McLaren S M 1996 Mobility and support. In: Hinchliff S M, Montague S E, Watson R (eds) Physiology for nursing practice. Baillière Tindall, London, pp 261–319
An excellent modern text that includes the physiology of mobility, related problems and application to nursing. Excellent colour diagrams supplement the text.

Minister for Disabled People 1996 The Disability Discrimination Act. Booklets DL60, DL70, DL80, DL90, DL100, DL110 and DL120. HSSS JO3-6299JP.100m. HMSO, London
A government reference source describing concisely all parts of the Disability Discrimination Act 1995.

Mulley G (ed) 1991 More everyday aids and appliances. British Medical Journal, London
Both texts are important for those embarking on a nursing career that involves substantial mobility assistance.

Social Security 1998 The disability handbook, 2nd edn. HMSO, London
A handbook of the care needs and mobility requirements likely to arise from various disabilities and chronic illnesses.

Taylor S, Field D 1993 Sociology of health and health care. Blackwell, Oxford, pp 79–132
These two chapters concentrate upon the experience of health and illness in a social context – an important dimension.

http://www.agepositive.gov.uk
Tackling discrimination and promoting diversity in the workplace.

http://www.disabilitynet.co.uk
Route to other websites regarding information on various subjects including policies.

http://www.disability.gov.uk
http://www.disbility.gov.uk/dda/index.html
Information regarding the Disability Discrimination Act 1995.

http://www.disability.gov.uk/drc/index.html
Website of the Disability Rights Commission: eliminating discrimination against disabled people.

http://www.dlcc.demon.co.uk/homepage.html
Local centres offering help, advice and information for users and carers.

http://www.dlabb.org.uk
Website of the Disability Living Allowance Advisory Board.

http://www.doh.gov.uk/olderpeople.htm
This is the online source of the National Service Framework for Older People.

http://www.doh.gov.uk/Research
Information on research being carried out by the Department of Health.

http://www.dptac.gov.uk
Advice on access to buildings and transport.

http://www.drc-gb.org/drc/InformationAndLegislation/page3D.asp
Scotland Disability Awareness Survey 2002 report.

http://www.eurag-europe.org/emobility55.htm
Project dealing with 'Mobility in Europe and active citizenship for the elderly'.

http://www.humanrights.gov.uk
Online text of Human Rights Treaties, including Article 8: 'Respect for family and private life'.

http://www.independentliving.org
Website containing views, experiences and articles dealing with disability issues such culture as disability.

http://www.learnwell.org
A useful website covering ethical aspects of health care.

http://www.Motability.co.uk
Motability is an organization that helps people with disabilities and their families with mobility.

http://www.mobility.Unit.dft.gov.uk
Department of Transport website, dealing with issues of mobility and inclusion.

http://www.preventinghomefalls.gov.uk
A campaign by the Department of Trade and Industry to prevent accidental falls in the home.

http://www.prs.1tsn.ac.uk/access/discussions/dact2001.html
Discussion on the Special Educational Needs and Disability Act 2001.

http://www.remploy.co.uk
Job opportunities for people with disabilities.

http://www.swap.ac.uk/Widen/DisabilityIT.asp
Website providing information about organizations and resources relating to disability.

http://www.who.ch/
International classification of impairments, activities and participation.

References

Abbruzzese L D 1998 The Tinetti Performance Orientated Mobility Assessment Tool. American Journal of Nursing 98(12):16J–L

Adams L 1995 How exercise can help people with mental health problems. Nursing Times 91(36):37–39

Armstrong L 1993 Promoting physical activity in schools. Health Visitor 66(10):362–364

Banyard P, Hayes N 1994 Psychology, theory and application. Chapman & Hall, London

Barker P J, Davidson B 1998 Psychiatric nursing: ethical strife. Edward Arnold, London

Batehup L, Squires A 1991 Mobility. In: Redfern S J (ed) Nursing elderly people, 2nd edn. Churchill Livingstone, Edinburgh, pp 135–136

Beauchamp T L, Childress J F 1995 Principles of biomedical ethics, 4th edn. Oxford University Press, New York

Beresford B 1994 Positively patients: caring for a severely disabled child. HMSO, London

Bond J, Coleman P, Peace S (eds) 1993 Ageing in society: an introduction to social gerontology. Sage, London

Brunner L S, Suddarth D S 1989 Rehabilitation concepts. The Lippincott manual of medical–surgical nursing, 2nd edn. Harper & Row, London, pp 9–42

Buckwalter K, Smith M, Martin M 1993 Attitude problem. Nursing Times 89(5):55–57

Comfort A 1977 A good age. Mitchell Beazley, London

Consumer Protection Act 1987 HMSO, London

Department of Health 2001 The National Service Framework for older people. HMSO, London

Department of Trade and Industry 2002 Home Safety Network. Online. Available: http://www.dti.gov.uk/homesafetynetwork/

Disability Discrimination Act 1995 HMSO, London

Disability Rights Commission Act 1999 HMSO, London

Dowswell T, Towner E, Cryer C et al 1999 Accidental falls: fatalities and injuries. An examination of the data sources and review of the literature on preventive strategies. Report for the Department of Trade and Industry. DTI URN 99/805

French S 1994 In whose service? A review of the development of the services for disabled people in Great Britain. Physiotherapy 80(24):200–204

Galley P M, Forster E L 1987 Human movement: an introductory text for physiotherapy students, 2nd edn. Churchill Livingstone, Edinburgh

Herbert R A, Alison J A 1996 Cardiovascular function. In: Hinchliff S M, Montague S E, Watson R (eds) Physiology for nursing practice, 2nd edn. Baillière Tindall, London, pp 445–447

Hinchliff S M, Montague S E, Watson R (eds) 1996 Physiology for nursing practice, 2nd edn. Baillière Tindall, London

Jones L 1994 The social context of health and health work. Macmillan, London

Jones L, Cribb A 1997 Ethical issues in health promotion. In: Katz J, Peberdy A Promoting health: knowledge and practice. Open University, London

Judd M 1989 Mobility: patient problems and nursing care. Heinemann Nursing, Oxford

McLaren S M 1996 Mobility and support. In: Hinchliff S M, Montague S E, Watson R (eds) Physiology for nursing practice, 2nd edn. Baillière Tindall, London, pp 309–319

Mahoney F I, Barthel D W 1965 Functional evaluation: the Barthel Index. Maryland State Medical Journal 14:61–65

Makin C (ed) 1991 Collins English Dictionary, 3rd edn. HarperCollins, Glasgow

Masterson A 1995 Mobility and immobility. In: Heath H B M (ed) Potter and Perry's Foundations in nursing theory and practice. Mosby, London, pp 481–504

Morris J 1993 Independent lives: community care and disabled people. Macmillan, London

National Health Service and Community Care Act 1990 HMSO, London

Nursing and Midwifery Council 2002 Code of professional conduct. Nursing and Midwifery Council, London

Office of Population Censuses and Surveys 1995 General household survey No. 24. HMSO, London

Office of Population Censuses and Surveys 2000 The national time use survey. HMSO, London

Office of Population Censuses and Surveys 2001 Census 2001. Online. Available: http://www.statistics.gov.uk/census2001/demographic_uk.asp

Ogden B 1992 Moving and lifting. In: Brown H, Benson S (eds) A practical guide to working with people with learning disabilities. Hawker, London, pp 123–146

Schwarz C (ed) 1995 Chambers Dictionary. Harrap, Edinburgh

Scottish Executive 2003 Let's make Scotland more active: a strategy for physical activity. Stationery Office, Edinburgh. Online. Available: http://www.scotland.gov.uk

Special Educational Needs and Disability Act 2001 HMSO, London

Taylor A 1995 Debilitating discrimination. Nursing Times 91(44):38–40

Taylor S, Field D 1993 Sociology of health and health care. Blackwell, Oxford

Thapa P B, Gideon P, Fought R L et al 1994 Comparison of clinical and biomechanical measures of balance and mobility in elderly nursing home residents. Journal of the American Geriatrics Society 42(5):439–500

Tortora G J, Grabowski S R 1996 Principles of anatomy and physiology, 8th edn. John Wiley & Sons, Chichester

Webb R, Tossell D 1991 Social issues for carers: a community care perspective. Edward Arnold, London

Windmill V 1990 Ageing today: a positive approach to caring for elderly people. Edward Arnold, London

Chapter 18

Continence

Alison Kelley

KEY ISSUES

SUBJECT KNOWLEDGE
- Definition of continence and incontinence
- Biology of the urinary system
- The process of defaecation
- Different types of incontinence and their causes
- Effects of the ageing process on continence
- Psychological and environmental causes of incontinence
- Behavioural problems caused by or causing incontinence
- The stigma of incontinence

CARE DELIVERY KNOWLEDGE
- Nursing assessment of urinary and faecal incontinence
- Ways of promoting urinary and faecal continence
- Aids and appliances used to manage incontinence

PROFESSIONAL AND ETHICAL KNOWLEDGE
- The effect of national policies on the Continence Advisory Service
- Education for continence promotion
- Quality assurance of continence care
- The rights of clients to quality continence care

PERSONAL AND REFLECTIVE KNOWLEDGE
- Empathy with the incontinent client
- Consolidation of knowledge through case studies

INTRODUCTION

People have the right to be continent whenever that is achievable. When true continence is not achievable, people have the right to the highest standards of continence care and incontinence management, to enable social continence and maintenance of the individual's dignity: this is the philosophy of the Association for Continence Advice, as given in their *Guidelines for Continence Care* (Association for Continence Advice 1993).

Urinary incontinence is a distressing condition causing the patient and carer to feel shame and embarrassment. Faecal incontinence is seen as less socially acceptable. Often incontinence is considered unacceptable by society, causing the sufferer to feel like an outcast (Mitteness 1992). However, 'Incontinence is a treatable condition' (Department of Health 2000). The nurse should not only be proactive in providing appropriate physiological and psychological intervention to help a client achieve continence but should also provide good health education to the general public to dispel negative and misguided attitudes.

This chapter aims to explain the reasons elimination problems occur and to introduce you to the knowledge and skills you will need to assess clients with continence difficulties and to plan their care. It also discusses the impact national policies have to ensure this care is of a high standard.

The exercises used throughout the text are designed to help you develop a thorough understanding of how continence is maintained and how problems, physical, psychological and social, can cause incontinence in clients in all branches of nursing. They are also designed to help you to reflect on this care in practice and guide you in developing your portfolio around this subject.

OVERVIEW

Subject knowledge

This section covers the normal anatomy and physiology of micturition and defaecation, how continence is gained, and then shows how alterations from the normal can give rise to incontinence. It explores how continence is affected when ability to cope with activities of daily living change, and examines how society and its attitudes can affect elimination behaviour.

Care delivery knowledge

The section on care delivery knowledge outlines the skills needed to assess clients' problems, ways of promoting continence, how to manage incontinence and additional treatments that can be offered by referring clients to the continence advisor and the multidisciplinary team. These principles can be applied to clients of all ages in all branches of nursing, whether the client is being cared for in hospital or at home.

Professional and ethical knowledge

This part of the chapter discusses how the importance of promoting and managing continence has been highlighted in the last few years. The responsibilities of the continence advisor, the nurse and the multidisciplinary team and the way it is envisaged the integrated services will run are also covered. Educational needs and ethical issues of continence will also be discussed.

Personal and reflective knowledge

The aim of the exercises is to help you use the knowledge gained and develop them for your portfolio.

On pages 419–420 there are four case studies, each one relating to one of the branch programmes. You may find it helpful to read one of them before you start the chapter and use it as a focus for your reflections while reading as part of your portfolio development.

SUBJECT KNOWLEDGE

BIOLOGICAL

Continence is a skill gained when a person learns to recognize the need to pass urine and/or bowel motion, has the ability to reach an acceptable place to void, is able to hold on until they reach there and is able to void/eliminate effectively on reaching that place (Association for Continence Advice 1993). The International Continence Society Committee on Standardization of Terminology defines urinary incontinence as 'The involuntary loss of urine which is objectively demonstrable and a social or hygiene problem' (Anderson et al 1988).

The document *Good Practice in Continence Services* (Department of Health 2000) suggests that urinary incontinence may, in the general population, be as high 1 in 10 to 1 in 5 women over 65 years old and 1 in 14 to 1 in 10 males

over 65 years old, and this may rise to 1 in 2 in homes caring for the infirm elderly. It also suggests that about 500 000 children suffer from bed-wetting.

The first section examines the physiological mechanism used to achieve continence and then how it may fail and cause urinary and faecal incontinence. Other types of physiological failures that may cause problems with elimination are also considered.

ANATOMY AND PHYSIOLOGY OF THE LOWER URINARY TRACT

The urinary system consists of two kidneys, two ureters, a bladder and a urethra. Urine is made in the kidneys when the blood is filtrated to remove waste products and keep water and electrolytes balanced in the body. Antidiuretic hormone (ADH) will decrease urine production, and will normally rise at night to decrease the amount of urine produced (Asplund & Aberg 1991). Urine passes down the ureters from the kidneys and it is important that it does not reflux back to the kidneys, causing renal damage. This is prevented by the angle at which the ureters enter the

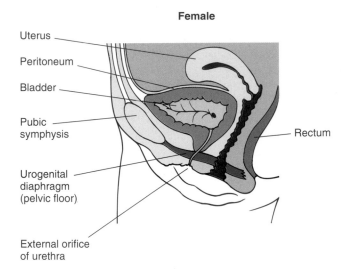

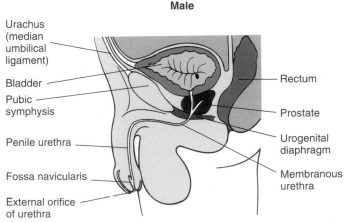

Figure 18.1 Anatomy of the urethra. (From Hinchliff et al 1996.)

bladder, peristalsis in the ureters causing urine to flow towards the bladder and the narrowing along the ureter.

To understand continence fully it is important to know about the organs involved in storage and evacuation (bladder and urethra) and how they relate to the lower bowel and the male and female reproductive organs (Fig. 18.1).

The bladder is made of four layers of tissue:

- an inner layer of transitional epithelium
- a connective tissue layer
- smooth muscle
- an outer coating covering the upper surface, the peritoneum (Fig. 18.2)

The epithelial layer has the ability to stretch and it also produces mucus to protect the tissues from the acidity of the urine. The smooth muscle is known as the detrusor muscle and is made up of layers of longitudinal and circular muscle to allow it to both expand and contract. Stretch receptors monitor the fullness of the bladder and are found throughout this muscle, but are concentrated in the sensitive trigone, a triangular area between the ureters and the urethra. Urine enters the bladder through the ureters and leaves through the urethra (see Fig. 18.2) (Colborn 1994).

The urethra is a tube running from the bladder and is 3–5 cm long in the female and 18–22 cm long in the male. It has a thick mucosal lining containing mucus-producing cells, and is folded to enhance the watertight seal of the bladder. At the bladder neck the smooth muscle passes from the bladder to the urethra, forming the internal closing mechanism. This is more distinct in men than women, being found just above the prostate gland (Fig. 18.3).

The external sphincter is made of voluntary muscle and in men it is a separate ring just below the prostate gland. This allows the sphincters to work independently so during ejaculation the bladder is closed but the urethra can be open (Fillingham & Douglas 1997). In women the internal closing mechanism is less distinct and the external sphincter surrounds this. It is also sensitive to oestrogen levels. These factors may give rise to an incompetent sphincter (discussed later in the chapter).

The pelvic floor is a muscular sling supporting the abdominal organs. It is pierced by the rectum posteriorly and the vagina and urethra anteriorly. It is very important in continence, contracting to maintain urinary and faecal continence, but relaxing to allow expulsion of urine and faeces (Lewis Wall 1994). The bladder and the proximal urethra sit well supported above the pelvic floor, a position needed to maintain continence (Fig. 18.2).

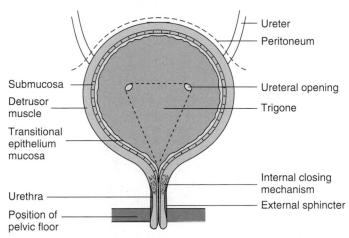

Figure 18.2   Cross-section of urinary bladder (female). (After Cheater 1992b.)

Labels: Ureter, Peritoneum, Ureteral opening, Trigone, Internal closing mechanism, External sphincter, Submucosa, Detrusor muscle, Transitional epithelium mucosa, Urethra, Position of pelvic floor

Decision making exercise

The co-ordination of bladder emptying is controlled by nerve pathways. Damage to these pathways can upset their balance and cause incontinence.

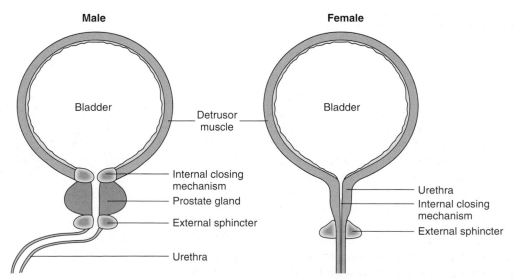

Figure 18.3   The sphincters of the bladder.

Male / Female. Labels: Bladder, Detrusor muscle, Internal closing mechanism, Prostate gland, External sphincter, Urethra, Internal closing mechanism, External sphincter

- How will damage in the following areas affect the micturition process?
    - the frontal lobe
    - the midbrain or pons
    - the cervical spine
    - the lumbar spine
    - the sacrum
    - the nerves forming the spinal reflex arc.
- Compare your answers with the problems described in the following discussion of altered physiology.
- As you gain nursing experience, list the conditions caused by damage to the central nervous system or spinal cord and look at the patient's subsequent continence.

The bladder is controlled by both the somatic and the autonomic nervous system, which allows it to store urine and expel it at a suitable time. The sympathetic system innervates the detrusor muscle of the bladder, allowing the bladder to relax during its filling phase while the sphincters remain closed. It allows filling up to approximately 300 mL without registering changes of pressure. This is known as compliance. Once this volume is reached the sensory parasympathetic nerves transmit impulses to the sacral area of the spinal cord (S2–S4). A spinal reflex arc is completed allowing impulses to pass back to the bladder through the parasympathetic motor nerves, causing the muscle to contract and the sphincter to open, resulting in micturition (Fig. 18.4).

The voluntary control works in an inhibitory manner: sensory impulses are sent through the pudendal nerve to the cortical micturition centre in the frontal lobe of the brain saying bladder is full. Inhibitory impulses are passed back to the sacrum to prevent the sacral reflex arc initiating micturition. When the individual is ready to pass urine, the inhibition is lifted (Fig. 18.4). These voluntary nerve pathways pass through the pons in the midbrain and it is thought that this area ensures that the sphincters opening and the bladder contraction are coordinated (Andrews & Hussman 1997). The reflex arc action occurs in babies, and the inhibitory process begins to develop in infants from the age of 18 months as the central nervous system matures.

ALTERED PHYSIOLOGY OF THE LOWER URINARY TRACT

Four main types of incontinence result from an alteration of the normal physiology described above. These are:

- stress incontinence
- detrusor instability
- reflex incontinence
- voiding difficulties.

The conditions will be discussed separately so that you can understand the different symptoms of each type. This is

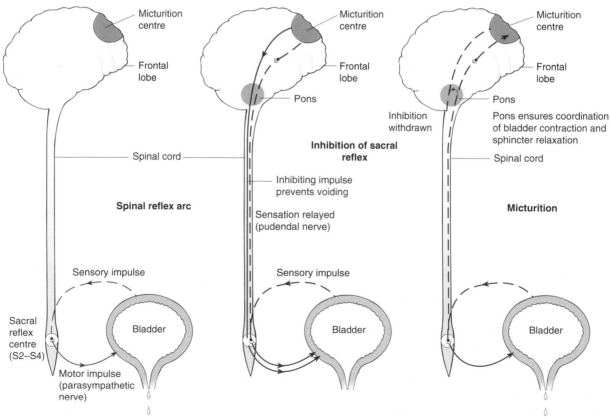

Figure 18.4   Involuntary and voluntary control of micturition.

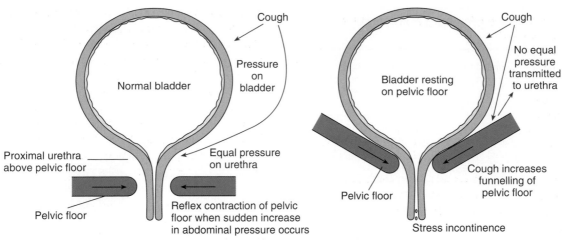

Figure 18.5 Diagram showing the relationship between the bladder and the pelvic floor for continence, and how a lax pelvic floor causes stress incontinence.

important when you assess patients as some clients may have more than one condition causing their continence difficulties.

Stress incontinence

Stress incontinence is the most common form of incontinence in women (Hill 1997). It is defined as an involuntary loss of urine during increase in intra-abdominal pressure caused by laughing, sneezing or lifting. It occurs during the filling phase of the bladder causing leakage of urine (Laycock et al 2001). When the bladder is held in the correct position by the pelvic floor the inner closing mechanism and the external sphincter of the bladder prevent leakage (Fig. 18.5). If the pelvic floor is weak the bladder prolapses downwards and there is no compensatory pressure helping to counteract the pressure on the bladder and leakage may occur (Fig. 18.5); this is made worse if the urethral closing mechanism is also weak, for example when oestrogen levels are low (Dolman 2003). Table 18.1 lists the common causes of stress incontinence.

Overactive bladder

Overactive bladder (detrusor instability) is characterized by involuntary bladder contractions during its filling phase (Wells 1996) and produces symptoms of urgency, frequency, urge incontinence, nocturia and nocturnal enuresis (Table 18.2). Simply explained, the inhibition impulse from the cortical micturition centre of the cortex is not sufficient to prevent the sacral reflex action occurring, so the bladder starts to contract and voiding begins. This may be due to damage to the central nervous system, for example a cerebrovascular accident (stroke), tumours, spinal cord injuries or malfunction of the conduction of the nerve impulses, as seen in multiple sclerosis (MS) and Parkinsonism. Local bladder factors may be responsible for causing spasm that overrides cortical

Table 18.1 Common causes of stress incontinence

Mechanism	Cause	Reference
Weakness of pelvic floor muscles (due to muscle or nerve damage)	Pregnancy Childbirth Trauma during child-birth (vaginal delivery) Forceps delivery Obesity	Wilson 1996 Sultan et al 1993 Bump et al 1991
Increased abdominal pressure	Chronic cough Prolonged lifting of heavy weights Childbirth	
Oestrogen deficiency (oestrogen receptors are found in pelvic floor, bladder and bladder neck, thus there is good muscle tone in the presence of oestrogen)	Pregnancy Last part of menstrual cycle Menopause	Hill 1997

inhibition, for example caffeine (Creighton & Stanton 1990), urinary tract infections, concentrated urine or external factors such as prostatic enlargement or constipation. Overactive bladder may occur in the absence of any detectable pathology (Fig. 18.6) (Getliffe & Dolman 2003).

Reflex incontinence

If there is damage between the sacral area of the spinal cord (S2–S4) and the higher centres, there is no inhibition and the reflex arc action occurs so the client experiences a full and uncontrollable void with no prior warning. The sensation of fullness is also missing. This is seen in clients with paraplegia, or some patients after a stroke (Colborn 1994).

Table 18.2   Definitions of terms used in connection with incontinence

Urgency	The need to pass urine in a great hurry
Sensory urgency	Urgency in the absence of unstable bladder contractions; the bladder is hypersensitive
Frequency	Visiting the toilet to pass urine more often than is acceptable to the patient; this usually means more than seven times during the day and more than once at night
Urge incontinence	While experiencing urgency the patient may not be able to get to the toilet in time and is therefore incontinent
Reflex incontinence	Urine loss due to detrusor hyperreflexia (or involuntary urethral relaxation) when there is a neuropathic absence of sensation
Hesitancy	Difficulty in initiating voiding
Dribbling	Dribbling of urine after voiding, due to pooling of urine in the urethra between internal and external sphincter
Nocturia	Waking at night to pass urine
Nocturnal enuresis	Bed-wetting while asleep
Passive incontinence	Wetting at rest without any coincident activity or sensation
Dysuria	Pain or burning while actually passing urine
Haematuria	Blood in the urine

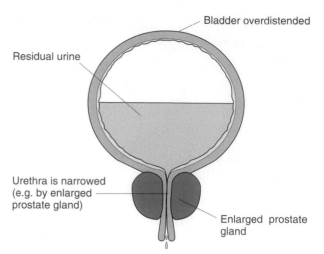

Figure 18.7   Obstruction with overflow incontinence. (Reproduced with kind permission of Coloplast Ltd.)

Voiding difficulties

There are two reasons for voiding difficulties and each is described in the following section.

Outflow obstruction

In some people the outlet of the bladder becomes blocked; this occurs mostly in men with prostatic enlargement and in clients with urethral narrowing (stricture) following infections or previous instrumentation. The narrowing can also be due to congenital causes. When these conditions occur, emptying of the bladder is impeded (Fig. 18.7). Outflow obstruction causes a variety of symptoms including hesitancy, poor stream due to the narrowing, frequency and urgency because the bladder is never completely emptied resulting in a residual volume of urine being left in the bladder. All these symptoms cause overflow incontinence (Getliffe & Dolman 2003). The residual volume also causes recurrent urinary tract infections, a further indication of this problem. The detrusor muscle of an obstructed bladder often becomes very powerful and hypertrophied in an attempt to overcome the high outflow resistance, and may cause secondary detrusor instability and urge incontinence. If the obstruction is long-standing, the bladder may eventually give up and become hypotonic.

Detrusor hypoactivity

In some cases the detrusor muscle is not able to contract effectively to empty the bladder (Fig. 18.8). This may be due to muscle weakness, as seen in some elderly clients (Swaffield 1996), damage to the spinal cord for example in MS and Parkinsonism, cerebral damage as in a stroke (Brittain et al 1998), or peripheral neuropathy associated with diabetes mellitus (Wells 1996). A residual volume will build up and cause symptoms similar to outflow obstruction; some clients may also complain of having to strain to

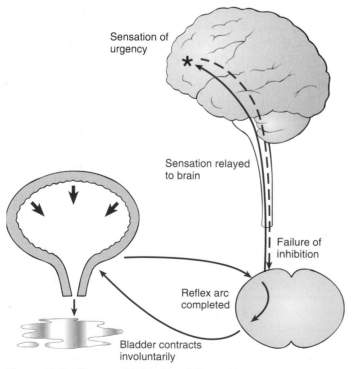

Figure 18.6   The unstable bladder: failure of inhibition of detrusor contraction. (Reproduced with kind permission of Coloplast Ltd.)

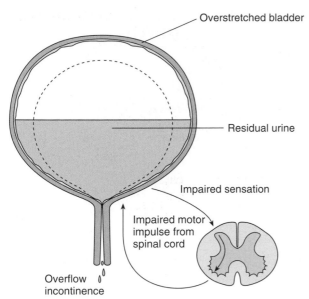

Figure 18.8 The underactive detrusor. (Reproduced with kind permission of Coloplast Ltd.)

pass urine. This is known as a hypotonic bladder. When the residual volume is more than 100 mL, it is considered significant and should be treated (Getliffe 2003). Urinary tract infections are often a presenting sign. Infection symptoms can cause bladder spasm, increasing urgency and thus frequency and overactive bladder may be wrongly diagnosed.

If the pons area of the midbrain is damaged then the control of the micturition cycle may be disrupted, i.e. the sphincters staying contracted (instead of relaxed) when the detrusor is contracting. The client may feel an urgent desire to pass urine but is unable to do so when sitting on the toilet. This is known as detrusor sphincter dyssynergia, and will cause incomplete emptying, leaving a residual volume. Clients with MS (Fowler 1996) or who have had a stroke (Brittain et al 1998) may exhibit this type of bladder dysfunction.

If the nervous control is completely damaged, as seen in some children with spina bifida, the bladder cannot empty at all and this is known as atonic bladder.

Evidence based practice

Wynd et al (1996) designed a study to identify factors contributing to urinary retention immediately following orthopaedic surgery. There are links between retention, anaesthetic, postoperative analgesia, the amount of intravenous fluid given in 24 hours postoperatively, age and history of past urinary problems. If this is not recognized early, continence difficulties may occur postoperatively or following discharge. Wynd et al (1996) recommend that early assessment should alleviate the problem and prevent prolonged hospitalization.

Influences on bladder function

There are other influences on the normal functioning bladder that may cause incontinence: these are fluid intake, urinary tract infection, drugs and constipation. The last two will be discussed later.

Norton (1996) states that a fluid intake of approximately 1500 mL is an appropriate daily amount for an adult. Many clients will cut down their fluid intake mistakenly believing it will reduce their incontinence. Concentrated urine will encourage bladder spasm and thus cause urgency and frequency (Norton 1996). This problem is also found in young children especially when starting school, unless encouraged. They may drink minimal amounts, which may cause some girls to exhibit daytime wetting. This may also be a factor in children who wet the bed (Butler 1994). The opposite problem sometimes occur in clients with learning disabilities who drink excessive amounts of water and produce large volumes of urine, causing frequency. Urinary tract infection will also cause bladder spasm giving urgency and frequency and may exacerbate urinary problems (Wells 1996).

Reflection and portfolio evidence

Drugs are useful in the promotion of continence. However, there are medications that may influence bladder function in some way and cause incontinence or retention of urine. Sedatives and antidepressants may have this action as a side effect. Using the *British National Formulary* (British Medical Association and Royal Pharmaceutical Society of Great Britain 2003), look up examples of these drugs and their side effects. From this information work out how they cause continence problems.

When in your mental health placement/s note how many clients this may affect.

- Describe how you would recognize they may be having elimination difficulties.
- Discuss with your mentor how to best deal with this problem, e.g. reduce the drug dose or commence continence promotion intervention.
- Record your thoughts on the ethical dilemma caused by the action of the drugs.

ANATOMY AND PHYSIOLOGY OF THE LOWER BOWEL

'Faecal incontinence is the most embarrassing, socially unacceptable and demoralizing of symptoms' (Irvine 1996: 226). Looking after a person with faecal incontinence is poorly tolerated by carers and frequently leads to the discontinuation of community care. Faecal incontinence is not as widespread as urinary incontinence. The Department of Health (2000) estimates a prevalence of faecal incontinence of 1% among total population of adults, rising to 17% in the very elderly.

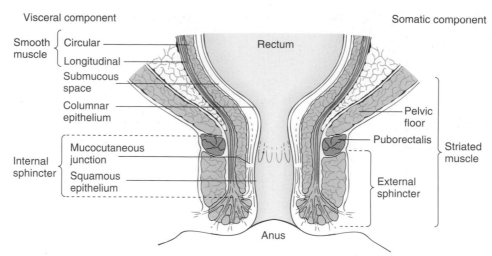

Figure 18.9 Section through the lower rectum and anus. (From Bendall 1989.)

The large intestine consists of the caecum and colon and terminates with the rectum and anal canal. It receives 600 mL of chyme from the small intestine daily and reduces it to 150–200 mL of faeces by reabsorbing water from the chyme as it travels through the colon. Faeces are stored in the rectum and eliminated though the anal canal (Hinchliff et al 1996). The rectum has a mucosal lining (i.e. columnar epithelial), which produces mucus to lubricate the passage of stool. The anal canal has a squamous epithelial lining, which is dry and very sensitive and can distinguish between flatus and stool, allowing flatulence to escape to relieve gaseous distension, but retaining faeces. The muscle layer of the rectum is smooth involuntary muscle and contains specialized stretch receptors, which monitor the fullness of the rectum. In the anal canal the smooth involuntary muscle thickens to form the internal sphincter, which is surrounded by a layer of voluntary muscle, the anal sphincter (Fig. 18.9) (Bendall 1989).

Faeces formed by the large bowel enter the rectum by a series of peristaltic movements known as the gastrocolic reflex, which is stimulated by physical activity and ingestion of food (Barrett 1992). Once 150 mL or more of stool is in the rectum, the individual gets a feeling of fullness and impending defaecation and the internal anal sphincter relaxes and allows the stool to enter the anal canal. If defaecation is not convenient, the external sphincter remains closed and the faeces return to the rectum (Edwards et al 2003). However, if it is appropriate, the external sphincter relaxes and defaecation occurs. This is most efficiently achieved in a squatting position as pressure from the abdominal muscles will cause the external and internal anal sphincters to relax, the pelvic floor will drop down to form a funnel, and the bowel will empty easily (Chiarelli & Markwell 1992).

The nervous control is a reflex action involving the myenteric plexus and stimulated by a full rectum. The internal anal sphincter is controlled by the autonomic nervous system and the external sphincter is controlled by the somatic nervous system (pudendal nerve).

If the defaecation mechanism is working properly the individual should be able to pass 150–200 mL of formed but soft stool regularly. However, the frequency of defaecation varies between individuals, ranging from three times a day to once in three days (Chiarelli & Markwell 1992). The consistency of the stool may show individual differences; these can be assessed using the Bristol Stool Scale, 3 and 4 on this scale being considered to be preferable (Fig. 18.10).

The pelvic floor is responsible for keeping the rectum in the correct position. The muscle of the pelvic floor, which anchors the rectum to the pubis (i.e. the puborectalis), is of great importance in maintaining faecal continence. The puborectalis maintains an angle of 60 to 105 degrees between the rectum and the anal canal. This angle acts as a flap valve, which closes when abdominal pressures rise, for example due to sneezing or lifting, preventing leakage through the canal (Fig. 18.11). During defaecation the pelvic floor relaxes increasing this angle allowing easy passing of stool (Fig. 18.11). The nerve supply of the pelvic floor is innervated by the same nerve as the external sphincter, the pudendal nerve. This nerve synapses with the autonomic system at S2–S4.

ALTERED PHYSIOLOGY OF THE LOWER BOWEL

Faecal incontinence is defined as involuntary and/or inappropriate passing of liquid or solid stool (Cook & Mortenson 1998). Barrett (1992) classifies the causes of faecal incontinence under five headings as follows:

- faecal impaction
- neurological – dementia, unconsciousness, behavioural, brain damage
- anorectal incontinence
- colorectal disease
- immobility (discussed in section on general altered physiology, below).

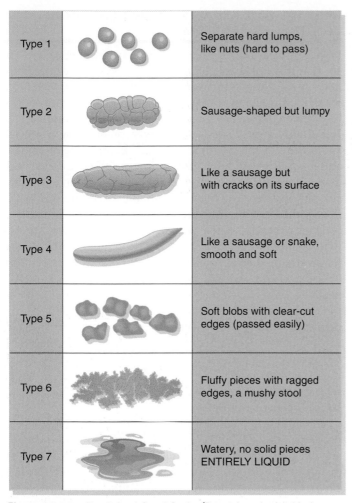

Figure 18.10   The Bristol Stool Scale. (Reproduced with kind permission of Norgine Ltd.)

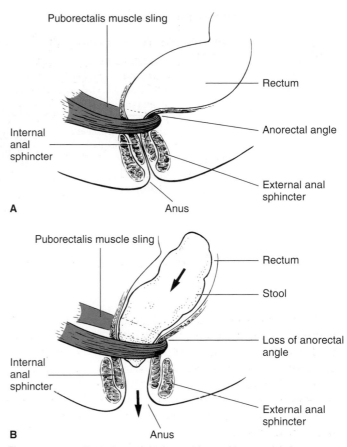

Figure 18.11   Faecal continence and incontinence and the anorectal angle.

Faecal impaction

Faecal impaction can be the result of chronic constipation (Table 18.3). If the constipation is rectal, it may exert pressure forcing the faecal matter through the anal sphincter. Colonic constipation, however, can also cause leakage of liquid stool (Colborn 1994). This may be a seepage of liquid waste from above the obstruction or the result of bacterial breakdown of the hard faeces resulting in a slimy liquid with extra mucus (i.e. a foul smelling spurious diarrhoea). There are many causes of constipation and a complete list is given in Table 18.3.

Thompson et al (1992) defined constipation as demonstrating two of the following symptoms: straining at stool; lumpy hard stools; sensation of incomplete emptying; and fewer than two bowel movements a week.

However, faecal impaction may not always be due to large amounts of small hard stool but large amounts of soft faeces. This type of client may be unable to completely empty their bowel despite daily bowel movement and this can also cause faecal incontinence; thus the term 'faecal loading' may be the best term for this type of bowel problem

(Barrett 1992). There is a higher prevalence of this problem in the frail elderly due to weaker peristaltic movements and weak sphincter muscles.

Neurological causes

Irvine (1996) says that any disorders in the higher cortical centres of the brain impair the ability of an individual to recognize or inhibit defaecation; for example, in paraplegics, in multiple sclerosis and in some cases of peripheral neuropathy this may cause faecal incontinence. Damage in the spinal area of S2–S4, for example, due to spina bifida or low spinal cord damage, can result in uncontrollable bowel evacuation (Glickman & Kamm 1996).

Anorectal incontinence

Anorectal incontinence results from weakness of the pelvic floor, particularly the puborectalis muscle, and as a result, the anorectal angle and therefore the flap valve are lost. Faecal incontinence may then occur when abdominal pressure increases, for example when sneezing or lifting (Fig. 18.11). This muscle weakness may result from damage to the nerves supplying the pelvic floor by chronic straining at stool. In the elderly, anorectal angle changes may be exacerbated by nerve degeneration and muscle weakness (Barrett

Table 18.3 Causes of constipation

Mechanism	Causes
Insufficient material in the bowel	Lack of fibre in the diet Poor fluid intake
Abnormal neurological control	Spinal or nerve injury affecting autonomic nervous system Hirschsprung disease (a condition where there is an absence of nerves in the wall of the bowel) Psychological factors, by an inhibitory effect on autonomic innervation
Obstruction	Tumours Diverticular disease Haemorrhoids Congenital abnormalities
Pregnancy	High progesterone levels causing decrease in motility of the gastrointestinal tract
Metabolic causes	Diabetes mellitus Hypothyroidism Dehydration
Drugs	Aluminium (antacids) Anticholinergics Diuretics Iron Analgesia opiates Verapamil
Laxative abuse	Overuse of laxatives can cause damage to the nerves in the colon, resulting in atonic bowel
Environmental	Anything preventing defaecation, e.g. lack of privacy, dirty toilets, insufficient toilets
Immobility	Lack of exercise means the bowel itself is less active. The client may have difficulty reaching the toilet

1992). Damage to the internal or external anal sphincters (or both) due to forceps delivery or perineal tears during childbirth are often responsible for faecal incontinence in younger women (Sultan et al 1993). If the external sphincter is damaged, women may experience urgency, while damage to the internal sphincter may cause faecal seeping (Johanson & Lafferty 1996).

Colorectal disease

A bad attack of diarrhoea may cause faecal incontinence, especially in those who are very ill, bed bound or have mobility problems. This may be due to infection or gastrointestinal disease. Severe and prolonged attacks of diarrhoea should have a medical referral as should rectal bleeding (Spiller & Farthing 1994).

GENERAL ALTERED PHYSIOLOGY CAUSING CONTINENCE PROBLEMS

If we return to the original definition of continence, we can see that physiological changes in other systems of the body may affect the continence state of the client. For example when identifying the place for elimination the client needs to be orientated. We may get confused when in unfamiliar surroundings, as may some clients, who on entering a strange environment, for example hospital, become disorientated and unable to find the toilet (Stokes 1987). Clients with dementia, confusion or disorientation may become incontinent simply because they are unable to locate the toilet (Swaffield 1996). Finding the correct receptacle may also be a problem: the demented patient may confuse washbasins with urinals. To locate a toilet, a person needs to be able to follow a signed route, which can be difficult in dim corridors or if the person is blind or partially sighted. The sign also needs to be recognizable, because notices in small print or the modern stylized pictures may not be obvious to the disorientated. A sign only saying 'toilets' is also unsuitable, causing discomfort to people who fear sharing facilities with the opposite sex. People may have to ask for the toilet, which can be embarrassing for some, but very difficult for clients with communication problems due to physical illness (e.g. stroke) or mental illness (e.g. depression).

The ability to reach the toilet is essential and clients with problems like stiff joints or poor balance may find this difficult. In addition this effort may tire them, resulting in an incontinent episode before they reach the toilet (Norton 1996). Obstacles en route such as stairs, narrow passages, sharp corners, loose mats and heavy doors can also hamper the journey to the toilet. Memory loss causes problems as the client may forget what their goal is after setting out to go to the toilet and wander around until it is too late (Stokes 1987). On reaching the toilet itself the client needs dexterity to remove clothing before eliminating; inappropriate clothing may slow the client so much that they may begin to void or defaecate too soon and incontinence may occur (Fader & Norton 1994). To complete the toileting sequence a person must be able to squat, or for men have the stability to stand to urinate, and this may cause problems for the disabled.

Ageing

Any of the general physiological factors discussed above may be a problem for the elderly, but they are not inevitable (Brocklehurst 1984). The ageing process may affect continence in many other ways and the following factors are some of the important ones.

- Circulatory changes and kidney deterioration mean that urine production is less efficient; this results in larger amounts of urine being produced during the night, 35% of the 24-hour volume as opposed to 20% in younger adults (Weiss & Blaivas 2000).

- Hormonal change in that the amount of oestrogen circulating in a woman's body decreases. As a result, the soft convoluted tissue of the vagina and urethra become less elastic with less pronounced folds, resulting in the loss of the watertight seal in the urethra. This deficiency also causes the pelvic floor muscle tone to become lax, and may lead to stress incontinence (Bidmead & Cardosa 1998). Antidiuretic hormone also decreases at night; this may cause nocturnal polyuria (Mattiasson 1999).
- The elderly man has a tendency towards prostatic enlargement and therefore overflow incontinence (Fillingham & Douglas 1997).
- The muscle tone of the bladder can become more lax, the bladder may not empty completely so that a residual volume builds up in the bladder (Hald & Horn 1998).
- Deterioration of nerves occurs so that the sensation of bladder fullness becomes less acute, and the older person will feel the urge to urinate when the bladder is 90% full, and not 50%, as in the younger person. There is also a tendency towards an overactive bladder in the elderly due to neural changes (Hald & Horn 1998).
- The immunological system becomes less efficient thus increasing the incidence of infections (Herbert 1991). This coupled with a residual volume of urine in the bladder increases the likelihood of urinary tract infections. Roe & Williams (1994) list infections as one of the factors that can cause transient incontinence in the elderly.

In summary, often continence difficulties in the elderly are multifactorial; for example, nocturia may be due to less efficient urine production, decreased antidiuretic hormone, less elastic bladder, increased bladder spasm or a combination of all of these (Fonda 1999).

PSYCHOSOCIAL

DEVELOPMENT OF CONTROL

To acquire continence the child needs to develop physically, mentally and socially. During the first 18 months of life bladder emptying is purely a reflex action. The child then becomes aware of the urge sensation of passing urine and wanting to defaecate, associating this with feeling wet or soiled. The ability to control the bladder and anal sphincters, also the pelvic floor is developed (Dobson 1996). The sequence of developing control of elimination is normally bowel control when asleep, followed by the child being clean during the day, then the child gaining urinary continence during the day and finally becoming dry at night (Rogers 1995). The child can be as old as 5 years prior to gaining full control (Blackwell 1989). There are other skills that a child needs to gain to become successfully toilet trained: gross motor skills of sitting and walking, the fine motor skills involved in dressing and undressing, and the ability to sit on the 'potty' for a few minutes (Dobson 1996). Communication skills to alert their parent or carer that they need to go to the toilet are essential (Wong 1993). For children with special needs, this signal may be a non-verbal cue or a type of behaviour. In a survey of two special schools, Bliss & Watson (1992) found if a child could communicate in some way they had a greater chance of being continent. Social skills include knowing where the action should take place (Lukeman 2003).

All these factors must be mastered to make 'potty training' successful. When the child has developed these diverse skills and is interested in using the toilet, they are ready for toilet training. Time should be given by the parent or carer to help the child get used to the potty or toilet, giving praise and encouragement when the child is successful (Dobson 1996). Toilet training takes time and accidents can occur, especially if the child is engrossed in play. This may upset the child and the parent.

Physical problems (illness) and emotional worries (parents' divorce, starting school, etc.) may prolong toilet training, or even cause a child already trained to regress and start wetting again.

Nocturnal enuresis can be defined as involuntary voiding during sleep (Butler 2000a). Children who have never been dry at night are classed as having primary nocturnal enuresis where as those who have been previously dry for 6 months or more are classed as having secondary nocturnal enuresis. Between the ages of 5 and 12, boys are much more

Reflection and portfolio evidence

In 2001 there was a national campaign to improve children's access to fresh drinking water in schools. (A pack on the *Water in Schools* campaign has been produced by ERIC, the Enuresis Resource and Information Centre. See the website: Wateriscoolinschool.org.uk.) This was because small levels of dehydration adversely effect children's health, not only causing urinary problems mentioned in the text but also affecting mental performance in class. Studies showed that the water supplies were often inadequate (one or two drinking fountains per primary school), inaccessible (the tap in the classroom surrounded by paints) or unpalatable (the taps were dirty and the drinking fountains placed in the toilet area).

We have seen throughout this chapter that drinking adequate amounts is essential to prevent urinary tract infections and other continence problems, not only in children but adults as well.

- Through your allocations in hospital, community and in everyday life assess how easy it is to have access to clean drinking water.
- Write up your findings and comment critically on what needs to be done to maintain or improve the current situation.

likely to experience bed-wetting than girls but by adolescence the rates have evened out (Butler 1994).

It is thought that bed-wetting may be multifactorial (Enuresis Resource and Information Centre 2002) arising from the following conditions:

- lack of antidiuretic hormone production at night resulting in high night-time urine production (Medel et al 1998).
- bladder (detrusor) instability which causes bladder spasm and a low bladder capacity which will need emptying at night.
- lack of arousal from sleep; being unable to wake from sleep when the bladder is full (Neveus et al 1999).

There is evidence to suggest that causes of nocturnal enuresis may be hereditary (Eisberg 1995). Harai & Moulden (2000) found a 5-year-old may have a 77% risk of being enuretic if both parents had bed-wetting problems and Norgaard et al (1985) found 60% of children with nocturnal enuresis had a family history of decreased antidiuretic hormone (Butler 2000a).

BEHAVIOURAL FACTORS

Incontinence in an individual cannot always be explained by physical factors alone (Norton 1996). The emotional and mental state of the individual, along with his or her attitude, will also have a bearing on the problem. In children, regression may occur when a sibling is born, while in an adult the beginning of continence problems can sometimes be traced to emotional traumas, for example bereavement, rejection or moving to a new place (Stokes 1987). Many people become incontinent on admission to residential care or soon after, and this may be related to the loss of independence and personal responsibility and a decreasing sense of self-worth.

Incontinence may be an expression of anger, as one of the few weapons available to the individual against his or her carers, not only getting their own back, but also gaining attention. In some cases, incontinence can become rewarding since it gains attention and creates fuss, especially in understaffed institutions where a one-to-one relationship is only available during toileting or when an incontinence episode occurs.

Continence is an acquired habit, and the motivation to be continent can be diminished in the apathetic or confused elderly person; for example, if a toilet is cold, unpleasant or a distance away, the call to micturate or defaecate may be ignored. Confused or demented people are very dependent upon familiar stimuli in order to maintain their activities. Most people have a lifetime of conditioned reflexes to pass urine while seated with no clothing over the genital areas on a toilet in privacy and with the sensation of a full bladder. If an individual is taken to the toilet or sat in a chair with a bare bottom on an underpad, confused messages are given as to where and when urine should be passed and may cause urination in inappropriate places.

Reflection and portfolio evidence

Most wards and units have staff toilets and patient toilets.

- Comment on why do you think this is so.
- List what makes a toilet acceptable to you.
- During your allocations reflect on what makes the patient toilet unacceptable to you.
- If the patient toilet is unacceptable to you, reflect on how an ill or frail person must feel using it.
- Discuss and record how we can make toilets acceptable to all individuals in the ward.

STIGMA AND INCONTINENCE

Eliminating both urine and stool are very personal functions of the human body and one of the few things we do alone. We tend to be embarrassed about it, using euphemisms for passing urine and defaecating. The definition of incontinence is 'lacking restraint or unable to retain control; unable to control excreta' (*Concise Oxford English Dictionary* 1978), a definition that implies clients with elimination difficulties are unclean and lax.

It was during the Victorian era that it was realized that poor sewage facilities and bad hygiene led to the spread of disease. The water closet was developed, giving a definite area for eliminating, and a system created to remove this waste from living areas. General standards of hygiene were improved and at the same time strict rules on self-discipline and sexual conduct were expected. The smell caused by wetting and soiling went against the Victorian ideal that cleanliness is next to godliness. Therefore during the Victorian era to admit to incontinence was a great social stigma. The elderly patients we nurse today will have been raised by parents who were born in the Victorian times and who will have instilled in them their values. Many myths are found around continence; for example, having children causes incontinence, and incontinence is an inevitable part of ageing. Thus incontinence is not be mentioned in the public arena and clients expect to suffer in silence with no hope of cure.

Passive acceptance coupled with extreme embarrassment means people often cope by adapting their lifestyle to hide their incontinence by not going out with friends or to social functions and giving up playing sport. Outings by bus or car can be an ordeal because of worrying about being able to get to a toilet when needed, and staying overnight with friends can be out of the question in case of wetting beds or furniture. This shame may go further than leading to social restriction and affect the individual's relationship with those closest to them. Some people find telling their spouses that they are incontinent is impossible. The guilt, shame, frustration and feelings of the hopelessness of a situation that does not seem to have a solution can then lead to depression. Therefore a problem that appears to be physical can cause severe social and psychological problems.

The sexuality of the individual is also affected by incontinence. There is a high correlation with impotence, and it has been shown that stress incontinence is associated with sexual dysfunction among middle-aged women (Association for Continence Advice 1995). The feeling of being unclean or smelly, and perhaps wearing incontinent aids will hamper a person's self-image and may cause them to question their sexual attractiveness. Sex is regarded as a private and personal matter and like incontinence is also taboo. Discussing this dual problem needs to be conducted with delicacy. It is important to remember that clients who have to rely on pads or catheters may still wish to have a sex life, and if these are causing problems, help and counselling should be sought from a specialist.

Reflection and portfolio evidence

- List the skills required by a healthy person for voiding or defaecating, from intially recognizing the need to actually passing urine or stool in the toilet and returning to their original activity.
- From this list, identify individuals who may have difficulty with any of these factors due to physical disease or disability, mental health problems or learning disabilities.
- You will notice that different clinical areas need different resources to deal with their clients' toileting needs. When in practice placements observe how nurses use this knowledge in helping clients with their toileting needs.
- Ask those nurses you observe to explain the reasons for their particular actions.
- Record your learning in your portfolio.

CARE DELIVERY KNOWLEDGE

ASSESSMENT OF URINARY INCONTINENCE

Care pathways are vehicles for planning care and these are being developed in continence care (Fig. 18.12). Bayliss et al (2000) suggest that good care pathways will direct health professionals with insufficient knowledge of continence promotion to provide quality care for clients with elimination difficulties. Care pathways develop a process of patient focused care which specifies tests and assessment to produce suitable outcomes for care within the limits of available resources (Wilson 1992). Each individual has a right to a full continence assessment and appropriate care (Association for Continence Advice 1993). Understanding the principles behind the assessment and interventions, the nurse can ensure the pathway is suitable for each individual.

Accurate assessment of the individual with incontinence is essential to ensure that the reason for incontinence is found so a pathway with suitable interventions where there is an identified need for medical referral can be followed (see Fig. 18.12 care pathway). Ideally the assessment will be multidisciplinary, involving doctors, nurses, physiotherapists and occupational therapists (Association for Continence Advice 1993).

When assessing and caring for a client with elimination difficulties nurses need to understand how the client and carer feel, and also to be aware of their own feelings towards the situation, so that negative attitudes are not transferred from the assessor to the client. The environment where the assessment takes place should be private and provide a relaxed atmosphere. It should not be done in a rush, making the client feel uncomfortable and the nurse should always use mutually understood terminology. The assessment should be holistic to include the influencing and functional factors of incontinence as well as the urinary symptoms and specific physical examination.

Holistic assessment

A holistic assessment (Table 18.4) is needed to assess if there are any functional problems as correcting these may be all that is needed for the client to regain continence. This should be followed by an in-depth assessment of any elimination difficulties found.

Assessment of urinary problems

The assessment should cover:

- Urinary symptoms
- Baseline chart
- Urinalysis
- Post-void residual volume
- Vaginal examination
- Rectal examination.

Urinary symptoms

It is important to gain the client's perspective in order to determine the severity of the problem. Wetting a teaspoonful a day into a panty liner may not seem much, but to certain individuals this loss of control can be devastating, both psychologically and socially.

Assessing the bladder symptoms and questioning should establish what type of urinary symptoms the client has. Firstly, an overall picture is needed, for example:

- How often do you pass urine? (frequency)
- How long can you hold following the desire to pass urine? (urgency)
- Do you wet before you reach the toilet? (urge incontinence)
- Is it painful to pass urine? (dysuria)
- Do you wake at night to pass urine? (nocturia)
- Do you strain to pass urine?
- Do you have to wait to start? (hesitancy)
- Do you gush or dribble? (poor stream)

Questions to ask at general assessment
- Do you have to go to the toilet frequently at night (i.e., more than twice)?
- Do you have to go to the toilet frequently during the day (i.e., more than 6–7 times per day)
- Do you have to rush to the toilet?
- Do you leak urine at any time?
- Do you have accidents with your bowel at any time?
- Do you have to take laxatives?

NO identified problems
- Give advice about fluid intake, i.e. 8–10 drinks per day and prevention of constipation

If answer is **YES** to any of these questions, the following assessment **MUST** be undertaken
- Commence continence assessment (see text)
- A baseline chart to be completed for 3 days
- Urinalysis for leucocytes, nitrites, protein, blood, pH, ketones, glucose SG – if **any** of first 4 positive, send midstream specimen urine
- Use bladder scanner to check post-void residual volume
- Assess for constipation
- Check BNF for any medication that may be affecting the bladder

Causes of incontinence
Having completed the assessment form, identify the possible cause of incontinence and plan care appropriately

Stress	Detrusor instability	Outflow obstruction Atonic bladder	Functional
No residual Wetting on exertion	No residual Frequency	Residual Hesitancy wetting (prostate enlargement) Poor stream (prostate enlargement)	Poor mobility Poor dexterity
Poor pelvic floor tone	Urgency, urge incontinence	May have frequency urgency	Clothing
Small wetting episodes	Nocturia Large wet episode	Nocturia Dribbling or large voids Recurrent UTIs	Environment

Stress	Detrusor instability	Outflow obstruction Atonic bladder	Functional/ miscellaneous
Using a diagram, explain normal bladder function; explain cause of bladder problems Advise about fluid intake, i.e. 8–10 drinks per day unless contra-indicated Advise types of drinks, i.e. decaffeinated tea and coffee, cranberry juice, prune juice Advise the prevention of constipation			
Consider:			
Pelvic floor exercises	Pelvic floor exercises (to aid bladder training)	In men, consider prostate enlargement/discuss with GP, otherwise	Consider is environment conducive to continence
Treatment of atrophic vaginitis – local oestrogen	Bladder training	Review medication – not causing incomplete emptying	Discuss with OT undressing, aids, etc. Consider use of urinals, sheaths, etc.
	Consider medication	If residual above 100 mL, discuss double voiding Consider a QSBS	Discuss with physio mobility, transfer, etc.
		If residual over 150 mL, consider intermittent catheterisation	Review medication, i.e. diuretics, e.g. alter timing
Consider referral to continence advisor	Consider referral to continence advisor	Consider referral to continence advisor or urologist	Consider referral to continence advisor

Figure 18.12 Continence care pathway. (With kind permission of Sue Brown, Continence Advisor, Nottingham.)

Table 18.4 Components of a holistic assessment of a client presenting with incontinence

Mobility	Difficulty in walking to or sitting on the toilet
Dexterity	Problems with opening doors or removing clothing
Communication	Problems with sight or hearing, speaking
Diet and fluids	Amount and type of fluid drunk, type of diet especially the amount of fibre eaten (see Ch. 7 on nutrition)
Elimination	The client's view of the problem, constipation history
Sleep	Tiredness may indicate lack of sleep due to nocturia
Psychological	Memory loss, confusion making finding the toilet difficult, behaviour associated with wanting to pass urine, any anxiety or depression caused by the incontinence
Environmental	Information about the toilet facilities at the client's home, location of toilet, up or down stairs, height of toilet, handwashing facilities, privacy
Recreational	To what extent has the problem affected their lives, socially, at work, their family, sexual relationships
Past medical history	Neurological, urological, and gynaecological problems. In women, details of menstrual cycle/menopause, obstetric history: number of children, weight of babies, type of delivery, were forceps used. In men, prostate history

- Does your bladder empty without warning? (decreased sensation)
- Do you leak when you cough or laugh? (stress incontinence)

Charting

To confirm the urinary symptoms, a chart should be filled in, usually by the patient or a carer (Fig. 18.13). The chart is the most useful nursing tool in assessing incontinence as part of a baseline assessment and a record of progress during treatment (Norton 1996). A well-kept chart will show times of voiding and episodes of incontinence. If the bladder capacity is needed the volume of urine is also recorded. The fluid intake may also need monitoring if the nurse needs to assess whether the client is drinking enough and has a balanced input and output.

Urinalysis

A specimen of urine should be taken for testing. If this shows protein or blood, infection may be indicated which might be exacerbating the urinary problems, in which case a specimen should be sent for culture and sensitivity. If the urine testing sticks are able to identify nitrates then the presence of infection is 90% certain; if no nitrates are present there is no infection (Evans 1990).

Residual volume

A post-void residual volume of urine should be determined using an ultrasound scanner (Addison 2000) or by intermittent catheterization. The post-void residual volume must be determined on initial assessment as the symptoms of a client with an increased residual volume may mimic the symptoms of detrusor muscle instability. If there is a residual volume and inappropriate treatment is commenced, e.g. drug therapy for bladder spasm, this may cause the volume to become greater and eventually cause hydronephrosis and severe kidney damage (Fillingham & Douglas 1997).

Physical examination

A nursing assessment should include a physical examination of the client, but the nurse must remember that the patient may find this embarrassing. The perineal area should be examined for signs of infection, prolapse, vaginitis and urethritis. A vaginal examination may need to be done by an experienced nurse if stress incontinence is suspected so the strength of the pelvic floor can be assessed and the ability of the client to identify her pelvic floor muscles (Bump et al 1991).

A digital examination of the rectum may be necessary to diagnose if a man has prostate enlargement; again this should only be done by a nurse specialist or a doctor (Addison 1995).

PROMOTING URINARY CONTINENCE

Once you have completed your assessment you should be able to use the information to identify the specific causes of the client's incontinence (see Fig. 18.12, Care Pathway). If you follow the pathway you will see that it indicates general nursing interventions that will benefit the client whatever their problem, followed by the specific treatment for each type of incontinence.

BLADDER CHART
showing stress incontinence
Week commencing: 05/04/03   Name: A. Smith

> Please tick in the **plain** column each time you pass urine

> Please tick in the **shaded** column each time you are wet

Special instructions : Chart for 1 week. Please measure the amount of urine passed.
Please state if wet on exertion with an E, e.g. getting out of bed, coughing, laughing, lifting, etc.

	Monday		Tuesday		Wednesday		Thursday		Friday		Saturday		Sunday	
Midnight													150	✓E
1a.m.														
2														
3														
4														
5														
6														
7	550	✓E	500	✓E			500	✓E	550					
8					600	✓E								
9										✓E				
10				✓E	300		250	✓E	300		600	✓E	500	✓E
11	300				300									
Noon								✓E				✓E	200	✓E
1p.m.			350	✓E	200				300		300			
2							350			✓E			300	
3	300													
4		✓E			200			✓E			300	✓E		✓E
5			300			✓E	300							✓E
6					200				300		350			
7		✓E		✓E				✓E				✓E		
8	450						300				450		200	
9									150	✓E				✓E
10	200		450	✓E	300	✓E	150	✓E						✓E
11									300	✓E	200		250	✓E
Totals	5	4	5	4	6	4	6	5	4			5	7	7

BLADDER CHART
showing possible overactive bladder
Week commencing: 05/04/03   Name: A. Smith

> Please tick in the **plain** column each time you pass urine

> Please tick in the **shaded** column each time you are wet

Special instructions: Chart for 5 days. Please measure the amount of urine passed.

	Monday		Tuesday		Wednesday		Thursday		Friday		Saturday		Sunday	
Midnight	50		50		50									
1a.m.							100		50					
2	100				50									
3			50						50					
4					50		100							
5			100						50					
6	300	✓												
7	100		100	✓	200	✓	150		200	✓				
8			50		50		50	✓						
9	100								50					
10	50	✓	50		100		50		50	✓				
11	50				50	✓	50	✓						
Noon			100	✓			50		30	✓				
1p.m.	50		80						50					
2	40		100		30	✓	100		100					
3	30	✓	40	✓			30	✓						
4														
5	100	✓	60		100		50		30	✓				
6	50		30	✓	50		30	✓	40	✓				
7														
8			100		50	✓	100		60					
9	100	✓			50				50	✓				
10	60		100	✓			150							
11			50		50	✓	100							
Totals	14	5	13	5		4	14	5	14	6				

Figure 18.13   Charting.

General nursing interventions

Information

If the client understands their problem the reasons for the treatments will be clear and their compliance and motivation should improve.

Fluid intake

Ensuring suitable fluid intake is important for a healthy bladder. This should be around 1500 mL a day for an adult. Abrams & Klevmar (1996) suggest this is dependent on weight, e.g. a client weighing 57 kg (9 stone) needs 6 mugs of fluid (1750 mL) while a client of 68 kg (11 stone) needs 7–8 mugs (2200 mL). This ensures that the bladder is expanded and the urine is not concentrated. Drinks that cause bladder spasm, e.g. alcohol or caffeine, should be avoided (Creighton & Stanton 1990). This intervention is particularly important for clients with an overactive bladder, and improvements in the clients' symptoms are often seen following this simple treatment (Dolman 2003).

Prevention of constipation

The pressure on the bladder and urethra will cause differing urinary problems, for example bladder spasm due to irritation caused by a rectum filled with hard stool. The nursing intervention will be discussed later.

Specific nursing interventions

Stress incontinence

The first line of treatment for women with genuine stress incontinence should be conservative and starts with strengthening the pelvic floor (Bo & Talseth 1994). The pelvic floor exercises regime should be individualized depending on the client's pelvic floor tone found on vaginal examination. Bo & Talseth (1994) demonstrated that patients with these individual programmes had a much greater cure rate.

If little or no pelvic floor tone is found on vaginal examination referral to a continence advisor or physiotherapist for electrostimulation may be beneficial. This technique involves a vaginal probe which is used to pass electrical impulses through the pelvic floor. These excite the motor and sensory nerve fibres to produce muscle contraction, leading to strengthening of the pelvic floor (Dolman 2000).

Pelvic floor exercises may take weeks before real improvements show, so motivating the client is important. Biofeedback monitors the pelvic floor strength giving feedback of progress to the client. This can be done by measuring the pelvic floor squeeze regularly with a vaginal probe that measures pressure (periometer). This is used on its own or as part of a computer assisted biofeedback machine (Smith & Newman 1994).

Reflection and portfolio evidence

This exercise for private work is physical, rather than the reflection in most such exercises.

Using the anatomy and physiology information discussed earlier, locate the pelvic floor.

- Identify the pelvic floor muscles around the anus by imagining you are holding back flatulence. You should be able to use these muscles without clenching your buttocks, sitting, lying, or standing, in fact anywhere.
- Repeat the previous action by imagining you need to pass urine, but you are in an inappropriate place: feel the muscles that inhibit this action.
- A typical regimen used for continence promotion could be to tighten the muscles around the vagina and anal sphincter, hold for a count of 5–10, then slowly release; repeat four times regularly throughout the day. This exercise is for 'slow twitch' (support) muscles of the pelvic floor. Fast tightenings (tighten and release immediately) are also needed to exercise the 'fast twitch' muscles.

Bayliss (1996:137–139) gives a detailed explanation of these exercises.

Research has shown that in motivated women, with no obvious prolapse, experiencing small to moderate leakage of urine, there is an 80% success rate using pelvic floor exercises (Norton 1996). Pelvic floor exercises can also be used for men following prostate surgery (Roe & Williams 1994). Men can check that they are using the correct muscles by cupping a hand under the scrotum while exercising: the scrotal sac will rise and fall slightly with each contraction.

Another way of improving the pelvic floor tone is using a vaginal cone. These are weights, the size of a tampon. Once in place, the pelvic floor contracts automatically to hold them. These should be held in place for 10–15 minutes; once this is achieved the weight of the cone is increased and the woman will aim to hold this in place. The increasing weights will strengthen the muscle tone.

Oestrogen therapy can be used in menopausal and postmenopausal women to help stress incontinence. It is thought to increase the activity of the alpha receptors found in the lower bladder and allows sphincters to work more effectively and prevent leaking (Miodrag et al 1988). Oestrogen is also used to treat symptoms of urgency and frequency (Drug and Therapeutic Bulletin 1999). Research for both uses are inconclusive (Cardosa et al 2000); however, topical oestrogen cream is effective for older women with atrophic vaginitis and urethritis, where urinary leakage may be a problem (Fonda 1999).

Evidence based practice

Chiarelli & Cockburn (2002) conducted a randomized controlled trial of 676 women who had experienced traumatic childbirth, e.g. forceps delivery, a large baby or long labour. They were put in two groups: one group had normal postnatal care while the other group were seen by a physiotherapist, taught pelvic floor exercises and followed up at home. The second group showed a greatly reduced prevalence of urinary incontinence.

Overactive bladder

The main choices for treatment of the overactive bladder are bladder retraining or medication. However, the appropriate fluid intake should be encourage from the outset.

Evidence based practice

Bryant et al (2002) built on the work done by Creighton & Stanton (1991) and looked at the effect of caffeine on the bladder. Using a randomized control trial of 95 clients with symptoms of an overactive bladder they were able to show a 57% reduction in urgency and frequency when their caffeine intake was reduced.

Bladder training The principles of bladder training are based on suppressing the urinary urge and extending the intervals between voiding to re-establish a normal pattern. There are different ways of doing this. Firstly, encourage the patient to hold on between voids and gradually increase the time intervals (Anders 1999). Secondly, provide a toileting regime giving specific times of voiding; again the time intervals are increased. Finally, use the techniques of habit training and prompted voiding, which are regimes particularly useful for confused clients (discussed later). Bladder retraining may take a long time and the nurse needs to be supportive through this process.

Table 18.5   Drug treatment for incontinence

Drug	Dose	Side effects
For detrusor instability *Anticholinergic (antagonizes the parasympathetic action decreasing bladder spasm)* (NB Antispasmodics should not be given to client with or a history of glaucoma)		
Oxybutynin (Cystrin, Ditropan)	2.5–5.0 mg bd–tds Start with minimum dose for the elderly For children 5 years and above 2.5 mg bd	Dry mouth with foul taste Constipation
Slow release oxybutynin (Ditropan XL)	Start with 5 mg daily, increase 5 mg per week up to 30 mg daily	As above but less of a dry mouth
Tolterodine (Detrusitol)	2 mg bd, 1 mg in liver failure	More bladder specific anticholinergic Similar side effects, less of a dry mouth
Trospium chlorine (Regurin)	20 mg bd	As above
Anticholinergic and calcium antagonist (prevents the uptake of calcium by muscle thus reducing muscle spasm)		
Propiverine (Detrunorm)	15–30 mg bd or tds low dose for the elderly	As oxybutynin
Tricyclic (prevents reuptake of noradrenaline (norepinephrine))		
Imipramine	50–75 mg nocte For nocturnal enuresis only use for 3 months at a time, rarely used for children now	Dry mouth Blurred vision Postural hypotension
Synthetic antidiuretic hormone		
Desmopressin	20–40 µg nasally	Do not use if client has water retention
Desmotabs	200–400 µg nocte	Do not use if client has water retention
For outflow incontinence *Alpha blockers (block action of noradrenaline (norepinephrine) to relax smooth muscle in the prostatic urethra)*		
Indoramin	20 mg nocte to 20 mg bd	Headache Drops blood pressure
Tamsulosin	0.4 mg daily	Minimal as drug is prostate specific
5 Alpha reductase inhibitors (androgen deprivation, shrinks benign hyperplastic tissue of prostate)		
Finasteride	5 mg daily	Decreased libido

Drug therapy   Detrusor instability is one cause of incontinence that maybe helped with drug therapy. In a literature review, Kennedy (1992) found that the success rate of a combination of bladder retraining and drug therapy was acceptable, but Burgio (1998) found that the elderly benefit less from drug therapy and that bladder retraining should be well established before medication is introduced. The aim of drug therapy is to decrease bladder spasms and thus urgency and frequency. Anticholinergic drugs, for example oxybutynin, antagonize the parasympathetic neurotransmitter acetylcholine, decreasing its action of bladder emptying. Tricyclic drugs, such as imipramine, have the action of prolonging the action of the sympathetic neurotransmitter noradrenaline (norepinephrine), allowing the bladder to relax (Table 18.5) (Drug and Therapeutic Bulletin 1999).

Voiding difficulties

Although outflow obstruction and detrusor hypotrophy show similar symptoms the underlying causes will eventually need different approaches to treatment.

Outflow obstruction   A client with an enlarged prostate gland will probably need it removed eventually; however, until such time, drug therapy can be used to improve the problem by relaxing the prostatic urethra. Alpha blockers, for example indoramin, will block the noradrenaline sites which activate the sympathetic nerves and thus relax the smooth muscle of the prostatic urethra thus sphincter, reducing resistance to the urine flow. Finasteride (5 alpha reductase) can also be used as this antagonizes testosterone, a hormone which encourages prostate enlargement.

Detrusor hypotrophy (atonic bladder)

- Double voiding. This is when the client voids, then stands up and sits down again to urinate; this technique helps to empty the bladder completely.
- Queens Square stimulator. This is a hand-held vibrating device which if put on the abdomen over the bladder may trigger a bladder contraction and initate voiding (Dasgupta et al 1997).
- Intermittent catheterization. This is the treatment of choice for residual volumes (Barton 2000), although on rare occasions an indwelling catheter may need to be used (see discussion in managing incontinence).

The final column in the Care Pathway (Fig. 18.12) suggests ways of overcoming functional incontinence; these you will be able to follow using the overall information of the chapter.

Promoting continence without treatments

Although the Care Pathway (Fig. 18.12) guides the nurse through the main promotion of continence nursing interventions, there are two areas that also need to be explored: (1) how to promote continence in those unable to cope with treatments, i.e. the confused on demented, or the client with learning disabilities, and (2) how to help the child with nocturnal enuresis. These areas will now be discussed.

Toileting programmes

Toileting programmes can be used in areas where incontinence has been found to be related to the behaviour of the client, or for clients who are unable to ask to be taken to the toilet. It is useless to toilet a patient every 2 hours without having a prior knowledge of their voiding habits. For example, a client may require the toilet more often in the morning if he/she has taken diuretic tablets and less during the rest of the day when the effect has worn off. Charting is a very good method of ensuring the correct toileting pattern is found and toileting is carried out at the necessary times. The individual needs to be encouraged to go to the toilet to pass urine either at the same time as they passed urine on the previous days or when they were incontinent of urine. Rigid regimens, such as everyone is toileted after meals, are best reserved for those people, usually the very demented, for whom all efforts at retraining have failed and where incontinence is intractable. In the demented or clients with learning disabilities, communication may be the problem. Charting should be used not only to find out when the client is wet or dry but also if there are any associated behaviour patterns. This allows an individual toileting programme to be written (Stokes 1987). In some cases confused clients may just be unaware they need to go, and regular prompting in line with information from a baseline chart may be the answer (Anders 1999).

Nocturnal enuresis

Children with nocturnal enuresis should be assessed holistically and individually by the multidisciplinary team, so if there are physical problems they can be referred on. As this problem may be multifactoral a thorough assessment of urinary symptoms is needed including a baseline chart, showing fluid input as well as urinary output, bladder capacity, number and type of wet episodes, and urinalysis. From this information, the cause of the problem can be diagnosed and treated (Table 18.6) (Butler 2000b). Throughout all treatments regular reviews should take place to monitor progress and praise for improvement (Enuresis Resource and Information Centre 2002). A positive attitude from the parents is essential to prevent negative feeling being transferred to the child (Dobson 1996). It must be remembered that 2% of adults also suffer from nocturnal enuresis (Ouslander et al 1993) and similar interventions will be needed to help them.

> ### Evidence based practice
>
> Rogers (1998) reported on a national investigation of the difficulties of toilet training for children with Down syndrome. Five thousand questionnaires were sent out and 198 returned. From this 63 girls and 75 boys between the age of 3 and 12 years were included in the study. The results showed a wide range for achieving bladder and bowel control. Some became toilet trained at the same age as non-disabled children, while many showed delayed development, becoming continent at the age of 7–8 years. Rogers suggested that an assessment tool should be used for such children, to ensure they were ready for toilet training. This included four areas of development: language, mobility, cognitive development and toilet awareness. The tool is explained in Rogers (1995).

Sines (1996) suggests that parents of a child with learning disabilities begin toilet training at the same time as a normal child despite the fact that the child may be developmentally slow. Rogers (1998) showed this to be the case in her study of toilet training for children with Down syndrome. It is often other factors, for example difficulties in walking, balance and dexterity, that hamper the client gaining continence. The process of normalization and establishing the social role of a client is easier if the client has achieved continence (Boulter 1995). Individual learning programmes can be introduced using the principles of behaviour modification. The programme must be tailored to the client; it needs to be broken into a series of smaller skills with suitable rewards identified for successfully achieving the skill

Table 18.6 The 'Three Systems': signs and symptoms and treatment of choice

Signs	Symptoms	Treatment of choice
Nocturnal polyuria due to lack of ADH (vasopressin)	Wet soon after sleeping Large wet patches Dilute urine Sleep through wetting Dry if wake to go to the toilet	Desmopressin: • can be used long term (Moffat et al 1993) • best response with older children with primary enuresis (Butler 2002) • needs structural withdrawal using reward charts
Low bladder capacity and bladder instability	Urgency Frequent small voids during day Varying sizes of wet patches Wet more than once a night Wake during or immediately after voiding	Encourage regular intake (6–7 cups a day) avoiding fizzy drinks and caffeine (Enuresis Resource and Information Centre 2002) Regular voiding through the day (6–7 times) Avoid delaying going to the toilet Medication: oxybutynin (Neveus 2001) Relax
Inability to arouse from sleep	Sleep through wetting Difficult to wake even in response to loud noises	Alarms (sensor paced in child's pyjamas or on the bed, this is attached to an alarm and will make a noise when urine wets the sensor) (Butler 2001)

(Smith & Smith 2003). Full involvement of the clients, their carers and key workers ensures a consistent approach to the plan (Boulter 1995).

ASSESSMENT OF FAECAL INCONTINENCE

This assessment will follow a similar pattern to that discussed for urinary incontinence, especially the questions relating to mobility, environment, dexterity, psychological factors, fluid intake and diet. Those areas that differ are discussed below.

Main complaint

The following key issues are important:

- Discover what term the client uses for defaecation, and also what he or she understands by diarrhoea and constipation. People vary enormously in what they consider as a normal bowel action, both in terms of frequency and consistency (Edwards et al 2003).
- The client's normal defaecation pattern should be noted: the frequency of passing stool, at what time of day and if

there are any associated habits (e.g. reading the newspaper, smoking a cigarette).
- The client's perspective of the problem.

Defaecation history

This needs to include:

- using the Bristol Stool Scale (Fig. 18.10) ask the patient to identify which is their type and consistency of stool
- amount
- ease of passing stool
- whether the client gets rectal sensation of the need to defaecate
- whether the client needs to strain or has pain on passing faeces
- whether the client has noted any differences in the stool such as a change in colour or consistency or in the normal eliminating pattern (a black stool indicates gastrointestinal bleeding, pale stool indicates bilary problems, excess pus or mucus indicates inflammation, for example ulcerative colitis or Crohn disease, altered bowel function may be due to a tumour).

Faecal incontinence history

This needs to include:

- a description of how bad the incontinence is (staining, light soiling, liquid stool, etc.)
- how often the incontinence occurs
- whether the client is aware that it is happening
- whether the incontinence is due to urgency, and not being able to reach the toilet in time
- any foods that may cause constipation, diarrhoea, wind or stomach cramps.

Medication history

A list of the client's drugs should be made as they may be responsible for constipation or diarrhoea. For example opiates taken for pain will cause constipation. Record any drugs taken for a bowel problem such as laxatives; the assessor should note whether there is any laxative abuse as the colon may have become resistant to their effect or even atonic (Curry 1992).

Physical examination

The perineum should be observed for signs of prolapse or haemorrhoids. A rectal examination, by an experienced nurse, will show if the rectum is empty or full of hard soft or loose stool. This nursing assessment will give a good picture of the problem and following the doctor's examination can be used to plan the management of the client. A good example of an assessment chart summarizing the above points can be found in Irvine (1996).

The commonest causes of soiling in children is constipation with faecal loading, leading to overflow (Bracey 2002). A similar in-depth assessment needs to be performed, especially in respect of the diet, but the causes may be more complex including psychological problems and difficulties within the family.

MANAGEMENT OF FAECAL INCONTINENCE

If the incontinence is due to impaction of faeces, the aim of treatment is twofold: firstly, to empty the rectum and colon; secondly, to avoid constipation and keep the rectum empty (Roe & Williams 1994).

If the impaction is due to hard faeces, the rectum should be empted from below by giving daily enemas, either phosphate or micro-enemas. Softener laxatives (Table 18.7) may be prescribed to treat the impaction from above. If the impaction is soft then any softening agent will give very loose stools and exacerbate the incontinence, so a micro-enema should be used with a stimulant laxative if necessary (Barrett 1992). If the impaction is great, sodium picosulphate, a strong stimulant laxative, or manual evacuation may be suggested, as a last resort. There are serious risks associated with manual evacuation, for example stimulation of the vagus nerve causing dysrhythmias, and perforation of the colonic wall (Addison 1995). Recently the development of a laxative with polyethylene glycol as a component has been developed; this is reported to clear faecal impaction using a high oral dose (Medicines Resource Centre 1999, Ungar 2000) and may eventually reduce the need for invasive treatments.

Simple improvement to a client's lifestyle may be enough to keep the bowel empty. The nurse has an important role in educating the patient in good dietary habits, including an intake of sufficient roughage (Edwards et al (2003)

recommend 30 g daily) and a good fluid intake, e.g. 2000 mL per day (Norton 1996). Bracey (2002) suggests that a child's fibre intake should be equal to age +5 in grams and the fluid intake is calculated by weight as follows:

- 1–3 years: 95 mL per kg
- 4–6 years: 85 mL per kg
- 7–10 years: 75 mL per kg
- 11–14 years: 55 mL per kg.

Too much bran should not be eaten without a good fluid intake as this may increase faecal loading in the elderly (Ardron & Main 1990). The ways in which the client could increase their exercise can be discussed. If these changes are not enough for a client prone to constipation to produce a regular motion, then a suitable laxative may be needed (see Table 18.7).

Those people who are unable to identify when their rectum is full, i.e. those with spinal injuries or demented clients, are managed by planned constipation and evacuation. Constipation is drug induced using codeine phosphate or loperamide, and the bowel is then evacuated by laxatives or enemas.

Restoring the anorectal angle to improve incontinence can be a more difficult problem, and surgery may be needed. Strengthening of the puborectalis and thus the anal sphincters can be done by pelvic floor exercises concentrating on the anal area (Edwards et al 2003). Electrical stimulation can also help (Barrett 1992). If diarrhoea is causing incontinence, this can be treated by drugs, if investigations show this is appropriate (Table 18.7).

For both urinary and faecal incontinence it must be remembered that very simple actions like being near to a toilet, a suitably placed commode, or an adapted bedpan or bottle and clothes that are easily removed can promote continence in clients where the problem is functional.

Table 18.7 Drug therapy for faecal incontinence: (a) in treating constipation and (b) in treating diarrhoea

Name	Dose	Starts working after	Action	Side effects and contraindications
(a) Constipation treatments				
Osmotic laxative				
Lactulose	10–15 mL bd children 5–10 years 5 g bd	Up to 2 days	It attracts water as it passes through the gut, softening the stool	Nausea and vomiting and problems with flatus
Fletchers' phosphate enema	1 × 128 mL enema	30 minutes	Increases water content causing rectal distension which stimulates motility	Local irritation; avoid long-term use; contraindicated in Hirschsprung disease
Micro-enemas (sodium citrate), e.g. Micolette, Micralax, Relaxit		30 minutes	Allows water to penetrate and soften the stool thus stimulating defaecation	Local irritation; avoid long-term use contraindicated in inflammatory bowel disease
Movicol	1–3 sachets daily 8 sachets in 1 litre daily for faecal impaction		Isotonic laxative which does not lose water if client is dehydrated	Abdominal distension and nausea; caution in pregnancy, women breast-feeding, cardiac patients, intestinal obstruction; not licensed for children
Stool softeners				
Arachis oil retention enema	Single dose enema		Covers the stool with a hydrophobic coat softening the stool and retaining water; the colon is also lubricated	Made from peanuts; be careful in clients with nut allergy
Stimulant laxative				
Senna	2–4 tablets nightly, children over 6 years half adult dose	24 hours plus	Increases rectal motility, i.e. increases peristalsis	Abdominal cramps; may colour the urine red; do not use in intestinal obstruction
Dantron (Co-danthramer)	1–2 capsules nightly or suspension 5–10 mL at night	6–12 hours	As above	Abdominal cramps; may colour the urine red; may cause cancer thus only use in elderly, or the terminally ill
Docusate sodium	Up to 5 × 100 mg capsules daily in divided doses	24 hours plus	Changes the surface tension of the stool allowing water to enter and soften it; this also has a stimulant effect	Abdominal cramps; do not use over a long period of time, or in intestinal obstruction
Bisacodyl tablets	10 mg nightly	10–12 hours	Increases rectal motility	Abdominal discomfort; avoid prolonged use; do not take at the same time as antacids
Bisacodyl suppositories	10 mg in the morning	20–60 minutes	As above	
Fletchers' Enemette (docusate)	5 ml	20–30 minutes	As above	As above
Picolax (sodium picosulphate)	10 mg sachet	3 hours	as above	Do not use in gastrointestinal obstruction on congestive cardiac failure
Bulking agents				
Bran		Up to 4 days	Attracts water, increasing faecal mass and thus stimulating peristasis	Flatulence, abdominal distension, intestinal obstruction; adequate fluids are essential
Ispaghula husk, e.g. Fybogel	1 sachet bd	As above	As above	As above
Regulan	1 sachet 1–3 times a day, for children over 6 years 1/2 to 1 level 5 mL spoon	As above	As above	As above
(b) Antidiarrhoeal agents				
Codeine phosphate	15–30 mg tds-qds		Stimulates opium receptors to decrease the gastrointestinal transit time	Short-term use only; may produce morphine-like dependence; not recommended for children
Loperamide	2 mg capsules after each loose stool, up to 8 mg max		Synthetic opiate inhibits relaxation of the anal sphincter thus retaining liquid stool	Short-term use only. Do not use in liver disease, inflammatory disease, and children under 12 years

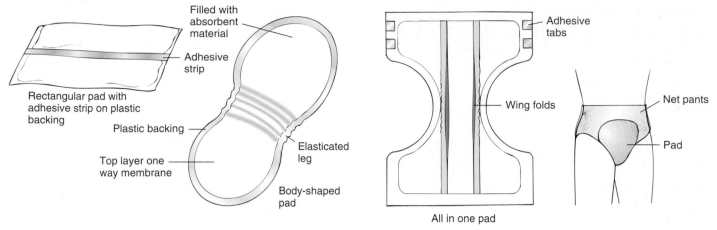

Figure 18.14   Types of disposable body worn pads.

GENERAL MANAGEMENT OF INCONTINENCE

There are clients who despite all efforts to regain continence never achieve it and clients who are too ill or frail to benefit from or indeed manage the treatment programmes recommended. The aim of management should be to ensure that the client keeps their dignity and self-esteem and that the client is socially acceptable by using pads, sheaths or catheters. Aids must prevent leakage of urine, faeces or any smell, be discreet under clothing and be comfortable to wear.

Absorbent products

These fall into three designs:

- body worn pads, all in one or fitted with pants (Fig. 18.14)
- pads built into the gusset of normal style pants
- pads placed on the bed or chair.

All these products may be disposable or reusable (White 1995). There is a range of pads, those absorbing small amounts (up to 80 mL) to suit mild stress incontinence or dribbling to those absorbing large amounts (up to 1000 mL) for heavy incontinence (White 1995).

Pad type depends upon patient preference; some people may prefer the safety of large pads, while others choose a slimmer one because of the appearance. The exact size of the pad is important as if it has too small capacity for the amount of urine passed it will leak, where as using one with a too large capacity is not cost effective. To confirm the capacity an assessment should be done by strict charting or weighing a wet pad (1 g = 1 mL). The client should be using about five pads a day and each pad may need to be of different capacities at different times of day, e.g. a larger one at night.

When applying a pad, the client should empty their bladder, so residual volumes are prevented from being left in the bladder. Pads should be applied from front to back, preventing contamination of the urethra by bowel flora.

The pad should be folded to form a valley shape to channel urine to the absorbent part of the pad.

Reusable pads are environmentally friendly, less bulky than disposables, easier to apply, and can be washed frequently (McKibben 1995). They also look like normal underwear, which is preferred by some clients. However, they are not suitable for faecal incontinence or heavy urinary incontinence.

Disposable underpads or bedpads are possibly one of the least effective and most misused of all items. Disposable pads were designed to protect chairs and beds, and well-applied body worn pads render these redundant.

Sheaths

Men, in preference to pads, often use sheaths. They are made of latex or silicone in different sizes, according to the diameter of the penis. The sheath is held in place by an adhesive which lines the sheath and is then connected to a drainage bag. Fitting correct sized sheaths is important as a device that is too small can restrict the blood flow to the penis, while one that is too large will fall off when urine is passed. When applying a sheath, space (2–3 cm) must be left between the penis and outflow tube, as this prevents backflow and leaking (Pomfret 1996). This type of aid can be used continually or intermittently and is suitable if the client is sexually active. It is unsuitable for men with a retracted penis, symptomatic urinary tract infection or outflow obstruction.

Catheters

A catheter is a hollow tube used for draining urine. Two types of catheter are used in practice: intermittent and indwelling. An intermittent catheter is a simple plastic tube with inlet holes at the tip and no balloon (a Nélaton catheter). An indwelling catheter is a more flexible tube with a balloon to hold it in place and another lumen to allow the balloon to be inflated (a Foley catheter).

Intermittent catheters

According to O'Hagan (1996), the biggest single advance in the management of neurogenic voiding difficulties has been the introduction of intermittent catheterization. The catheter is introduced periodically into the bladder to remove residual volumes greater than 100 mL in clients experiencing problems of overflow incontinence or recurrent urinary tract infection.

Intermittent catheterization is used in all areas of nursing where patients have problems with residual volumes of urine, for example people with spinal injury or peripheral neuropathy, children with spina bifida, the elderly with hypotonic bladder tendencies and postoperatively.

The frequency of intermittent catheterization will depend on the size of the residual volume of urine found in the bladder. The client with an atonic bladder may need to be catheterized four to six times a day. If the problem is due to a hypoactive detrusor, the client will still be voiding and the residual volume may build up slowly. Catheterization may only be needed two or three times a week just to ensure the detrusor muscle is not over-stretched making it more lax. Bladder volume equals void plus residual volume and should not be more than 500 mL (Winder 1992).

Many clients self-catheterize and for this they need good dexterity, motivation and understanding of the procedure; if they are unable to do it, a carer can be taught.

Evidence based practice

Wyndale & Maes (1990) conducted a follow up of 50 patients; some had begun intermittent self-catheterization 12 years before (the average time was 7 years). It showed that 92% were continent using this method. Although some clients had asymptomatic bacteraemia they did not need treatment. Wyndale & Maes (1990) also postulated from the results that infection rates were lower than clients managed with indwelling catheters.

Bakke et al (1997) studied 170 patients (equal numbers of men and women) to look at the possibility of stricture formation and found none. The average time a client had been completing self-catheterization was 8.8 years. To evaluate the long-term problems with intermittent catheterization it is suggested that these studies should last at least 5 years.

Indwelling catheters

Indwelling (or Foley) catheters may be used for a client with chronic incontinence after all alternative methods of management have been unsuccessful or are inappropriate.

Catheter management

Long-term indwelling catheters can have serious complications; one of the main ones is that the risk of catheter

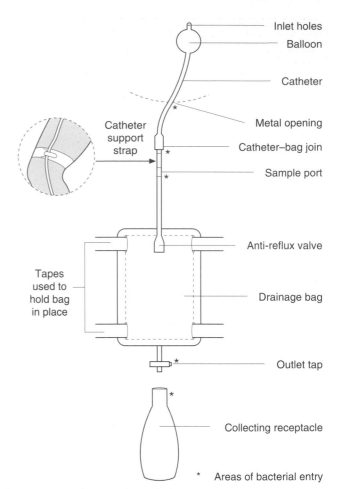

Figure 18.15 Closed urinary drainage system.

associated infection increases 5–8% per day the catheter is *in situ* (Mullhall et al 1988) and thus the care of a client with a catheter is focused on prevention of infection.

It is important to ensure a correct type and size of catheter and a suitable drainage system is chosen (Fig. 18.15). The length of time a catheter will be *in situ* will determine the most appropriate catheter material, i.e. either latex or Teflon-coated latex for short-term catheterization (up to 4 weeks), and silicone or hydrogel-coated for long-term catheterization (12 weeks) (Getliffe 2003).

Catheters come in two lengths: 25 cm for women and 45 cm for men, and with differing diameters, which are measured in Charrières (ch) (0.3 mm = 1 ch). Size 10–12 ch should be used for female clients, 12–14 ch for males and 6–10 ch for children. The smallest catheter possible should be used as one that is too large can cause bladder irritability, occlude urethral glands and cause ulceration of the bladder or urethra or strictures (Getliffe 2003). The catheter is held in place by a catheter balloon; due to the drainage eyelets position above the balloon a small residual volume will collect in the bladder. The inflated balloon will sit next to the sensitive trigone and may cause irritation and bladder spasm; thus a 10 mL balloon is used for most adults (Getliffe 2003). A 30 mL

Table 18.8 Some complications of catheterization

Problem	Cause	Action	Reference
Catheter associated infection	Microorganisms introduced by: (a) poor catheterization technique (b) migration between urethra and catheter (c) migration within the closed system by: • break in closed system • poor emptying technique (d) poor fluid intake	Improve aseptic technique Daily metal cleansing using clean water Use specimen port to take urine specimens Change drainage bag every 7 days Empty bag when two-thirds full Wash hands before and after emptying and use clean gloves Empty into disposable receptacle or receptacle that is used for an individual client and can be hot washed Increase to 1500 to 2000 mL a day Introduce cranberry juice as a prevention of urinary tract infection	DoH 2001d Stamm 1991 Wilson 1997a DoH 1990 Winson 1997 Gould 1994 J. Wilson 1997 Avorn et al 1994
Catheter not draining urine	Kink in tubing Drainage bag positioned above bladder Drainage bag too full Inadequate fluid intake Constipation Encrustation/blocked catheter	Check tubing and reposition as necessary Reposition drainage bag below the bladder Empty regularly as per procedure Increase to approx. 10 drinks per day Clear constipation (see text) See below	 Getliffe 2003
Urine bypassing catheter (a) While catheter is still draining (b) When there is no drainage from the catheter	Detrusor spasm due to: • too large a catheter • too large a balloon • concentrated urine Debris Encrustation	Recatheterization with smaller catheter Recatheterization with smaller balloon Increase fluid intake Anticholinergic medication Bladder washouts not recommended Intermittent bladder washouts Change catheter and observe tip for encrustation. If this is an ongoing problem planned catheter changes should be adopted	Getliffe 2003 Wilson 1997b Fillingham & Douglas 1997 Rew 1996 Getliffe 1994
Bladder expelling the catheter	Balloon deflation Detrusor spasm Poor support of drainage system Self-removal by client Inflammation around catheter	Replace catheter Anticholinergic medication Check tapes etc. holding the catheter bag Check for pain and discomfort Remove to allow inflammation to subside, check catheter material	 Getliffe 2003
Haematuria	Trauma Infection	Monitor by observation; if bleeding becomes heavy seek medical advice immediately Urinalysis, urine sample for culture	

balloon should only be used following bladder surgery to minimize bleeding (Fillingham & Douglas 1997).

The natural defences against urinary tract infection include the tightly closed folds of the urethra and the bladder's flushing action caused by regular emptying. The invasive nature of catheterization compromises these defences and infection is an inevitable consequence (Getliffe 2003). The ways in which catheter-associated infection occurs and means of preventing them are shown in Table 18.8.

A major complication in up to 50% of clients with long-term catheters is encrustation (Getliffe 2003). This forms when urine becomes infected with urease-producing microorganisms, e.g. *Proteus mirabilis* or *Staphylococcus aureus*. These organisms produce a biofilm covering the catheter. Their action is to split the urinary urea to release ammonia which in solution makes the urine alkaline. This encourages mineral salts to precipitate, thus encrusting the surface of the catheter (Getliffe 2003). Catheter maintenance solutions may be of benefit for these patients (Table 18.9); however, identifying when the catheter blocks and planning catheter changes accordingly may be the best answer (Getliffe 2003).

Table 18.9 Catheter maintenance solutions (Rew 1996)

Solution	Content	Action
Suby G (pH 4)	3.23% citric acid + magnesium oxide (to decrease tissue irritation)	Reduces encrustation by keeping pH low (acidic)
Solution R (pH 2)	6% citric acid solution + magnesium carbonate	Aims to dissolve encrustation
Mandelic acid (pH2)	Acidic solution	Aims at inhibiting growth of urease producers
Saline	Antiseptic solution	For removing debris and clots only

---

Reflection and portfolio evidence

Sometimes patients are discharged from hospital with little information about their catheter, making ordering difficult for the district nurse. If a client has a long-term catheter and is admitted to hospital similar information is also needed. More worryingly, it sometimes happens that there are clients who have a catheter and the nurse cannot find the reason for it being put in originally. It is then a decision making issue on whether the catheter should be removed or not.

'Thorough documentation is important to ensure patient safety, consistency in delivery of high quality care and effective monitoring' Getliffe (2003: 297).

In your practice placement, check the care plans of your catheterized patients and see what information has been documented.

- Can you see clearly when the catheter is due out, to be changed or to be evaluated?
- Find out the type of catheter: its material, size, length, and its balloon size.
- Find out which drainage system is being used.
- Do you understand the rationale for the client's catheterization?
- Obtain a company name, batch number, expiry date so that you can lodge a complaint if there is a problem with the patient's catheter.
- Write up your experiences with critical commentary and add to your portfolio.

The most suitable drainage system selected for a client using a catheter for incontinence is a body worn drainage bag with a capacity of 350–750 mL, as it will allow more independence (Getliffe 2003). For the dexterous client with good cognitive function, and who does not have uncontrolled

bladder spasm, a catheter valve may be used as an alternative to a leg bag (Getliffe 2003). Tissue damage can be caused by full catheter bags pulling on the catheter if they are not firmly secured to the leg, so a further support in the form of a catheter support strap around the thigh should also be used.

Indwelling catheters can be urethral or suprapubic, with the latter becoming more popular. The suprapubic catheter (usually a Foley type, size 16 ch) is inserted through a small cut in the abdominal wall just above the pubic bone and drains into an ordinary catheter bag (Iacovou 1994). This method is used for clients with urethral problems, those who wish to be sexually active and wheelchair bound individuals who find this site easier when self-caring.

PROFESSIONAL AND ETHICAL KNOWLEDGE

This part of the chapter will give an outline of recent national policies, how they impinge on continence care and the way the future service will become integrated. This should allow you to identify the role that nurses will have as part of a multidisciplinary framework needed to care for clients with elimination problems.

THE CONTINENCE ADVISORY SERVICE

Promoting continence is a relatively new nursing specialty. The first continence advisor was employed in 1974 by the Disabled Living Foundation, and since then the aim of care has moved from coping with the problem to actively promoting continence. Rhodes (1995) found that there was no universal job description for continence advisors, and that the quality of the service provided was patchy. Roles depended on their employers, i.e. advisors were attached to urology services or to the community and might have responsibilities district-wide or for one hospital unit. In 1991 an *Agenda for Action on Continence Services* report (Sanderson 1991) showed good practice in many areas but emphasized the need for a seamless integrated service. A report by the Royal College of Physicians (1995) identified the extent of the problem for all the healthcare professionals, showing that there was a need for a national strategy for continence promotion as opposed to just providing containment products. For this they suggested all members of the multidisciplinary team needed better education. In 1998 a review of the continence service was conducted which showed great geographical differences, e.g. in the number of staff involved in the service, the amount of education and training, the involvement or otherwise of users and carers, and the number of pads provided to clients with similar continence difficulties (Anthony 1998).

The above reviews led to a working group producing the document *Good Practice in Continence Services* (Department of Health 2000) which gave national guidelines on how continence services should be delivered. However, these guidelines were only recommendations, and needed some key government policies to influence the development of the suggested continence strategies. The National Service Framework for Older People (Department of Health 2001a) outlines the importance of continence in Standard Two of the framework. In the same year *Essence of Care* (Department of Health 2001b) was published; this outlines a benchmarking programme which focuses on essential aspects of care. It identifies eight areas of concern of which bladder and bowel care are one. The *Good Practice in Continence Services* (Department of Health 2000) document is aimed at anyone in the general population so that as frameworks for other groups of clients are written and implemented, e.g. *Valuing People: A New Strategy for Learning Disabilities* (Department of Health 2001) and the National Service Framework for Children, these should also influence the use of the continence services guidelines.

The *Good Practice in Continence Services* document (Department of Health 2000) states that continence services should be integrated and work at different levels. Firstly, there should be a level at which staff are responsible for identifying clients with continence difficulties, doing an initial assessment, planning care where appropriate and referring on where necessary. This group of people includes all community nurses and other community health professionals, the staff of residential and nursing homes whether private or public (run by the NHS or Social Services department of local authorities) and hospital nurses. The next tier provides more specialized interventions through continence advisors, specialist nurses both adult and paediatric, physiotherapists, and investigation services; this group will see clients who need further treatments. From here referrals are made to local specialist medical and surgical units and the final tier to be developed will be national centres of excellence.

Evidence based practice

Flemming et al (2000) were concerned about the care and management of catheterized clients in a rehabilitation and long-term care hospital, and the knowledge of the trained staff nursing them. A questionnaire was sent to 60 qualified staff, and 39 were filled in. The questions covered indications of use of catheters, catheter selection, care of the catheter and drainage system and management of problems caused by indwelling catheters. When tabulating the results, the knowledge scores were below what the researchers considered reasonable. The authors concluded that despite promoting evidence based nursing, it was not being embedded in nursing practice and good pre- and postregistration education is essential.

EDUCATION FOR CONTINENCE PROMOTION

The guidance in *Good Practice in Continence Services* expects all nurses and other health professionals to assess and identify clients with continence problems, and to do this successfully the nurse needs the appropriate knowledge and skills. Work by Cheater (1992a) and Palmer (1995) has shown that good-quality care for these clients is hampered by lack of knowledge. Laycock (1995) found that an average of 9.4 hours was devoted to continence in preregistration nursing programmes and much of this was in the clinical area. Thus education is essential for the seamless framework to be successful. In-service training should be developed by NHS Trusts and Primary Care Trusts in the UK (Department of Health 2000). It is recommended that the service provider should work closely with higher education institutes to provide valid educational programmes to both pre- and postregistered nurses that reflect continence care as a specialty.

Education is also deemed important in benchmarking required in the document *Essence of Care* (Department of Health 2001b). For example, good practice benchmark 5 looks at what education assessors and care planners have

---

Reflection and portfolio evidence

The first factor to be benchmarked for the section 'Continence and bladder and bowel care' of *Essence of Care* (Department of Health 2001b: 98) reads 'Information for patients/clients/carers'. And the benchmark of best practice reads:

'Patients/clients/carers have free access to evidence based information about bladder and bowel care that has been adapted to meet individual patient/client needs and/or those of their carer.'

With this in mind, when on placement decide what areas of bladder and bowel care are most essential, for example:

In gynaecological wards or mother and baby units, pelvic floor re-education may be appropriate; in mental health wards where there are depressed patients, there may be a high rate of constipation; in health care of the elderly in hospital and in the community, prevention of urinary tract infections may be important.

- Find out what information there is on the ward.
- If you consider more is needed, think of where you may get more information, e.g. websites, health promotion units.
- Then pick a client and using this information, make it relevant to that individual and help in his/her continence health promotion.
- Add your learning to your portfolio.

received for their role and benchmark 8 is concerned that the carer has been given suitable training to undertake the continence care needed by their charges.

QUALITY ASSURANCE OF CONTINENCE CARE

The *Good Practice in Continence Service* guidelines suggest targets for all areas of the health service and the use of performance indicators and audits to monitor progress. When implemented this should ensure equality of service nationally. In 1998, a survey of provision of continence supplies in 173 NHS Trusts was commissioned by the self-help group Incontact (Continence Foundation 2000). This found no equity between the Trusts. The Department of Health (2000) suggests that no products should be given without assessment and that the type must be determined for appropriateness not cost. The Continence Foundation in 2000 estimated that an average Primary Community Group would spend £737 000 a year on incontinence including drugs, appliances, pads and surgery; however, the biggest cost was staff time. They concluded that large savings could not be made but that the money should be used wisely to ensure quality care.

National integrated services are being commissioned but a survey undertaken by the Royal College of Nursing and the Continence Advisory Service during 2001 and 2002 (Continence Foundation 2002) showed that although work had begun in many places that there is still much to be done.

ETHICAL CONSIDERATIONS

Some areas of continence assessment and care give rise to ethical dilemmas for the nurse. One such area is digital rectal examination and manual evacuation. 'Many nurses are confused about the professional and legal aspects of digital rectal examination and manual evacuation of faeces' (Royal College of Nursing 2000: 1).

The intimate and invasive nature of these procedures make nurses worry that they may be accused of abuse. Recent cases of professional misconduct where inappropriate digital rectal examination and manual evacuations were used with frail elderly people has increased this dilemma (Willis 2000). In the past digital rectal examination and manual evacuation were skills that had to be picked up with experience (Willis 2000). The Royal College of Nursing (2000) guidelines consider there is a need for these procedures, in certain cases, but that they must be carried out by a competent practitioner, who has the knowledge to judge the appropriateness of their action. It is recommended that employers also have procedures in place that will guide and support their employees in this practice. These Royal College of Nursing guidelines identify key issues for the nurse to follow: she/he must have a suitable rationale for using the procedures; and have received instruction and training in performing the technique. Most importantly there needs to be consent of the client to permit the procedure; consent can only be given when the client is in full knowledge of the facts. This will still cause dilemmas in caring for the demented clients who may need this procedure.

Digital rectal examination and manual evacuation are not the only invasive and embarrassing interventions needed to care for a client with continence problems. Vaginal examination and urodynamics investigations are also invasive and compromise the client's dignity, so the same principles of good practice should be followed. Clients should always be fully involved with their care (White & Dolman 2003). The Charter for Continence states that clients have a right to clear explanation of their treatment and full information about available products, and the right to participate fully in the discussions of care. The nurse should take this into account when planning care, making certain that it is what the client wants and not what is the most convenient to the nurse. For example pressures on a busy ward may mean an indwelling catheter instead of regular intermittent catherization is used to save time, or the client who needs a different type of pad or appliance that is not the one supplied by the Trust may cause difficulties. The nurse needs to use the Charter for Continence and the Nursing and Midwifery Council's *Code of Professional Conduct* (Nursing and Midwifery Council 2002) to ensure she/he is providing the best possible continence care.

PERSONAL AND REFLECTIVE KNOWLEDGE

EMPATHY WITH THE INCONTINENT CLIENT

Reflective and decision making exercises have been provided throughout the chapter. By completing these exercises and also keeping a reflective journal of your practice learning, you will build up your knowledge base and expertise, and develop empathy with the incontinent client.

CASE STUDIES IN THE MANAGEMENT OF INCONTINENCE

In this final part of the chapter, case studies are presented with related decision making questions in order for you to consolidate the knowledge you have gained from this chapter and your experiences in the practice setting.

Case study: Adult

Mr Jones is a 70-year-old man who lives with his wife in a semi-detached house in the middle of a small town. He is a retired builder but is still fit and does odd jobs for his neighbours. He is an avid football fan and travels to away matches on the supporters' coach. Recently he has stopped going to matches too far away because he finds he can't always 'last' until he reaches the football ground.

He eats and drinks well, really enjoying a cup of tea and a pint or two at his local two or three nights a week. He has stopped going to the pub recently as he thinks his drinking might be causing him to pass urine so often. His wife wants him to see someone because he is waking her two or three times a night when he gets up to pass urine.

- Using the assessment tool described in the chapter try and identify Mr Jones' problems.
- A frequency/volume chart showed that Mr Jones was passing urine approximately 14 times a day (two to four times were at night) and was drinking six cups of fluid, mostly tea, and only half a pint of beer if he went to the pub.
- What may be the cause of Mr Jones' problem, and what advice would you give him?

Case study: Learning disabilities

Susan is a 26-year-old woman with moderate learning difficulties. She lives in a supervised bungalow and goes out to work each day to a local hotel where she cleans. She is taken there by bus. At the bungalow she is able to make her bed and help in the kitchen making simple meals under supervision.

Susan has had no continence problems since she came to the bungalow 6 years ago, but over the last 6 months she has started to wet once she has got to work.

- List all the reasons you can think of for Susan wetting at work and what assessments you could carry out with her.
- When a baseline chart was completed by the home staff, it showed a good fluid intake of 10 cups of fluid a day but the urinary output was high. What reasons can you give for this pattern? (*Clue:* the staff only charted the drinks they gave Susan)

Case study: Mental health

Mrs Jones is 79 years old, a widow with no family, is mildly demented and lives in a nursing home which specializes in the elderly with mental health problems. She is mobile, drinks well and usually eats a well-balanced diet. Although she tends to wander she is usually amicable.

Lately she has been wandering much more and appears quite agitated. The care assistants report that she is having trouble using the toilet as occasionally her underclothes are damp with urine. This morning she has become very aggressive and appears to be running a temperature.

- Why do you think Mrs Jones is aggressive?
- What do you think is causing her continence difficulties?
- Do you think the two are related?
- What might you find if you do a continence assessment?
- What treatment will Mrs Jones need?
- What ethical issues may this cause?

Case study: Child

Alex is a 4 years old and attends a local primary school every morning; he lives with his mother and older brother John who is 7. His parents split up 18 months ago and his father now lives with a new partner; the brothers stay with father at weekends. The split was acrimonious, and both parents have accused the other of mistreating the boys. The mother finds it difficult to cope in the mornings as she has to drop the children with a childminder early to get to work on time.

The school nurse is concerned as the teaching staff suggest he has a soiling problem. Mother reports that Alex has always had a problem and was prescribed laxatives in the past which he would not take. She also reports that she and John only have their bowels open once a week.

The reception class staff revealed later that Alex has been found on a couple of occasions attempting to open his bowels where he happens to be (he has been seen squatting and straining while playing with other children). They have removed him to the toilets when this has occurred. Mother reveals he still wears nappies at home and has never sat on the toilet to open his bowels.

- What issues, physical, psychological and social, may contribute to Alex's problem?
- List the types of management that may be needed to help Alex.
- What health messages do you need to get over to Alex's mother?

Summary

In order to be an effective decision maker in relation to continence care you need knowledge and skills in continence promotion and the management of incontinence. This chapter has included:

1. An outline of the normal and altered anatomy and physiology of related organs.
2. Information on the psychosocial pressures and the many causes of urinary and faecal incontinence in all age groups.
3. A comprehesive overview of assessment of urinary and faeceal incontinence.
4. Information on promotion of continence and management of incontinence.
5. An outline of current national guidelines on continence care.
6. A review of ethical issues related to continence care.

Annotated further reading and websites

Button D, Roe B, Webb C et al 1998 Continence promotion and management by the primary health care team: consensus guidelines. Whurr, Gateshead

An overview of continence problems with guidelines for suitable interventions for clients of all ages. It gives principles of good practice well backed with evidence.

Cardoza L, Staskin D, Kirby M 2000 Urinary incontinence in primary care. ISIS Medical Media, Oxford
A reference guide covering reasons for incontinence, investigations that are performed, clear interventions for these clients along with tips for care and some coping strategies. It has good clear pictures and diagrams to illustrate key points.

Colburn D 1994 The promotion of continence in adult nursing. Chapman & Hall, London
A good textbook that covers ways of promoting continence and managing incontinence in the adult. Particularly useful for adult branch students.

Getliffe K, Dolman P 2003 Promoting continence, 2nd edn. Baillière Tindall, London
This is a very informative book. A full discussion on catheters and their drainage systems is found in Chapter 9. An in-depth chapter on the elimination problems of the elderly and clients with neurological disabilities is in Chapter 6; Chapter 5 (Mainly children: childhood enuresis and encopresis) is useful for child branch students; and Chapter 10 is useful for nurses from the learning difficulties branch.

Norton C 1996 Nursing for continence, 2nd edn. Beaconsfield Press, Beaconsfield
This book covers most areas of incontinence. There are chapters suitable for child branch (Ch. 5) and learning disabilities branch (Ch. 4) and continence care for people with physical disabilities (Ch. 13), all of which are very readable.

Stokes G 1987 Incontinence and inappropriate urination: common problems with the confused elderly. Winslow Press, Bicester
This book is useful for all nurses who are caring for confused or demented clients, giving an overview of the types of incontinence they may suffer, and offering outlines on managing incontinence.

http://www.bowelcontrol.org.uk
A website provided by St Mark's Hospital giving practical advice for clients and information for professionals.

http://www.eric.org.uk
Site of the Enuresis Resource and Information Centre, where parents and clients can get information on day time wetting, bed-wetting, soiling and constipation. Questions and expert answers displayed.

http://www.continence-foundation.org.uk/
For people with bladder and bowel problems. The Continence Foundation gives information about causes, symptoms, treatments and products. Useful information for professionals.

http://www.incontinencesupport.org
Information for carers, products, information, etc.

Acknowledgements

The author wishes to thank: Sue Brown, senior continence advisor, Nottingham; Fiona Saunders, continence advisor, Mansfield; Ruth Wint, continence advisor (learning disabilities), Mansfield; Jackie Bracey, school nurse; and Anita Counsel, continence nurse specialist.

References

Abrams P, Klevmar K 1996 Frequency volume charts: an indispensable part of lower urinary tract assessment. Scandinavian Journal of Urology and Nephrology (Suppl.) 179:47–53

Addison R 1995 Continence care forum: the role of the nurse in digital rectal examination and manual evacuation. Royal College of Nursing, London

Addison R 2000 A guide to bladder ultra sound. Nursing Times 96(40):14–15

Anders K 1999 Bladder retraining. Professional Nurse 14(5):14–16

Anderson J, Abrams P, Blaivas J G et al 1988 The standardization of terminology of the lower urinary tract function. Scandinavian Journal of Nephrology (Suppl.) 114:5–19

Andrews K, Hussman D 1997 Bladder dysfunction and management in multiple sclerosis. Mayo Clinic Proceedings 72(12):1176–1183

Anthony B 1998 Provision of continence supplies by NHS trusts. Middlesex University, London

Ardron M E, Main A N H 1990 Management of constipation. British Medical Journal 300:1400–1402

Asplund R, Aberg H 1991 Diurnal variations in the levels of antidiuretic hormone in the elderly. Journal of Urology 82 (Suppl.):18–25

Association for Continence Advice 1993 Guidelines for continence care. Association for Continence Advice, London

Association for Continence Advice 1995 Sexuality and incontinence: professional issues. Association for Continence Advice, London

Avorn J, Monane M, Gurwitz J et al 1994 Reduction in bacteriuria and pyuria after ingestion of cranberry juice. Journal of the American Medical Association 271(10):751–754

Bakke A, Digranes A, Hoister P 1997 Physical predictors of infection in patients treated with clean intermittent catheterisation: a prospective 7-year study. British Journal of Urology 79(1):85–90

Barrett J 1992 Faecal incontinence. In: Roe B H (ed) Clinical nursing practice. the promotion and management of continence. Prentice-Hall, Hemel Hempstead, pp 196–219

Barton R 2000 Intermittent self-catheterization. Nursing Standard 15(9):47–52

Bayliss V, Cherry M, Lock R et al 2000 Pathway for continence care: background and audit. British Journal of Nursing 9(9):590–596

Bayliss V 1996 Female urinary incontinence. In: Norton C (ed) Nursing for continence, 2nd edn. Beaconsfield Press, Beaconsfield, pp 123–152

Bendall M J 1989 Faecal incontinence: teaching pack for continence advisors. Wallace, Colchester

Bidmead L, Cardosa L 1998 Pelvic floor changes in older women. British Journal of Urology 82(Suppl.):18–25

Blackwell C 1989 A guide to enuresis UK. Enuresis Resource and Information Centre, London

Bliss J, Watson E 1992 A basis for change. Nursing Times 88(13):69–70

Bo K, Talseth T 1994 Five-year follow up of pelvic floor muscle exercise treatment for stress urinary incontinence: clinical and urodynamic assessment. Neurology and Urodynamics 13(4):374–376

Boulter P 1995 Increasing independence. Nursing Standard 10(4):18–20

Bracey J 2002 Solving children's soiling problems. Churchill Livingstone, Edinburgh

British Medical Association and Royal Pharmaceutical Society of Great Britain 2003 British national formulary, No. 45. British Medical Association, London

Brittain K, Peat S, Castleden C 1998 Stroke and incontinence. Stroke 29(2):524–528

Brocklehurst J C 1984 Urinary incontinence in the elderly. The Practitioner 228:275–282

Bryant C, Dowell C, Fairbrother G 2002 Caffeine reduction education to improve urinary symptoms. British Journal of Nursing 11(8):560–565

Bugio K, Locher J, Goodwin P et al 1998 Behavioural versus drug therapy for urge incontinence in older women: a randomized trial. Journal of the American Medical Association 280(23): 1995–2000

Bump R, Hurt W, Fantl J et al 1991 Assessment of Kegel pelvic floor exercises performed after brief verbal instruction. American Journal of Obstetrics and Gynaecology 165(2):322–329

Butler R 1994 Nocturnal enuresis: the child's experience. Butterworth-Heinemann, London

Butler R 2000a A fresh approach to understanding childhood nocturnal enuresis. Urology News 4(2):29–32

Butler R 2000b The three systems approach. Ferring, London

Butler R 2001 Management of nocturnal enuresis. Current Paediatrics 11:126–129

Butler R, Holland P, Robinson J 2001 An examination of structural withdrawal programme to prevent relapse in nocturnal enuresis. Journal of Urology 166:2463–2466

Cardosa L, Staskin D, Kirby M 2000 Urinary incontinence in primary care. ISIS Medical Media, Oxford

Cheater F M 1992a Nurses' education, preparation and knowledge concerning continence promotion. Journal of Advanced Nursing 17:328–338

Cheater F M 1992b The aetiology of urinary incontinence. In: Roe B (ed) Clinical nursing practice: the promotion and management of continence. Prentice-Hall, Hemel Hempstead, pp 20–40

Chiarelli P, Cockburn J 2002 Promoting urinary continence in women after delivery: a random trial. British Medical Journal 324:71–78

Chiarelli P, Markwell S 1992 Let's get things moving: overcoming constipation. Neen Health Care, Dereham

Colborn D 1994 The promotion of continence in adult nursing. Chapman & Hall, London

Concise Oxford English Dictionary 1978. Clarendon Press, Oxford

Continence Foundation 2000 Making a case for investment in continence services. Continence Foundation, London

Continence Foundation 2002 Good, better and best practice. Continence Foundation, London

Cook T, Mortensen N 1998 Prevention of faecal incontinence of obstetric origin. Trends in Urology, Gynaecology and Sexual Health 3(7):37–40

Creighton S, Stanton S I 1990 Caffeine: does it affect your bladder? Journal of Urology 66:613–614

Curry T 1992 Drugs and constipation: a view from pharmacy. Prescriber May:53–55

Dasgupta P, Haslam C, Goodwin R et al 1997 The Queen's Square stimulator, a device for assisting in emptying a neurogenic bladder. British Journal of Urology 81:234–237

Department of Health 1990 Drug Tariff. HMSO, London

Department of Health 2000 Good practice in continence services. HMSO, London

Department of Health 2001a National Framework for older people. HMSO, London

Department of Health 2001b Essence of care: patient focused benchmarking for healthcare professionals. HMSO, London

Department of Health 2001c Valuing people: a new strategy for learning disabilities. HMSO, London

Department of Health 2001d Guidelines for preventing infections associated with the insertion of short term indwelling urethral catheters in acute care. Journal of Hospital Infection (Suppl.) 47:39–46

Dobson P 1996 Childhood enuresis. In: Norton C (ed) Nursing for continence, 2nd edn. Beaconsfield, Beaconsfield Publishers, pp 102–118

Dolman M 2000 Electro stimulation for urinary incontinence: Levator 100. British Journal of Community Nursing 5(5):294–220

Dolman M 2003 Mostly female. In: Getliffe K, Dolman P (eds) Promoting continence, 2nd edn. Baillière Tindall, London, pp 185–227

Drug and Therapeutic Bulletin Review 1999 Managing incontinence due to detrusor instability. Drug and Therapeutic Bulletin 39(8):59–63

Drug and Therapeutic Bulletin 2000

Edwards C, Dolman M, Horton N 2003 Down, down and away: an overview of adult constipation and faecal incontinence. In: Getliffe K, Dolman P (eds) Promoting continence, 2nd edn. Baillière Tindall, London, pp 185–227

Eisberg H 1995 Assignment of dominant inherited nocturnal enuresis (ENURI) to chromosome 13q. Nature Genetics 10(3):354–356

Enuresis Resource and Information Centre 2002 Bed-wetting: treating the underlying problem. Ferring, London

Evans P 1990 Urinary tract infection in the elderly. In: Newell R, Howell R (eds) Clinical urinalysis. Ames Division Miles Ltd, Stoke Poges, pp 104–108

Fader M, Norton C 1994 Caring for continence: a care assistant's guide. Hawker Press, London

Flemming A, Day J, Glanfield L 2000 Registered nurses' management of urinary catheters in a rehabilitation, long term hospital. International Journal of Nursing Practice 6:237–240

Fillingham S, Douglas J 1997 Urological nursing. Baillière Tindall, London

Fonda D 1999 Nocturia: a disease or normal aging? British Jounal of Urology 84(Suppl. 1):11–13

Fowler C 1996 Bladder dysfunction in multiple sclerosis. Multiple Sclerosis Journal 1(3):99–107

Getliffe K 1994 The characteristics and management of patients with recurrent blockage of long-term urinary catheters. Journal of Advanced Nursing 20:140–145

Getliffe K 2003 Catheters and catheterization. In: Getliffe K, Dolman P (eds) Promoting continence, 2nd edn. Baillière Tindall, London, pp 259–303

Getliffe K, Dolman M 2003 Normal and abnormal bladders. In: Getliffe K, Dolman P (eds) Promoting continence, 2nd edn. Baillière Tindall, London, pp 21–53

Glickman S, Kamm M 1996 Bowel dysfunction in spinal cord injury patterns. Lancet 347:1651–1653

Gould D 1994 Keeping on tract. Nursing Times 90(40):58–64

Hald T, Horn T 1998 The human bladder in ageing. British Journal of Urology 82(Suppl. 1):59–65

Havari M, Moulden A 2000 Nocturnal enuresis: what is happening? Journal of Paediatric and Child Health 36(1):78–81

Herbert R A 1991 The biology of human ageing. In: Redfern S (ed) Nursing elderly people. Churchill Livingstone, Edinburgh, pp 39–66

Hill S 1997 Genuine stress incontinence. In: Cardosa L (ed) Urogynaecology. Churchill Livingstone, Edinburgh

Hinchliff S, Montague S, Watson R (eds) 1996 Physiology for nursing practice, 2nd edn. Baillière Tindall, London

Iacovou J W 1994 Suprapubic catheterization of the urinary bladder. Hospital Update March:159–161

Irvine L 1996 Faecal incontinence. In: Norton C (ed) Nursing for continence, 2nd edn. Beaconsfield Press, Beaconsfield, pp 226–254

Johanson T, Lafferty C 1996 Fecal incontinence. American Journal of Geriatrics 111:1–32

Kennedy A P 1992 Bladder re-education for the promotion of continence. In: Roe B H (ed) Clinical nursing practice: the promotion and management of continence. Prentice-Hall, Hemel Hempstead, pp 77–93

Laycock J 1995 Must do better: survey of continence education in schools of nursing, medicine, physiotherapy and GP training. Nursing Times 91(7):64

Laycock J, Brown J, Cusack C et al 2001 Pelvic floor re-education for stress incontinence: comparing three methods. British Journal of Community Nursing 6(5):230–234

Lewis Wall L 1994 Anatomy and physiology of the pelvic floor. In: Laycock J, Wyndale J L (eds) Understanding the pelvic floor. Neen Health Books, Dereham, pp 35–42

Lukeman D 2003 Mainly children: childhood enuresis. In: Getliffe K, Dolman P (eds) Promoting continence, 2nd edn. Baillière Tindall, London, pp 21–53

McKibben E 1995 Pad use in perspective. Nursing Times 91(24):61–62

Mattiasson A 1999 Nocturia: current knowledge and future directions. British Journal of Urology 84(Suppl. 1):33–35

Medel R, Dieguez S, Brindo M et al 1998 Monosymptomatic primary enuresis: differences between patients responding or not responding to oral desmopressin. British Journal of Urology 81:46–49

Medicines Resource Centre 1999 The management of constipation. MeReC Bulletin 10(9)

Miodrag A, Castleden M, Vallance T 1988 Sex hormones and the urinary tract. Drugs 36:491–504

Mitteness L S 1992 Social aspects of urinary incontinence in the elderly. AORN Journal 56(4):731–737

Moffat M E, Harlos S, Kirshen A J et al 1993 Desmopressin acetate and nocturnal enuresis: how much do we know? Journal of Paediatrics 92(3):420–425

Mulhall A, Chapman R, Crow R 1988 Bacteriuria during indwelling catheterization. Journal of Hospital Infection. 1:253–262

Neveus T 2001 Oxybutynin, desmopressin and enuresis. Journal of Urology 166:1459–2462

Neveus T, Lackgren G, Tuverno T et al 1999 Osmoregulation and desmopressin: pharmcokinetics in enuretic children. Paediatrics 103:65–70

Norgaard J, Pederson E, Djurhua J 1985 Diurnal antidiuretic hormone levels in enuretics. Journal of Urology 134:1029–1031

Norton C (ed) 1996 Nursing for continence, 2nd edn. Beaconsfield Press, Beaconsfield

Nursing and Midwifery Council 2002 Code of Professional Conduct. Nursing and Midwifery Council, London

O'Hagan M 1996 Neurogenic bladder dysfunction. In: Norton C (ed) Nursing for continence, 2nd edn. Beaconsfield Press, Beaconsfield, pp 170–191

Ouslander J, Palmer M, Ravner B et al 1993 Urinary incontinence in nursing homes. Journal of American Geriatrics Society 88(4):440–445

Palmer M 1995 Nurses' knowledge and beliefs about continence interventions in long-term care. Journal of Advanced Nursing 21:1065–1072

Pomfret I 1996 The use of continence products. In: Norton C (ed) Nursing for continence, 2nd edn. Beaconsfield Press, Beaconsfield, pp 335–364

Poulton A, Thomas S 1999 The cost of constipation. Primary Health Care 9(9):17–20

Rew M 1996 Use of catheter maintence solutions for long-term catheters. British Journal of Nursing 8(11):10–13

Rhodes P 1995 The postal survey of continence advisors in England and Wales. Journal of Advanced Nursing 21:286–294

Roe B, Williams K 1994 Clinical handbook for continence care. Scutari Press, London

Rogers J 1995 A user friendly approach to toilet training children with special needs. Child Health 3(3):115–117

Rogers J 1998 Lessons in control. Nursing Times 94(6)(Suppl.):1–3

Royal College of Nursing 2000 Digital rectal examination and manual removal of faeces: guidance for nurses. Royal College of Nurses, London

Royal College of Physicians 1995 Incontinence causes and management and provision of services. Royal College of Physicians, London

Sanderson J 1991 Agenda for action on continence services. Department of Health, London

Sines D 1996 Acquiring continence: supporting people with learning disabilities. In: Norton C (ed) Nursing for continence, 2nd edn. Beaconsfield Press, Beaconsfield, pp 317–334

Smith D, Newman D 1994 Basic elements of biofeedback therapy for pelvic floor muscle rehabilitation. Urological Nursing 14(3):130–135

Smith P, Smith L 2003 Continence training in intellectual disability. In: Getliffe K, Dolman P (eds) Promoting continence, 2nd edn. Baillière Tindall, London, pp 303–337

Spiller R, Farthing M 1994 Diarrhoea and constipation. Science Press, London

Stamm W 1991 Catheter associated urinary tract infection: epidemiology, pathogenesis, and prevention. Journal of the American Medical Association 91(Suppl. 3B):65–71

Stokes G 1987 Incontinence and inappropriate urination: common problems with the confused elderly. Winslow Press, Bicester

Sultan A, Kamm M, Hudson C et al 1993 Anal sphincter disruption during vaginal delivery. New England Journal of Medicine 329(26):1905–1911

Swaffield J 1996 Continence in older people. In: Norton C (ed) Nursing for continence, 2nd edn. Beaconsfield Press, Beaconsfield, pp 170–191

Thompson W, Creed F, Droosman D et al 1992 Functional bowel disease and functional abdominal pain. Gastroenterology International 5:75–91

Ungar A 2000 Movicol: its treatment of constipation and faecal incontinence. Hospital Medicine 61(11):37–40

Weiss J, Blaivas J 2000 Nocturia. Journal of Urology 163(1):5–15

Wells M 1996 The development of urinary continence and the causes of incontinence. In: Norton C (ed) Nursing for continence, 2nd edn. Beaconsfield Press, Beaconsfield, pp 12–16

White H 1995 In control with incontinence aids. British Journal of Nursing 4(6):334–338

White H, Dolman M 2003 Incontinence in perspective. In: Getliffe K, Dolman P (eds) Promoting continence, 2nd edn. Baillière Tindall, London, pp 303–337

Willis J 2000 Bowel management and consent. Nursing Times 96(6):6–7

Wilson L 1992 An introduction to multidisciplinary pathway care. Northern Region Health, Cambridge

Wilson J 1997a Control and prevention infection in catheter care. Community Nurse 3(5):39–40

Wilson M 1997b Infection control and drainage bag design. Professional Nurse 11(14):245–250

Winder A 1992 Intermittent catheterization. In: Roe B (ed) Clinical practice: the promotion and management of continence. Prentice-Hall, Hemel Hempstead, pp 157–175

Winson L 1997 Catheterization: extending scope of practice. British Journal of Nursing 6(21):1229–1231

Wong D L 1993 Essentials of paediatric nursing. Mosby, London

Wynd C, Wallace M, Smith K 1996 Factors influencing postoperative urinary retention following orthopaedic surgical procedures. Orthopaedic Nursing 15(10):43–46

Wyndale J, Maes D 1990 Clean intermittent self-catheterisation: a 12-year follow up. Journal of Urology 143:904–908

Chapter 19

Rehabilitation

Janet Barker

KEY ISSUES

SUBJECT KNOWLEDGE
- The social and political context of rehabilitation
- Social roles
- Labelling and stigma
- Altered body image
- Loss and grieving
- Motivation
- Management of change
- Promoting effective communication
- Teams and leadership

CARE DELIVERY KNOWLEDGE
- Assessment in rehabilitation
- Goal setting
- The nurse as an educator or facilitator of change

PROFESSIONAL AND ETHICAL KNOWLEDGE
- Impact of health and social policy on the provision of care
- Social exclusion
- The nurse as a member of the multidisciplinary team
- Ethical considerations

PERSONAL AND REFLECTIVE KNOWLEDGE
- Rehabilitation in professional practice

INTRODUCTION

There has been a shift from custodial care to rehabilitation in a variety of contexts ranging from the care of the elderly to children's disorders and from physical disorders to enduring mental illness. Indeed health policy over a decade ago in the form of *The Health of the Nation* (Department of Health 1991) identified rehabilitation as a key area in the strategy for health. Rehabilitation has become an area of increasing importance and is likely to remain so.

Various definitions of rehabilitation are available, but Waters' definition (1994: 239) is the most comprehensive, suggesting the term relates to

> the whole process of enabling and facilitating the restoration of a disabled person to regain optimum functioning (physically, socially and psychologically) to the level they are able or motivated to achieve.

The word 'process' in the above definition suggests an activity that moves forward through a series of actions aimed at achieving an identified result. Williams (1993: 67) asserts that

> rehabilitation is a process not an end in itself, where the greatest steps are usually the smallest, sometimes literally, and every day gives the opportunity to see someone win a major victory over his or her own body or mind.

Gibbon & Thompson (1992) found that nurses had difficulty in defining their role in the process of rehabilitation. Although they thought they made a contribution this was usually in collaboration with other members of the care team such as occupational therapists and physiotherapists. They concluded from this that nurses should recognize their own role in rehabilitation and develop the confidence to implement their own rehabilitation programmes rather than taking their lead from other disciplines. Rehabilitation is seen by Doughty (1991) as not only the province of the old, immobile or physically disabled, but for all who experience health problems, both acute and chronic. She suggests that whenever it is necessary for choices to be made relating to the achieving of a full, active, healthy lifestyle following illness, a rehabilitation process is necessary. If this is so, rehabilitation is therefore an aspect of every nurse's practice and as such warrants close consideration.

OVERVIEW

This chapter addresses the various factors that may have a bearing on the process of rehabilitation. It is divided into four main parts.

Subject knowledge

The first section, Subject Knowledge, develops the scope of rehabilitation. Rehabilitation is undertaken in a wide range of settings and as such it would be impossible to address all care groups here. However, the social, psychological and health policy aspects are common and have great relevance to all forms of rehabilitation and for this reason form a large section of this part. Interpersonal aspects of care provision are also discussed in relation to communication between nurses and clients and interprofessionally. The development of such skills is central to professional practice in the rehabilitation setting.

Care delivery knowledge

The second section of the chapter, Care Delivery Knowledge, looks at the nurse's role in the process of rehabilitation through assessment, goal setting and health education. The use of decision making exercises and suggestions for portfolio work help to promote consideration and development of knowledge essential to the provision of nursing care.

Professional and ethical knowledge

The third section of the chapter, Professional and Ethical Knowledge, focuses on three main issues: the impact of health policy, the nurse's membership of a multidisciplinary team and ethical issues in rehabilitation.

Personal and reflective knowledge

Finally, in Personal and Reflective Knowledge, the main points of the chapter are revisited both through the use of case studies and in providing suggestions for portfolio evidence. You may find it helpful to read one of the case studies on pages 441–442 before you start the chapter and use it as a focus for your reflections while reading.

SUBJECT KNOWLEDGE

> **Evidence based practice**
>
> In investigating access to cardiac rehabilitation, Tod et al (2002) found the following issues impeded clients' ability to access:
>
> - absence of services
> - long waiting lists
> - poor communication
> - lack of understanding of cardiac rehabilitation process
> - services not appropriate for all individuals' needs.
>
> They suggest that without substantial investment in cardiac rehabilitation the needs of many will not be met.

THE SOCIAL AND POLITICAL CONTEXT OF REHABILITATION

Social policy relates to central and local government activities associated with the provision of services related to health, education, housing and social services, including social security and income support. It addresses questions concerning how much welfare the state should provide and how this is to be funded. Health policy, as one aspect of this, is of particular interest to those involved in the delivery of care. Scott (2001) argues that the overlapping of health policy with nursing policy requires nursing to have an understanding of how one impacts on the other and the implication of this for care delivery.

Developed countries are viewed as having a mixed economy of welfare made up of:

- state sector
- private sector
- voluntary sector
- informal carers.

The term 'welfare state' is used to describe the type of society that developed in the UK after 1945. Successive governments have intervened positively in the economic and social interests of the general public with a view to achieving a minimum standard of living for all. This approach grew out of a distinct set of social ideas – ideology – known as 'collectivism' where all individuals have certain social, economic and political rights. Before this the ideology had been that of *laissez faire* associated with minimal state interference in social and economic affairs.

The growth of the welfare state continued from 1940s until the late 1970s, supported by what is known as consensus politics. Here political parties have a basic agreement about the desirability of a welfare state. This consensus broke down in the late 1970s due to a growing dissatisfaction with the welfare state as it became seen as ineffective and expensive to maintain.

The Thatcherite years (1979–1990) saw the introduction of what was known as the 'New Right' ideology which introduced general management into healthcare provision, advocating the creation of an 'internal market' where patients were to be seen as consumers. Various agencies within the National Health Service were to assess local need and purchase care on their behalf, whilst others were to provide the services needed. Emphasis was placed on care in the community. This approach was driven by economics and an attempt to control increasing healthcare costs and culminated in the NHS and Community Care Act 1990.

The election of the 'New Labour' government in 1997 saw the abolition of some aspects of the internal market with the introduction of the white paper *The New NHS: Modern and Dependable* (Department of Health 1997). Here it was identified that National Service Frameworks (NSFs) were to be developed which set national standards and identified models of care for particular care group and/or clinical specialties. At present NSFs for Mental Health, Coronary Heart Disease, Cancer, Older People and Diabetes are available. Others are in preparation for Renal Services, Children's Services and Long-Term Conditions. *A First Class Service* (Department of Health 1998) introduced the concept of Clinical Governance with the stated intention of improving the quality of services and promoting evidence based practice. These issues are re-emphasized in *The NHS Plan* (Department of Health 2000) whilst advocating various changes in service delivery and promising that the NHS will provide a 'comprehensive range of services' including rehabilitative ones.

SOCIAL ROLES

The social and political context explains how a society views rehabilitation. To explore what it actually means for individuals requires an understanding of how individuals interact within society.

Individuals and society interact through taking various social roles. This provides a sense of purpose and belonging for all individuals within society and allows the individual to develop a concept of self. A loss of social role can occur following illness or disability or as a result of the often prolonged process of rehabilitation. In enabling an individual to achieve their optimum level of functioning, Smith & Clark (1995) suggest that within the rehabilitation process an individual's ability to resume his or her normal social role is of great importance. This is supported by McGrath & Davis (1992), who also propose that a major aim of rehabilitation is to enable individuals to resume valued social roles. An understanding of social roles is therefore central to planning rehabilitation programmes.

Social roles are associated with the individual's status within his or her society. Status relates to things such as:

- gender (e.g. male or female)
- occupation (e.g. nurse, farm worker, tailor)
- family relationships (e.g. daughter, brother, parent).

Table 19.1	Role of the nurse
Status	**Nurse**
Norms	Knowledge of illness
	Cares for people
	Gentle and kind
Role	Wears a uniform
	Practical
	Busy

Status is culturally defined and may be either:

- fixed or ascribed (e.g. gender or caste)

or

- achieved (e.g. marital status or class).

For each status there are identifiable expected and acceptable ways of behaving. These are known as 'norms'. The group of norms attached to a particular status is a 'role'. Therefore each status is accompanied by a role, which shapes and directs social behaviour. Individuals then perform this role in relation to one another (Table 19.1). This enables individuals to interact with one another, predict how each other will behave and have a clear idea of what is expected in terms of their own and related roles. For example, in the interaction between nurse and client, each knows what is expected of them and how the other should respond. Both nurse and client can then concentrate on the situation they are in without being inhibited by other aspects of their lives.

When someone becomes ill they may not be able to fulfil their normal roles and this affects their perceived status and self-esteem. For example, if a woman experiences a stroke that affects her ability to do domestic chores, she may feel that this affects her role as a provider of care for her husband. This may have an impact on the way the husband and wife interact and their expectations of each other.

So far it seems that social roles and obligations are clearly identified and explicit. Such a view of role is adopted by a particular perspective in sociology known as 'functionalism'. An alternative theoretical stance is that of 'interactionism'.

From an interactionist perspective the idea of role is less defined. Although roles are viewed as a part of the social system, role is seen as a set of general guidelines, which allows negotiation between two individuals. A role is not fixed, but fluid and changeable. Therefore there is no script as to how a student nurse should behave; rather this is negotiated between students and their teachers, ward supervisor and clients. This negotiation occurs in relation to an individual's understanding of the role and their beliefs.

Sick role

From all sociological perspectives individuals have a variety of roles, which are culturally defined and carry obligations.

Table 19.2 The sick role (after Parsons 1951)

Right or obligation	Provisos
Two rights	
The sick person is exempt from performing his or her usual social role	This exemption is relative to the severity of the illness
	It must be legitimized by others – often the doctor is the legitimizing agent
The sick person is not responsible for his or her illness	The person is not expected to 'pull themselves together'
	As he or she is exempt from responsibility, there is an expectation of 'being taken care of'
Two obligations	
The sick person must get better as soon as possible	Being ill is unacceptable and the person must be motivated to get well
The sick person must seek medical advice and comply with the treatment prescribed	Help must be sought from a competent and acceptable source in relation to the severity of the illness

Reflection and portfolio evidence

Think of a client in whose care you have recently been involved during a clinical placement.

- Identify the various roles that individual may have.
- How might their illness or disability affect these roles?
- How could the nurse help the client adjust to the new role demands in the short term?
- What long-term role adjustments might this client have to make?
- On your last practice placement, did the clients meet Parsons' (1951) criteria for the sick role (Table 19.2)?
- If they did, how?
- Have you ever taken the sick role?
- Did you fulfil the demands and obligations?
- What problems are there in applying the sick role to individuals with mental health problems who do not comply with medical advice?

When people become ill, they are unable to continue their normal roles. In a definitive analysis on the impact of illness on social status, Parsons (1951) suggested that this inability of sick people to perform their usual social roles is viewed as deviant behaviour and requires some form of regulation. Normally within a society any behaviour that is viewed as deviant and is preventable is regulated through sanctions such as the imprisonment imposed on those who commit crimes. As illness cannot be prevented, Parsons suggested regulation is achieved through a socially prescribed role to control the behaviour of the sick person (i.e. a defined sick role). This sick role contains four expectations, consisting of two rights and two obligations (Table 19.2).

The granting of the rights of the sick role is dependent upon the individual fulfilling the obligations. If a person fails to meet the obligations the rights may be suspended and the individual is seen as responsible for his or her illness. The sick role is viewed as a temporary role with the main function of minimizing the disruptive effect of illness on society and ensuring that individuals return to a healthy state as soon as possible. This is very limiting and various criticisms are therefore levelled at Parsons' (1951) proposed sick role:

- people with minor illnesses are not expected to adopt the sick role
- the sick role usually applies only to acute physical illnesses
- people with mental illness are often reluctant to adopt the sick role
- the sick role is seen as non-applicable to chronic illnesses as these are not temporary and the individual may not be able to return to previous roles.

LABELLING AND STIGMA

Becoming ill can be viewed as deviant and the sick role offers a way of describing how behaviour is regulated. An alternative way of viewing this is through labelling theory. This offers an interactionist view of society and an explanation as to how a client's role is negotiated and maintained.

Lemert (1951) suggested two forms of deviation: primary and secondary. Primary deviation relates to acts that an individual may engage in before being publicly labelled as deviant. These acts are seen as relatively unimportant as they have little impact on an individual's self-concept. What is important is society's response to the individual. Public recognition and labelling of deviant behaviour coupled with the consequences of such identification produces a response from the individual. This response is the secondary deviation. Society's reaction to the individual assigns a new role and status, which has an impact on the individual's self-concept and future actions. The transformation from primary deviance to secondary deviance occurs when an individual labelled deviant accepts the 'new' social status and role.

Williams (1987) discusses primary deviance in relation to a medical diagnosis. Secondary deviation occurs where the diagnosis is accepted and associated with a negative social status. As a result of illness or surgery, labels such as diabetic, schizophrenic or amputee may be applied. Therefore the labelled individual is marked as different from the rest of society and may invoke negative social reactions. 'Stigma' is the term applied to such responses.

The classic work on stigma was produced by Goffman (1963), who identified various sources and attributes in relation to this phenomenon (Table 19.3). The negative social

Table 19.3   Sources and attributes of stigma
(after Goffman 1963)

Sources	Abominations of the body	Physical disabilities
	Blemishes of character	Mental illness, sexual deviance
	Tribal stigmas	Race, nation, religion
Attributes	Discreditable	Those that are not visible or known and are therefore only potentially stigmatizing such as epilepsy, acquired immunodeficiency syndrome (AIDS), diabetes mellitus
	Discrediting	Known, visible and provoking a reaction in others, for example facial disablement or deformities, symptoms of mental illness

Table 19.4   Responses to stigma (after Goffman 1963)

Passing	Tries to conceal attribute and pass as normal (e.g. an individual not disclosing a history of mental illness to an employer)
Covering	Tries to reduce the significance of the condition (e.g. attempts to resume 'normal behaviour')
Withdrawal	Opts out of social interaction with 'normal' people (e.g. all social activities involve others with a similar disorder)

Table 19.5   Components of body image (after Price 1990)

Reality	As it really is: tall/short, fat/thin, dark/fair Norm for race and relative to wider social group Not a constant state, dependent upon age and physical changes
Presentation	Dress and fashion Control of functions, movement and pose How others receive us
Ideal	How a body should look and act (culturally determined and includes size, proportion, odours and smells) Personal norm for personal space Body reliability, which may be unrealistic Applied not only to self, but to those around us

responses to conditions that attract stigmas are related to feelings such as fear or disgust associated with certain labels and the attributing of stereotypical traits to individuals. Therefore people in wheelchairs are often viewed as both mentally and physically disabled, while someone with a mental illness is considered to be potentially violent.

Reflection and portfolio evidence

On your last clinical placement:

- What diagnostic labels were attached to clients?
- What effect did the diagnostic label have on the client? – the client's family? – the care team?
- How can the nurse minimize the negative effects of stigmas attached to diagnostic labels?

Stigmatized ideas are culturally determined, that is they are based on the society's norms and values, which are learned early in life and reinforced through everyday conversations and the media. Individuals with stigmatizing illnesses may be viewed as socially inferior and may also be subject to discrimination and socially disadvantaged. The imposing of such social disfavour may result in poor self-concept and identity. Goffman (1963) suggests that the stigmatized individual may adopt various responses when interacting with a non-stigmatized individual (Table 19.4).

ALTERED BODY IMAGE

Many stigmatizing illnesses have an impact on the way an individual perceives his or her body and therefore his or her body image. Body image is a much-used term that has wide applications in holistic care. Body image affects the social, spiritual, physical and psychological aspects of well-being, and as such, an understanding of this subject is vital to the provision of care. Price (1990) suggests that a client's body image has an impact on the process of rehabilitation, having consequences for and affecting the client's well being. He identifies three components to body image:

- how individuals perceive and feel about their bodies (body reality)
- how the body responds to commands (body presentation)
- how the first two components compare with an internal standard (body ideal).

Throughout life there is an attempt to achieve and maintain a balance between the three elements (Table 19.5).

Body image depends not only upon the individual's response to his or her own body, but also upon the appearance, attitude and responses of others. This is important for nurses to remember when delivering care, as their own responses may have a great impact on how clients perceive themselves.

Body image and self-image are interconnected, self-image being central to an individual's confidence, motivation and sense of achievement. It is a product of an individual's personality, being moulded by socialization and represents an assessment of self-worth (Price 1990). There is a high valuing of attractiveness within developed

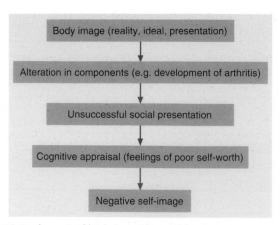

Figure 19.1   Impact of body image on self-image.

countries, with an associated stereotyping of beautiful as good (Bercheid & Walster 1974). When the three elements of body image are in a state of equilibrium, meeting both personal and social expectations and therefore enabling a successful presentation of self, there is a corresponding positive self-image. If, however, changes occur that result in an alteration of one or more of the body image components, a negative self-image may follow (Fig. 19.1).

Altered body images can arise from two sources:

- open (i.e. visible) as with arthritis
- hidden (i.e. not readily observable) such as a colostomy.

Personal responses to altered body image will arise from the interaction of a variety of factors, including:

- visibility
- associated shame or guilt
- significance for the future – work, social life, personal
- support during transition
- personal coping strategies
- stage of the grieving process.

In discussing the types of problems that an individual with spinal injuries may encounter in relation to altered body image, Brennan (1994) identifies three main areas of concern as physical, psychological and social (Table 19.6).

Decision making exercise

Gareth Pearce, aged 23, is developing his career as a professional footballer. He played for a third division team when he was spotted by a scout for a premier league team, who subsequently signed him on. He appeared to have a promising career ahead of him. However, in his fourth match in the first team, as a result of a bad tackle, Gareth finds himself in the Accident and Emergency department with a fractured left tibia and fibula. He is accompanied by his wife and young son. The orthopaedic surgeon informs Gareth that he will not be playing football again for the rest of the season and that the

fracture is so severe that at this stage he is uncertain whether Gareth will be able to play football again.

- What losses might Gareth and his family experience as a result of the accident and during his hospitalization?
- What responses or behaviour could this evoke?
- How might a knowledge of the grief reaction help the nurse to support Gareth and his family over the immediate crisis?

(For further information on the grief reaction see Ch. 12 on death and dying.)

Table 19.6   Problems related to altered body image in people with spinal injuries following surgery (after Brennan 1994)

Physical	Problems arise from altered body reality related to reduced ability to care for self and presence of inhibiting factors such as catheter, sutures, drains
Psychological	The extent to which the body reality deviates from the body ideal will have a psychological impact on the individual
	These problems may arise from a sense of loss related to appearance, ability and function, resulting in the person experiencing the grieving process Self-esteem may be lowered
Social	Body presentation is altered through the use of equipment (e.g. wheelchair, cervical collar, walking frame)
	This may cause anxiety relating to how the person thinks he or she will be viewed by others and in turn this has an impact on self-image and confidence Social isolation can result

Table 19.7   Stages of grief (after Kubler Ross 1975)

Stage of grief	Features
Denial	Feeling that 'This can't be true', emotions are not expressed and the person tries to continue as if nothing has happened
Anger	Following acknowledgement of the reality an individual may express anger; this may be directed at themselves, friends, family, carers, God, everyone or everything in general
Bargaining	The person seeks to avoid the inevitable by proposing 'bargains' such as becoming a good person or going to church regularly if only they are allowed to live longer or have less pain; these 'bargains' are made privately or silently
Anger, depression	As the individual begins to feel that bargaining is futile they may lapse into depression or revert to their anger, questioning 'Why me?' For the person to feel this way there has to be a certain element of acceptance
True acceptance	Or resignation to their fate

LOSS AND GRIEVING

The concept of grief is usually associated with death and dying, but it can also be examined in terms of loss in more general ways. Costello (1995) suggests that grief relates to the feelings evoked through the loss of something valued, and as proposed by Sheppard (1994), individuals requiring rehabilitation have to come to terms with many losses. These losses relate to things such as lifestyle changes, altered physical or psychological functioning and loss of body parts. This can give rise to the grieving process.

In her work with terminally ill people and their families Kubler Ross (1975) identified a number of emotional stages experienced by people faced with death (Table 19.7). She suggests that not all individuals will go through all these stages, that some may never reach acceptance, and that individuals may move to and fro between the stages. Although this process is viewed in terms of the individual's impending 'loss' through their own death, it can also have relevance to losses experienced from illness and disability.

MOTIVATION

One of the most important factors in the process of rehabilitation is that of the client's motivation. Where a client's physical ability is present, but motivation is lacking, rehabilitation becomes a most frustrating experience for those providing care. There is a need to understand what motivates people and why some individuals appear more motivated than others.

Atkinson et al (1993) suggest that three different types of motives drive behaviour:

- survival needs – related to those activities necessary to ensure the individual's survival such as eating and drinking, and having a biological basis
- social needs – may have a biological basis, but require interaction with others, for example sexual drives where the need to reproduce the species has a biological basis, but the behaviour is culturally determined in terms of what is acceptable or not
- the need to satisfy curiosity.

Various theories of motivation have been put forward and Sternberg (1995) suggests that the concept has captured the imagination of psychologists from varying academic backgrounds. The theories are classified into three general approaches:

- physiological approaches, which address the relationship between the central nervous system and behavioural aspects of motivation
- clinical approaches, which consider the relationship between personality and motivation
- cognitive approaches, which are viewed as examining the thought process underlying behaviour.

Examples of these various approaches are given in Table 19.8. As Sternberg (1995) identifies, an individual's physiology, personality and cognitive processes cannot be examined in isolation as each interacts with the others. Therefore

Table 19.8 Examples of different approaches to motivation

Approach	Features and example
Physiological approach, e.g. arousal theory	Activity in the central nervous system dictates level of arousal (cited in Sternberg 1995) Each person has their optimum level of arousal Individuals perform most efficiently at the optimum arousal level Low levels of arousal result in boredom, inactivity and poor motivation High levels of arousal result in anxiety and tension
Clinical approach, e.g. Maslow's hierarchy of needs	Needs are hierarchical in nature, having the following seven levels of needs (Maslow 1970): 1. Food, water, air 2. Safety, shelter 3. Belonging, love, companionship 4. Self-esteem 5. Cognitive needs – knowledge 6. Aesthetic needs – goodness, beauty 7. Self-actualization. Each level of need (beginning with physiological) must be satisfied before moving onto the next. Having achieved or satisfied one level individuals are motivated to satisfy the next level of need
Cognitive approach, e.g. intrinsic and extrinsic	Intrinsic motivators come from within – doing things because they are interesting and important to the individual motivators (cited in Sternberg 1995) Extrinsic motivators come from outside the individual in the form of perceived rewards or punishments Motivation results from either one or a combination of both intrinsic or extrinsic factors

it may be necessary to adopt an integrated approach to the understanding of motivation.

MANAGEMENT OF CHANGE

The alteration of an individual's health status may necessitate lifestyle changes to reduce risk factors associated with particular disorders. The rehabilitation process therefore involves the developing of skills, attitudes and norms in individuals to enable the achievement of optimum well-being. For example, someone with hypertension may be asked to stop smoking, lose weight, take up an exercise routine and reduce their stress. Such a regimen involves major lifestyle changes, an increased knowledge relating to diet and exercise and the development of alternative coping skills.

Change is described by Keyser (1986: 103) as 'an attempt to alter or replace existing knowledge or skills, attitudes, norms, and styles of individuals or groups'.

To facilitate change the nurse must adopt the role of 'change agent'. A change agent is someone who creates an environment conducive to change, overcomes resistance to change, understands how to encourage acceptance of the need for change, generates ideas and implements and evaluates the process. Lancaster & Lancaster (1982) identified specific skills that are required to successfully facilitate change:

- communication
- group process
- self-awareness
- interpersonal
- assertiveness
- assessment
- planning
- implementation
- evaluation
- prioritizing.

People prefer the familiar and often show resistance to change, seeing it as a threat. This may relate to the nature of the change or beliefs (real or imagined) about what the change will mean. The anxiety invoked by change may be related to:

- fear of the unknown
- uncertainty
- lack of knowledge or skills to achieve change
- low confidence
- feelings of powerlessness
- resentment of the need for change.

Resistance to change manifests itself in a variety of ways as the experience is a personal one, but there are some common responses (Table 19.9).

The process of change also provokes an emotional response in those involved, which has been described as 'the emotional cycle of change' (Table 19.10) (Kelley & Connor 1979). Here individuals experience a variety of highs and

Table 19.9 Common resistance to change behaviours (after Vaughan & Pillmoor 1989 by kind permission)

Lip service	Individuals listen to suggestions, agree while change agent is present, but do not undertake proposed action or behaviour in their absence
Aggression	Person displays aggressive behaviour, which results in them not having to face or undertake the change
Destruction	In an attempt to reduce feelings of anxiety individuals may demonstrate destructive behaviour (e.g. a family member may encourage the client not to adhere to a diet when trying to lose weight or to have a cigarette when attempting to give up smoking)
Lack of continuity	Individuals may find excuses not to do certain things – 'I'm too busy today to do my exercises'; the excuses increase until the proposed change is shelved completely

lows as change occurs, and the process ends in 'the glow' of satisfaction (Vaughan & Pillmoor 1989).

To summarize so far, then, to reduce resistance to change and to help individuals through the cycle of change, a change agent must:

- communicate effectively – this includes listening
- develop trust among all participants
- clearly identify goals, plans, priorities and problems
- ensure necessary resources are available
- define responsibilities of others, allowing individuals freedom to do their part
- evaluate at regular intervals to review provide feedback on progress (Lancaster & Lancaster 1982).

In selecting the appropriate strategy to facilitate change, two criteria are essential (Haffer 1986). Firstly, it is necessary

Evidence based practice

Davis et al (1992) implemented changes to working practice in a rehabilitation centre where they moved from a multidisciplinary to an interdisciplinary approach. This led to the adoption of a more client-centred method of care, which was directed by a specific 'care coordinator'. They described the process of change and highlighted the problems that occurred. From the experience they identified that:

- the terminology used by all involved on the process of change must be clearly defined and understood
- aims and objectives must be clearly stated
- sufficient time must be given for the change to occur
- records should be kept throughout the process and should include all successes and failures
- evaluation must occur.

Table 19.10 Stages of the emotional cycle of change (after Kelley & Connor 1979 by kind permission of John Wiley & Sons)

Stage	Features	Individual experiences
Uninformed optimism (certainty)	Ideas look good Obstacles are trivial Morale at its peak	Highs
Informed pessimism (doubt)	Problems occur Energy wanes Solutions difficult to identify Why did I ever start this?	Lows
Hopeful realism (hope)	Deals with emotions and doubts Modifies goals	
Informed optimism (confidence)	Individual gains confidence in abilities to succeed Encouragement, recognition and support are needed	
Rewarding completion (satisfaction)	Successful implementation of change	Glows

Table 19.11 Implementing change requires the following elements (after Lancaster & Lancaster 1982)

Element	Features
Involvement	Of all individuals who will be affected, professionals and carers
Motivation	Valuing of everyone's contribution Listening to and respect for all involved
Planning	Must be flexible
Legitimization	Sanctioned or owned by those involved
Education	Individuals have the necessary skills or knowledge
Management	Aimed at developing the necessary skills
Expectations	To expect the unexpected To respect other's experiences
Nurturance	Recognition of individuals' needs Support
Trust	

to focus on an appropriate goal. Secondly, the individual should be both willing and able to make the change. For example if implementing a fitness regimen the goal of walking 10 miles every day may not be appropriate for an 80-year-old woman. She may be neither willing nor physically able to undertake such a proposal. To implement change successfully, then, a variety of factors must be considered and used effectively (Table 19.11). Without these elements in place change is unlikely to occur.

PROMOTING EFFECTIVE COMMUNICATION

To communicate is generally taken to mean to 'impart', 'transmit' or 'share'. Thurgood (1990) states that communication is central to the rehabilitation programme, as without good communication the client ultimately suffers. From Thurgood's perspective, effective communication is essential to the rehabilitation process, ensuring that all involved – nurse, client, family, friends and members of the multidisciplinary team – are fully aware of and can participate in the process. Tod et al (2002) identify that poor communication is one of the barriers to people accessing cardiac rehabilitation programmes effectively. Therefore a general understanding of the factors that promote and hinder the process of effective communication is essential (see also Ch. 1).

Decision making exercise

Your client, George Rowe, appears to be distressed. Following a road traffic accident in which he sustained a severe head injury George has become dysphasic. You think that his distress may be related to his concern about his wife's ability to care for herself in his absence.

- How would you encourage George to discuss his feelings?
- What questions would it be appropriate to ask?
- What aids to communication would you consider using?
- Some people are perceived by others as 'easy to talk to'. What particular communication skills do you think these people possess?

To communicate effectively various skills need to be developed. These include:

- active listening
- awareness of non-verbal communication
- use of appropriate questioning.

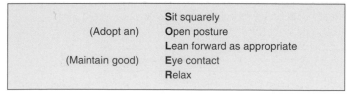

	Sit squarely
(Adopt an)	**O**pen posture
	Lean forward as appropriate
(Maintain good)	**E**ye contact
	Relax

Figure 19.2   SOLER to convey interest and promote active listening. (After Egan 1986.)

Active listening

Active listening or attending is more than hearing what an individual says. It involves showing people that you are interested in them and that you value what they have to say, and encouraging the disclosure of information and expression of feelings. This is achieved through the use of both verbal and non-verbal strategies and observing individual behaviour to pinpoint meanings behind words.

Awareness of non-verbal communication

The listener must be aware of his or her own body language. People believe what they say is most important, but up to 80% of communication is via body language. If verbal and non-verbal communications are not synchronized, non-verbal communication will take priority. It is easy to convey lack of interest through simple gestures. The listener may say verbally 'I'm interested', but if their body language is saying 'I haven't got time for this' (e.g. looking at the time, wringing hands, glancing towards paperwork), the 'talker' will pay more attention to the body language and communication will stop.

The use of non-verbal prompts such as nods and smiles and paralinguistic communication such as 'mmms' and 'uh huhs' can also encourage an individual to continue talking.

To convey interest and promote active listening you might consider the use of Egan's (1986) acronym SOLER (Fig. 19.2). Responding in this manner conveys interest and suggests active listening.

Observing the talker's non-verbal and paralinguistic behaviours can provide the nurse with important cues about the talker's feelings. For instance in response to 'How are you?' the client may say 'I'm fine' while his or her facial expression suggests distress and hunched shoulders, a bowed head and a low and anguished tone of voice suggest that all is not well. Recognizing these cues enables the listener to adopt appropriate interventions.

Appropriate questioning

Skilled questioning is essential in communication. Questioning can serve many functions, for example:

- to encourage conversation
- to promote information gathering
- to clarify issues, feelings or beliefs

Table 19.12   Examples of open and closed questions

Type of question	Example
Open	How did you sleep?
	Tell me how you feel?
	What would you like to have for your dinner today?
Closed	What is your name?
	Are you feeling OK?
	Did you sleep well?

- to identify problems
- to check the listener's understanding of issues
- to focus the discussion on specific issues.

There are two main types of questions: open and closed. Closed questions restrict the possible responses to either yes or no or the giving of direct information. Such questions are useful in obtaining specific information or facts, but do not allow for the expression of feelings, thoughts or opinions. Open questions encourage the expression of thoughts and feelings, place no restrictions on the responder and usually begin with 'How', 'What', 'Where', 'When', and 'Why'. Table 19.12 gives examples of open and closed questions. Both types of questions have their uses, but open questions promote the disclosure of issues most relevant to an individual and offer the individual some control over his or her response.

Barriers to communication

Communication between client, family and care team sometimes goes wrong. Reasons for poor communication are wide ranging, but some of the factors involved are examined here.

Physiological factors

A variety of physical problems can act as barriers to communication. A visual or hearing impairment can reduce an individual's ability to communicate with others unless appropriate strategies are used. Touching a person who is blind makes them aware of your presence and allows the person to orientate towards communication. Similarly someone with hearing difficulties may have problems if the communicator does not face them or is unable to use sign language or if hearing aids are appropriate, but are not used.

Neurological damage following stroke or head injury can give rise to dysphasia, poor concentration, confusion or memory impairment, all of which can serve as barriers to communication.

Cognitive factors

Cognitive barriers relate to those factors that affect processes such as attention, perception, thinking, problem solving, reasoning, memory and language. Neurological damage can give rise to problems in some of these areas, as can some mental health problems and learning disabilities. For example, someone with schizophrenia may have a poor attention span resulting from altered perceptions and thought disorder.

Stress and anxiety can have an impact on all cognitive processes. Individuals who are only just beginning to come to terms with an illness or new situation may have high levels of stress and anxiety. In such situations the individual's perception of information being given and interpretation of things said can be affected (see Ch. 8 on stress, relaxation and rest).

In health care medical jargon is common, but can appear as a foreign language to someone receiving care. Use of words that are not within the client's own vocabulary generally results in misunderstandings and poor communication.

Environmental factors

Trying to talk to someone in a noisy environment where there are continual interruptions leads to frustration, lack of understanding and poor concentration. Similarly individuals are often disinclined to discuss personal information or the expression of strong emotions if they can be overheard or seen.

Other environmental factors may relate to time available to talk. Nurses often feel under pressure to 'get the job done' and their workloads may either inhibit clients ('I don't want to bother the nurses, they're so busy') or result in the nurse communicating poorly because of pressure of work.

Personal factors

Individual nurses may lack the knowledge, experience and skills to promote effective communication. There is a belief that communication is just about talking, but effective communication requires the learning of skills, practice and confidence (refer also to Ch. 1).

TEAMS AND LEADERSHIP

A rehabilitation programme requires the involvement of a variety of healthcare professionals in the bid to return the client to their optimum level of functioning. Multidisciplinary involvement necessitates a coordinated approach to ensure that the needs of the client are addressed. This is best achieved through teamwork.

A team is a group of people working together; it is more than an aggregate of individuals, but rather what Huczynski & Buchanan (1985) describe as a 'psychological group' where individuals have a sense of collective identity and interact in a significant way. A multidisciplinary team is also a 'formal group'. It is created by an organization to achieve specific goals related to identified tasks.

Groups do not come into being fully formed and functional; they grow and develop over time. Groups form by passing through sequential steps – forming, storming, norming, performing (Table 19.13).

Table 19.13 Group formation and stages of group development (after Tuckman 1965)

Forming	Feelings of uncertainty, anxiety and looking for leadership
Storming	People try to find a role within the group, and conflict and competition arise as bids for dominance are made
Norming	Group identity emerges – there is an acceptance of common rules and a sense of belonging
Performing	Solidarity, commitment to group goals, individual responsibility for work, agreed objectives

Table 19.14 Leadership styles and their characteristics

Autocratic	Defensive, restrictive, fearing, obedience, punishment, reward, threat, constant surveillance
Democratic	Open, accepting, trusting, recognition, satisfaction, self-discipline, challenge
Laissez faire	Permissive, abdicating, indifferent, self-direction, differences, ultraliberal, equality

Argyle (1969) suggests that in all groups a hierarchy appears with a leader at the top. In formal groups, such as teams, this leader is either formally appointed or becomes the person with the highest status. Leadership is concerned with the guiding, directing and influencing of others towards an identified goal or result. In a formally appointed leader, control is based upon power and the leader is able to exert power to influence the group. This is not the same for all leaders, however, and styles of leadership can vary (Table 19.14).

The ability of the leader to influence others in the group relates to the power structure within the group, which may stem from a variety of sources. The way in which communication occurs within a group will vary according to the group structure and the style of leadership. With autocratic leadership communication tends to go in one direction – from the leader to the other members. The democratic style encourages multidirectional communication that flows between group members and the leader. Communication within a group with laissez faire leadership only occurs when the leader is asked to provide information. The different styles of leadership and communication structures are appropriate to use in particular situations.

CARE DELIVERY KNOWLEDGE

ASSESSMENT IN REHABILITATION

Assessment is often described as the first stage of the nursing process. This suggests that it is a one-off activity that only occurs within the nursing domain. Such an assumption is inappropriate in the sphere of rehabilitation where the emphasis is placed on continuous multidisciplinary assessment, with Nazarko (2001) proclaiming assessment as a 'crucial' aspect of rehabilitation. The process of rehabilitation requires an assessment of multiple factors in an effort to ensure an individual's needs and abilities are fully identified. This allows for rehabilitation to be ability-led and therefore reflect the needs of the individual. Wing (1983: 55) suggests that:

> the value of assessment is to determine the severity and the chronicity of disablement and its main causes, to discover what talents might be developed, to lay down a plan of rehabilitation, to allocate the appropriate professional help to the client and relatives, and to monitor progress and update the plan as necessary.

Although Wing (1983) is referring to the assessment of individuals with schizophrenia, this statement applies to all aspects of rehabilitation. It is only through rigorous assessment that an appropriate rehabilitation programme can be developed. Within such a programme reassessment to monitor progress is essential. One-off assessment only tells how an individual functions at a particular time. On-going assessment allows identification of changes in the client's status.

Assessment is also essential to provide a baseline from which to measure improvement and rehabilitation success. This should include identification of an individual's capabilities before the illness episode to provide a true picture of what is achievable. Often the client's family and friends will be involved in the assessment if this does not compromise confidentiality. This information is helpful to identify the client's previous level of social, cognitive and practical skills.

Assessment requires the collection of data based on:

- direct observation
- interviews
- assessment tools.

The focus of observations and interviews and the types of assessment tools used will be dictated by the individual's illness or disorder. For example, Appleton (1994) suggests that in the rehabilitation of children with head injuries a strong emphasis should be placed on emotional, intellectual and cognitive needs as well as physical requirements. The National Service Framework for Older People (Department of Health 2001a) advocates a multidisciplinary assessment using shared documentation.

Although particular illnesses or disorders may require specific assessment criteria, the basic principles of data collection and assessment skills remain the same. When considering the role of mental health nurses, the Department of Health (1994) identified skills of assessment (Table 19.15). These are relevant to all areas of rehabilitation and cannot be emphasized too strongly.

Reflection and portfolio evidence

Think of a client you have recently been involved in caring for.

- What data would you need to collect to develop a rehabilitation programme?
- How could these data be collected?
- Identify specific assessment tools to aid this process.

Table 19.15 Assessment skills (Reproduced by kind permission of Department of Health 1994)

Skill	Associated activities
Self-awareness	Own values, attitudes, prejudices and their management; motives and needs; competence and limitations; non-verbal communication; effect on others
Observing	Verbal and non-verbal communication; group and family dynamics; interaction with others
Data collection	Recognize sources; identify factors that may affect data collection; acknowledge range of observations available in relation to activities of living; ability to identify relevance or validity of data; awareness of policies and procedures; present data in a logical manner
Interviewing	Formulate strategies in relation to individual differences; consider environment, time, individual needs; communication skills – for example listening and attending, questioning, paraphrasing; being non-judgemental
Identifying needs	Identify factors influencing need; classify need; prioritize need
Diagnosing problems	Independence or dependence level; consider motivation, level of cooperation and possible constraints; base judgements on available data; identify problems; identify areas for nursing intervention and those requiring interventions from other agencies
Recording and disseminating information	Assemble, document, process and organize data accurately; comply with legal requirements; formulate a nursing history; maintain confidentiality; disseminate information quickly

The development of a trusting relationship is also central to assessment. Without such a relationship with both the clients and their families the gathering of relevant information becomes difficult, if not impossible. To facilitate this, good communication skills are essential, and as identified earlier, those factors that promote and act as barriers to communication must be considered.

GOAL SETTING

Goals are viewed as facilitating communication interprofessionally and between health professionals, clients and informal carers. Goals also have a motivational aspect, giving a sense of direction, and when achieved, increasing self-esteem and feelings of satisfaction. Scut & Stam (1994) identify that goal setting in rehabilitation is an essential prerequisite to effective teamwork, and promote a problem solving approach to care.

There are two different types of goals, long-term and short-term. The overall goal of a rehabilitation programme may be to restore an individual to a certain level of functioning. This is a long-term goal. Rehabilitation is often a lengthy undertaking and the daily grind of working towards a too distant goal is demoralizing and demotivating. To maintain a sense of progress there is a need to identify smaller goals that are attainable in a shorter space of time. Short-term goals provide the means of evaluating the rehabilitation programme. This is essential both from the clients' perspective – to enable clients to see their own improvement – and from the formal and informal carers' view to determine whether the care they are giving is appropriate.

Goals are an expression of desired outcomes or objectives that identify the direction of care. The rehabilitation process can be said to stand or fall on the quality and relevance of the goals set, and the importance of this aspect of rehabilitation cannot be emphasized too strongly.

Goal setting is not without its problems; these have been listed by McGrath & Davis (1992) as follows:

- incompatibility of goals (within a discipline, between disciplines, between patient and professionals, between patient and family or friends)
- setting appropriate time scales
- setting the goal at an appropriate level.

When identifying goals it must be remembered that what is important to the nurse or carer may not be so to the client, therefore mutual goal setting is essential. To this end, it is useful to remember the findings of Lewinter & Mikkelsen (1995). They interviewed individuals who had undergone rehabilitation following a stroke. Generally, the physical retraining aspects of the rehabilitation programmes were evaluated well. However, they found that the care programmes failed to address psychological and social needs, in particular counselling and group support. Individuals were also critical of the lack of sexual counselling (a topic that staff evaded) and cognitive training. If a goal is viewed by anyone involved in the rehabilitation process as irrelevant, the motivation to achieve the goal will be lacking and difficulties will arise (see Table 19.9 for those behaviours associated with resistance to change), whereas goals that are too complex will act as a disincentive if they are beyond the client's ability. There is a need for discussion, negotiation, and at times, compromise between all involved.

Goals also need to be set in order of priority. In addition, different members of the multidisciplinary team may have conflicting views about what is essential for the rehabilitation of an individual and the priority each goal should take. Additionally, what is a priority to the team may not be so for the client. If the priorities of goal setting are not universally agreed, there may be a resistance to change and the rehabilitation plan may well be undermined. It is essential therefore that all individuals communicate effectively and openly in the setting and prioritizing of goals.

The goal should express what is to be accomplished rather than describing what is to be done to or by the individual. Goals should also be phrased in a positive manner, proposing the outcome to be achieved, for example 'Be able to make a cup of tea unaided' as opposed to 'Reduce dependency upon others'. This approach puts the process in a positive framework and clearly states what is expected as opposed to identifying what is not wanted. If this is coupled with the writing of goals in behavioural terms, for example stating what is to be observed if the goal is achieved and when it is expected to be achieved by (Table 19.16), goals become well defined, unambiguous and easy to evaluate (Binnie et al 1984).

Table 19.16 All behavioural goals must contain the five elements listed here with examples

Behavioural goal	Evelyn is becoming mobile following a hip replacement and will walk for 30 m using a walking frame without sitting down twice daily for 5 days
1. Who will demonstrate behaviour?	Evelyn
2. What will he or she do?	Walk 30 m
3. Under what conditions?	Using her walking frame
4. To what standard?	Without sitting down
5. Expected time or interval by which?	Twice a day for 5 days

THE NURSE AS AN EDUCATOR OR FACILITATOR OF CHANGE

An integral part of rehabilitation is the education of individuals in terms of health promotion and self-care. This includes the identification of risk factors associated with certain illnesses or disorders and the facilitating of changes to reduce such risk factors and adopt healthier lifestyles. This aspect of rehabilitation helps to reduce the dependency of an individual on others and encourages the client to take responsibility for his or her own well-being. Individuals must accept such responsibilities if they are to become more than passive consumers of care. Successful rehabilitation programmes require active client participation.

Healthcare professionals have a responsibility to promote health through increasing awareness of risk factors and facilitating appropriate changes in lifestyles. This is enabled by the acquisition of skills relevant to risk assessment identified by Priest & Speller (1991):

- knowledge relating to risk factors
- awareness and understanding of an individual's attitudes to the identified health problem
- ability to apply knowledge and skills to facilitate change.

Goeppinger (1982: 373) identified that:

life-style factors are amenable to change only by individuals who understand the rationale to change and are sustained in their efforts by strong family ties, assistance of friends, community support systems, and relevant social policy.

This is echoed by Sheppard (1994) who suggests it is imperative that nurses educate clients about the meaning of rehabilitation and what it entails. This is not only to enable the individual to take part more fully in the process, but also to allow a full understanding of the various responsibilities of those involved. The nurse must, however, beware of prescribing lifestyles; informed choice is the most appropriate intervention. An example of the aims of a health education programme is given in Figure 19.3.

Evidence based practice

Ostir et al (2002) investigated the impact of premorbid emotional health on recovery of functional ability in people who had experienced stroke, heart attack or hip fractures. They found that those who had depressive symptoms prior to the disabling event were less likely to recover functional ability than those who had positive emotional health. It is suggested that depressive symptoms reduce the individual's motivation to maintain rehabilitation regimes and are related to poor lifestyles – inactivity, poor nutrition, smoking, lack of social interaction, increased feelings of helplessness and hopelessness.

- An understanding of their physical capabilities and the knowledge to maintain a reasonable level of fitness
- An awareness of the adverse effects of smoking, obesity, poor diet, lack of exercise and stress
- An appreciation of the benefits of a healthier way of life
- An ability to identify individual risk factors and take measures to modify them

Figure 19.3 Example of aims for participants in a cardiac rehabilitation programme. (After Doughty 1991.)

Table 19.17 Health belief model (after Mainman & Becker 1974)

Health related behaviour is related to:
How much the health goal is valued by individual
The strength of belief that a change will result in avoidance of ill health

The ramifications of these are:
The client's perceived susceptibility: 'Will it happen to me?'
The client's perceived severity: 'How badly will it affect me?'
Perceived benefits for the client: 'What do I get out of changing?'
Perceived barriers for the client: 'Is it worth the discomfort?'

Table 19.18 Stages of change model (after Priest & Speller 1991 by kind permission of Radcliffe Medical Press)

Stage	Description
Precontemplation	'There is no problem for me, why change?'
Contemplation	'OK so it's a problem but I'm not sure if I'm ready to do anything about it'
Action	'I'm ready to do something now'
Maintenance	'I'll keep going even though it's difficult'
Relapse	'I didn't really want to change, I'll go back to the old behaviour'

Priest & Speller (1991) suggest the use of the 'health belief model' (Table 19.17) and the 'stages of change model' (Table 19.18) to structure nurse interventions with the individuals when identifying lifestyles, risk factors and areas for change. This enables the identification of beliefs related to risk factors and the individual's readiness to change.

PROFESSIONAL AND ETHICAL KNOWLEDGE

IMPACT OF HEALTH AND SOCIAL POLICY ON THE PROVISION OF CARE

The implementation of the NHS and Community Care Act 1990 reflected health policy aimed at pushing people through the hospital system as quickly as possible with the aim of returning them to the community. However, 'return to the community' often meant placement in private healthcare facilities, nursing homes or care being provided by family members or neighbours. The rising tide of people presenting with long-term health needs, and increasing longevity in society as a whole, have caused such initiatives to falter and required a rethink of how best to provide for the healthcare needs of those in need of rehabilitation services.

The NHS Plan (Department of Health 2000) introduced the idea of 'intermediate care'. Here it is envisaged that a new form of services will be developed to reduce the pressure placed on acute services by those with subacute and longer term/rehabilitation needs. Intermediate care is a major tenet of the National Service Framework for Older People (Department of Health 2001a). It is proposed that intermediate care can improve recovery rates and increase patient satisfaction, whilst at the same time reducing cost incurred through inappropriate admissions to NHS services (such as acute units) and private sector facilities (nursing/residential homes). Units specializing in rehabilitation are viewed as enabling people to regain physical functioning at a faster pace and promoting early discharge enabling people to stay in their own homes for longer. Although much that has been written regarding intermediate care relates to physical disorders, such models may also be of benefit in the mental health setting.

The Department of Health (2001b) identifies three issues as central to the successful implementation of these services:

- consultation with service users and carers
- mapping of local need
- development of care pathways.

Nursing is seen to play a large role in the development of intermediate care, with a number of nurse-led units being planned.

The success of a rehabilitation programme depends upon the availability of support and resources in the individual's own home. Where resources are limited it is essential that needs are prioritized to ensure that the individual receives the optimum level of care available. Williams (1993) suggests that the success of rehabilitation rests on the ability to maintain and support individuals in the community. However, Nazarko (2001) suggests that intermediate care models are based on the premise that care in the community is in place and able to meet the demands placed on it by the new initiatives. This she proposes is not so and may result in rehabilitation services failing to meeting the demands placed on them.

SOCIAL EXCLUSION

Social exclusion is said to affect a wide range of social groups – low income families, those in care, ex-prisoners, ethnic minorities, those with mental health problems, people with disabilities and older people (Social Exclusion Unit 2001). These groups are often at risk of falling into poverty, discriminated against in the job market and prevented from participating in normal social activities due to lack of mobility either as a result of their disability/age or lack of money to enable use of transport. Such discrimination often leads to depression, loneliness and poor morale. The costs of social exclusion to the individual are:

- financial
- poor access to services
- stress
- poor health
- lack of hope.

The Social Exclusion Unit (2001: 51) sees poor health and disability as one of the 'key causes of social exclusion' and proposes a number of initiatives aimed at addressing inequalities in health and supporting those with long term health needs and/or disabilities. These include focusing health services to ensure those in most need receive appropriate care interventions.

THE NURSE AS A MEMBER OF THE MULTIDISCIPLINARY TEAM

Most literature relating to the nurse's role within the rehabilitation team suggests that the nurse has a vital part to play. The Royal College of Nursing (1991) sees the 24-hour presence of nurses during the individual's stay in hospital as a significant aspect of the nurse's role in rehabilitation. This is echoed by Williams (1993), who identifies that no other health professional has such close and continuous contact.

Long et al (2002) identify six interlinking roles for nurses in the rehabilitation setting:

- assessment – identifying actual and potential problems
- coordination and communication
- technical and physical care
- therapy integration and therapy carry on – ensuring the environment is conducive and treatment regimes maintained
- emotional support
- involving the family.

Evidence based practice

Sheppard's work (1994) identifies that the client often perceives the nurse in a stereotypical way as a provider of physical care undertaking tasks such as taking temperatures and checking pulse and respiration rates, and therefore fails to recognize the nurse's role of educator or facilitator. This indicates that there may be a need for nurses to clarify their role with the client.

Compare this with the work of Easton et al (1995) who looked at the role of the advanced practice nurse (APN) working with clients discharged from a rehabilitation unit. Using an experimental design they demonstrated that the

> group who received follow-up care from the APN developed considerably more effective and positive coping strategies. They concluded that the APN was an extremely effective part of the rehabilitation programme for providing psycho-educational support to clients.

Long et al (2002) suggests there may be a tension for nurses between their traditional role of 'caring' which is often seen as 'doing for' the patient and 'rehabilitation therapy' which demands a standing back and encouraging independence.

The key role of ensuring effective communication between members of the multidisciplinary team, health professionals and clients and their families is viewed by Williams (1993) as falling within the domain of nurses. The relationship between the nurse and client is central to a therapeutic programme, with O'Connor (1990) suggesting that the nurse should match interventions with the physical, psychological and emotional needs of the individual. This ensures that the rehabilitation process keeps pace with the client's needs and progress. This aspect of the nurse's role is essential in ensuring the rehabilitation process takes account of the client's current and changing needs.

The process of rehabilitation often begins in hospital, but as Appleton (1994) proposes, it is continued in the community taking days or months depending upon the severity of problem. Although Appleton referred to children with head injuries, this principle is true of most aspects of rehabilitation. In mental health, for example, rehabilitation is often conducted over a number of years with a gradual reintroduction of the individual into the community. This blend of hospital and community care underlines the need for nurses in both settings to develop skills and knowledge related to the process of rehabilitation.

how people should and should not act. The promoting of individual responsibility for health is central to rehabilitation, but as Goeppinger (1982) suggested, such an approach may give rise to dilemmas, which grow out of differing political ideologies. On one side the responsibility of individuals for their own health is seen as paramount. Therefore if individuals do not reduce identified risk factors in their lifestyles they are viewed as responsible for their own ill health. The opposing argument suggests that there are extraneous factors that make it difficult for individuals to adopt healthy lifestyles, such as poverty and media pressure. Added to this is the suggestion that although the correlation between healthy lifestyles and good health outcomes is strong, it is not conclusive. Social factors, for instance, may have a large part to play in health. From this perspective the emphasis on individual responsibility is seen as making a scapegoat of the sick and blaming them for their own misfortune. Such a debate has implications for the allocation of resources.

Associated with the dilemma relating to the allocation of resources is a suggestion that changes in social policy relating to resourcing of services and the prioritizing of need have a profound impact on those requiring rehabilitation programmes. Elliot (1995) talks of the stresses experienced by health carers in the conflict between the identification of those in greatest need when allocating resources and the belief in the right to equal assess to care and treatment and provision of resources to all in need.

Within the general sphere of health care the individual's right to choose how his or her care is managed and the possible lack of clarity as to the right or wrong of a situation (for example, whether or not to provide care for someone with heart disease who continues to smoke) may leave the practitioner unsure about how to act and moral dilemmas

ETHICAL CONSIDERATIONS

Ethics is said to be about the 'rights and wrongs' of a situation, the value judgements and decisions made relating to

---

Decision making exercise

Should people with cardiac problems be admitted to a rehabilitation programme if they continue to smoke?

- Should scarce resources be allocated only to those who show a willingness to adapt their behaviour or does everyone have a right to treatment regardless of their lifestyle?
- Is it possible to deliver a rehabilitation programme when care is based on availability of resources rather than the needs of patients?
- What should be the nurse's response in such circumstances?

Decision making exercise

Gordon Hill is a 29-year-old sales representative. Recently, following a road traffic accident, he has become severely disabled. He sees life as worthless and a rehabilitation programme to maximize his abilities and independence as useless. The nurse, believing that disability does not devalue the individual, views the development of skills to promote independence as vital.

- Why do you think that Gordon feels this way?
- Gordon and the nurse have differing views on rehabilitation. What are the consequences of accepting each view?
- How might the nurse acknowledge Gordon's feelings, but also encourage him to take a more positive outlook?
- Devise a plan to reinforce Gordon's self-esteem by using appropriate goals?

arise. The same is true in the arena of rehabilitation, particularly in relation to goal setting. There may be times when the goals of the health professional and those of the client are diametrically opposed. Kuczewski & Fiedler (2001) identify the individual's right to self-determination and thus the right to refuse treatment or to participate in rehabilitation programmes. Thus informed consent is central to the process of rehabilitation, all information being made available to the individual allowing them to weigh the pros and cons and make informed decisions.

PERSONAL AND REFLECTIVE KNOWLEDGE

REHABILITATION IN PROFESSIONAL PRACTICE

Rehabilitation is a complex activity. It requires an understanding of the psychological and social impacts illness has on an individual and how these can influence a client's progress to optimum functioning. The nurse must also consider policy issues in relation to the provision of care and address ethical dilemmas. The role of the nurse within the rehabilitation process is therefore multifaceted and requires a dynamic approach. The nurse must draw on wide ranging knowledge to promote the well-being of clients, facilitate multidisciplinary teamwork and deliver individualized care.

Case studies in rehabilitation

Four case studies now follow, one from each branch of nursing. Use the knowledge you have gained from this chapter to answer the questions set in each.

Case study: Mental health

Kevin is 20 years old and has been diagnosed as schizophrenic. He is an only child, has very few friends and normally lives with his parents. Kevin was attending university, but had to leave because of his illness. He has had a number of admissions to his local acute psychiatric unit, usually when his parents feel they can no longer cope with his 'odd' behaviour. Following his most recent admission he has been referred to the rehabilitation team with a view to placing him in a rehabilitation hostel. It is hoped to enable Kevin to live independently in the community.

- What are the immediate problems that confront Kevin and the rehabilitation team?
- Consider the examples of motivation theories and suggest how these could be used to motivate Kevin to participate in his rehabilitation programme.
- Select one of the problems you have identified and construct a rehabilitation programme encompassing short-term and long-term goals.

Case study: Adult

Edna is 64 years old and lives with her 72-year-old husband, Sidney. They have three daughters, June aged 44 years, Mary aged 42 years and Joan aged 40 years, all of whom are married and live some distance away. Edna is the main carer for her husband who has dementia. She suffers a severe stroke and is admitted to hospital with a left-sided hemiplegia. Initially she is very reliant on the nursing staff for many of the basic requirements to sustain life. Gradually her condition improves.

- Identify the changes in body image Edna may experience following her stroke.
- What sort of labels may be applied to Edna and what impact could these have on her self-concept?
- What impact may the recent developments in welfare provision have on the planning of a rehabilitation programme for Edna?
- Identify and prioritize the services that Edna may require to enable her to live in her own home following her recovery.

Case study: Learning disabilities

John is 45 years old, has a moderate learning disability and lives in a staffed group home with three other residents. Before this he lived in the local large institution, which closed 7 years ago. He is a popular member of the home, and takes part in many social activities. John is overweight, having a 'sweet tooth' and taking very little exercise. While attending the social education centre John has a heart attack and is admitted to hospital.

- What personal characteristics may be attributed to John and how might these affect his care?
- What changes might John need to make because of his myocardial infarction?
- How could you use change theory to facilitate John's well-being?
- John is to undertake a fitness regimen. Identify a possible long-term goal and the sequential short-terms goals to meet such a requirement.

Case study: Child

Susan is 8 years old and is the middle child of three.
Her family live in a three-bedroom semi-detached house on the outskirts of the city. Both her parents work: her father Paul is a police officer, her mother Sarah works part time as a nurse. While on her way home from school Susan is knocked down by a car. As she has suffered severe head injuries she is transferred

from the local hospital to the nearest neurosurgical ward some 40 miles away.

- What barriers to communication may be present for Susan and how could you overcome these?
- Susan is referred to a rehabilitation team. What data would be needed to develop her rehabilitation programme and how could these be collected?
- Identify a selection of assessment tools that will aid this process.

Summary

The main points covered in this chapter were as follows:

1. Rehabilitation is a process aimed at enabling an individual to gain his or her optimum level of functioning through a multidisciplinary approach.
2. The nurse's role is multifaceted and requires a breadth and depth of knowledge relating to clients' physical, social and psychological needs and care management and delivery issues.
3. Communication is a central factor in the effectiveness of rehabilitation programmes.
4. Integral parts of the nurse's role are those of health educator (this includes the identification of risk factors associated with various disorders) and of facilitator of change.
5. Rigorous assessment is essential in providing a baseline from which to work, identifying what is achievable and in monitoring progress.
6. Appropriate goal setting is a prerequisite to the identification of desired outcomes of care, ensuring effective communication, teamwork and the maintenance of client and carer motivation.
7. Social and psychological issues have a profound influence on the individual's experience of illness, provision of services and delivery of care.

Annotated further reading and websites

Brennan J 1994 A vital component of care: the nurse's role in recognizing altered body image. Professional Nurse February:298
This paper offers the reader insight into the nurse's role in caring for clients with altered body image.

Haynes S 1992 Let the change come from within: the process of change in nursing. Professional Nurse July:635–638
This provides an insight into change theory and a comprehensive discourse on the management of change and nursing practice.

Long A, Kneafsey R, Ryan J et al 2002 The role of the nurse within the multiprofessional rehabilitation team. Journal of Advanced Nursing 37(1):70–78
This article describes a qualitative investigation into the role of the nurse in the rehabilitation setting.

Scut H A, Stam H J 1994 Goals in rehabilitation teamwork. Disability and Rehabilitation 16(4):223–226
This article contains an in-depth discussion of goal setting in the rehabilitation setting.

Worden J W 1991 Grief counselling and grief therapy, 2nd edn. Routledge, London
Every change involves a loss and many people grieve or mourn, because of change. This is an area where people may be helped through the process of change. Worden identifies four tasks of mourning that must be completed for successful resolution. Although this was written with the bereaved in mind the principles may be applied to most loss. By identifying that a person may be grieving we may assist them through the grieving process and consequently facilitate their successful adaptation to change.

http://www.rethink.org/index.html
The homepage of Rethink, a UK based organization that supports people who suffer from schizophrenia, and their carers. Formerly named the National Schizophrenia Fellowship (changed following the introduction of National Service Frameworks – both were abbreviated to NSF!), this organization is an excellent resource for suffers and professionals. Of particular relevance to this chapter is a section on returning to employment.

http://www.radar.org.uk
The website of RADAR, the disability network. The site is designed for service users; however, there is much of interest for service providers. It is an excellent resource for information and there is a comprehensive library of links to relevant sites.

http://www.dialuk.org.uk/
A website focusing on disability, run by the DIAL organization. Provides information and advice on welfare benefits, community care, equipment, independent living, mobility, discrimination and holidays. Contains numerous factsheets that are useful for service users and practitioners.

http://www.drc-gb.org/
The Disability Rights Commission (DRC) is an independent body, established by Act of Parliament, to eliminate discrimination against disabled people and promote equality of opportunity. Despite legislation being introduced to support the rights of disabled people, many find it hard to take part in day-to-day life and are denied the opportunities available to non-disabled people. The role of the DRC is to act as their advocate. This site has a considerable amount of information and relevant links.

References

Appleton R 1994 Head injury rehabilitation for children. Nursing Times 90(22):29–31

Argyle M 1969 Social interaction. Methuen, London

Atkinson R L, Atkinson R G, Smith E E et al 1993 Introduction to psychology, 11th edn. Harcourt Brace, London

Bercheid E, Walster E M 1974 Physical attractiveness. In: Berkowitz L (ed) Advances in experimental social psychology. Academic Press, New York

Binnie A, Bond S, Law G et al (1984) A systematic approach to nursing care. Open University Press, Milton Keynes

Brennan J 1994 A vital component of care: the nurse's role in recognizing altered body image. Professional Nurse 9(5):298

Costello J 1995 Helping relatives cope with the grieving process. Professional Nurse 11(2):89–92

Davis A, Davis S, Moss N et al 1992 First steps towards an interdisciplinary approach to rehabilitation. Clinical Rehabilitation 6:237–244

Department of Health 1991 The health of the nation. HMSO, London

Department of Health 1994 Working in partnership: a collaborative approach to care. HMSO, London

Department of Health 1997 The new NHS: modern, dependable. HMSO, London

Department of Health 1998 A first class service. HMSO, London

Department of Health 2000 The NHS plan. HMSO, London

Department of Health 2001a National Service Framework for older people. HMSO, London

Department of Health 2001b Intermediate care: HSC2001/01/LAC(2001) 1. HMSO, London

Doughty C 1991 A multidisciplinary approach to cardiac rehabilitation. Nursing Standard 5(45):13–15

Easton K L, Rawl S M, Zemen D et al 1995 The effects of nursing follow-up on the coping strategies used by rehabilitation patients after discharge. Rehabilitation Nursing Research 4(4):119–127

Egan G 1986 The skilled helper: a problem-management approach to helping. Brooks/Cole, Pacific Grove

Elliot M 1995 Care management in the community: a case study. Nursing Times 91(48):34–35

Gibbon B, Thompson A 1992 The role of the nurse in rehabilitation. Nursing Standard 6(36):32–35

Goeppinger J 1982 Changing health behaviours and outcomes through self-care. In: Lancaster J, Lancaster W (eds) Concepts for advanced nursing: the nurse as a change agent. Mosby, St Louis, pp 372–387

Goffman E 1963 Stigma: notes on the management of a spoiled identity. Prentice-Hall, Englewood Cliffs

Haffer A 1986 Facilitating change. Journal of Nursing Administration 16(4):18–22

Huczynski A, Buchanan D 1985 Organizational behaviour: an introductory text, 2nd edn. Prentice-Hall, London

Kelley D, Connor D R 1979 The emotional cycle of change. In: Jones J E, Pfeiffer J W (eds) Annual handbook for group facilitators. University Associates, San Diego

Keyser D 1986 Using nursing contracts to support change in nursing organizations. Nurse Education Today 6(3):103–108

Kubler Ross E 1975 Death: the final stage of growth. Prentice-Hall, London

Kuczewski M, Fiedler I 2001 Ethical issues in rehabilitation: conceptualizing the next generation of challenges. American Journal of Physical Medicine and Rehabilitation 80(11):848–851

Lancaster J, Lancaster W (eds) 1982 Concepts for advanced nursing: – the nurse as a change agent. Mosby, St Louis

Lemert E 1951 Social pathology. McGraw Hill, New York

Lewinter M, Mikkelsen S 1995 Patients' experience of rehabilitation after stroke. Disability and Rehabilitation 17(1):3–9

Long A, Kneafsey R, Ryan J et al 2002 The role of the nurse within the multiprofessional rehabilitation team. Journal of Advanced Nursing 37(1):70–78

McGrath J R, Davis A M 1992 Rehabilitation: where are we going and how do we get there? Clinical Rehabilitation 6:225–235

Mainman L A, Becker M H 1974 The health belief model: origin and correlation in psychological theory. Health Education Monograph 2:336–353

Maslow A H 1970 Motivation and personality, 2nd edn. Harper & Row, New York

Nazarko L 2001 Rehabilitation. Part 1: The evidence base for practice. Nursing Management 8(8):14–18

NHS and Community Care Act 1990 HMSO, London

O'Connor S 1990 Removing barriers to communication. Nursing Standard 6:26–27

Ostir G, Goodwin J S, Markides K et al 2002 Differential effects of premorbid physical and emotional health on recovery from acute events. Journal of the American Geriatrics Society 50(4):713–718

Parsons T 1951 The social system. Routledge & Kegan Paul, London

Price B 1990 Body image: nursing concepts and care. Prentice-Hall, London

Priest V, Speller V 1991 The risk factor manual. Radcliffe Medical Press, Oxford

Royal College of Nursing 1991 The role of the nurse in rehabilitation of elderly people. Scutari, London

Scott C 2001 Nursing in the public sphere: health policy research in a changing world. Journal of Advanced Nursing 33(3):387–395

Scut H A, Stam H J 1994 Goals in rehabilitation teamwork. Disability and Rehabilitation 16(4):223–226

Sheppard B 1994 Client's views of rehabilitation. Nursing Standard 9(10):27–29

Smith D S, Clark M S 1995 Competence and performance in activities of daily living of clients following rehabilitation from stroke. Disability and Rehabilitation 17(1):15–23

Social Exclusion Unit 2001 Preventing social exclusion. Social Exclusion Unit, London

Sternberg R J 1995 In search of the human mind. Harcourt Brace, London

Thurgood A 1990 Seven steps to rehabilitation. Nursing Times 86(25):38–41

Tod A M, Lacey E A, McNeill F 2002 'I'm still waiting …': barriers to accessing cardiac rehabilitation services. Journal of Advanced Nursing 40(4):421–431

Tuckman B W 1965 Developmental sequences in small groups. Psychological Bulletin 63:384–399

Vaughan B, Pillmoor M 1989 Managing nursing work. Scutari, London

Waters K R 1994 Getting dressed in the early mornings: styles of staff/client interaction on rehabilitation hospital wards for elderly people. Journal of Advanced Nursing 19:239–248

Williams J 1993 Rehabilitation challenge. Nursing Times 89(31):67–70

Williams S 1987 Goffman, interactionism, and the management of stigma in everyday life. In: Scambler G (ed) Sociology theory and medical sociology. Tavistock, London

Wing J 1983 Schizophrenia. In: Watts F N, Bennet D H (eds) Theory and practice of psychiatric rehabilitation. John Wiley, Chichester, pp 45–67

Glossary

Ablution   The act of washing or cleansing, especially the washing of hands.

Abrasion   A superficial wound in the skin, where damage has been caused by some kind of scraping.

'Adverse event'   In health care, any act or omission that leads to unintended or unexpected harm, loss or damage. Compare **Near miss**.

Advocacy   Active support or representation. Advocacy is the expression of support for or opposition to a cause, argument or proposal. Advocacy may include influencing laws, legislation or attitudes. A nurse may act as the client's advocate, representing their interests and interpreting wishes to others involved in their care.

Aetiology   The cause(s) or origin(s) of a disease. (Note that the US spelling is etiology.)

Ageism   Prejudice and discrimination against elderly people solely on the grounds of their age.

Aggression   A hostile or destructive attitude to other persons or objects, and which can include verbal attacks or physical violence.

Allograft   A graft of tissue between individuals of the same species; in the medical context, between two humans. The tissue donor might be a cadaver, or might be a living person, related or unrelated. Compare **Autograft**, **Xenograft**.

Amino acid   An organic compound containing an amino (-NH$_2$) and a carboxyl (-COOH) group. Amino acids are combined into proteins and are thus an important element of the diet. See also **Essential amino acid**.

Analgesia   The relief of pain without loss of consciousness.

Androgen   Any of several steroid hormones produced in the testes (or synthetically), and promoting male secondary sexual characteristics.

Angiogenesis   The development of blood vessels. This can be in the embryo and foetus during development, or during the growth of a tumour. It also occurs during a stage of wound healing.

Antibiotic   A chemical substance produced by a microorganism or made synthetically, that inhibits or destroys other microorganisms.

Antidepressant   Any drug that stimulates the mood of a depressed patient, e.g. amitriptyline or fluoxetine.

Antipsychotic   A drug used to treat psychotic disorders such as schizophrenia.

Anxiolytic   Any drug that reduces anxiety; the most usual ones are in the benzodiazepine group, e.g. diazepam.

Arousal   The state of responsiveness to sensory stimuli.

Asepsis   The absence of microorganisms.

Assertiveness   Confidently but sensitively claiming one's position or stating one's point of view.

Autograft   A graft of tissue between one part of a patient's body to another. Compare **Allograft**, **Xenograft**.

Biofeedback   A technique for controlling one's own body state, e.g. anxiety, by the aid of electronic devices that monitor and report functions increasing self-awareness of the body's response to stress, such as pulse rate, respiration rate or blood pressure.

Burnout   A condition that occurs following prolonged exposure to high levels of stress, characterized by emotional numbing and changes to personality that result in the individual becoming isolated and acquiring an overwhelming cynical attitude that belittles the achievement of self and others.

Carbohydrate   Any of a large group of organic compounds having the general formula $C_m(H_2O)_n$. It includes the sugars (e.g. glucose) and polysaccharides (e.g. starch), which are important energy producing foods.

Catheter   A tube that is inserted into the body to introduce or remove fluid.

Charting   The technique of recording at regular time intervals aspects of a patient's state, e.g. fluid intake/urinary output.

Chemoreceptor   A sensory receptor in a cell membrane which receives molecules from the external environment and gives rise to the sensation of smell or taste.

Chemotherapy The treatment of a disease with a chemical substance.

Circadian rhythm The pattern of biological processes that occur regularly at 25-hour intervals. These patterns persist even in the absence of environmental cues, e.g. in crews of spacecraft.

Circumcision Male – removal of foreskin; female – removal of clitoris (and sometimes also the labia majora and labia minora).

Clinical audit Examination or measurement of clinical practice quality standards and associated outcomes.

Clinical governance An initiative of the Department of Health begun in 1997 and defined by them as 'a system through which NHS organizations are accountable for continuously improving the quality of their services and safeguarding high standards of care by creating an environment in which excellence will flourish'.

Commensal Two different species of organisms that live together without one of them being dependent on the other or one being parasitic on the other.

Complementary medicines Treatments taken by patients that are not prescribed through conventional medical sources, but may complement such treatments; they are not alternative, as they do not replace medical treatments.

Compliance The act of obeying. In health care, compliance refers to the patient/client's conduct in carrying out the agreed treatment or regime, e.g. by taking the medications prescribed or by adhering to diet.

Compression Depression of the chest by a rescuer to 'squeeze' the heart between the sternum and spine as a means of emptying the heart of blood to pump the blood around the circulation.

Confidentiality The understanding that no information relating to a patient, e.g. personal or clinical details, may be divulged to unauthorized individuals or data sites without their consent.

Confusion Disturbance of a person's orientation as to place or time or their own personhood.

Consciousness The state of being aware of oneself, one's environment and one's physical and mental condition. Immediate knowledge or perception of the presence of any object, state, or sensation.

Consent Agreement with a client/patient for a procedure to be undertaken or withheld. For the consent to be valid it is important that the client/patient has been fully informed of all relevant factors, is not under some form of coercion, and is mentally fit to grant consent. In the UK the age at which a client/patient may give consent is 16.

Coroner In England and Wales, the public official responsible for the investigation of unexplained deaths, be they sudden, violent, or otherwise suspicious. The coroner is usually, but need not be, medically qualified.

Cosmopolitan Occurring worldwide, or nearly so.

Counselling Support offered to a person who is trying to overcome a psychosocial problem. Broadly defined, it includes both 'therapy and psychotherapy'. Counselling is a developmental process, in which one individual (the counsellor) provides to another individual or group (the client), guidance and encouragement, challenge and inspiration in creatively managing and resolving practical, personal and relationship issues, in achieving goals, and in self-realization. Counsellors are nowadays usually professionals specializing in particular problem areas, e.g. bereavement.

Cytoplasm The protoplasm of a cell, i.e. everything within the cell membrane except the nucleus. It consists of a fluid (the cytosol) in which are suspended the various cell organelles.

Deciduous Of teeth, the non-permanent of the infant and child, colloquially known as 'milk teeth'.

Decontamination Removal of a contaminant or pollutant.

Defibrillation A method of sending a controlled electrical shock through the chest wall to terminate a chaotic cardiac rhythm, allowing, when possible, the heart's own electrical conduction system to regain control. It does not 'restart' the heart.

Dehydration The condition resulting from excessive loss of body water.

Delirium A transitory state of disturbed consciousness, which can be caused by various factors including fever, brain injury or drug intoxication.

Dementia A clinical state characterized by progressive deterioration or impairment of brain function. Dementia is the mental deterioration (loss of intellectual ability) that is associated with old age. Two major types of senile dementia are identified: those due to generalized atrophy (Alzheimer type) and those due to vascular problems (mainly strokes).

Dependency Over-reliance by a person on some external form of support, most commonly some other person, or something that is psychologically or physically habit-forming (especially alcohol or narcotic drugs).

Deviation Behaviour that does not conform to what is considered acceptable, especially sexual behaviour.

Disinfection A process which reduces the number of microorganisms to a level at which they are no longer harmful.

Diuretic An agent that promotes the excretion of urine.

Dizygotic twins Non-identical twins, resulting from the separate fertilization of two ova by two spermatozoa; in effect brothers/sisters born at the same time. Compare **Monozygotic twins**.

Duty of care The legal or moral obligations that a person has to perform actions for another's welfare.

Electrolyte   A chemical compound that when in solution dissociates into ions.

Elimination   The act of clearing waste from the body, including both urination and defaecation.

Emollient   Any substance, especially an ointment, that has a softening effect when applied to the skin.

Emulsion   A mixture in which both constituents are liquids.

Endemic   The usual level or presence of an agent or disease in a defined population during a given period.

Endorphins   Various polypeptides that occur naturally in the brain and can bind to pain receptors (**nociceptors**) thus blocking off the sensation of pain.

Energy   The capacity to do work: in the body, it takes two forms, heat and chemical energy. It is measured in joules or calories.

Epidemic   An unusual higher than expected level of infection or disease in a defined population in a given period.

Ergonomics   The science that tries to adapt the task, the equipment and the working environment to suit the worker(s).

Essential amino acid   One of the nine amino acids that cannot be synthesized in the human body so must be taken in the diet.

Ethics   Moral standards and criteria for conduct. The socially agreed rules and principles that should be applied in decisions about actions towards others. Ethics is the field of study that is concerned with questions of value, that is, judgements about what human behaviour is 'good' or 'bad'.

Ethnicity   The sense of belonging to a particular cultural or racial group, with its own customs, practices and beliefs.

Ethology   The study of the behaviour of non-human animals in their natural habitats.

Euthanasia   The practice of 'mercy killing', i.e. painlessly ending the life of a person with an incurable illness. It is not legal in the UK.

Exudate   Matter that oozes from a blood vessel into surrounding tissues, usually as a result of inflammation.

Fat   A non-technical term for the component in the diet more properly called lipids. In the diet these are mostly triglycerides, which consist of three fatty acids and a glycerol molecule.

Feedback loop   A closed pathway in which the input signal directly controls the output. In positive feedback higher input leads to higher output. In negative feedback increased input results in a reduction of output, which is a common mechanism of **homeostasis**.

Fulcrum   Of a lever, the point about which a lever turns.

Goal setting   A technique in rehabilitation in which the patient and nurse agree step by step projects within a timeframe, to recover as much as possible of normal function.

Hazard   An event or situation that has the potential to cause harm.

Heimlich manoeuvre   Action taken by a rescuer when the victim has a partial or complete obstruction of the upper airway by standing behind the victim, forming hand into a fist, covering it with the other hand and applying pressure to the upper abdomen. The action should push upwards against the diaphragm so increasing the pressure in the chest cavity under the obstruction helping to move it upwards.

Holistic   A system of treatment that takes into account the whole person, i.e. their physical, psychological and social aspects.

Homeostasis   A tendency to stability in the body's metabolism; the maintenance of a constant internal environment. It is achieved by a system in which the negative **feedback loop** is the basic mechanism.

Homeothermy   The maintenance of a constant internal body temperature.

Homophobia   Fearing or disliking of homosexual people or homosexuality. There are four basic levels of homophobia: (1) the fear and hatred of gays and lesbians, (2) the fear of being perceived as gay or lesbian, (3) the fear of one's own sexual or physical attraction for same-sex individuals, and (4) the fear of being gay or lesbian.

Hospice   A nursing home that specializes in the care of the dying, either full-time as a place for the patient to die or part-time to give respite to the caring family.

Hydrotherapy   The application of water in the treatment of disease, especially the use of swimming as therapeutic exercise to strengthen weak joints and wasted muscles.

Hygiene   Strictly, the science of health, and its maintenance, but more generally used to mean the practices of bodily cleanliness that promote health.

Hypoallergenic   Made of substances known to be unlikely to provoke an allergic reaction.

Immunity   The ability of an organism to resist infection by means of circulating antibodies.

Immunocompromised   Having impaired immune response that renders the host particularly susceptible to an infection.

Indemnity insurance   Insurance that covers a professional person for damages resulting from being sued by a patient, colleague or member of the public.

Infection   An invasion of the body by pathogenic microorganisms, or the disease resulting therefrom.

Infestation   An invasion of the body by parasites, usually insects. Compare **Infection**.

Inflammation   The self-protective reaction of tissue to infection or injury, the signs of which are swelling, redness, heat and pain.

Learning disabilities The arrested or incomplete development of mind or significant impairment to intellectual, adaptive or social functioning. The dimensions of this term are defined by the World Health Organization as: (1) a state of arrested or incomplete development of mind; (2) significant impairment of intellectual functioning; (3) significant impairment of adaptive/social functioning. One of the four branches of nursing concerns the care of clients with learning disabilities.

Lesion Any injury or ailment involving direct damage to tissue or loss of a body part.

Libido The urge towards sexual activity.

Living will A form of advance directive which can be verbal to something more formal as found in the USA in which the patient/client expresses what should happen within certain situations, e.g. refusal of resuscitation or life-prolonging treatment in the case of serious incapacity. The validity of a living will is recognized under UK common law.

Malnutrition Any disorder of nutrition. Although used most commonly referring to an insufficient quantity of nutrition, it can also mean oversupply of nutrition, or dietary imbalance.

Marginalization The act of relegating a person or group to the fringes of society, owing to some perceived shortcoming, e.g. disability or age.

Menopause The ending of menstruation in a woman's life cycle, either naturally at the age of about 50, or as the result of surgical intervention (e.g. hysterectomy).

Menstruation The cyclic discharge of blood through the vagina in a non-pregnant woman of childbearing age.

Metabolism The chemical processes that drive the machinery of the body, giving rise to growth, movement and elimination of waste.

Microorganism Any organism of microscopic size, e.g. a virus, bacterium or protozoan. It may or may not be a **pathogen**, i.e. capable of causing a disease.

Mobilism Prejudice and discrimination against people with impaired mobility.

Monozygotic twins Identical twins, resulting from the fertilization of a single ovum by a single spermatozoon, with subsequent division of the early zygote into two independent embryos. Compare **Dizygotic twins**.

'Near miss' In health care any act or omission that could have led to unintended or unexpected harm, loss or damage but did not actually do so. (If it had done so it would have been an **adverse event**.)

Necrosis Death of a group of cells or part of a structure or organ, often resulting from failure of blood supply.

Negligence A civil wrong in which the defendant has breached a duty of care which has caused some injury, loss or damage to the claimant of a type that the law acknowledges.

Neurotransmitter A chemical by means of which a neurone passes on a message to another neurone or a muscle.

Nociceptor A receptor for pain. The stimulus may be either physical (e.g. heat, a blow or electric shock) or chemical (presence of a toxin).

Nomogram Graphical representation of relationship between two or more variables.

Non-verbal communication Communication by means other than speech, i.e. facial expressions, gestures, posture, non-word sounds, or non-verbal aspects of speech such as tone of voice, accent, pace of speaking. It may be both intentional and unintentional.

Norm An established standard of behaviour applicable to and upheld by a social group.

Nosocomial An infection that is acquired or occurring in hospital.

Oedema Swelling caused by accumulation of fluid in the intercellular spaces of tissue. (Note that US spelling is edema.)

Off-label The unlicensed use of a medication with a client group who are not included in the licensing criteria, or (off-licence) are given in a manner not included in the licensing criteria, e.g. an alternative route is used.

Oscillation A regular fluctuation above or below a mean value.

Palliation Any system of care that aims to provide relief from pain rather than cure.

Pathogen A microorganism that is capable of causing a disease.

Pathway In metabolism, a series of reactions that converts one biological substance to another.

Phagocytosis The process by which a white blood cell ingests objects such as microorganisms or foreign bodies.

Pharmacodynamics A study of the mechanism of a drug in relation to cellular physiology and biochemistry.

Pharmacokinetics A process of drug movement through the body; this includes phases of absorption, distribution, metabolism and excretion where drug action may take place.

Photoageing The process of premature ageing of the skin due to the action of sunlight.

Physiotherapy The use of physical means such as exercise, massage, or manipulation in the treatment of musculoskeletal problems.

Pigmentation Coloration in the skin or other tissue caused by the presence of pigments such as melanin in the cells.

Polypharmacy The practice of treatment with more than one prescribed medicine simultaneously.

Postmortem The examination (including dissection and possibly also tissue culture) of a dead body to ascertain the cause of an otherwise unexplained death.

Prognosis The prediction of the likely outcome of a disease, injury or inborn disorder.

Protein A chain of amino acids joined by peptide bonds and folded into a three-dimensional shape typical for each protein. Proteins are found in all cells of the body; some from the basic components of tissue, some functions as enzymes, hormones or antibodies.

Psychoanalysis A method, pioneered by Sigmund Freud, of treating patients with psychological disorders based on investigating and bringing to light the unconscious and repressed processes of the mind.

Puberty The phase of maturation at which the sex glands become functional and the secondary sexual characteristics develop. In boys, spermatogenesis begins and the voice 'breaks'; in girls, menstruation commences.

Recumbency The state of being unable to maintain any body posture other than lying down.

Rehydration The restoration of normal body fluid content. This may be done orally, by feeding tube or intravenously.

Respiration Breathing, i.e. the process of exchange of air between the lungs and the external environment; it includes inspiration, breathing in, and expiration, breathing out. Breathing is known as external respiration, while internal respiration refers to the exchange of oxygen and carbon dioxide at cellular level.

Resuscitation Action taken to restore breathing and normal heart rhythm in a person in whom these have ceased.

Risk The possibility that a **hazard** will cause harm.

Risk assessment The science of assessing (1) the probability of a harmful outcome in any situation, and (2) the extent of the harm resulting.

Risk management The control of hazards in any situation so as to minimize the possibility of a harmful outcome and limit its extent.

Sociobiology The study of social behaviour in animals and humans, especially with a view to interpreting the evolutionary advantage of particular behaviours.

Stereotype A way of judging a person by simplistic (usually derogatory) generalizations about the group of which they are or are supposed to be a member.

Sterilization A process that completely removes or destroys all microorganisms.

Stigmatization The act or practice of marking out a person or group as being inferior due to some perceived failing, either mental, physical or social.

Stressor Any stimulus to which an individual responds either physically or psychologically.

Surveillance The systematic collection, collation, interpretation and dissemination of information essential to identifying outbreaks and trends of infectious disease.

Suture Anything used to secure the edges of a wound together to promote healing. Formerly always done with silk thread, now often metal clips are used, or absorbable threads that are dissolved by enzymes and do not need removal.

Thermogenesis The production of heat by body processes. Shivering, producing heat by activity in the muscles, is a form of thermogenesis.

Thermoregulation The control of body heat. Warm-blooded animals (including humans) maintain a constant internal body heat despite fluctuations of external environmental temperature.

Trauma In psychology, an event causing a powerful shock that has long-lasting effects on the personality. In pathology, any injury or wound.

Ulceration The formation of an ulcer, i.e. a hole in the surface of a tissue or an organ due to **necrosis**.

Ultrasound Sound waves above the audible range (above 20 kHz) used for viewing internal structures of the body, or the fetus *in utero*.

Unlicensed Drugs that have no product licence, and no data sheet/product specification.

Urinalysis Chemical analysis of the urine to test for signs of disease or malfunction.

Vaccination The process of inducing immunity by the giving of a vaccine which is an inactivated microbial toxin or microbial antigen.

Ventilation Movement of air in and out of the lungs either by the individual (self-ventilating) or by another person, e.g. a first-aider (mouth to mouth), or by artificial means using a machine.

Vitamin A general term for a number of unrelated organic substances that are essential in small quantities for the normal functioning of the body. Some can be synthesized in the human body, but others must be taken in the diet. Vitamins may be either water-soluble or fat-soluble.

Vocabulary The stock of words that a person has at their disposal; also the system of techniques or symbols serving as a means of expression. The number of words understood is always greater that the number that a person will themselves use in speech or writing.

Xenograft A graft of tissue between different species. Compare **Allograft**, **Autograft**.

Zeitgeber A stimulus that affects an organism's biological clock, e.g. a change in the level of light.

Zero tolerance The policy of applying penalties to even minor offences in order to enforce the overall principles of a code of behaviour.

Index

Page numbers in **bold** refer to illustrations and table.

A

ABC approach, resuscitation, 54–57
Abdominal thrust (Heimlich manoeuvre), 59, **60**, 62
Abduction, joint movement, **371**
Absorbent products, incontinence, 413, **413**, 418
Abuse
    communication by victims of, 7
    and continence care, 418
    of elderly people, 361
    of patients, 19, 114
Accidents, 30, 42
    emergency care *see* Resuscitation and emergency care
    falls, 119, 375, 380
    major wounds, 319–320
    with medications, 208, 216
    monitoring, 118
Accountability
    nursing observations, 147
    nutritional care, 171
    resuscitation and emergency care, 65–70
Acetylcholine, 372
Acidity, and infection control, **79**
Acinetobacter, **77**
Acne, 283
Activities of daily living (ADL), 377
Acupressure, 235
Acupuncture, 235
Adduction, joint movement, **371**
Adenosine diphosphate (ADP), 155–156
Adenosine triphosphate (ATP), 155–156
Adipose tissue
    lipid storage, 157
    thermogenesis, 130, 131
Adolescents *see* Children
Adrenaline (epinephrine), resuscitation, 64
Advance directives, 71, 275
Advanced cardiac life support (ACLS), 45, 62–63, **64**, 69–70
Advanced practice nurses, 325, 437–438

Adverse events
    drug-related *see* Medicines, adverse effects
    investigation, 35
    learning from, 34–35
    patient handling, 118
    reporting, 34–35, 39
Advocacy, 19–20
    infection control, 97
    mobility care, 384
Aged people *see* Elderly people
Ageing effects
    continence, 400–401
    sexuality, 334–335, 344, 345–346
Ageing process, 264, 308
Ageism, 361, 376
Aggression, 245–259
    assault cycle, 250–251, **250**
    assertiveness, 249, 255
    biological theories, 246–247
    bullying, 246, 248, 249
    care delivery knowledge, 245, 248–256
    case studies, 258–259
    community nurses, 258
    definitions, 246
    employers' responsibilities, 256–257
    ethological theories, 247
    forms of, 248
    harassment, 246, 248, 249
    legal issues, 256–258
    management, 250–255
        after the incident, 251–253
        communication skills, 253–255
        debriefing, 252
        immediate response, 250
        incident containment, 250–251
        incident review, 252–253
        support for staff, 252
    minimizing risk of, 249–250
    number of incidents, 253
    personal knowledge, 245, 258–259
    prediction, **249**
    prevention, 255–256
    professional knowledge, 245, 256–258
    psychosocial factors, **249**
    psychosocial theories, 247–248
    reflective knowledge, 245, 258–259
    risk management, 255–256

    self-defence, 257
    and stress, 180
    subject knowledge, 245, 246–248
    warning signs, 250
    Zero Tolerance campaign, 257–258
Aids
    bathing, 291, **291**
    mobility, 380–382, 384, 385
Air, environmental safety, 27
Airway obstruction (choking), 59–62
Airway opening, resuscitation, 55, **56**
    altered anatomical airways, 59
    children, 50
    choking, 59–62
    spine injuries, 58
Alcohol misuse
    and homeopathy, 236
    intoxication, 355
    stress, 190
Alcohol solutions, **82**, 90, **90**, 91
Alkalinity, infection control, **79**
Allergies
    to drugs, **206**
    food, 170
    latex, 94, 312
Alpha blockers, incontinence, **408**
Alternative therapies, 208–209
Alzheimer disease, 356, 359, 360
Ambulance service, 64
Amino acids, 157, 158
Anal canal, defaecation, 398, **398**
    anorectal incontinence, 399–400, **399**, 411
Analgesia, 226, 228, 232–233, 238
    in palliative care, 275
    patient controlled (PCA), 233
    xerostomia with, **293**
Anger, and sexual response, 340
    see also Aggression
Angiogenesis, 309
Anorectal incontinence, 399–400, **399**, 411
Anorexia nervosa, 169–170, 172
Antibiotics
    resistance to, 75, 80, 96, 97
    wound healing, 318
    xerostomia with, **293**
Anticholinergics, **293**, 408, **408**
Antidepressants, 190, **293**, **343**

Antihistamines, **293**, **343**
Antipsychotics, **293**, **343**
Antiseptics, **90**, 318
Anxiety
  change management, 430
  communication barriers, 433
  and sexual response, 340
Anxiety management groups, 189
Anxiolytics
  to aid sleep, 191
  and sexual activity, **343**
  stress management, 190
Apnoea, 146
Apocrine glands, 283
Appetite, 154
Aprons, 93, 94
Aromatherapy, 235
Arousal theory, **429**
Ascorbic acid (vitamin C), **159**
Aseptic technique, 95–96
  wound care, 318, 319, 320
Assault *see* Aggression
Assertiveness, and aggression, 249, 255
Assertiveness groups, 189
Assessment skills, 434, **434**
Atropine, resuscitation, 64
Axillary thermometry, 139, 140–141, **140**

B

Babies *see* Children
Back injury, 105, 108–110, 118, 119
  avoidance of *see* Handling and moving
    patients
  first aid process, 55, 58, **58**
Bacteria, 76, 77–78
  carriers, 80, 96, 97
  catheter encrustation, 415
  classification, 77, **78**
  dental hygiene, 286
  diseases caused by, 77, 78, 80
  eye care, 287
  growth requirements, **79**
  immune response to, **81**
  infection control *see* Infection control
  skin care, 282–283, 289
Balance, mobility, 379–380, 381–382
Basal metabolic rate (BMR), 162, 164
Basic life support (BLS), 45, 53–62, **65–68**,
  69–70
Bathing, 287–288, 289, 290–292, 297, 298
Bed bathing, 289, 290
Bed sores *see* Pressure sores
Bed-wetting *see* Nocturnal enuresis
Behavioural assessment, 358
Bereavement, 50–51, 180–181, 267–270,
  273–274, 429
Beta blockers, sexual activity, **343**
Biofeedback, 189–190, 407
Biotin, **159**
Bladder, 393–394
  atonic, 397, 409
  detrusor muscle, 393, **394**
    ageing effects, 401

drug treatment, 408, **408**
  hyperactivity, 394, 395, **396**, 407–408
  hypoactivity, 396–397, **397**, 409, 414
  and fluid intake, 406
  hypotonic, 397
  influences on function, 397
  nerve supply, 394, **394**, 395, 401
  pelvic floor, 393, 395, **395**, 406–407
  retraining, 407, 408
  stress incontinence, 395, 407
  voiding difficulties, 396–397, 401, 408–409
Bleach (hypochlorites), **82**, 92
Blindness *see* Eyesight, impaired
Blood–brain barrier, 204
Blood cells
  immune response, 81
  oxygen transport, 136
Blood dyscrasias, drug-related, **206**
Blood pressure
  balance, 132–134
  diastolic, 132, **133**, 143, **143**, 144
  high (hypertension), 129, **142**, 144–145
  Korotkoff phases, 143, **143**
  low (hypotension), **142**, 145
  measurement, 142–144, 147–148
  pulse, 133–134
  systolic, 132, **133**, 143, 144
Blood spills, disposal of, 92
Blood supply
  muscle, 372, 373
  wounds, 309, 310
Bobath method, 382
Body alignment, mobility, 379
Body image, 311, 427–428
Body language, 254–255, 432
Body levers, 372–373
Body mass index (BMI), 164, **165**
Body odour, 283, 287–288
Body piercings, 312
Body surface area (BSA), **201**
Body temperature *see* Temperature, body
Body weight, 161, 164, **165**, 168–170
Bone
  effects of immobility, 374
  microscopic structure, 369, **369**
Bovine spongiform encephalitis, 356
Bowel, lower, 398–400
  see also Faecal incontinence
Bradycardia, 134
Bradypnoea, 146
Brain
  aggression, 246, **246**
  appetite, 154
  communication barriers, 432, 433
  criteria for death, 265–266
  dementia, 356
  drug distribution, 204
  homeostatic mechanisms, 128
    blood pressure, 133
    respiration, 136
    thermoregulation, 128, 130, 131
  language areas, 5–6, **6**
  pain transmission, 223
  physical damage to, 356
Brain stem death, 265

Breastmilk, 161, 204
Breath sounds, 146–147
Breathing
  assessment, 145–147
  dying patients, 146, 271, 272
  physiology of, 135–136
Brown fat, thermogenesis, 130, 131
Buildings, safety, 28
Bulimia nervosa, 169–170
Bullying, 246, 248, 249
Bureaucracy, and mobility, 375–376
Burnout, 182, 193–194

C

Calciferol (vitamin D), **158**, 161, 308
Calcium, dietary importance, **160**, 161
Calcium antagonists, incontinence, **408**
Campylobacter, **77**
Cancellous bone, 369
Cancer cells, lifespan, 264
Candida albicans, **77**, 78, **79**
Carbohydrates, 154–156, 168, 169
Carbon dioxide
  partial pressure (pCO_2), 135, **137**
  respiratory homeostasis, 135–136, **137**, 146
Cardiac arrest, resuscitation
  advanced life support, 62–63, **64**, 69–70
  basic life support, 45, 53–62, **65–68**, 69–70
  chain of survival, 48–49
  children, 49, 50, 62–63, **64**
  detecting impending, 46
  heart rhythms, 47–48
  near death experiences, 266
  pregnant women, 58
Cardiac chest compressions, 56, 57, 58–59,
  61, 62
Cardiac output, 133
Cardiopulmonary resuscitation *see*
  Resuscitation and emergency care
Cardiorespiratory death, 265
Cardiovascular system
  dying patients, 271
  effects of immobility, 374
  exercise, 373
  see also Cardiac arrest; Heart; Heart disease
Care, duty of, 39, 66–69
Care institutions *see* Institutional care
Care Standards Act (2000), 40
Carers, informal *see* Informal carers
Catheters, 409, 413–416, 417
Cells, 264
  bone, 369
  skin, 282, 306–307, 308
Cellulose, 155
Ceruminous glands, 307
Chain of survival, 48–49
Change, 430–431, **430**, 436
  emotional cycle, 430, **431**
  stages, **436**
Chemicals
  for disinfection, **82**, 83, 92
  hazards of, 29, 37–38
  for sterilization, **82**, 83

Chest compressions
  choking *see* Chest thrusts
  first aid, 56, 57, 58–59, **61**, 62
Chest thrusts, choking, 59, **60**, **61**, 62
Cheyne–Stokes respiration, 146, 271
Childbirth, and continence, 400, 407
Children
  abuse of, 320
  aggression, 248, **249**
  analgesia, 226, 232, 238
  back pain, 109, 121
  basal metabolic rate, 164
  bereavement, 269–270
  blood pressure, **133**, 142, 145
  body temperature, 130, 131, 132, 138,
    140, 141
  bruising, 313
  choking, 59–62
  communication, 3, 5, 6–7, 21–22
  consent to treatment, 41, 71
  death of, 51, 268, 269, 271
  dive reflex, 132
  drinking water, 397, 401
  eating disorders, 161–162, 169–170
  faecal continence, 401, 411
  fever, 141
  grieving by, 269–270
  handling, 115–116, **116**, 120–121
  hygiene care
    bathing, 290, 291
    eyes, 286–287, 296
    hair, 284, 296
    head lice, 296
    nails, 284, 290
    needs assessment, 288
    perineal, 290
    privacy, 288
    psychosocial aspects, 287
    safety, 291
    sebaceous glands, 283
    teeth, 285, 286, 292, 293, 294
  hypothermia, 132
  infection control
    cultural behaviour, 85
    hand hygiene, 89
    immunization, 84
    infection risk, **83**
    patient advocacy, 97
  language acquisition, 6–7, **6**
  medicines
    administration, 211–212, 215, 232
    analgesia, 226, 232, 238
    in breastmilk, 204
    excretion, 204
    licences, 215
    metabolism, 204
    poisoning, 207–208
  mobility care, 374–375
  non-accidental injuries, 320
  nutrition, 159, 161–162
  obesity, 161, 169
  pain, 225–226, 231, 232, 234, 238
  physical activity, 373
  poisoning, 207–208
  puberty, 332, 336, 344, 346

pulse, 133, 134, **134**
respiration, 50, 145, **145**, 146
resuscitation
  advanced cardiac life support, 62–63, **64**
  airway opening, 50
  anatomy, 50
  causes of collapse, 48, 49–50
  chest compressions, 57, **61**
  choking, 59–62
  consent, 71
  defibrillation, 49
  mouth-to-mouth ventilation, 56, 57
  oxygen administration, 62
  Resuscitation Council guidelines,
    67–68
safety and risk, 27, 28, 29, 41, 291
sexuality, 346–347
  development, 332, 344
  gender roles, 331, 337
  sexual identity, 335–336, 337
  sexual norms, 337
skin, 308, 313, 314
sleep patterns, **184**
suicide, 268
terminal care, 271
thermogenesis, 130, 131
thermoregulation, 130, 131, 132, 138
toilet training, 401, 409–410
urinary continence
  catheters, 414
  causes of incontinence, 409, **410**
  development, 401–402
  nocturnal enuresis, 401–402, 409–410
  water intake, 397, 401
Chlamydia, **77**, 287
Chlorhexidine
  dental hygiene, 294, **295**
  disinfection with, **82**
  hand hygiene, 90, **90**
Chlorine, dietary importance, **160**
Choking, management of, 59–62
Cholesterol, 156
Chronic obstructive pulmonary disease
  (COPD), 62
Circadian rhythm, 184
Circumcision, 85
Circumduction, joint movement, **371**
Clean technique, wound care, 319
Cleaning, infection control, 81–83, 112
  blood spills, 92
  dry method, **82**
  wet method, **82**
Clifton Assessment Procedures for the Elderly
  (CAPE), 357–358
Climate change, 129
Clinical audit, 87, 97
Clinical Governance, 25–26, 40, 41, 425
Clinical Negligence Scheme for Trusts
  (CNST), 40
Clinical nurse specialists, pain, 238
Clinical supervision, 191–192, 274
Clinical waste, disposal, 29, 91–93, 98
Clostridium, **77**, 79
Clothing
  footwear, 109–110

and hygiene care, 288
non-accidental injuries, 320
protective, 93–95
uniforms, 93, 94, 96
Cochlear implants, 6
Code of Professional Conduct
  complementary therapies, 235
  confidentiality, 98
  consent, 147–148
  emergencies, 69
  extended practice, 324–325
  homeostasis assessment, 147
  infection control, 96, 97, 98
  medicine administration, 214
  mobility care, 384
  nutritional care, 171
  pain management, 235, 237
  patient handling, 117
  safety and risk, 39, 42
  substance misuse, 209
Cognitive assessment, 357–358
Cognitive barriers, communication, 432–433
Cognitive behavioural therapy (CBT), 188
Cognitive dissonance, 310
Cognitive theories, motivation, 429–430, **429**
Cold-related deaths, 129, 132
Collectivism, 424
Colon, 398
Colorectal disease, 400
Comfort Talk Register, 9
Commission for Health and Audit
  Improvement (CHAI), 40
Commission for Health Improvement
  (CHI), 40
Communication, 1–22
  aggressive incidents, 253–256
  assessment process, 13–14, **14**
  barriers, 432–433
  biological basis, 4–6, 432
  body language, 254–255, 432
  breaking bad news, 270–271
  care delivery knowledge, 2, 12–17
  case studies, 21–22
  closure, 13
  complaints about, 19
  counselling, 12–13
  and culture, 10–12
  deafness, 5, 6, 16–17, 432
  discussing sexuality, 341–342, 344
  elderly patients, 9, 10, 13
  empathy, 12
  environmental factors, 433
  ethical knowledge, 2, 17–20
  graphical, 7
  health care advice, 33
  health promotion, 14, 33
  and ideology of nursing, 9
  impairments, 5, 6, 16–17, 21–22, 357,
    432–433
  information provision, 14
  institutional care, 10
  interagency, 13
  interviewing, 13–14
  language acquisition, 6–7, **6**
  language of health care, 8–12, 20–22

Communication (*contd*)
learning disabled people, 5, 16, 21–22
legal aspects, 17–19
listening, 12, 432
message interpretation in brain, 5–6
models of, 2–4
narratives of health/illness, 10–12, 21
negative use of, 9–10
non-verbal, 5, 7, 254–255, 432
paraphrasing, 12
patient advocacy, 19–20
personal knowledge, 2, 20–22
power relations, 8, 9
professional knowledge, 2, 17–20
psychosocial aspects, 8–12, 431–433
questions, 13, 432
rapport building, 12
records, 14–16, 17–19
reflection, 12
reflective knowledge, 2, 20–22
for rehabilitation, 431–433
self-identity, 17
sensory impairments, 5, 6, 16, 357, 432
sign language, **5**
speech mechanisms, 4–6, 16
stroke patients, 16, 17
styles of, 8, 9, 10
subject knowledge, 2–12
teams, 433
therapeutic relationship, 12–13
through drawing, 7
visual impairment, 5, 432
writing skills, 16
Community care, 192–193
and aggression, 258
dying patients, 273
elderly confused people, 358, 361–363
hygiene care, 298–299
mobility impairment, 384
rehabilitation, 436–437, 438
Compact (Haversian) bone, 369
Complaints, about communication, 19
Complementary therapies, 208–209
pain management, 235–236
Computer based records, 15–16, 17
Conduction, for thermoregulation, 130
Confidentiality
infection control, 97–98
records, 18–19
Confusion, 353–364
assessment, 357–358
attitudes to, 360–361
care delivery knowledge, 353, 357–360
care planning, 358–360, 362–363
case studies, 363–364
causes, 354–356
community care, 358, 361–363
and continence, 400, 402
definition, 354
environmental factors, **354**, 356, 358
ethical knowledge, 353, 360–363
personal knowledge, 354, 363–364
physiological factors, 354–355, **354**, 357, 359
professional knowledge, 353, 360–363
psychological factors, **354**, 356, 357–358
reality orientation, 359, 360

reflective knowledge, 354, 363–364
reminiscence therapy, 359–360
subject knowledge, 353, 354–356
translocation syndrome, 358
types of, 354
validation therapy, 360
Conjunctivitis, 287, 296
Consent
continence care, 418
hygiene care, 298
to medication, 215–216
for observations, 147–148
rehabilitation, 439
resuscitation, 51, 70–71
safety and risk, 41
wound management, 325
Constipation, 272, 399, **400**, 406, 410, 411
Continence, 391–419
assessment, 403–405, 410–411
care delivery knowledge, 392, 403–416
case studies, 418–419
environmental factors, 400
ethical knowledge, 392, 418
faecal, 391, 397–400, 402, 410–412, 413, 416–419
management, 411–412, 413–416, 418
personal knowledge, 392, 418–419
physiology of, 392–401
professional knowledge, 392, 416–418
promotion of, 405–410, 416–418
psychosocial aspects, 400, 401–403
quality assurance of care, 418
reflective knowledge, 392, 418–419
subject knowledge, 391–403
urinary, 391, 392–397, 400–410, 413–419
Continence Advisory Service, 416–417
Control of Substances Hazardous to Health
(COSHH) Regulations (1988), 37–38, 139
Controlled drugs, 213
Controls Assurance, 40
Controls Assurance Unit (CASU), 36–37
Convection, thermoregulation, 130
Coronary heart disease (CHD)
government policy, 129
and hypertension, 144–145
stress, 177–178
ventricular fibrillation, 47–49
Coroners, 274
Corticosteroids, **293**, **343**
Cortisol, stress response, 177
Cosmetics, 311
Coughing, 147
Counselling
bereavement, 274
burnout, 182
communication in, 12–13
stress, 183, 188
Creutzfeld–Jakob disease (CJD), 78
variant (vCJD), 356
Crutches, 380, 381–382, **381**, **382**, 385
Cultural aspects
ageism, 361
communication, 10–12
homeostasis, 128–129
hygiene care, 287–288, 295
infection control, 85

nutrition, 159–160, 164
pain, 227–228
physical appearance, 311–312
risk perception, 31
sexuality, 337
Cyanocobalamin (vitamin B$_{12}$), **159**
Cyanosis, 147, 313
Cytotoxics, **293**, **343**

D

Dandruff, 282
Deafness, 5, **5**, 6, 16, 357, 432
Death and dying, 263–277
advance directives, 71, 275
'appropriate' death, 267–268
attitudes to, 266–268
bereavement, 50–51, 180–181, 267–270, 273–274
biology of, 264–266, 271
brain stem death, 265
breaking bad news, 270–271
cardiorespiratory death, 265
care delivery knowledge, 264, 270–272
case studies, 277
Cheyne–Stokes respiration, 146, 271
cortical brain death, 265–266
diagnostic criteria, 265–266
doctrine of double effect, 275
effects of sudden, 50–52, 267–268, 269
ethics, 264, 274–276
euthanasia, 275–276
fear of, 185–186, 267
grief, 50–51, 268–270, 273–274, 429
legal issues, 274–275, 276
living wills, 71, 275
location of, 272–273
near death experiences, 266
nurses' grief, 273–274
ontological death, 266
organ donation, 276
pain, 271
palliative care, 263, 275
personal knowledge, 264, 276–277
process of, 270, 271
professional knowledge, 264, 272–274
psychosocial aspects, 50–52, 180–181, 185–186, 266–270, 273–274
reflective knowledge, 264, 276–277
religious beliefs, 267, 268
spiritual needs, 186, 267
subject knowledge, 264–270
suicide
grief of families, 268
overdoses, 208, 238
physician assisted, 276
tasks of mourning, 269
terminal care, 263, 271–272
withholding treatment, 274–275
Debriefing, aggressive incidents, 252
Decubitus ulcers *see* Pressure sores
Defaecation *see* Faecal incontinence
Defence mechanisms, mental, 179–180, **179**
Defibrillation, 47–49, 57
Delirium, 354

Dementia
  confusion with, 354, 356, 359–360
  and continence, 400, 402, 409
  iatrogenic, 355
  nutrition, 162, 172
  therapy, 359–360
Denial, stress, **179**
Dental caries, 286
Dental hygiene, 285–286, 292–295
Dentures, care of, 294–295
Depression
  or confusion, 357–358, 359
  and rehabilitation, 436
  and sexual response, 340
Dermatitis, prevalence, 314
Dermis, 282, 283, 307
Detrusor hyperactivity, 394, 395, **396**, 407–408
Detrusor hypoactivity, 396–397, **397**, 409, 414
Detrusor sphincter dyssynergia, 397
Diabetes mellitus, 168
  and confusion, 354
  foot care, 290
  infection control, **83**
  obesity, 161
  Type 2, 161, 168
Diagnoses
  delivery of, 4, 270–271
  labelling theory, 426–427
Diarrhoea, 400, 411, **412**
Diet see Food and nutrition
Digestion
  carbohydrates, 155
  fats, 156–157
  proteins, 158
Digestive system see Gastrointestinal system
Digital rectal examination, 405, 410, 418
Digital thermometers, 139, 140–141, **140**
Disability
  bathing aids, 291, **291**
  definition, 368
  legal aspects, 119, 375, 383–384
  mobility see Mobility care
Disability Discrimination Act (1995), 375, 383–384
Disabled Living Centres, 384
Disaccharides, 154–155
Discharge planning, medicines, 211
Disfigurement, exposure therapy, 311
Disinfection, 81, **82**, 83
  blood spills, 92
Displacement, stress, **179**
Diuretics, **293**, **343**, 354–355
Dive reflex, 132
Doctrine of double effect, 275
Documentation see Records
Drainage tubes, surgical wounds, 320
Drawing, communication through, 7
Dressings, wounds, 309, 318, 319, 320
Drugs
  illegal, 208
    causing confusion, 355–356
    and stress, 190
    use by nurses, 209
  medicinal see Medicines
Dry mouth (xerostomia), 293, **293**

Duodenum, immune response, **81**
Duty of care, 39
  emergencies, 66–69
Dying see Death and dying
Dyspnoea, 147
Dysuria, **396**

E

Ear
  anatomy, **5**
  balance, 379–380
  cochlear implants, 6
  hearing impairment, 5, 6, 16, 357, 432
  processing of sound, 5
  tympanic thermometry, 139, 140–141, **140**, **141**
Eating, difficulties with, 164, 166
Eating disorders, 161–162, 169–170, 172–173
Eccrine glands, 283
Economic factors
  employment conditions, 193
  health policy, 424, 425
  homeostasis, 129
  informal care, 192–193
  resource allocation, 438
  stress, 194
Ecstasy (MDMA), 355–356
Eczema, 310, 314
Education
  health see Health education
  nurses see Education and training
Education and training
  continence care, 417–418
  resuscitation skills, 70, 71
Elderly people
  abuse of, 361
  attitudes to, 361, 376
  care services, 192–193, 361–363
  cold-related deaths, 129, 132
  communication with, 9, 10, 13
  confusion
    assessment, 357–358
    attitudes to, 361
    causes, 354–355
    community care, 358, 361–363
    informal carers, 358, 361, 362–363
    therapy, 359–360
  depression, 357–358
  domiciliary services, 361
  faecal incontinence
    causes, 399
    digital rectal examination, 418
    manual evacuations, 418
    prevalence, 397
    stigma, 402
  falls, 375, 380
  handling and moving, 121–122
  heat-related deaths, 129, 131–132
  hygiene care
    bathing, 297
    dentures, 295
    eyes, 297
    feet, 290
    gender aspects, 298
    oral, 293, 295

hyponatraemia, 354–355
hypothermia, 129, 132
infection control, **83**
informal carers of, 192–193, 358, 361, 362–363
malnutrition, 355
medicines
  confusion related to, 355
  excretion, 204
  polypharmacy, 205
mobility care, 368–369, 375
  assessment, 377
  and eyesight, 379
  falls, 375, 380
nutrition, 162, 355
residential care, 361–362
safety and risk, 42
sexuality, 345–346
skin, 308, 314
sleep patterns, **184**
temperature measurement, 139, **140**
thermoregulation, 130, 131–132
urinary incontinence
  behavioural factors, 402
  catheters, 414
  drug therapy, 407, 408
  physiology, 396, 400–401
  stigma, 402
Electrolyte imbalance
  confusion with, 354–355
  with immobility, 374
Electromagnetic radiation, 29
Electronic records, 15–16, 17
Electronic thermometers, 139, 140–141, **140**
Emergency care see Resuscitation and emergency care
Empathy, in communication, 12
Employment-related stress, 193–194
Endocrine system
  and confusion, 354
  and continence, 401
  effects of immobility, 374
  and sexuality, 332, **332**, 333, 334, **343**, 344
  see also Sex hormones
Enemas, 411, **412**
Energy balance, 154
Energy producing foods, 154–158
  see also Carbohydrates; Fats; Proteins
Energy supplements, elderly people, 162
Entamoeba, **77**
Enteral feeding, 166, 167, 172
Enterococci, **77**, 80
Enterovirus, **77**
Environmental factors
  communication, 433
  confusion, **354**, 356, 358
  homeostasis, 129
  incontinence, 400
  mobility, 378, **379**
Environmental hazards, 27–30, 31–33, 42
  infection control, 100
Environmental health, 99–100
Enzymes
  carbohydrate digestion, 155
  protein digestion, 158
  shape, 157

EPIC project, 88, 92
Epidemiology
    back injury, 108
    infection control, 85–86
Epidermis, 282, 306–307
Epinephrine (adrenaline), resuscitation, 64
Epstein–Barr virus, **77**
Equipment, 29–30, 34, 37
    blood pressure measurement, 142–143
    body temperature measurement, 139–140
    defibrillation, 49
    for handling patients, 111–114, 120, 122, 123
    infection control
        cleaning, 81–83, 112
        disinfection, **82**, 83
        protective clothing, 93–95
        sterilization, **82**, 83
    oxygen administration, 62
    personal protective, 93–95
    respiration assessment, 145, 146
Ergonomics, 106, 117
Escherichia coli, 77, **77**, 79
Ethics
    communication, 2, 17–20
    continence care, 392, 418
    death and dying, 264, 274–276
    handling and moving patients, 118–119
    hygiene care, 297–299
    infection control, 97–98
    medication, 213–216
    mobility care, 384–385
    nursing observations, 147–148
    nutritional care, 171–172
    pain management, 238–239
    principles of, 384
    rehabilitation, 438–439
    resuscitation, 70–71, 275
    safety and risk, 26, 38–41
    sexuality, 347–348
    skin care, 324–325
    stress, 192–194
    whistleblowing, 41
Ethnic minority groups
    death and dying, 267
    hair care, 295
    harassment of nurses from, 249
    pain, 227–228
    skin colour assessment, 313
Ethological theories, aggression, 247
European Union
    back injury, 108
    handling patients, 117, 119
    infection control, 96, 97
    safety directives, **39**
Euthanasia, 275–276
Evaporation, thermoregulation, 130
Eversion, joint movement, **371**
Evolutionary biology, 336
Exercise, 169, 187, 373, 382–383
Exposure therapy, 311
Extended practice, 324–325, 437–438
    see also Specialist nurses
Extension, joint movement, **371**
Eye contact, aggressive situations, 255
Eyes
    hygiene care, 286–287, 296–297
    immune response, **81**

protective equipment, 93, 94–95
    stress reaction, **178**
Eyesight, impaired, 5, 379, 432

F

Faecal impaction, 399, 411
Faecal incontinence, 391
    anorectal, 399–400, **399**, 411
    assessment, 410–411, 418
    case studies, 418–419
    causes, 398–400
    colorectal disease, 400
    Continence Advisory Service, 416–417
    definition, 398
    digital rectal examination, 410, 418
    environmental factors, 400
    ethics, 418
    faecal impaction, 399, 411
    management, 411, **412**, 413
    manual evacuation, 411, 418
    neurological causes, 399
    nurse education, 417–418
    physiology, 397–400
    prevalence, 397
    psychosocial aspects, 401, 402, 403
    quality assurance of care, 418
    stigma, 402
Fallopian tubes, 333
Falls, 119, 375, 380
Families
    bereavement, 50–51, 180–181, 267–270
    hygiene care, 287
    stress in, 180–181, 186
    see also Informal carers
Fasting, 159–160
Fats, 156–157, 161, 168, 169
Fatty acids, 156, 157
Feeding patients, 166–168, 172
Feet, hygiene care, 290
Femininity, 331, 345
Fever (pyrexia), 131, 141, **141**, 142
Fibre, dietary, 158, 411
First aid, 53–62, 66–69, 319–320
Flexion, joint movement, **371**
Flossing, dental care, 294
Fluid intake, continence, 397, 401, 406, 411
Fluoride, dental care, 294
Foam swabs, dental hygiene, 294, **295**
Foley (indwelling) catheters, 413, 414–416, 417
Folic acid (folacin), **159**, 161
Food and nutrition, 153–173
    adults, 162
    appetite, 154
    babies, 161
    benchmarks of good practice, 154
    biology, 154–158
    carbohydrates, 154–156, 168, 169
    care delivery knowledge, 154, 160–170
    case studies, 172–173
    dental hygiene, 286
    diabetes mellitus, 161, 168
    dying patients, 272
    eating difficulties, 164, 166
    eating disorders, 161–162, 169–170, 172–173
    elderly people, 162, 355

energy producing foods, 154–158
    see also Carbohydrates; Fats; Proteins
    enteral feeding, 166, 167, 172
    ethical knowledge, 154, 171–172
    fats, 156–157, 161, 168
    feeding patients, 166–168, 172
    fibre, 158, 411
    fluid intake, 397, 401, 406, 411
    food safety, 28, 100, 161, 170–171
    government recommendations, 162
    and infection control, **79**, 170–171
        cultural behaviour, 85
        environmental health, 100
        health behaviour, 84
        pregnant women, 161
    lactating women, 161
    legal aspects, 170, 172
    malnutrition, 162, 355
    mealtimes, 166
    minerals, 158, **160**, 161
    muscle activity, 372
    non-energy producing foods, 158
        see also Minerals; Vitamins
    nursing interventions, 166
    obesity, 161, 168–169
    older people, 162
    overweight, 168, 169
    parenteral feeding, 167–168
    patient assessment, 162–164
    personal knowledge, 154, 172–173
    planning, 164–166
    in pregnancy, 160–161
    professional knowledge, 154, 170–172
    proteins, 157–158, 161, 162
    psychosocial factors, 158–160
    reflective knowledge, 154, 172–173
    schoolchildren, 161
    stress, 187
    subject knowledge, 154–160
    teenagers, 161–162
    tube feeding, 166, 167, 172
    vitamins, 158, **158**, **159**, 161
    weight loss diets, 164, 166, 169
    wound healing, 171, 320–321
Food poisoning, 170–171
Food Safety Act (1990), 170
Foods Standards Act (1999), 170
Foot drop, 374
Footwear
    back injury, 109–110
    infection control, 93, 95
Foreign bodies
    choking on, 59–62
    in wounds, 310, 320
Frames, walking, **380**, 381, **381**
Freud, S, psychoanalytic theory, 247–248, 335–336
Frustration–aggression hypothesis, 248
Functionalism, 425
Fungi, 76, **77**, 78, **79**, **82**

G

Gait, 379, 381–382, **381**
Gargles, **295**
Gas, for sterilization, **82**, 83

Gaseous exchange, respiration, 134–136, **137**, 145, 146
Gastrointestinal system
  carbohydrate digestion, 155
  defaecation, 398
    see also Faecal incontinence
  drug-related reactions, **206**
  effects of immobility, 374, **400**
  immune response, **81**
  lipid digestion, 156–157
  oral cavity, 285, **285**
  protein digestion, 158
  stress reaction, **178**
Gastrostomy, 167
Gate theory, pain, 223, **224**
Gender aspects, hygiene care, 297–298, 345
Gender differences
  homosexuality, 338, 339
  pain perception, 228
  sexual behaviour, 338–339
  sexual identity, 335–337
  sexual norms, 337
  speech styles, 8
Gender roles, 331, 337, 345
General adaptation syndrome, 177, **178**
Genetic factors
  aggression, 247
  blood pressure, 144
Genitalia
  development of, 332–333
  hygiene care, 284, 290
Gibson Spiral Maze, 357, **357**
Gingivitis, 286
Glass and mercury thermometers, 139, 140–141, **140**
Gloves, protective, 93–94
Glucagon, 155
Glucocorticosteroids, **293**, **343**
Glucose, 154, 155, 156, 158
Glycaemic index, 168
Glycogen, 155
Goal setting, rehabilitation, 435, 439
Gowns, infection control, 93, 95
Graphical communication, 7
Grief, 50–51, 268–270, 273–274, **428**, 429
Group supervision, 192
Group therapy, stress management, 188–189
Groups, development of, 433
Guedal airway, 62
Gums, hygiene care, 286, 294
Gutter frames, **380**, 381

H

Haematuria, **396**, **415**
Haemoglobin, 136
Hair, 283–284, **284**, 288, 295–296
Halitosis, 286, 293
Hand hygiene, 83, 84, 88, 89–91
Handling inanimate objects, 115, **115**
Handling and moving patients, 105–123
  accident monitoring, 118
  adverse incidents, 118
  assessment for, 110–112, 116–117
  back injury, 58, 105, 108–110, 118, 119
  behavioural issues, 109

biology, 106–108
care delivery knowledge, 106, 110–116
case studies, 119–123
children, 115–116, **116**, 120–121
community care plan, **112**
in confined spaces, 115
coordinating strategy for, 114
cumulative strain, 108, 110–111
disabled people's rights, 119
in emergencies, 117
epidemiology, 108
ergonomics, 106, 117
ethics, 106, 118–119
falling patients, 119
handling equipment, 114
hoists, 113–114, 115, 122, 123
leg lifting equipment, 113
legal aspects, 116–117, 118, 119
lifting equipment, 113–114, 115, 116, 122, 123
monkey poles, 113
optimum height for, 114–115
outcome evaluation, 116
personal knowledge, 106, 119–123
plan implementation, 114–116
planning, 112–114, 116
in pregnancy, 111
principles of, 110
professional knowledge, 106, 116–119
psychosocial aspects, 108–110
record keeping, 116, 118
reflective knowledge, 106, 119–123
and resuscitation, 117
risk assessment, 110–112, 116–117
sliding equipment, 113, 114, 122, 123
spinal cord, 106–108
subject knowledge, 106–110
terminal care, 272
TILER method, 115
transfer equipment, 113, 120
turning equipment, 113
Harassment, 246, 248, 249
Hats, infection control, 93, 95
Haversian (compact) bone, 369
Head lice, 296
Healing, wounds see Wounds, healing
Health
  cultural narratives, 10–12
  environmental factors, 129
  and stress, 177–179, 185–186, 194
Health Act (1999), 193
Health behaviour
  back injury, 109
  infection control, 84–85, 86
  risk taking, 33, 38
Health beliefs, 86, **436**
Health education
  communication, 14, 33
  hand hygiene, 91
  infection control, 86, 91
  medicines, 211
  rehabilitation, 436
Health inequalities, 129
Health policy, 192–193, 424–425, 436–437
  see also Political factors
Health promotion
  communication, 14, 33
  hygiene care, 286, 287

infection control, 86
medicines, 209, 238
nursing observations, 148
political factors, 129
rehabilitation, 436
skin, 323–324
Health and safety see Safety and risk
Health and Safety at Work Act (1974), 37, 38–39
  aggression, 257
  handling patients, 117, 118
  infection control
    personal protective equipment, 93
    political issues, 98
    waste disposal, 92, 98
Hearing impairment, 5, 6, 16, 357, 432
Heart
  arrest see Cardiac arrest
  asystole, 47, 48
  pulse rates, 133–134
  pulse rhythm, 47, 134
  pulseless electrical activity, 48
  pulseless ventricular tachycardia, 48
  sinus rhythm, 47
  structure, 47, **47**
  ventricular fibrillation, 47–49
Heart disease
  government policy, 129
  and hypertension, 144–145
  infection risk, **83**
  stress and, 177–178
  ventricular fibrillation, 47–49
Heat
  for disinfection, **82**, 83
  as physical hazard, 29
  for sterilization, **82**, 83
  washing of laundry, 93, 96
Heat exhaustion, 132
Heat-related deaths, 129, 132
Heat stroke, 131–132
Heimlich manoeuvre, 59, **60**, 62
Helicobacter pylori, 77
Hepatitis A, **77**
Hepatitis B, **77**
  carriers, 80, 96
  immunization, 96, 97
Hepatitis C, **77**
  infection control, 84, 85, 96
Herbal preparations, stress management, 190
Herpes (type 1 and type 2), **77**
HIV see Human immunodeficiency virus (HIV)
Hoists, for lifting patients, 113–114, 115, 122, 123
Home care
  dying patients, 272, 273, **273**
  elderly confused people, 358, 361, 362–363
  rehabilitation, 437
  safety, 258
Homeopathy, 235–236
Homeostasis, 26–27, 127–149
  blood pressure, 129, 132–134, 142–145, 147–148
  body temperature, 128, 129–132, 137, 138–142, 147–148
  care delivery knowledge, 128, 136–147
  case studies, 148–149
  coronary heart disease, 129, 144–145
  ethical knowledge, 128, 147–148

Homeostasis (*contd*)
external influences on, 128–129
mechanisms in, 128
negative feedback loop, 128, **128**
personal knowledge, 128, 148–149
professional knowledge, 128, 147–148
reflective knowledge, 128, 148–149
respiratory, 135–136, **137**, 145–147
screening changes in, 136–148
subject knowledge, 127–136
thermoregulation *see* Homeostasis, body
temperature
Homosexuality, 337–338, 339
Hospice care, 273, **273**
Hospital acquired infections (HAIs), 76
antimicrobial resistance, 80, 96
clinical audits, 87
hand hygiene, 84, 89
hospital cleanliness, 98
infection control teams, 99
policies, 97
political issues, 98
vulnerable patients, 83
Hospital Anxiety and Depression Scale, 357
Housing, safety, 28
Human immunodeficiency virus (HIV), **77**
infection control
behavioural factors, 85
drug-resistant tuberculosis, 80
ethics, 97–98
first-aiders, 53
healthcare staff, 92–93, 96, 97
sharps injuries, 92–93
Human Rights Act (1998)
aggression against staff, 257
disabled people, 119
risk management, 41
Hydration
and continence, 397, 401, 406, 411
dying patients, 272
skin, 313
Hygiene care, 281–301
bathing, 287–288, 289, 290–292, 297, 298
bathing aids, 291, **291**
bed bathing, 289, 290
body odour, 283, 287–288
care delivery knowledge, 282, 288–297
case studies, 300–301
consent, 298
cultural aspects, 287–288, 295
dentures, 294–295
dignity, 298
ethical knowledge, 282, 297–299
eyes, 286–287, 296–297
feet, 290
gender aspects, 297–298, 345
goals of, 289
hair, 283–284, **284**, 288, 295–296
medicated baths, 291
mouth, 284–286, 292–294
nails, 284, 290
needs assessment, 288–289, 292–293
nursing activities in, 291–292
perineal area, 284, 290
personal knowledge, 282, 299–301
political aspects, 298–299

principles, 291–292
privacy, 288, 297, 298
professional knowledge, 282, 297–299
psychosocial aspects, 287–288
reflective knowledge, 282, 299–301
registered nurse role, 291–292, 297, 299
ritualization, 297
skill mix debate, 291–292, 297, 299
skin, 282–283, 289, 290
soaps, 290
spiritual aspects, 287–288
subject knowledge, 282–288
teeth, 285–286, 292–295
therapeutic baths, 290–291
towel bathing, 289, 290
Hypericum perforatum, 190
Hypertension, 144–145
associated symptoms, **142**
government policy, 129
Hypnotherapy, 236
Hypnotics, to aid sleep, 191
Hypochlorites, disinfection with, **82**, 92
Hyponatraemia, 354–355
Hypotension, **142**, 145
Hypothalamus
appetite, 154
thermoregulation, 128, 130, 131
Hypothermia, 129, 132, 141–142
Hypoxia, 147

I

Iatrogenesis, 207
Identity, self *see* Self-identity
Ideology, nursing, 9
Illness
cultural narratives, 10–12, 21
environmental factors, 129
sick role, 425–426, **426**
and stress, 177–179, 185–186, 194
Immobility *see* Mobility care
Immune response
fever, 131
infection control, 80–81
Immune system, stress, 177–179
Immunizations, 81
health behaviour, 84, 86
for nurses, 96, 97
political issues, 98–99
Immunosuppressed patients, infections, **83**
Incontinence *see* Faecal incontinence; Urinary
incontinence
Indwelling (Foley) catheters, 413, 414–416, 417
Infants *see* Children
Infection control, 75–101
antimicrobial resistance, 75, 80, 96, 97
aseptic technique, 95–96, 318, 319, 320
assessment in, 87
behavioural factors, 84–85, 86
biology, 76–84
body systems, 80–81
care delivery knowledge, 76, 86–97
carriers, 80, 96, 97
case studies, 100–101
chain of infection, 77, **77**, 79–80

cleaning, 81–83, **82**, 92, 112
clinical audit, 87, 97
clinical waste, 91–93, 98
in the community, 76
disinfection, 81, **82**, 83, 92
environmental health, 99–100
EPIC project, 88, 92
epidemiology, 85–86
ethical issues, 76, 97–98
first-aider safety, 53
food safety, **79**, 84, 85, 100, 161, 170–171
growth requirements of organisms, 79
hand hygiene, 83, 84, 88, 89–91
health promotion, 86
hospital acquired infections *see* Hospital
acquired infections (HAIs)
hospital cleanliness, 98
hosts, 79–80
immune response, 80–81
immunization, 81, 84, 86, 96, 97, 98–99
implementation, 88
indwelling catheters, 415, **415**
infective agents, 76–78
see also Bacteria; Fungi; Prions; Protozoa;
Viruses
linen, 93
maggot therapy, 316, 325
national targets, 99
nurses' personal care, 96, 97, 320
outcome evaluation, 96–97
personal knowledge, 76, 100–101
personal protective equipment, 93–95
physical, 81–83
physiological, 80–81
planning, 87–88
political issues, 98–99
principles of, 89–96
problem solving approach, 87–88, 96–97
professional issues, 76, 97
psychosocial factors, 84–86
reflective knowledge, 76, 100–101
and risk of infection, 81–83, 87
routes of spread of infection, 79–80
sterilization, 81, **82**, 83
subject knowledge, 76–86
surveillance, 87, 97, 99–100
teams for, 99
uniforms, 93, 94, 96
Universal Precautions, 88–89
vulnerable patients, 81, 83, 87, 97, 100–101
wounds, 316, 318–319, 320
Infections
confusion caused by, 354
control of *see* Infection control
Informal carers
clean technique, 319
of the confused elderly, 358, 361, 362–363
hygiene care, 299
stress, 192–193, 359, 362
support for, 362–363
Information provision, 14, 33
Informed consent *see* Consent
Institutional care
communication, 10
disabled people, 375
safety, 28

Insulin
    carbohydrate metabolism, 155
    diabetes mellitus, 168
Integrated care pathways, 324
Intellectualization, stress, **179**
Intensive care patients, infection risk, **83**
Interactionism, 425
    labelling theory, 426
Intermediate care, 437
Intermittent catheterization, 409, 414
Internal market, 425
International Classification for Nursing
        Practice (ICNP), 18
Interprofessional working
    change management, 430
    communication in assessment process, 13
    consent to treatment, 41
    infection control, 97, 99
    safety and risk, 38, 41
    see also Multidisciplinary teams
Interviews, 13–14
    aggression prevention, 256
Intravenous feeding, 167–168
Intravenous infusion rate, 202
Inversion, joint movement, **371**
Iodine, dietary, **160**
Iron, dietary, **160**, 161
Irradiation see Radiation
Ischaemic heart disease (IHD), 47–49

J

Jejunal feeding, 167
Joints, 370–372, **371**, 374, 378–379

K

Keratin, 282, 306–307
Kidneys see Renal system
Korotkoff phases, 143, **143**

L

Labelling theory, 426–427
Lactating women, 161
Langerhans' cells, 307
Language
    acquisition, 6–7, **6**
    awareness of use of, 20–22
    brain function, 5–6
    in discussing sexuality, 341–342
    of health care, 8–12, 20–22
    health/illness narratives, 10–12, 21
    models of communication, 2–4
    need for monitoring, 19
    psychosocial factors in communication, 8
    records, 14–15, 16, 18
Larval therapy, 316, 325
Latex allergy, 94, 312
Laundry, 93, 96
Laxatives, **412**
    electrolyte imbalance, 355

and incontinence, 410, 411
Leadership, 433
Learning, health promotion, 14
Learning disabilities, people with
    communication, 5, 16, 21–22
    handling and moving, 120
    infection control, 84, 97
    nocturnal enuresis, 409–410
    pain
        assessment, 231
        behavioural responses, 225–226
    sexuality, 22, **343**, 346
    toileting programmes, 409–410
Learning environments, patient safety,
        34–35
Leg lifting equipment, 113
Leg ulcers, 321
Legal aspects
    aggression, 256–258
    consent to treatment, 41
    continence care, 418
    death and dying, 274–275, 276
    disability, 375
    employment, 193, 194
    food and nutrition, 100, 170, 172
    illegal substances, 208
    infection control, 92, 93, 96, 97, 98, 100
    medicines, 200, 213–216
    mobility care, 375, 383–384
    negligence, 39, 40, 69
    non-accidental injuries, 320
    patient handling, 116–117, 118, 119
    record keeping, 17–18, 19
    resuscitation and emergency care, 66–69
    safety, 26, 37–39, 40, 41, 92, 100
    sexuality, 346, 347–348
    stress, 193, 194
    waste disposal, 92, 98
Legionella, **77**
Levers, body, 372–373
Lice, head, 296
Life crisis, situational, 50–51
Life events, stress, 178–179, 180–181
Life expectancy, 264
Life quality, 30, 323
Lifestyle factors
    infection control, 84
    rehabilitation ethics, 438–439
Lifting equipment, 113–114, 115, 116, 122, 123
Light, infection control, **79**
Linen, infection control, 93
Lipids (fats), 156–157, 161, 168, 169
Lipoproteins, 157
Listening, communication, 12, 432
Listeria, **77**, 161
Litigation, negligence, 39, 40, 69
Liver
    deamination, 158
    drug metabolism, 204
    glycogen storage, 155
    lipid metabolism, 157
Living wills, 71, 275
Loss, 429
    see also Bereavement
Lungs, respiration, 135
Lymphocytes, 81

M

Machinery, safety and risk, 29–30, 37
    see also Equipment
Macmillan nurses, 273
Maggot therapy, 316, 325
Magnesium, dietary, **160**
Malaria, 78
Malnutrition, 162, 355
Management of Health and Safety at Work
        Regulations (1999), 39
Manual evacuations, 411, 418
Masculinity, 331, 345
Masks, infection control, 93, 94
Maslow's hierarchy of needs, **429**
Massage, 189, 234
MDMA (ecstasy), 355–356
Mealtimes, 166
Medical records see Records
Medicines, 199–218
    absorption, 203
    administration
        children, 211–212, 215
        doctrine of double effect, 275
        eight rights of, 211, **212**
        error management, 216
        euthanasia, 275
        local policies, 214–215
        mentally ill clients, 215–216
        nurse's role, 209–212
        nursing care evaluation, 212–213
        organizing, 209
        professional standards, 214
        recording of, 210
        routes of, 202, **203**, 232, 233
    adverse effects, 205–207, **206**
        see also side effects below
    alternative, 208–209
    biology, 200–207
    and brain stem death tests, 265
    care delivery knowledge, 200, 209–213
    care planning, 210
    case studies, 217–218
    classification, 200–201, **201**, 213
    clients' rights, 215–216
    complementary, 208–209, 235–236
    controlled drugs, 213
    definition, 200
    discharge planning, 211
    distribution, 203–204
    dose calculation, 201–202, **201**, **202**, 205
    errors, 208, 216
    ethical knowledge, 200, 213–216
    excretion, 204–205
    faecal incontinence, 410, 411, **412**
    half-life, 204
    health promotion, 209, 238
    iatrogenesis, 207
    intentional overdose, 208, 238
    interactions, 205
    intravenous infusion rate calculation, 202
    legal considerations, 200, 213–216
    licensing, 200, 215
    metabolism, 204
    names of, 200

Medicines (*contd*)
  non-prescribed substances, 207–209
  nurse prescribing, 213–214
  pain relief, 226, 228, 232–233, 238, 275
  palliative care, 275
  personal knowledge, 200, 217–218
  pharmacist's role, 206
  pharmacodynamics, 205
  pharmacokinetics, 203–205
  poisoning, 207–208
  polypharmacy, 205–206
  professional knowledge, 200, 213–216
  psychosociology, 207–209
  reflective knowledge, 200, 217–218
  safe administration, 211
  and sexual function, 343–344, **343**
  side effects
    confusion, 355
    constipation, **400**, 410
    sexual function, 343–344, **343**
    urinary incontinence, 397
    xerostomia, 293, **293**
    see also adverse effects *above*
  subject knowledge, 199–209
  teratogenesis, 206–207
  in terminal care, 272
  therapeutic dose, 205
  topical, 203, 211
  urinary incontinence, 408–409
  withdrawal of, 216
Meditation, 189
  pain management, 234
Melanocytes, 307, 308
Men
  hygiene care, 297–298, 345
  reproductive system, 332–333, **332**, 393
  see also Gender differences; Gender roles
Menopause, 334, 344
Menstrual cycle, 333–334
Mental ill health
  confusion *see* Confusion
  depression, 340, 357–358, 359, 436
  and grief, 269
  people with
    consent to treatment, 41
    handling and moving, 122–123
    hygiene care, 289, 293, 298
    infection control, 84
    living wills, 275
    medicines, 215–216
    nutrition, 162
    safety and risk, 41
    sexuality, **343**, 347
Mental pain, 227
Mercury sphygmomanometers, 143
Mercury thermometers, 139, 140–141, **140**
Metabolism, effects of immobility, 374
Metaphors of illness, 11
Methicillin resistant *Staphylococcus aureus*
    (MRSA), 80, 96, 97
Micro-enemas, 411, **412**
Micturition *see* Urinary incontinence
Milk, babies' requirements, 161
Minerals, 158, **160**, 161
Mirroring, aggressive situations, 254–255
Mitochondria, glucose metabolism, 156

MMR vaccine, 85, 86
Mobilism, 376
Mobility care, 367–387
  aids, 380–382, 384, 385
  balance, 379–380, 381–382
  biology, 369–374
  body alignment, 379
  bureaucracy and, 375–376
  care delivery knowledge, 367–368, 377–383
  case studies, 386–387
  community facilities, 384
  definition, 368
  demographic trends, 368–369
  disability factors, 378, **379**
  Disabled Living Centres, 384
  environmental factors, 378, **379**
  ethical knowledge, 368, 384–385
  exercise, 373, 382–383
  gait, 379, 381–382, **381**
  and incontinence, 400
  legal aspects, 375, 383–384
  management of care, 378–383
  mobility triad, 378, **378**, **379**
  multidisciplinary assessment, 377
  musculoskeletal system, 369–373
  patient advocacy, 384
  patients' rights, 383
  personal factors, 378, **379**
  personal knowledge, 368, 385–387
  physical effects of immobility, 373–374
  prevalence, 368
  professional knowledge, 368, 383–384
  psychosocial aspects, 374–377
  public places, 375, 383–384, 385–386
  range of movement, 370–372, 378–379
  reflective knowledge, 368, 383–384
  schools, 375
  sitting to standing, 382
  stigmatization, 376–377
  subject knowledge, 367, 368–377
Monosaccharides, 154–155
Mood, and sexual response, 340
  see also Depression
Mood matching, aggressive situations, 254
Moral issues *see* Ethics
Morbidity, government policy, 129
Mortality, government policy, 129
Motivation, 429–430
Mourning, tasks of, 269
Mouth
  immune response, **81**
  oral hygiene, 284–286, 292–294
  oral thermometry, 139, 140–141, **140**
  structure, **285**
Mouth-to-mouth resuscitation, 53, 56, 57
Mouthwashes, **295**
Movement, normal range of, 370–372
  see also Mobility care
Moving patients *see* Handling and moving
    patients
Multidisciplinary teams
  change management, 430
  development, 433
  mobility assessment, 377
  pain management, 237–238
  pressure sore management, 322–323

  rehabilitation, 437–438
  see also Interprofessional working
Multidrug-resistant tuberculosis (MDRTB), 80
Muscle relaxation, progressive, 189
Muscles, 372–373, **372**
  effects of immobility, 374
  see also Musculoskeletal system
Musculoskeletal system, 369–373
  disorders, and sexuality, **343**
  dying patients, 271
Mycobacterium tuberculosis, **77**

N

Nails
  colour, 313
  hygiene, 284, 290
Narcotic analgesics *see* Opioid drugs,
    analgesia
Narratives
  health/illness, 10–12, 21
  records, 15
Nasogastric tube feeding, 167
Nasopharynx, immune response, **81**
National Back Pain Association, 119
National Health Service and Community Care
    Act (1990), 193, 194
National Institute for Clinical Excellence
    (NICE), 40, 41
National Patient Safety Agency (NPSA), 34, 35
National Service Frameworks (NSFs), 425
Near death experiences (NDEs), 266
Needlestick injuries, 92–93
Negligence, 39, 40, 69
Neisseria gonorrhoea, **77**
Neisseria meningitidis, 80
Neisseria meningococcus, **77**
Neoanalytic theory, sexual identity, 336
Nerve supply
  bladder, 394, 395, 401
  muscles, 372
  pelvic floor, 398
Nervous system
  defaecation, 398, 399
  drug-related upset, **206**
  micturition, 394, **394**, 395, 397, 401
  pain transmission, 223
  see also Brain; Spinal cord
Neurotransmitters
  aggression, 246
  and MDMA, 355–356
  pain, 223, **223**
NHS Litigation Authority (NHSLA), 40, 41
Nicotinic acid (niacin), **159**
Nitrogen, proteins, 157, 158
Nociceptors, 223
Nocturia, **396**, 403
Nocturnal enuresis, **396**, 401–402, 409–410
Nomograms, **201**
Non-verbal communication, 5, 7, 254–255, 432
Noradrenaline (norepinephrine), 246
Norms, 425
  sexual, 337–338, 346
Nostrils, infection control, **81**
Nucidex (peracetic acid), **82**

Nursing
    extended practice, 324–325, 437–438
    as female profession, 297–298, 345
    models of, and sexuality, 340
Nursing beds, elderly people, 361–362
Nursing and Midwifery Council
    complaints, 19
    complementary therapies, 235
    confidentiality, 98
    consent, 147–148
    emergencies, 69
    extended practice, 324–325
    handling patients, 114, 117
    homeostasis assessment, 147
    infection control, 96, 97, 98
    medications, 205, 209, 211, 214, 215, 216
    mobility care, 384
    nutritional care, 171
    pain management, 235, 237
    record keeping, 17, 18
    safety and risk, 39, 42
    substance misuse, 209
Nursing records *see* Records
Nutrition *see* Food and nutrition

O

Obesity, 161, 168–169
Occupational Health departments, 42
    food poisoning, 171
    handling patients, 118
    infection control, 93, 96, 97
Oestrogen therapy, stress incontinence, 407
Older people *see* Elderly people
Ontological death, 266
Oocytes, 33
Ophthalmia neonatorum, 296
Opioid drugs
    analgesia, 232, 275, **293**
    antidiarrhoeal, **412**
Oral hygiene, 284–286, 292–294
Oral malodour (halitosis), 286, 293
Oral thermometry, 139, 140–141, **140**
Organ donation, 276
Orthopnoea, 146
Ovaries, 333
Overdoses
    accidental, 208, 216
    intentional, 208, 238
Overshoes, 93, 95
Overweight, 168, 169
Oximetry, 145, 147
Oxygen
    and infection control, **79**
    partial pressure (pO_2), 135, **137**
    respiratory homeostasis, 135–136, **137**, 145, 146, 147
    resuscitation and emergency care, 62
    transport, 136
    wound healing, 310

P

P-LI-SS-IT model, 344–345
Pads, incontinence, 413, **413**, 418

Pain, 221–241
    acute, 224
    assessment, 228–231
    behavioural responses, 225–227, 229, 231
    on breathing, 147
    care delivery knowledge, 222, 228–236
    chronic, 224
    definition, 225
    dying patients, 271
    ethical knowledge, 222, 238–239
    gate theory, 223, **224**
    management, 231–241
        acupressure, 235
        acupuncture, 235
        analgesia, 226, 228, 232–233, 238, 275
        aromatherapy, 235
        case studies, 239–241
        clinical nurse specialist, 238
        homeopathy, 235–236
        hypnotherapy, 236
        massage, 234
        meditation, 234
        multidisciplinary teams, 237–238
        non-pharmacological, 234–236
        nurse's role, 237, 238, 239
        reflexology, 235
        TENS, 234
        visual stimuli, 234
    mental, 227
    personal knowledge, 222, 239–241
    physiology of, 222–224
    professional knowledge, 222, 236–239
    psychiatric, 227
    psychogenic, 239
    psychosocial elements, 225–228, 229–230
    reflective knowledge, 222, 239–241
    subject knowledge, 222–228
    theories of, 222–223, **222**, **224**
    transmission, 223
Palliative care
    definition, 263
    doctrine of double effect, 275
    nutrition, 172
Pancreas, carbohydrate metabolism, 155
Pantothenic acid, **159**
Paracetamol, 238
Para-suicide, 208, 238
Parenteral nutrition (PN), 167–168
Partnership working, hygiene care, 298–299
Pathogens, definition, 77
    see also Infection control
Patient Advice and Liaison Services (PALS), 20
Patient advocacy, 19–20
    infection control, 97
    mobility care, 384
Patient-centred care
    assessment process, 13–14
    diet, 164, 166
    records, 15, 18, 19
Patient controlled analgesia (PCA), 233, 234
Patient handling *see* Handling and moving patients
Patient records *see* Records
Patient safety incidents, 34–35
Peak flow meters, 146, **146**
Pelvic floor

defaecation, 398, 399
    exercises, 406–407
    urinary continence, 393, 395, **395**, 405, 406–407
Penis, 332–333, **332**
    hygiene care, 284, 290
    sexual response, 334
Peracetic acid (Nucidex), **82**
Perineum
    hygiene care, 284, 290
    and incontinence, 405, 410
Periodontal disease, 286
Peripheral resistance, 133
Persistent vegetative state (PVS), 172, 265–266
Personal care
    back injury, 109–110
    infection control, 96, 97, 320
Personal hygiene *see* Hygiene care
Personality types
    communicative styles, 8
    stress, 182, 187, 189
Perspective Display Sequence, 4
pH, and infection control, **79**
Pharmacists, role of, 206
Pharmacodynamics, 205
Pharmacokinetics, 203–205
Pharynx, infection control, **81**
Phenolics, disinfection with, **82**
Phylloquinone (vitamin K), **158**
Physical exercise, 169, 187, 373, 382–383
Piercings, 312
Pituitary gland, homeostasis, 128
Plasmodium falciparum, **77**, 78
Poisoning, 207–208
    confusion with, 355–356
Political factors
    community care, 192–193, 361–362
    homeostasis, 129
    hygiene care, 298–299
    infection control, 98–99
    nursing as female profession, 345
    rehabilitation, 424–425, 436–437
    stress, 192–193
Polypharmacy, 205–206
Postoperative care, safety and risk, 34
Post-traumatic stress disorder (PTSD), 52, 183
Potassium, dietary, **160**
Power relations, communication, 8, 9
Pregnancy
    dental hygiene, 286
    female reproductive system, 333
    medicines in, 204, 207
    nutritional requirements, 160–161
    patient handling, 111
    resuscitation, 58–59
    skin changes in, 308
Premenstrual syndrome, 334
Prescribing, by nurses, 213–214
Pressure sores, 272, 315, **315**, 321–323, 324
Prevented patient safety incidents, 34–35
Prions, **77**, 78, 356
Privacy, hygiene care, 288, 297, 298
Private nursing beds, elderly people, 361–362
Progesterone, 333
Progressive muscle relaxation, 189
Projection, stress, **179**

Pronation, joint movement, **371**
Proprioceptors, 372
Protective clothing, 93–95
Proteins, 157–158, 161, 162
Protozoa, 76, **77**, 78
Protraction, joint movement, **371**
Pseudomonas, **77**
Psoriasis, 282, 310
Psychiatric illness *see* Mental ill health
Psychiatric pain, 227
Psychoanalytic theory
    aggression, 247–248
    sexual identity, 335–336
Psychogenic pain, 239
Psychological contracts, 194
Psychological stress *see* Stress
Psychosocial aspects
    back injury, 108–110
    communication, 8–12, 431–433
    confusion, 356, 357–358
    continence, 400, 401–403
    death and dying, 50–52, 180–181, 185–186,
        266–270, 273–274, 429
    homeostasis, 128–129
    hygiene care, 287–288
    infection control, 84–86
    male mid-life crisis, 334, 344
    medicines, 207–209
    menopause, 334, 344
    mobility care, 374–377
    nutrition, 158–160
    pain, 225–228, 229–230
    rehabilitation, 425–433
    resuscitation, 50–52
    safety and risk, 30–33
    sexuality, 335–338, 340, 347
    skin, 310–312, 315
    stress, 179–183, 184–185, 187–189
Psychosocial theories, aggression, 247–248
Puberty, 332, 336, 344, 346
Pulse, 47, 56, 133–134
Pyrexia (fever), 131, 141, **141**, 142
Pyridoxine (vitamin B₆), **159**

Q

Quality assurance, continence care, 418
Quality of life
    and the environment, 30
    pressure sores, 323
Quality systems of care, 324
Questioning, communication, 13, 432

R

Race factors, blood pressure, 144
    see also Ethnic minority groups
Racial harassment, 249
Radiation
    as physical hazard, 29
    for sterilization, **82**, 83
    for thermoregulation, 130
Rapport building, 12
Rashes, skin, 314

Rationalization, stress, **179**
Reaction formation, stress, **179**
Reality orientation, 359, 360
Records, 14–16
    aggressive incidents, 251, **252**
    blood pressure measurement, 143–144
    confidentiality, 18–19
    drug administration, 210
    of handling tasks, 116, 118
    legal aspects, 17–18, 19
    non-accidental injuries, 320
    patient access to, 19
    tissue viability, 325
Rectal thermometry, 139, **140**
Rectum
    defaecation, 398, **398**
    digital examination, 405, 410, 418
Red blood cells, oxygen transport, 136
Reflective practice, 252, 258, 326
Reflex incontinence, 394, 395
Reflexology, 235
Regression, stress, **179**
Rehabilitation, 423–440
    assessment, 433–435
    body image, 427–428
    care delivery knowledge, 424, 433–436
    case studies, 439–440
    change management, 430–431, 436
    communication, 431–433
    definitions, 423
    ethical knowledge, 424, 438–439
    goal setting, 435, 439
    grieving, **428**, 429
    intermediate care, 437
    labelling, 426–427
    leadership, 433
    loss, 429
    motivation, 429–430
    nurse's role, 423–424, 436, 437–438, 439
    personal knowledge, 424, 439–440
    political contexts, 424–425, 436–437
    professional knowledge, 424, 436–438
    reflective knowledge, 424, 439–440
    social contexts, 424–425, 436–437, 438
    social exclusion, 437
    social roles, 425–426
    stigma, 426–427
    subject knowledge, 424–433
    teams, 433, 437–438
Rehearsal technique, stress management, 188
Relatives *see* Families; Informal carers
Relaxation, 175–176, 177, 183, 189–190, 234
Religious aspects
    bathing, 287, 288
    death, 186, 267, 268
    nutrition, 159–160, 164
    pain, 227
    stress, 186, 188
Reminiscence therapy, 359–360
Renal system
    drug excretion, 204–205
    dying patients, 271
    urinary continence, 392–393
Reporting of Injuries, Diseases and
        Dangerous Occurrences Regulations
        (RIDDOR), 39

Repression, stress, **179**
Reproductive system
    female, 333–334, **333**
    male, 332–333, **332**, 393
Research, patient records for, 18–19
Residential care, elderly people, 361–362
Resource allocation, 438
Respiration, 135–136, **137**
    carbohydrate utilization, 155–156
    children, 50, **145**, 146
    dying patients, 146, 271, 272
    effects of immobility, 374
    measurement, 145–147
    stress reaction, **178**
Respiratory disease
    infection risk, 83
    oxygen therapy, 62
    and sexuality, **343**
Respiratory tree, infection control, **81**
Rest, 175–176, 177, 183
Resuscitation and emergency care, 45–72
    advance directives, 71, 275
    advanced life support, 45, 62–63, **64**, 69–70
    ambulance service, 64
    assessment, 53–55
    basic life support, 45, 53–62, **65–68**, 69–70
    biology, 46–50
    care delivery knowledge, 46, 52–65
    case studies, 72
    chain of survival, 48–49
    children, 48, 49–50, 56, 57, 59–63, **64**, **67–68**,
        71
    consent, 51, 70–71
    defibrillation, 47–49, 57
    detecting impending collapse, 46
    'do not resuscitate' orders, 70–71
    drugs, 64
    effects of sudden death, 50–52
    ethics, 46, 70–71, 275
    first aid process, 53–62
        ABC approach, 54–57
        airway opening, 50, 55, **56**, 58, 59–62
        chest compressions, 56, 57, 58–59, **61**
        children, 50, 56, 57, 59–62, **67–68**
        choking, 59–62
        circulation checking, 55, 56
        diagnosis, 54–55
        establishing priorities, 53–54
        getting help, 53–54
        major wounds, 319–320
        mouth-to-mouth ventilation, 53, 56, 57
        personal safety, 53
        pregnant women, 58–59
        Resuscitation Council guidelines, **65–68**
        spinal injury, 58, **58**
    handing over responsibility, 64–65
    legal issues, 66–69
    living wills, 71, 275
    major wounds, 319–320
    mechanisms of collapse
        cardiac, 47–49
        respiratory, 47, 49–50
    near death experiences, 266
    and patient handling, 117
    personal knowledge, 46, 71–72
    post-traumatic stress disorder, 52

presence of relatives during, 51
professional knowledge, 46, 65–71
psychosocial, 50–52
reflective knowledge, 46, 71–72
Resuscitation Council guidelines, 46, 47, 52, 60–62, 63, **65–68**, 71
subject knowledge, 46–52
supplementary oxygen, 62
training for, 70, 71
Retinol (vitamin A), **158**, 161
Retraction, joint movement, **371**
Riboflavine (vitamin B$_2$), **159**
Risk *see* Safety and risk
Risk assessment *see* Safety and risk, risk assessment
Risk management *see* Safety and risk, risk management
Risk Pooling Scheme for Trusts (RPST), 40
Rotation, joint movement, **371**
Royal College of Nursing (RCN)
    continence care guidelines, 418
    handling patients, 117
    Work Injured Nurses' Group, 119

S

Safety and risk, 25–43
    accidents, 30, 42, 118
    adverse events, 34–35, 39
    aggressive incidents, 250, 255–258
    air, 27
    bathing, 291
    biological basis, 26–30
    biological hazards, 29, 37–38
    care delivery knowledge, 26, 33–39
    care planning, 36
    case studies, 42
    chemical hazards, 29, 37–38
    Clinical Governance, 40, 41
    Clinical Negligence Scheme for Trusts, 40
    Commission for Health and Audit Improvement, 40
    Commission for Health Improvement, 40
    consent process, 41
    Controls Assurance, 40
    Controls Assurance Unit, 36–37
    and culture, 31
    environmental hazards, 27–30, 31–33, **32**
    equipment, 29–30, 34, 37, 93–95
    ethical knowledge, 26, 38–41
    external agencies, 39–40, 41
    first-aiders, 53
    food, 28, 100, 161, 170–171
    handling patients *see* Handling and moving patients
    hazard management, 32–33, 36–37, 42
    hazard–risk relation, 36
    health care advice, 33
    home visits, 258
    homeostasis, 26–27
    infections *see* Infection control
    interprofessional working, 38, 41
    latent risks, 31
    learning environment, 34–35
    legal aspects, 26, 37–39, 40, 41

medicine administration, 211
mobility aids, 381–382, 385
National Institute for Clinical Excellence, 40, 41
National Patient Safety Agency, 34, 35
NHS Litigation Authority, 40, 41
patient safety incidents, 34–35
personal knowledge, 26, 42
personal protective equipment, 93–95
physical hazards, 29–30, 32, 36
physiological needs, 27–28
postoperative care, 34
prevented patient safety incidents, 34–35
professional knowledge, 26, 38–41
psychosocial hazards, 30–33
reflective knowledge, 26, 42
risk assessment, 33–34, 35–36
    aggression, 255–256
    confused clients, 358
    infection control, 87
    mobility, 377
    patient handling, 110–112, 116–117
risk–hazard relation, 36
risk management, 31, 34, 36–38, 39–40, 41, 42
    aggression, 255–256
risk perception, 31, 32
Risk Pooling Scheme for Trusts, 40
risk taking behaviour, 33, 38
shelter, 28
stress, 182, 186, 191–192, 193–195
subject knowledge, 26–33
systems failures, 31
waste disposal, 29, 91–93, 98
water, 27–28, 100
whistleblowing, 41
St John's wort, 190
Saliva, oral hygiene, 286, 292, 293, **293**
Salivary glands, 285, **285**
Salmonella, **77**, 161
Sebaceous glands, 283, 307
Self-catheterization, 409, 414
Self-concept, social roles, 425–427
Self-defence, 257
Self-harm, overdoses, 208, 238
    see also Suicide
Self-help groups, 189
Self-identity
    communication, 17
    sexuality, 335–338, 344
Self-image, 310–311, 427–428
Semen, 332
Sensory impairments, 5, 6, 16–17, 357, 432
Sensory nerve fibres, muscle, 372
Sensory sensitivity, dying patients, 271
Serotonin
    aggression, 246
    and MDMA, 355–356
Sex hormones, 332, 333
    aggression, 246–247
    male mid-life crisis, 334, 344
    menopause, 334, 344
Sexuality, 329–349
    assessment, 341
    care delivery knowledge, 330, 340–345
    case studies, 348–349

children, 331, 332, 335–336, 337, 344, 346–347
defining, 330–331
discussing with clients, 341–342, 344
elderly people, 346–347
emotions and, 339–340
ethical knowledge, 330, 347–348
facilitated sex, 347–348
femininity, 331, 345
gender roles, 331, 337, 345
and health conditions, 342–343, **343**, 346
heterosexual behaviour, 338–339
history of, 330–331, 337–338
homosexual behaviour, 338, 339
and incontinence, 403
learning disabled people, 22, 346
legal issues, 346, 347–348
male mid-life crisis, 334, 344
masculinity, 331, 345
medications, side effects, 343–344
menopause, 334, 344
menstrual cycle, 333–334
mental health nursing, **343**, 347
models of nursing, 340
neoanalytic theory, 336
norms, 337–338, 346
nursing actions, 344–345
nursing as female profession, 345
P-LI-SS-IT model, 344–345
personal knowledge, 330, 348–349
problems related to, 342–345
professional knowledge, 330, 345–348
psychoanalytic theory, 335–336
reflective knowledge, 330, 348–349
reproductive system, 332–333
sexual behaviour, 85, 330–331, 338–339, 340
sexual development, 332–334, 344, 346–347
sexual health, 341, 348
    see also Sexually transmitted diseases
sexual identity, 335–338, 344
sexual response, 334–335, 339–340, 345–346
social learning theory, 337
sociobiological theories, 336
stereotypes, 330–331, 345
subject knowledge, 329, 330–340
Sexually transmitted diseases
    government policy, 341, 348
    infection control, 85
    and sexual behaviour, 339
    see also Human immunodeficiency virus
Sharps, disposal of, 29, 92–93
Sheaths, urinary incontinence, 413
Shelter, environmental safety, 28
Shivering, 138
Shoes
    back injury, 109–110
    infection control, 93, 95
Sick building syndrome, 28
Sick role, 425–426, **426**
Sight, impaired, 5, 379, 432
Sign language, **5**
Sitting to standing movement, 382
Situational life crisis, 50–51
Skeleton
    effects of immobility, 374
    functions, **369**
    see also Musculoskeletal system

Skin, 305–327
  ageing and, 308
  assessment, 312–314
    blemishes, 314
    colour, 313
    hydration, 313
    lesions, 314
    pressure sores, 321–322
    temperature, 313
    texture, 313
    turgor, 313
    wound sites, 315–316, **317**
    the wounded person, 315
  cancers, 307, 314
  care delivery knowledge, 305, 312–323
  case studies, 326
  changes in pregnancy, 308
  cosmetics, 311
  cultural aspects, 311–312
  discoloration with cyanosis, 147, 313
  drug-related reactions, **206**
  effects of disorders of, 310–311, 314, **343**
  ethical knowledge, 306, 324–325
  functions, 282, 307–308
  glands in, 283, 307
  grafts, 323
  health promotion, 323–324
  hygiene care, 282–283, 289, 290
  infection control
    immune response, **81**
    maggot therapy, 316, 325
    nurses' personal care, 96, 320
    wounds, 316, 318–319, 320, 325
  leg ulcers, 321
  normal flora (commensals), 282–283
  personal knowledge, 306, 326
  piercings, 312
  pigmentation, 307
  pressure sores, 272, 315, **315**, 321–323, 324
  professional knowledge, 306, 323–325
  psychosocial aspects, 310–312, 315
  quality systems of care, 324
  rashes, 314
  reflective knowledge, 306, 326
  self-image, 310–311
  stress reaction, **178**
  structure, 282, 306–307, **306**
  subject knowledge, 305, 306–312
  sun-bathing, 307, 308, 310
  sun damage, 307, 308
  tattoos, 311–312
  thermoregulation, 129–130, 138, 307
  tissue viability records, 325
  tribal markings, 312
  wounds
    classification, 314–315
    healing, 171, 308–310, 316, 318–319, 320–321, 322, 323
    management, 315–323, 324, 325
    quality systems of care, 324
    skin damage severity, 315
Sleep, 183–184, **183**, 187, 191
Sliding equipment, 113, 114, 122, 123
Smoking
  as cultural behaviour, 85
  government policy, 129

hypertension, 144
patient safety, 36
and stress, 190
Sneezing, 147
Soaps, 90, **90**, 91, 290
Social contexts
  rehabilitation, 424–425, 436–437, 438
  stress, 192–193
  see also Political factors; Psychosocial aspects
Social exclusion, 437
Social learning theory
  aggression, 248
  sexual identity, 337
Social readjustment rating scale, 180–182, **180**, 184–185
Social roles, 425–426
  see also Gender roles
Social services
  care of the elderly, 361
  partnership working, 298–299
Social skills groups, 189
Socialization, stress management, 187–188
Sociobiological theories, sexuality, 336
Sodium, **160**, 354–355
Sodium chloride solution, wound cleansing, 318
Specialist nurses, 238, 325
Speech mechanisms, 4–6, 16
Speech styles, 8, 9, 10
Sperm, 332
Sphygmomanometers, 143
Spinal cord, 106–108
  intervertebral discs, 106, 108, **108**
  movements, 106, **107**
  optimum height for patient handling, 115
  pain transmission, 223
  vertebrae, 106, **107**
Spinal injuries
  avoidance *see* Handling and moving patients
  body image, 428, **428**
  first aid process, 55, 58, **58**
Spiritual aspects
  death, 186, 267
  distress, 186, 188
  hygiene care, 287–288
  pain, 227–228
Sputum, 147
Staphylococcus aureus
  catheter encrustation, 415
  chemical disinfection, **82**
  diseases caused by, **77**, 80
  growth requirements, **79**
  methicillin resistant (MRSA), 80, 96, 97
Staphylococcus epidermidis, **77**
Starch, 155
Status, social roles, 425, 426
Sterilization (infection control), 81, **82**, 83
Steroid therapy, **293**, **343**
Stigmatization, 426–427
  immobility, 376–377
  incontinence, 402–403
  responses, **427**
  sources, **427**
Stoke beds, 113
Stomach, infection control, **81**

Stools
  consistency, 398, **399**
  formation, 398
  softeners, 411, **412**
  see also Faecal incontinence
Storytelling
  health/illness, 10–12, 21
  records, 15
Streptococci, **77**
  growth requirements, **79**
  shape, **78**
Stress, 31, 175–196
  arousal curve, 176
  assessment, 184–187
  burnout, 182, 193–194
  care delivery knowledge, 175, 184–192
  case studies, 195–196
  causes, 180–182, **180**, 185–186, 193
  communication barriers, 433
  definitions, 176
  ethical knowledge, 176, 192–194
  of failed resuscitation, 52
  financial costs of, 194
  general adaptation syndrome, 177, **178**
  healthcare workers, 52, 182, 186, 191–192, 193–195
  informal carers, 192–193, 359, 362
  legal aspects, 193, 194
  management, 187–192, 194–195
  measurement, 184–187
  negative (distress), 176–177, 184
  personal knowledge, 176, 194–196
  and personality, 182, 187, 189
  physiology of, 177–179, 184, 185
  positive (eustress), 176–177, 184
  post-traumatic stress disorder, 52, 183
  professional knowledge, 176, 192–194
  psychosociology of, 179–183, 187–189
  reflective knowledge, 176, 194–196
  social readjustment rating scale, 180–182, **180**, 184–185
  subject knowledge, 175, 176–184
Stress incontinence, 394, 395, **395**, 401, 405, 406–407
Stroke patients
  communication, 16, 17
  mobility, 382
Sublimation, stress, **179**
Substance misuse, 208
  analgesia, 238
  causing confusion, 355–356
  and homeopathy, 236
  by nurses, 209
  stress, 190
Sugars, 154–155, 168
Suicide
  grief of families, 268
  overdoses, 208, 238
  physician assisted, 276
Sun-bathing, 307, 308, 310
Supervision, clinical, 191–192, 274
Supination, joint movement, **371**
Surgical patients, infection risk, **83**
Surgical wounds, 320–321
Surveillance, infection control, 87, 97, 99–100
Sutures, 320

Swabbing, dental hygiene, 294, **295**
Sweat
    hygiene care, 283, 289
    skin assessment, 313
    thermoregulation, 130, 132, 307
Sweat glands, 283, 307
Sympathetic tone, 133
Sympatholytics, **343**
Synovial joints, 370–372, **371**, 378–379

T

Tachycardia, 134
Tachypnoea, 146
Tattoos, 311–312
Teaching, health promotion, 14
Teams, 433
    multidisciplinary see Multidisciplinary teams
Tears, eye hygiene, 286
Teeth, 285–286, **285**, 292–295
Tempadot thermometry, 140, **140**
Temperature
    body
        assessment, 137, 138
        balance, 128, 129–132, 138, 307
        fever, 131, 141, **141**, 142
        heat exhaustion, 132
        heat stroke, 131–132
        hypothermia, 129, 132, 141–142
        measurement, 137, 138–142, 147–148
        physical factors affecting, 131
    environmental, 129
        and infection control, **79**
        as physical hazard, 29
    and infection control, **79**
        disinfection, **82**, 83
        laundry washing, 93, 96
        sterilization, **82**, 83
    skin, 313
    for wound healing, 310
Teratogenic medicines, 206–207
Terminal care, 263, 271–272
Testes, 332
Testosterone, 332, 334
Therapeutic relationships, 12–13
Thermogenesis, 130, 131
Thermometers, 139–141
Thermoregulation, 128, 129–132, 138, 307
Thiamin (vitamin B$_1$), **159**
TILER method, patient handling, 115
Time management, 192, 194–195
Tinea, **77**, 78
Tocopherol (vitamin E), **158**
Toilet training, 401, 409–410
Toileting programmes, 409–410
Toilets, and continence, 400, 402
Tongue, 285
Toothbrushes/brushing, 294
Toothpaste, 294
Topical medications
    absorption, 203
    safety, 211
Touch
    aggressive situations, 255
    massage, 189, 234

Towel bathing, 289, 290
Toxoplasma gondii, 78
Training see Education and training
Transcutaneous electric nerve stimulation
        (TENS), 234
Transfer equipment, patient handling, 113, 120
Translocation syndrome, 358
Tribal markings, 312
Trichomonas vaginalis, **77**, 78
Tricyclics, incontinence, 408, **408**
Triglycerides, 156, 157
Tube feeding, 166, 167, 172
Tuberculosis
    infection control, 94
    multidrug-resistant (MDRTB), 80
Tympanic thermometry, 139, 140–141, **140**, **141**

U

UK Central Council
    complaints, 19
    successor see Nursing and Midwifery
        Council
Ulcers
    leg, 321
    pressure see Pressure sores
Unconscious patients, eye care, 296–297
Uniforms
    footwear, 109–110
    infection control, 93, 94, 96
Universal Precautions, 88–89
Ureters, 392–393
Urethra
    anatomy, **392**
    infection control, **81**
    urinary incontinence, 393, **393**, 395, 401
Urge incontinence, **396**, 403
Urinary incontinence, 391
    absorbent products, 413, **413**, 418
    ageing process, 400–401
    assessment, 403–405, **404**, **405**
        charting, 405, **406**
        physical examination, 405, 418
        residual volume, 405
        symptoms, 403, 405
        urinalysis, 405
    behavioural factors, 402
    case studies, 418–419
    catheterization, 409, 413–416, 417
    causes, 394–397, 400–402, 409, **410**
    Continence Advisory Service, 416–417
    definitions, 392, **396**
    detrusor hyperactivity, 394, 395, **396**,
        407–408
    detrusor hypoactivity, 396–397, **397**, 409, 414
    digital rectal examination, 405, 418
    dribbling, **396**, 403
    dysuria, **396**
    environmental factors, 400
    ethics, 418
    fluid intake, 397, 401, 406
    frequency, **396**, 403
    general management, 413–416, 418
    haematuria, **396**, **415**
    hesitancy, **396**, 403

nocturia, **396**, 403
    nocturnal enuresis, **396**, 401–402, 409–410
    nurse education, 417–418
    outflow obstruction, 396, **396**, 408–409
    passive, **396**
    physiology, 392–397, 400–401
    prevalence, 392
    promotion of continence, 405–410
    psychosocial aspects, 401–403
    quality assurance of care, 418
    reflex, 394, 395
    sensory urgency, **396**
    sheaths, 413
    stigma, 402–403
    stress, 394, 395, **395**, 401, 405, 406–407
    toileting programmes, 409–410
    urge, **396**, 403
    urgency, **396**, 403
    voiding difficulties, 394, 396–397, 401,
        408–409
Urine, infection control, **81**
Utilitarianism, 384–385

V

Vaccines, 81, 84, 86, 96, 97, 98–99
Vagina, 333
    infection control, **81**
    and urinary incontinence, 405, 407, 418
Vaginal cones, 407
Valerian, 190
Validation therapy, 360
Vasomotor activity, 133
Ventricular fibrillation (VF), 47–49
Ventricular tachycardia, pulseless, 48
Violence see Aggression
Viruses, 76–77, **77**, 78
    carriers, 80, 96
    growth requirements, **79**
    immunization, 81, 84, 86, 96, 97, 98–99
    see also Infection control; Prions
Visual impairment, 5, 379, 432
Visual stimuli, pain management, 234
Vital signs, 137
    see also Blood pressure, measurement; Pulse;
        Temperature, body, measurement
Vitamins, 158, **158**, **159**
    and confusion, 355
    in pregnancy, 161
    synthesis of vitamin D, 308
Voiding difficulties, 394, 396–397, 401, 408–409

W

Waiting times, 256
Walking
    aids, 380–382, 385
    style of, 379
Washing
    hands, 83, 84, 88, 89–91
    laundry, 93, 96
Waste, safe disposal, 29, 91–93, 98
Water
    drinking

Water (*contd*)
    and continence, 397, 401, 406, 411
       dying patients, 272
  environmental safety, 27–28, 100
  fluoridation, 294
  and infection control, **79**, 100
Weight, body, 161, 164, **165**, 168–170
Welfare state, 424
Wheelchairs, 385
Whistleblowing, 41
White blood cells, 81
Women
  hygiene care, 297–298, 345
  reproductive system, 333–334, **333**
  see also Gender differences; Gender roles
Work Injured Nurses' Group (WING), 119
Workplace safety *see* Safety and risk
Workplace stress, 193–194
Wounds
  accidental, 319–320

chronic, 314, 321–323, 324
classification, 314–315
cleansing, 318–319, 320
dressings, 309, 318, 319, 320
healing, 308–310
  blood supply, 309, 310
  debridement, 316, 323
  evaluation, 319
  facilitation of, 316, 318–319
  foreign bodies, 310
  maggot therapy, 316, 325
  moisture, 310
  necrotic tissue, 316, 325
  nutrition and, 171, 320–321
  oxygen, 310
  pressure sores, 322, 323
  by primary intention, 308–309, **309**, 320
  by secondary intention, 309, **309**
  temperature, 310
  tertiary, 309

infection control, 316, 318–319, 320
legal aspects, 320
management, 315–323, 324, 325
quality systems of care, 324
skin grafts, 323
surgical, 320–321
Writing skills, 16

X

X-rays, as physical hazard, 29
Xerostomia (dry mouth), 293, **293**

Z

Zero Tolerance campaign, 257–258
Zinc, dietary, **160**, 161